Lecture Notes of the Institute for Computer Sciences, Social Informatics and Telecommunications Engineering 666

The LNICST series publishes ICST's conferences, symposia and workshops.

LNICST reports state-of-the-art results in areas related to the scope of the Institute.

The type of material published includes

- Proceedings (published in time for the respective event)
- Other edited monographs (such as project reports or invited volumes)

LNICST topics span the following areas:

- General Computer Science
- E-Economy
- E-Medicine
- Knowledge Management
- Multimedia
- Operations, Management and Policy
- Social Informatics
- Systems

Atul Kumar · Shivam Verma ·
Somak Bhattacharyya
Editors

Body Area Networks

19th EAI International Conference, BODYNETS 2024
Varanasi, India, December 15–16, 2024
Proceedings, Part I

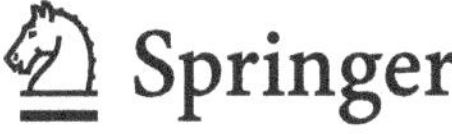

Editors
Atul Kumar
Department of Electronics Engineering
IIT(BHU)
Varanasi, Uttar Pradesh, India

Shivam Verma
Department of Electronics Engineering
IIT(BHU)
Varanasi, Uttar Pradesh, India

Somak Bhattacharyya
Department of Electronics Engineering
IIT(BHU)
Varanasi, Uttar Pradesh, India

ISSN 1867-8211 ISSN 1867-822X (electronic)
Lecture Notes of the Institute for Computer Sciences, Social Informatics and Telecommunications Engineering
ISBN 978-3-032-16098-0 ISBN 978-3-032-16099-7 (eBook)
https://doi.org/10.1007/978-3-032-16099-7

This Springer imprint is published by the registered company Springer Nature Switzerland AG
The registered company address is: Gewerbestrasse 11, 6330 Cham, Switzerland

Preface

We are pleased to present the proceedings of the 19th EAI International Conference on Body Area Networks (BODYNETS 2024), organized by the European Alliance for Innovation (EAI) and hosted by the Indian Institute of Technology (BHU), Varanasi, India, on 15–16 December 2024. Over the years, BODYNETS has established itself as a premier international forum that brings together researchers, developers, and practitioners from academia and industry to exchange knowledge, foster collaborations, and advance the field of body area networks and related technologies.

The technical program of BODYNETS 2024 featured oral presentations across four thematic tracks:

- Track A – Wireless Communications and Networking
- Track B – Wearable and Implantable Sensors
- Track C – Biomedical Signal Processing and AI-driven Healthcare
- Track D – IoT-based Monitoring and Next-Generation Applications

The 86 accepted papers were selected from 211 submissions. Each submission was reviewed following a single-blind process with a minimum of 3 reviews per paper. In addition to these high-quality paper sessions, the program included keynote addresses and invited talks by distinguished international experts, who offered valuable perspectives on the future of body area networks, healthcare IoT, and 6G-enabled pervasive sensing systems. Panel discussions and networking sessions further enriched the conference, fostering productive dialogue and inspiring future research directions.

We extend our heartfelt gratitude to the Steering Committee for their continuous guidance and support, and to the Technical Program Committee members for their diligent efforts in reviewing submissions and shaping a strong technical program. Our sincere appreciation also goes to the Organizing Committee, volunteers, and conference managers, whose commitment and hard work ensured the success of BODYNETS 2024. Above all, we thank the authors for their invaluable contributions, which have significantly enriched this volume and strengthened the BODYNETS community.

We believe that BODYNETS 2024 provided an excellent platform for presenting innovative ideas, addressing emerging challenges, and exploring cutting-edge solutions in the rapidly evolving field of body area networks. We are confident that the insights shared and contributions presented in this volume will inspire future research and technological progress, and we look forward to the continued growth and success of BODYNETS in the years ahead.

Atul Kumar
Shivam Verma
Somak Bhattacharyya

Organization

Steering Committee

Maurizio Magarini	Politecnico di Milano, Italy
Muralikrishnan Srinivasan	IIT (BHU) Varanasi, India
Atul Kumar	IIT (BHU) Varanasi, India

Organizing Committee

General Chair

Atul Kumar	IIT (BHU) Varanasi, India

General Co-chairs

Shivam Verma	IIT (BHU) Varanasi, India
Somak Bhattacharyya	IIT (BHU) Varanasi, India

TPC Chairs and Co-chairs

Chairs

Aditya K. Jagannatham	IIT Kanpur, India
Satyabrata Jit	IIT (BHU) Varanasi, India
Manoj Kumar Meshram	IIT (BHU) Varanasi, India
Vishwambhar Nath Mishra	IIT (BHU) Varanasi, India

Co-chairs

Matti Hämäläinen	University of Oulu, Finland
Lorenzo Mucchi	University of Florence, Italy
Maurizio Magarini	Politecnico di Milano, Italy
Kapal Dev	Munster Technological University, Ireland
Manoj Kumar Singh	IIT (BHU) Varanasi, India

Sponsorship and Exhibit Chairs

Sponsorship

Sonam Jain	IIT (BHU) Varanasi, India
Oppili Prasad L.	IIT (BHU) Varanasi, India
Ankit Arora	IIT (BHU) Varanasi, India

Local Chair

Atul Kumar	IIT (BHU) Varanasi, India

Workshops Chairs

Om Jee Pandey	IIT (BHU) Varanasi, India
Prodyut Dhar	IIT (BHU) Varanasi, India
Jaya Jha	IIT (BHU) Varanasi, India
Astha Sharma	Bharat 6G Alliance, India

Publicity and Social Media Chair

Muralikrishnan Srinivasan	IIT (BHU) Varanasi, India

Publications Chair

Atul Kumar	IIT (BHU) Varanasi, India

Web Chair

Ankur Pandey	Rajiv Gandhi Institute of Petroleum Technology (RGIPT), India

Panels Chairs

Sanjeev Sharma	IIT (BHU) Varanasi, India
Navin Singh Rajput	IIT (BHU) Varanasi, India
Amit Kumar Singh	IIT (BHU) Varanasi, India
M. Thottappan	IIT (BHU) Varanasi, India
Smrity Dwivedi	IIT (BHU) Varanasi, India

Tutorials Chairs

Priya Ranjan Muduli	IIT (BHU) Varanasi, India
Oppili Prasad L.	IIT (BHU) Varanasi, India

Technical Program Committee

Abhay Kumar Sah	IIT Roorkee, India
Amritanshu Pandey	IIT (BHU) Varanasi, India
Ankit Arora	IIT (BHU) Varanasi, India
Ashutosh Kumar Singh	Thapar Institute of Engineering and Technology, India
Jaya Jha	IIT (BHU) Varanasi, India
Kishor P. Sarawadekar	IIT (BHU) Varanasi, India
Muralikrishnan Srinivasa	IIT (BHU) Varanasi, India
Om Jee Pandey	IIT (BHU) Varanasi, India
Priya Ranjan Muduli	IIT (BHU) Varanasi, India
Prodyut Dhar	IIT (BHU) Varanasi, India
Ranjay Hazra	National Institute of Technology Silchar, India
Sanjeev Sharma	IIT (BHU) Varanasi, India
Shivam Verma	IIT (BHU) Varanasi, India
Somak Bhattacharyya	IIT (BHU) Varanasi, India
Sudhir Kumar	IIT Patna, India

Contents

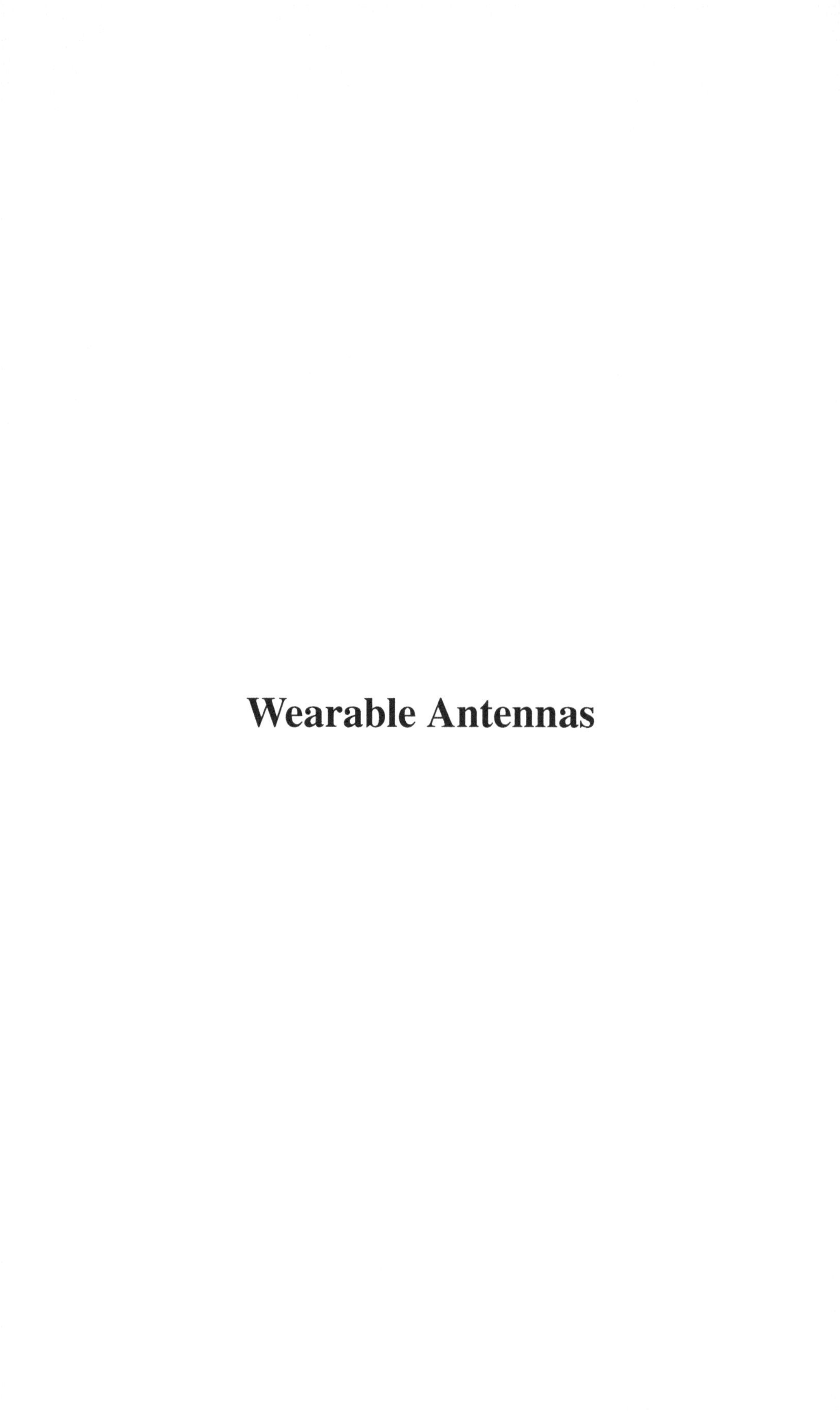

Wearable Antennas

A Multi-Band Wearable Textile Patch Antenna for ISM, IoT, C, X, and Ku Band Applications

Kamisetti Sasank[1](✉), Deepak Ram[3], Kalyani Kandiraju[2], and Somak Bhattacharyya[3]

[1] Vignan's Institute of Information Technology, Visakhapatnam 530 049, India
kamisettisasank681@gmail.com

[2] Sai Vidya Institute of Technology, Rajanukunte, Bangalore 560 064, India
kalyani.potturi@saividya.ac.in

[3] Indian Institute of Technology, Varanasi, Uttar Pradesh 221 005, India
{deepakram.rs.ece20,somakbhattacharyya.ece}@iitbhu.ac.in

Abstract. The paper introduces a multi-band wearable textile patch antenna tailored for operation across the ISM, IoT, C, X, and Ku bands. The antenna features a rectangular patch integrated with U-shaped, circular, and triangular slots to enhance performance. The antenna was crafted on a Jeans substrate with dimensions $0.6\,\lambda o \times 0.8\,\lambda o \times 0.01\,\lambda o\ mm^3$. The antenna has a notable -10 dB impedance bandwidths across 3.15 to 3.25 GHz, 4.04 to 4.17 GHz, 9.67 to 10 GHz, and 10.99 to 12.44GHz that ensure minimal signal loss and reliable performance across the target frequency ranges. The antenna achieves a maximum gain of 7.4 dBi at 12.1 GHz, 3.2 dBi at 9.8 GHz, 5.86 dBi at 4.1 GHz, and 3.58 dBi at 3.2 GHz. The proposed antenna is versatile in terms of frequency bands of operation and applications such as ECG monitoring, Industrial IoT, Wireless Body-Area Network (WBAN) implementations (3.1 GHz), telemetry systems to track the patient in real-time, 5G wireless communication (4.1 GHz), satellite downlinks and radar systems to capture high-resolution images as well as medical imaging and Augmented reality (7.25 GHz). This paper provides a comprehensive overview of the design process for the multi-band wearable textile patch antenna, emphasizing its potential applications and advantages in wearable technology.

Keywords: ISM · IoT · WBAN · Multi-band Antenna

1 Introduction

Wearable antennas have become increasingly important in the development of modern communication systems. The increasing demand for wearable antennas has spurred research into innovative solutions that provide enhanced performance in terms of bandwidth, gain, flexibility, and integration. These antennas integrated into clothing offer the advantage of continuous monitoring and real-time data transmission, making them essential for a wide range of applications, including healthcare monitoring, fitness tracking, military communications, and medical imaging [1, 2]. The Textile materials have a lower

K. Atul et al. (Eds.): BodyNets 2024, LNICST 666, pp. 3–10, 2026.
https://doi.org/10.1007/978-3-032-16099-7_1

value of dielectric constant and also improves the bandwidth of impedance [3]. In healthcare and fitness, for instance, they can support the simultaneous monitoring of different physiological parameters, multiband antennas enable real-time performance tracking, providing users with instant feedback on their physical activities across multiple devices and platforms. In military bases ability to function across diverse frequencies also makes them highly resilient to interference, ensuring continuous and reliable communication in challenging environments [4, 5]. In particular, the need for multiband wearable antennas has emerged as a critical factor in addressing the diverse frequency requirements of these applications [6]. Multiband antennas allow a single device to operate across multiple frequency bands. It enhances operational efficiency, reduces equipment weight, and improves mobility in the field. The multiband antennas becoming an essential component in advancing portable and high-performance communication systems for various practical applications such as Bluetooth, Wi-Fi, cellular networks, and military and healthcare applications [7, 8]. To achieve the multiband functionality include employing multiple resonant elements, such as slots, which are strategically placed to resonate at different frequencies. The fractal or meandered geometries, which allow a compact antenna structure to resonate at several distinct bands [9]. The impedance matching techniques, such as incorporating stubs or matching networks, are crucial for ensuring the antenna performs effectively across the targeted frequency bands [10].

Defended grounded structure is a popular technique for miniaturizing the antenna and achieving multiband behaviour while maintaining a low profile [11]. Reconfigurable antennas utilize tunable components, such as varactors, PIN diodes, or MEMS switches, to adjust the antenna's operating frequency dynamically by altering the antenna's configuration, the same structure can resonate at different frequency bands [12]. Metamaterials and Metasurfaces with unique electromagnetic properties can be integrated into the antenna design to create additional resonant bands [13]. By integrating different types of slots into wearable antennas, multiband functionality can be achieved. Each slot is designed to resonate at a specific frequency, enabling the antenna to operate across multiple frequency bands simultaneously. This technique allows for efficient use of space while maintaining a compact form factor, which is essential for wearable applications [14, 15]. This integration of slots enhances the versatility of wearable antennas, making them suitable for a wide range of applications where multi-frequency operation is crucial.

The proposed design a multiband flexible antenna has been designed on a textile material Jeans substrate with dimensions $0.6\lambda o \times 0.8\lambda o \times 0.01\ \lambda o\ mm^3$. The antenna dimensions are designed to be compact to ensure user comfort when worn on the body while ensuring excellent flexibility. The proposed antenna acquires multiple frequency bands with bandwidth coverage percentage, the first band from 3.15 to 3.25 GHz with 3.2%, the second band from 4.04 to 4.17 GHz with 2.92%, the third band with from 9.67 to 10 GHz with 3.4%, fourth band from 10.99 to 12.44 GHz with 13.01% that ensure minimal signal loss and reliable performance across the target frequency ranges. The antenna achieves a maximum gain of 7.4 dBi at 12.1 GHz, 3.2 dBi at 9.8 GHz, 5.86 dBi at 4.1 GHz, and 3.58 dBi at 3.2 GHz. The proposed prototype focuses on the development of a Multi-band flexible antenna designed specifically for wearable devices. The primary objective of this research is to achieve the multiple bands in the antenna and to improve its performance and functionality in the context of wearable applications.

2 Design Methodology

The design of the proposed multiband textile antenna is illustrated in Fig. 1. The antenna is constructed using a Jeans fabric substrate, which has a relative permittivity of 1.7 and a loss tangent of 0.02, providing a thickness of 1 mm. The patch incorporates a combination of U-shaped, circular, and triangular slots. Both the ground plane and the patch are fabricated from copper a material chosen for its excellent conductivity and efficiency in radiating signals.

(Designed parameters: $W_s = W_g = 90$ mm, $L_s = L_g = 86$ mm, $L_p = 40$ mm, $W_p = 48$ mm, $S_a = 2.5$ mm, $S_b = 5$ mm, $U_a = 22$ mm, $U_b = 38$ mm, $L_f = 23$ mm)

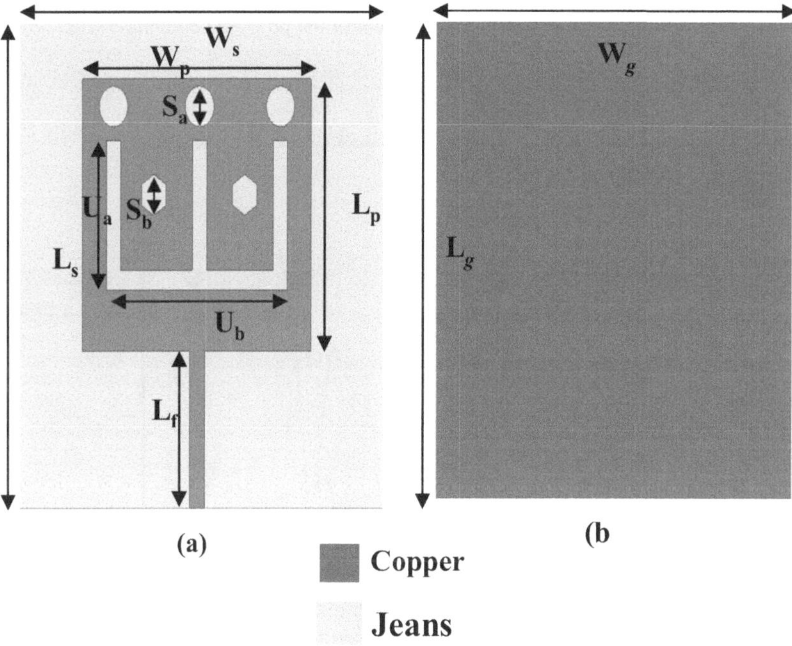

Fig. 1. (a) Top view and (b) bottom view of the proposed an- tenna (Designed parameters: $W_s = W_g = 90$ mm, $L_s = L_g = 86$ mm, $L_p = 40$ mm, $W_p = 48$ mm, $S_a = 2.5$ mm, $S_b = 5$ mm, $U_a = 22$ mm, $U_b = 38$ mm, $L_f = 23$ mm)

3 Results and Discussion

The proposed antenna was simulated using Ansys HFSS software. The reflection coefficient of the proposed antenna is illustrated in Fig. 2.

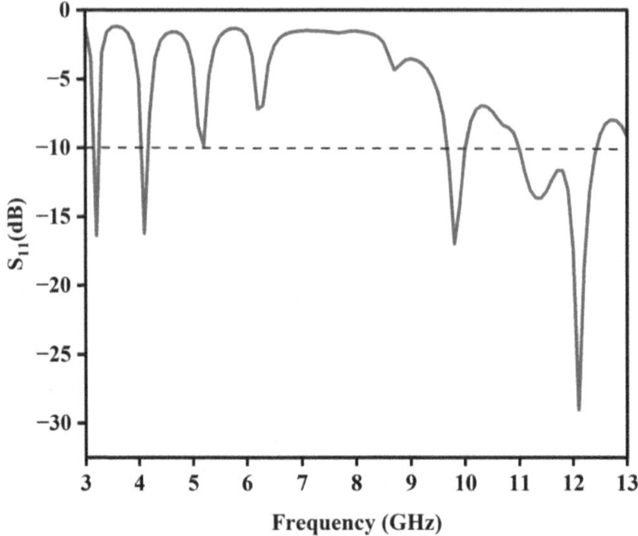

Fig. 2. Simulated reflection coefficient plot of the proposed antenna.

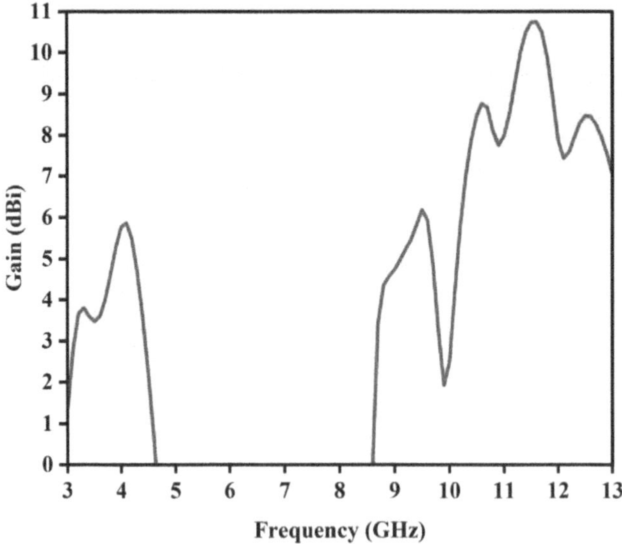

Fig. 3. Simulated gain vs frequency plot of the proposed antenna.

The four distinct frequency bands were identified with S11 values ≤-10 dB. These bands are observed in the ranges of 3.15–3.25 GHz, 4.04–4.17 GHz, 9.67–10 GHz, and 10.99–12.44 GHz. The corresponding return losses of 16.31 dB, 16.21 dB, 17 dB, and 29.3 dB were recorded for the first, second, third, and fourth bands, respectively. The antenna's gain performance across these frequencies, as depicted in Fig. 3, demonstrates maximum realized gains of 7.42 dBi at 12.1 GHz, 3.58 dBi at 3.2 GHz, 5.86 dBi at 4.1 GHz, and 3.23 dBi at 9.8 GHz. These results validate the proposed antenna's efficiency across the designated frequency bands.

The induced surface current distributions at 3.2 GHz, 4.1 GHz, 9.8 GHz, and 12.1 GHz are shown in Fig. 4. These distributions highlight the role of the slots in facilitating antenna radiation. The relatively uniform surface current observed on the patch suggests effective electromagnetic wave propagation, reduced impedance mismatches, and efficient energy transfer. These characteristics are crucial for ensuring stable antenna performance, particularly in wearable applications. The radiation patterns of the proposed dual-band antenna were evaluated at phi = 0° and phi = 90° for 3.2 GHz, 4.1 GHz, 9.8 GHz, and 12.1 GHz, as illustrated in Fig. 5(a)-(c). Across all frequencies, the patterns demonstrate their maximum radiation along the broadside direction.

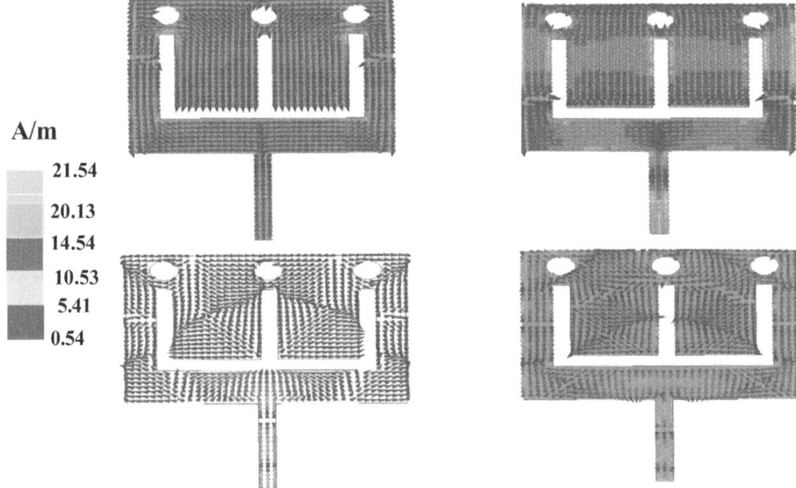

Fig. 4. Induced surface current distributions on the patch at (a) 3.2 GHz (b)4.1 GHz (c) 9.8 GHz and (d) 12.1 GHz.

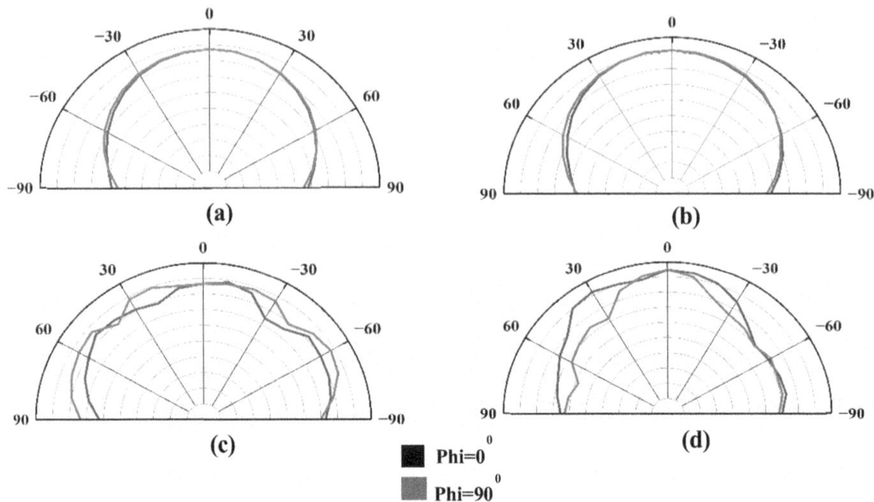

Fig. 5. Radiation patterns of the textile antenna at(a) 3.2 GHz (b) 4.1 GHz (c) 9.8 GHz (d) 12.1 GHz.

Table 1. Comparison of the proposed antenna with existing tri- band antennas

Ref.	3 Size (λo)	Freq. (GHz)	|S11|<-10dB Bandwidth	Peak Gain (dBi)	**Sub- strate**
[12]	0.64λo × 0.67λo × 1.1λo	2.42/4.2/6.8	16.2/23.7/34 1	2.09/3.8/ 5.05	Felt
[13]	0.88λo × 0.57λo × 0.04λo	2.45/5	25.7/32.5	5.1/5.5	PDMS
[14]	0.55λo × 0.65λo × 0.12λo	2.38/5.1/5.8	34.3/24.4/20 6	2.5/3.52/ 4.8	Polymi de
[15]	0.54λo × 0.53λo × 0.07λo	0.9/1.7/2.3/4.2	20.4/14.0/16 2/25.2	2.2/3.3/2.2 /3.8	E-fi- bers
This work	**0.6λo × 0.8λo × 0.01 λo**	**3.2/4.1/9.8/12 1**	**16.4/16/17.4/ 30.2**	**3.58/5.86/ 3.2/7.34**	**Jeans**

The proposed antenna not only exhibits flexibility but also demonstrates improved performance by providing higher gain across multiple frequency bands. Table 1 presents a detailed comparison between the proposed antenna and several existing multiband antennas from the literature. This enhanced functionality makes it a versatile option, particularly for applications requiring a flexible and efficient multiband operation.

4 Conclusion

This paper introduces a wearable multi-band antenna crafted on a jeans substrate that achieves impressive performance. The proposed antenna acquires multiple frequency bands with notable impedance bandwidth coverage percentage, the first band from 3.15 to 3.25 GHz with 3.2%, the second band from 4.04 to 4.17 GHz with 2.92%, the third band from 9.67 to 10 GHz with 3.4%, fourth band from 10.99 to 12.44 GHz with 13.01%. Additionally, the antenna delivers a maximum gain of 7.4 dBi at 12.1 GHz, 3.2 dBi at 9.8 GHz, 5.86 dBi at 4.1 GHz, and 3.58 dBi at 3.2 GHz. Notably, this design leverages a cost-effective textile substrate, offering enhanced performance over previous designs that used flexible substrates. The proposed multiband antenna is well-adapted for wearable applications including healthcare, IoT, ISM, and military applications.

References

1. Samal, P.B., Chen, S.J., Fumeaux, C.: Wearable textile multiband antenna for WBAN applications. IEEE Trans. Antennas Propag. **71**(2), 1391–1402 (2023). https://doi.org/10.1109/TAP.2022.3230550
2. Sasank, K., Yuvaraju, M., Samantaray, D., Swain, B.R., Ram, D., Bhattacharyya, S.: Metasurface-integrated flexible antenna with enhanced bandwidth for wearable IoT devices. In: 2023 8th International Conference on Computers and Devices for Communication (CODEC), Kolkata, pp. 1–2 (2023). https://doi.org/10.1109/CODEC60112.2023.10466101
3. Kaufmann, T., Fumeaux, C.: Wearable textile half-mode substrate-integrated cavity antenna using embroidered vias. IEEE Antennas Wirel. Propag. Lett. **12**, 805–808 (2013). https://doi.org/10.1109/LAWP.2013.2270939
4. Khan, U.R., Sheikh, J.A., Junaid, A., Amin, R., Ashraf, S., Ahmed, S.: Design of a compact hybrid moore's fractal inspired wearable antenna for IoT enabled bio- telemetry in diagnostic health monitoring system. IEEE Access **10**, 116129–116140 (2022). https://doi.org/10.1109/ACCESS.2022.3219442
5. Çelenk, E., Tokan, N.T.: All-textile on-body antenna for military applications. IEEE Antennas Wirel. Propag. Lett. **21**(5), 1065–1069 (2022). https://doi.org/10.1109/LAWP.2022.3159301
6. Zhang, C., Zhao, Z., Xiao, P., Liu, Q., Wang, N., Li, G.: A miniaturized wearable annular slot antenna based on designer LSPs for telemedicine communication. IEEE Trans. Antennas Propag. **72**(9), 7293–7298 (2024). https://doi.org/10.1109/TAP.2024.3415434
7. Li, H., Du, J., Yang, X.-X., Gao, S.: Low-profile all-textile multiband microstrip circular patch antenna for WBAN applications. IEEE Antennas Wirel. Propag. Lett. **21**(4), 779–783 (2022). https://doi.org/10.1109/LAWP.2022.3146435
8. Modak, S., Kaim, V., Khan, T., Kanaujia, B.K., Matekovits, L., Rambabu, K.: Design and performance measurement of worn-on-body instrumental ultra-miniaturized UWB wearable patch for e-health monitoring. IEEE Access **12**, 25719–25730 (2024). https://doi.org/10.1109/ACCESS.2024.3365938
9. Le, T.T., Yun, T.-Y.: Miniaturization of a dual-band wearable antenna for WBAN applications. IEEE Antennas Wirel. Propag. Lett. **19**(8), 1452–1456 (2020). https://doi.org/10.1109/LAWP.2020.3005658
10. Song, M., et al.: An energy-efficient antenna impedance detection using electrical balance for single-step on-chip tunable matching in wearable/implantable applications. IEEE Trans. Biomed. Circuits Syst. **11**(6), 1236–1244 (2017). https://doi.org/10.1109/TBCAS.2017.2771500

11. Ashyap, A.Y.I., et al.: Robust and efficient integrated antenna with EBG-DGS enabled wide bandwidth for wearable medical device applications. IEEE Access **8**, 56346–56358 (2020). https://doi.org/10.1109/ACCESS.2020.2981867
12. Yan, S., Vandenbosch, G.A.E.: Radiation pattern-reconfigurable wearable antenna based on metamaterial structure. IEEE Antennas Wirel. Propag. Lett. **15**, 1715–1718 (2016). https://doi.org/10.1109/LAWP.2016.2528299
13. Gao, G.-P., Meng, H.-J., Geng, W.-F., Dou, Z.-H., Zhang, B.-K., Hu, B.: A wideband metasurface antenna with dual-band dual-mode for body-centric communications. IEEE Antennas Wirel. Propag. Lett. **21**(1), 149–153 (2022). https://doi.org/10.1109/LAWP.2021.3121585
14. Yu, Z., et al.: A wearable self-grounding slit antenna for ISM/4G/5G/Bluetooth/WLAN applications. IEEE Access **11**, 87930–87937 (2023). https://doi.org/10.1109/ACCESS.2023.3305258
15. Wang, Z., Lee, L.Z., Psychoudakis, D., Volakis, J.L.: Embroidered multiband body- worn antenna for GSM/PCS/WLAN communications. IEEE Trans. Antennas Propag. **62**(6), 3321–3329 (2014). https://doi.org/10.1109/TAP.2014.2314311

A Tri-Band Wearable Textile Patch Antenna Designed for ISM, IoT and C Band Applications

Aritra Biswas[1], Nurhak Mondal[1], Deepak Ram[2], Ardhendu Kundu[1](✉), Sayan Sarkar[1], Gobinda Sen[1], and Somak Bhattacharyya[2]

[1] Institute of Engineering & Management, Salt Lake, Kolkata 700091, India
aritrabiswas1209@gmail.com, ardhendukundu.1989@gmail.com

[2] Indian Institute of Technology (BHU) Varanasi, Varanasi, Uttar Pradesh 221005, India

Abstract. The paper presents a tri-band wearable textile patch antenna designed for use in the ISM band, IoT band, and C band. The antenna is composed of a rectangular patch with pentagonal and rectangular slots to improve its performance. It is made on a wool substrate, which is chosen for its flexibility, comfort, and easy integration into wearable devices. The design provides competitive antenna performance along with mechanical flexibility. The antenna operates well across three distinct frequency bands, viz., 2.44 to 2.50 GHz, 4.81 to 4.88 GHz, and 7.04 to 7.44 GHz. The antenna achieves a maximum gain of 6.3dBi at 2.47 GHz, 2.66dBi at 4.88 GHz and 5.85dBi at 7.05 GHz. The proposed antenna is versatile in terms of frequency bands of operation and applications such as fitness monitoring for patients with chronic illnesses, real-time patient tracking, healthcare applications, Wireless Body-Area Network (WBAN) implementations (2.47 GHz), sub-5G wireless communication (4.85 GHz) as well as military satellite communication (7.25 GHz). By operating in these frequency bands, the antenna supports multiple wireless communication applications, ensuring compatibility and easy integration into existing and new wireless systems. This work outlines detailed design steps of the tri-band wearable textile patch antenna, highlighting its potential uses and benefits in wearable electronics.

Keywords: ISM Band · IoT · WBAN · Microwave · Tri-band Antenna

1 Introduction

Wearable antennas face unique challenges compared to conventional antennas, as they must be flexible, comfortable, and durable, while maintaining high efficiency [1]. Medical and IoT applications of wearable antennas, which focus on fitness monitoring for patients with chronic illness, patient tracking, and healthcare, commonly use the ISM (Industrial, Scientific, and Medical) bands due to its regulatory compliance, ability to mitigate interference, and broad acceptance across diverse technologies [2].The application of IoT technologies spans over a diverse range of fields, including healthcare systems for monitoring vital signs such as heartbeat and body temperature, to help soldiers communicate with other units on the battlefield, smart cities and homes for improved living

K. Atul et al. (Eds.): BodyNets 2024, LNICST 666, pp. 11–18, 2026.
https://doi.org/10.1007/978-3-032-16099-7_2

standards, and agricultural applications for optimizing farming practices [3, 4]. The need for wearable electronic devices with integrated antennas for monitoring patients' vital health parameters has now become an integral part of the healthcare system. These devices offer continuous real-time health monitoring, significantly improving patient care by using radio frequency (RF) waves to send and receive patient information. However, the RF radiation emitted by these devices raises concerns about tissue heating. Since the human body is composed of nearly 70% water, electrolytes, and ions, it can absorb RF energy – potentially causing biological consequences. Therefore, careful consideration of safety standards and regulations is essential in designing and deploying these devices in healthcare monitoring systems [5]. The ISM band (2.4–2.5 GHz) is widely used for Wireless Body-Area Network (WBAN) applications [6]. The International Telecommunication Union has assigned 7.25–7.75 GHz band for downlink satellite communication in particular for military applications [7]. Recently, the 4.85 GHz band has emerged as a preferable choice for the future 5G wireless communication system [8].

The bandwidth and gain enhancement of a conventional rectangular patch antenna has been achieved by incorporating various rectangular and pentagonal slots [9–11]. Inset feed is an efficient method for powering wearable antennas [12]. The full ground plane in a patch antenna enhances performance by reducing radiation losses, minimizing interference and providing greater stability and consistency in operation [13]. The low-profile antenna in [14] minimizes size and cost, making it an efficient and cost-effective solution for applications requiring compact and affordable antenna designs. Tri-band microstrip antennas enhance transceiver system performance through proper frequency band selection [15]. Similarly, reconfigurable antennas are advantageous as those allow a single antenna to serve multiple wireless communication systems [16, 17]. A lower Specific Absorption Rate (SAR) value of the wearable antenna minimizes its impact on the human body [18].

In this paper, a tri-band band flexible antenna has been designed on textile material wool substrate with dimensions $0.49\lambda_0 \times 0.37\lambda_0 \times 0.015\lambda_0$. The antenna dimensions are designed to be compact to ensure user-comfort when worn on the body, while ensuring excellent flexibility. It provides a -10dB impedance bandwidth ranging from 2.44 to 2.50GHz, 4.81 to 4.88GHz, and 7.04 to 7.44GHz, with respective center frequencies at 2.47GHz, 4.85 GHz and 7.23 GHz. In the three distinct bands, the antenna exhibits gain of 6.31 dBi, 2.66 dBi and 5.85 dBi at 2.47 GHz, 4.88 GHz and 7.05GHz respectively. The designed antenna is potentially useful for ISM, IoT band applications (2.47GHz), sub-5G wireless communication (4.85GHz), military satellite communication (7.25GHz) and other C band applications like wireless networks and remote sensing to name a few.

2 Design Methodology

The proposed tri-band textile antenna is depicted in Fig. 1. The antenna includes a wool substrate (relative permittivity = 1.2 and loss tangent = 0.02) with a thickness of 2 mm and a patch that is fed using inset feed. The patch incorporates rectangular and pentagonal slots to achieve the desired frequency and improve its performance. Both ground plane and the patch are made of copper.

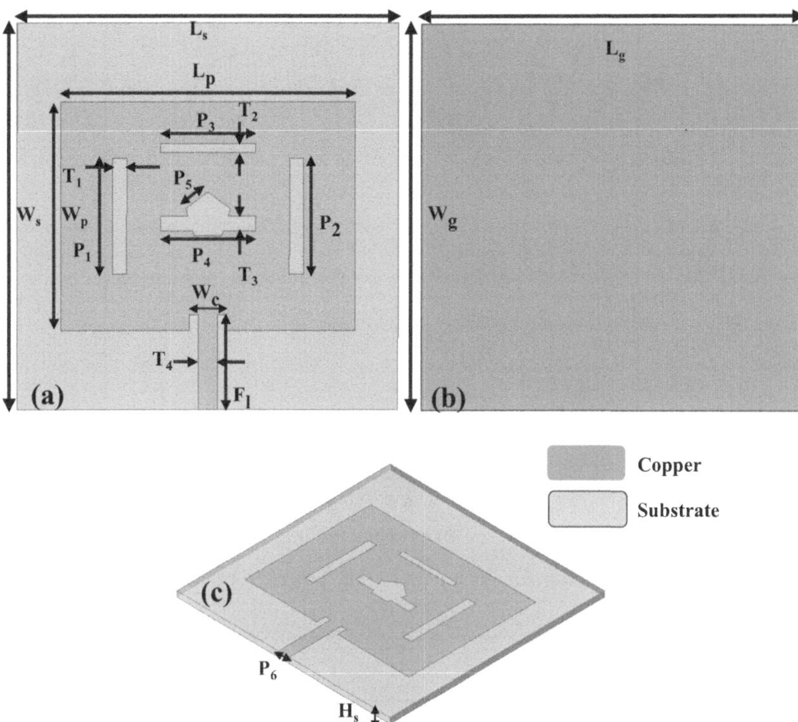

Fig. 1. (a) Top view and (b) bottom view and (c) Side view of the proposed antenna. (Designed parameters: Wp = 47.2mm, Lp = 61.6mm, Pl = P2 = 24mm, P3 = 20mm, P4 = 20mm, P5 = 5mm, P_6 = 3.75 mm, T1 = 3mm, T2 = 1.875mm, T3 = 3mm,T4 = 3.75mm, W_c = 7 mm, F1 = 20 mm, H_S = 2 mm, Wg = Lg = Ws = Ls = 80mm).

3 Results and Discussion

Frequency response of the simulated reflection coefficient plot for the proposed antenna design is shown in Fig. 2.

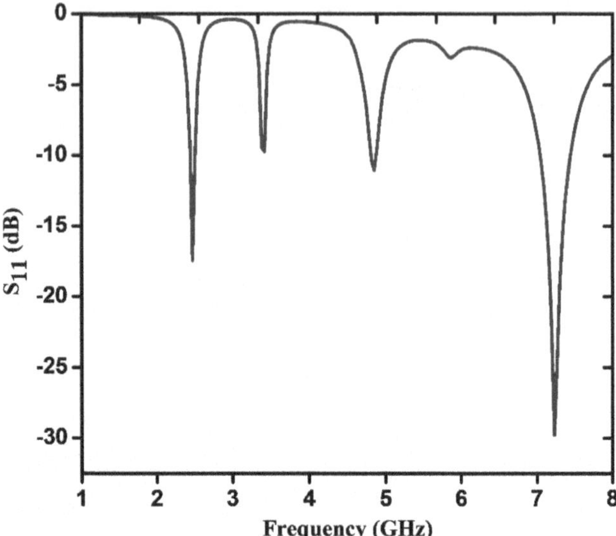

Fig. 2. Simulated reflection coefficient plot of the proposed tri-band textile antenna.

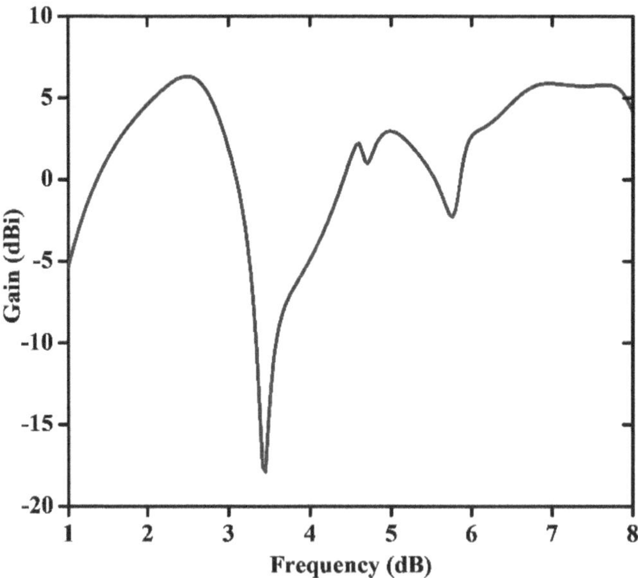

Fig. 3. Simulated gain vs frequency plot of the tri-band textile antenna.

Three distinct frequency bands have been observed with $S_{11} \leq$ -10dB as seen from Fig. 2. The first band lies within 2.44–2.50 GHz, while the second band lies within 4.81–4.88 GHz and the third band lies within 7.04–7.44 GHz. The return losses of

17.41dB, 11.08dB and 29.76dB have been observed within the first, second and third bands respectively. Analysis of the proposed antenna's gain with respect to frequency is illustrated in Fig. 3. It is observed that maximum realized gains of 6.31dBi, 2.66dBi and 5.85dBi have been achieved at 2.47 GHz, 4.88 GHz and 7.05 GHz respectively.

Induced surface current distributions within the structure at 2.47 GHz, 4.85 GHz and 7.25 GHz are illustrated in Figs. 4(a) to 4(c). It is clear that the slots are responsible for antenna radiation. Surface current distribution on the patch reveals a relatively uniform pattern, which is indicative of efficient electromagnetic wave propagation, minimal impedance mismatch, and optimal energy transfer – all of these are essential for maintaining consistent antenna performance in wearable applications designed for healthcare monitoring and fitness tracking.

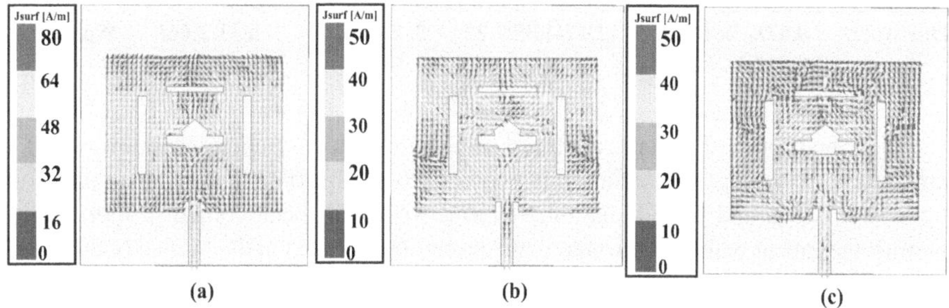

Fig. 4. Induced surface current distributions on the patch at (a) 2.47 GHz (b) 4.85 GHz and (c) 7.23 GHz.

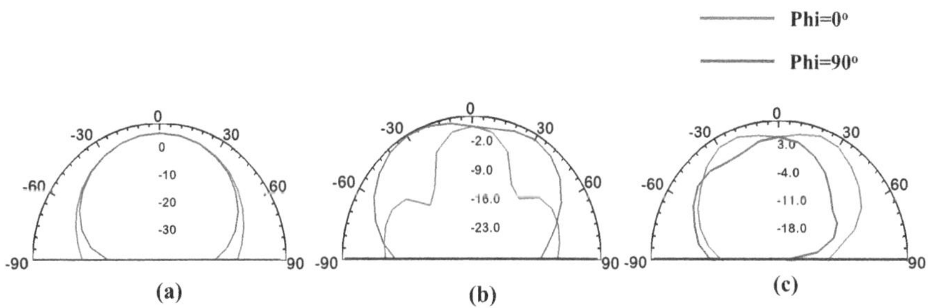

Fig. 5. Radiation patterns of the textile antenna at(a) 3.2 GHz (b) 4.1 GHz (c) 9.8 GHz (d) 12.1 GHz.

Radiation patterns of the proposed tri-band antenna have been analyzed at phi = 0^0 and phi = 90^0 at 2.47 GHz, 4.85 GHz and 7.05 GHz as shown in Figs. 5(a) to 5(c) respectively. All radiation patterns have their maxima along the broadside direction.

Table 1 provides a comparison between the proposed antenna and a few existing triple band antennas present in literature [19–22]. The proposed tri-band antenna is flexible in nature while offering enhanced gain in three frequency bands.

Table 1. Comparison of the proposed antenna with existing tri-band antennas

Ref.	Size (λ_0^3)	Freq (GHz)	$\|S_{11}\|$<-10dB Bandwidth	Peak Gain (dBi)	Substrate
[19]	$0.44\lambda_0 \times 0.33\lambda_0 \times 0.02\lambda_0$	3.5/5.5/9.1	35.5/4.2/34.1	3.09/2.8/5.05	FR4
[20]	$0.67\lambda_0 \times 0.67\lambda_0 \times 0.02\lambda_0$	2.4/3.5/4.6	11/7/5	1.1/0.9/2.1	Leather
[21]	$0.05\lambda_0 \times 0.05\lambda_0 \times 0.0006\lambda_0$	0.8/2.3/5.8	4.3/2.1/2.5	2.5/3.52/4.8	Rogers
[22]	$0.5\lambda_0 \times 0.5\lambda_0 \times 0.06\ \lambda_0$	2.45/3.0/3.45	4.4/4.0/6.2	4.2/6.6/5.0	Felt
This work	$\mathbf{0.67\lambda_0 \times 0.6\lambda_0 \times 0.012\ \lambda_0}$	**2.47/4.85/7.25**	**2.42/0.72/2.76**	**6.31/2.66/5.85**	**Wool**

When the proposed antenna is placed on a homogeneous human phantom model, a part of the electromagnetic radiation is expected to be absorbed in the human phantom due to side lobes and back radiation. A term 'SAR' has been coined in literature to quantify the rate at which electromagnetic energy is absorbed in the human body - SAR value must be restricted within 1.6 watts per kilogram, averaged over 1 g of contiguous human tissue [23–25]. SAR simulation was performed for the proposed wearable antenna on a flat body phantom model. To keep the SAR value within 1.6 W/kg, the maximum permissible power levels have been found to be 266 mW at 2.47 GHz and 325 mW at 4.88 GHz respectively. To further reduce SAR levels, a thin foam layer can be placed between the antenna's ground plane and the body phantom.

4 Conclusion

Wearable antennas are critical in advancing medical and IoT applications, particularly for healthcare monitoring, fitness tracking, and patients' health management. This paper details the design, development and applications of a tri-band flexible antenna crafted on wool substrate. The antenna has dimensions of $0.49\lambda_0 \times 0.37\lambda_0 \times 0.015\lambda_0$, providing a compact and highly flexible design that provides user comfort. It provides -10dB impedance bandwidth spanning over 2.44–2.50 GHz, 4.81–4.88 GHz and 7.04–7.44 GHz, with resonance frequencies at 2.47 GHz, 4.85 GHz and 7.23 GHz, respectively. The antenna achieves peak total gains of 6.31dBi at 2.47 GHz, 2.66dBi at 4.88 GHz, and 5.85dBi at 7.05 GHz. The antenna performance ensures its compatibility with ISM, IoT, and C-band applications, such as wireless networks and remote sensing. This novel tri-band flexible antenna design addresses the increasing need for efficient, low-profile, and cost-effective solutions in wearable technology, improving healthcare monitoring systems and other IoT applications.

References

1. Jiang, Z.H., Cui, Z., Yue, T., Zhu, Y., Werner, D.H.: Compact, highly efficient, and fully flexible circularly polarized antenna enabled by silver nanowires for wireless body-area networks. IEEE Trans. Biomed. Circuits Syst. **11**(4), 920–932 (2017)
2. Kaur, H., Chawla, P.: Design and performance analysis of wearable antenna for ISM band applications. Int. J. Electron. **110**(6), 986–1005 (2022)
3. Qian, Z., et al.: Development of a real-time wearable fall detection system in the context of Internet of Things. IEEE Internet Things J. **9**(21), 21999–22007 (2022)
4. Khalifeh, A., et al.: Wireless sensor networks for smart cities: Network design, implementation and performance evaluation. Electronics **10**(2), Article No. 218, 1–28 (2021)
5. Revilla, M., Titchenal, A., Calabrese, A., Gibby, C.: Human nutrition. In: Department of Human Nutrition, Food, and Animal Sciences, University of Hawaii at Manoa, vol. 3, pp. 1–20 (2019)
6. Arif, A., Zubair, M., Ali, M., Khan, M.U., Mehmood, M.Q.: A compact, low-profile fractal antenna for wearable on-body WBAN applications. IEEE Antennas Wirel. Propag. Lett. **18**(5), 981–985 (2019)
7. Rana, M.J., Mollah, M.A.S.: Numerical study of a loaded U-antenna for 3.5 GHz mobile WiMAX and 7.5 GHz military satellite communication applications. In: 16th International Conference on Computer and Information Technology, vol. 16, pp. 283–286. Khulna (2014)
8. Guo, Y.Q., Pan, Y.M., Zheng, S.Y., Lu, K.: A singly-fed dual-band microstrip antenna for microwave and millimeter-wave applications in 5G wireless communication. IEEE Trans. Veh. Technol. **70**(6), 5419–5430 (2021)
9. Shinde, P.N., Shinde, J.P.: Design of compact pentagonal slot antenna with bandwidth enhancement for multiband wireless applications. AEU-Int. J. Electron. C. **69**(10), 1489–1494 (2015)
10. Sreemathy, R., et al.: Design, analysis, and fabrication of dual frequency distinct bandwidth slot-loaded wash cotton flexible textile antenna for ISM band applications. Progress Electromagnetics Res. M **109**, 191–203 (2022)
11. Hossain, M.S., Rana, M.M., Anower, M.S., Paul, A.K.: Enhancing the performance of rectangular patch antenna using E shaped slot technique for 5.75 GHz ISM band applications. In: 5th International Conference on Informatics, Electronics, and Vision (ICIEV), pp. 449–453. Dhaka (2016)
12. Mathur, V., Gupta, M.: Comparison of performance characteristics of rectangular, square, and hexagonal microstrip patch antennas. In: 3rd International Conference on Reliability, Infocom Technologies, and Optimization, pp. 1–6. Noida (2014)
13. Hussain, N., Awan, W.A., Ali, W., Naqvi, S.I., Zaidi, A., Le, T.T.: Compact wideband patch antenna and its MIMO configuration for 28 GHz applications. AEU-Int. J. Electron. C. **132**, 1–10 (2021)
14. Wu, T.L., Pan, Y.M., Hu, P.F., Zheng, S.Y.: Design of a low profile and compact omnidirectional filtering patch antenna. IEEE Access **5**, 1083–1089 (2017)
15. Li, E., Li, X.J., Seet, B.C.: A triband slot patch antenna for conformal and wearable applications. Electronics **10**(24), Article No. 3155, 1–25 (2021)
16. Nasimuddin, et al.: Slotted microstrip antennas for circular polarization with compact size. IEEE Antennas Propag. Magazine **55**(2), 124–135 (2013)
17. Thaiwirot, W., Hengroemyat, Y., Kaewthai, T., Akkaraekthalin, P.: Analysis of flexible dual-band microstrip patch antenna for wearable applications. In: Research, Invention, and Innovation Congress: Innovative Electricals and Electronics (RI2C), pp. 9–12. Bangkok (2023)

18. Yin, B., Gu, J., Feng, X., Wang, B., Yu, Y., Ruan, W.: A low SAR value wearable antenna for wireless body area network based on AMC structure. Pro. Electromagnetics Res. C **95**, 119–129 (2019)
19. Shakib, M.N., Moghavvemi, M., Wan Mahadi, W.N.L.B.: Design of a tri-band off-body antenna for WBAN communication. IEEE Antennas Wireless Propag. Lett. **16**, 210–213 (2017)
20. Mandal, B., Parui, S.K.: Wearable tri-band SIW-based antenna on leather substrate. Electron. Lett. **51**(20), 1563–1564 (2015)
21. Sambandam, P., Kanagasabai, M., Natarajan, R., Alsath, M.G.N., Palaniswamy, S.: Miniaturized button-like WBAN antenna for off-body communication. IEEE Trans. Antennas Propag. **68**(7), 5228–5235 (2020)
22. Le, T.T., Kim, Y.-D., Yun, T.-Y.: A triple-band dual-open-ring high-gain high-efficiency antenna for wearable applications. IEEE Access **9**, 118435–118442 (2021)
23. Ali, I.H., Hamd, H.I., Abdalla, A.I.: Design and comparison of two types of antennas for SAR calculation in wireless applications. In: 2018 Advances in Science and Engineering Technology International Conferences (ASET), Dubai, Sharjah, Abu Dhabi, pp. 1–5 (2018)
24. Kundu, A., Patra, K., Gupta, B., Mallick, A.I.: A structured basis to determine equivalent dielectric properties of homogeneous phantom liquid representing multilayer biological tissues for SAR measurement. Progress Electromagnetics Res. B **108**, Article No. 24042703, 1–16 (2024)
25. Ghosh, S., Kundu, A., Gupta, B.: Slot-based miniaturized human body implantable antenna design at 2.45 GHz ISM band. In: 2022 IEEE Wireless Antenna and Microwave Symposium (WAMS), Rourkela Article No. 9848416, pp. 1–5 (2022)

Circular Shaped 6G Wearable Patch Antennas for Wireless Body Area Network

Siddalingappagouda Biradar[1(✉)] and G. S. Rajanna[2]

[1] Department of Electronics and Communication Engineering, Srinivas University, Mangalore, India
siddubbiradarr@gmail.com
[2] Srinivas University, Mangalore, India

Abstract. Wireless Body Area Network (WBAN) is an innovative network system, which consists of numerous wearable or implantable devices that monitors and transmits the physiological data. Designing a wearable patch antenna for WBAN is a challenging, because human body is a lossy medium which can absorb and scatter electromagnetic waves, thus leads to degrade of antenna performance. In this paper, we have designed a wearable 6G microstrip patch antennas with diamond (substrate plane) and gold material (ground plane), these antennas are very small and light weight with a flat surface, unlike traditional counterparts and these can be placed directly on a human body and are comfortable to wear for long periods. The antenna is designed, simulated, and analyzed using Computer Simulated Technology (CST) studio suite and the design consists of microstrip patch, substrate, feedline, and ground plane. The simulation parameters such as Return loss, Bandwidth, Gain, VSWR, Directivity, Efficiency and Far Field radiation is calculated. The simulation results show that, the antenna made with diamond material resonates at frequency of 2.09 THz, 3.94 THz, 7.47 THz and 8.8 THz performances better, when compared to antenna made with gold material resonating at frequency of 2.50 THz, 4.69 THz and 6.86 THz.

Keywords: Terahertz Frequency · 6G Wearable patch antenna · Diamond, and gold material · WBAN · CST Tool

1 Introduction

Imagine a scenario, where our health and overall wellness are constantly monitored in a real time manner without the hassle of carrying around bulky gadgets or having frequent medical examinations required. This vision is made possible by WBAN, a technology that enables direct connectivity to your body. Whether, it involves keeping tracks on our fitness, monitoring chronic ailments, or offering immediate medical updates and recommendations. WBAN systems are revolutionizing our perceptions of health and technology integration and they are like a group of wireless sensors positioned on or inside our body, that can communicate with each other and along other external devices. These sensors can be integrated into wearable devices, like a smart watches and fitness

K. Atul et al. (Eds.): BodyNets 2024, LNICST 666, pp. 19–30, 2026.
https://doi.org/10.1007/978-3-032-16099-7_3

trackers or even into clothing. They may also be placed beneath the skin for health monitoring. The purpose of this is to monitor our signs and movements, and the real-time data that can be used for everything from improving our workout to detecting health issues at early stage. WBAN are important because,

i. Continuous Health Monitoring: These advanced networks seamlessly track health parameters such as heart rate and blood pressure around the clock. Whether, we are at work or even asleep. Ensuring uninterrupted monitoring, for proactive healthcare management instead of reactive treatments.
ii. Personalized Fitness: For fitness enthusiasts, WBAN technology provides the ability to monitor everything from calorie burn to muscle activity in real time, Imagine exercising with equipment that provides real time feedback on our form, adjusts your routine based on how your body is responding, and even tells you when to hydrate or rest.
iii. Managing Chronic Conditions: For those with chronic health situations, individuals dealing with long term health issues or chronic conditions like diabetes or heart disease and respiratory problems can greatly benefit from WBAN. These networks constantly track health data, which in turn allows for the detection of possible health issues and timely alerts to healthcare professionals, for prompt interventions and improved management of these conditions.

In the paper referred [1], Microstrip Circular antenna is designed for different frequency bands of S, K, C, L, Ku, Ka bands, and 5G Wireless Applications. The proposed antenna is constructed at $(30\times40\times1.6)$ mm^3 with a thickness of 0.035 mm, substrate of FR-4, patch, and ground with copper material. So, four-band are achieved in the range from 1 GHz to 15 GHz, the bands at 3.07 GHz -3.34 GHz, 4.75 GHz-4.92 GHz, 5.83 GHz-5.96 GHz and 11.69 GHz-13.65 GHz. The reflection co-efficient at these frequencies is of - 29.454 dB, -23.199 dB, -17.254 dB and -35.248 dB. The 6G antenna design with measure of $(2.5 \times 2.5 \times 2)$ cm^3 is presented in [2]. The simulation is carried out using CST tool, the return loss is -54 dB, resonating frequency at 5.8GHz. In [3], the rectangular antenna is designed with an array pattern of $(2 \times 2 \times 2)$ mm^3, and 1×4 mm for 6G Applications using CST tool. The simulation results predict, VSWR value of 1.05, gain around 7.77 dBi and 8.18 dBi, return loss of -52.9 dB and 56.36 dB with bandwidth of 5.26 GHz and 16.26 GHz. The work carried out in the paper [4], the 'U' shaped design is proposed for terahertz communication systems, the simulation is performed using CST tool and the results are -19.5 dB of return loss, bandwidth of 44 GHz at resonating frequency of 0.8 THz. In the study provided [5], The planar microstrip patch antenna with triple-band for two different application and frequencies band such as WLAN, WiMAX and C-band, radar Ku-band. The proposed antenna has dimension of $(6\times38\times1.6)$ mm^3, CST tool is used for simulation and the performance of antenna is, gain of 2.8, 3.8, and 4.7 dBi, return loss of more than -10 dB and 87 % of total efficiency. In [6], A rectangular dual-band microstrip patch antenna for 5G Application is designed with dimension of $(9.08 \times 66.65 \times 0.16)$ mm^3. The simulation is done utilizing HFSS tool, The resonating frequency of 23.8 GHz with -27.5 dB reflection co-efficient, 0.7 GHz of bandwidth, and gain of 2.84 dB for first band and second band echoes at 37.5 GHz with S_{11}-parameter value of -28.87 dB, 1 GHz of bandwidth, and 3.33 dB of gain value. The design of body application, 5G microstrip patch antenna is represented in [7] using FEKO software and the simulation results shows 100% of total radiation efficiency, gain value of 10 dB, bandwidth of 1.63 GHz and return loss of -32.86 dB. In the paper [8], arc shaped microstrip patch antenna is designed for 5G application, shows good results at resonating frequency of 37 GHz and has return loss value of -36 dB with peak gain of 2.57 dBi. The discussion carried out in [9, 10], the split ring resonator microstrip antenna is designed a for sub-6 GHz applications using CST tool and fabricated, with measuring of $(22 \times 16 \times 1.6)\ mm^3$, ground and patch using copper material and FR-4 Substrate, the simulation results shows that the resonant frequency is of around 5.2 GHz, return loss of -32 dB and bandwidth of 1.8 GHz. The fractal antenna is designed for wideband application using CST tool and the design is fabricated with a height of 1.6 mm, substrate width, and length of 35 mm^2. The simulation result shows of resonance frequency are 10 GHz, the gain is 6 dB and the directivity is of 8.58 dB (Table 1).

Table 1. Comparison of the proposed antenna with design and performance parameters of antenna defined in the references section

Ref No	Design Area (L*W) mm	Resonating Frequency GHz	Gain dBi	BandwidthGHz	Substrate Material	Shape	Return Loss dB	Tool used
[11]	0.51×0.78	28	7.75	0.66	RT/Duroid 5880	Circular	-43.23	CST
[12]	7×6	26.84	9.24	2.1	RT/Duroid 5880	Circular	− 10	CST
[13]	$1.24 \times 0.6 \times 0.15$	28	3.87	4.1	FR-4	Circular	-26.96	CST
[14]	50×50	2.5	5.31	0.11	FR-4	Circular	-12.19	CST
[15]	10×10	32.7	3.28	7.74	Taconic RF-60A	Circular	-24.26	CST
[16]	5.6×4.65	28	6.63	0.97	RT/Duroid 5880	Circular	-32.21	CST
[17]	6×4	41.08	6.16	0.15	RT/Duroid 5880	Circular	-12.4	CST
[18]	33×36	3.5	5.11	0.16	FR-4	Circular	-42	CST
[19]	32×32	3.6	3.13	1.14	FR-4	Circular	-36.05	CST
[20]	21×18	28	7.19	1.13	FR-4	Circular	-24.51	CST
[21]	5.95×5.95	28	0.16	1.76	FR-4	Circular	-45.11	CST
[Proposed]	**37.58 μm × 37.58 μm**	**7.47 THz & 6.86 THz**	**6.72 & 5.62**	**650 & 820**	**FR-4 & Diamond, Gold & Copper (Ground)**	**Circular**	**-36.57&--23.46**	**CST**

2 Design and Simulation Parameters

The design of circular shaped 6G wearable patch antenna mainly consist of ground plane, substrate, patch antenna, feedline placed on human body tissues (Skin, Fat and Muscle Area). The front view of antenna and description of its part are shown in the Fig. 1 (Table 2).

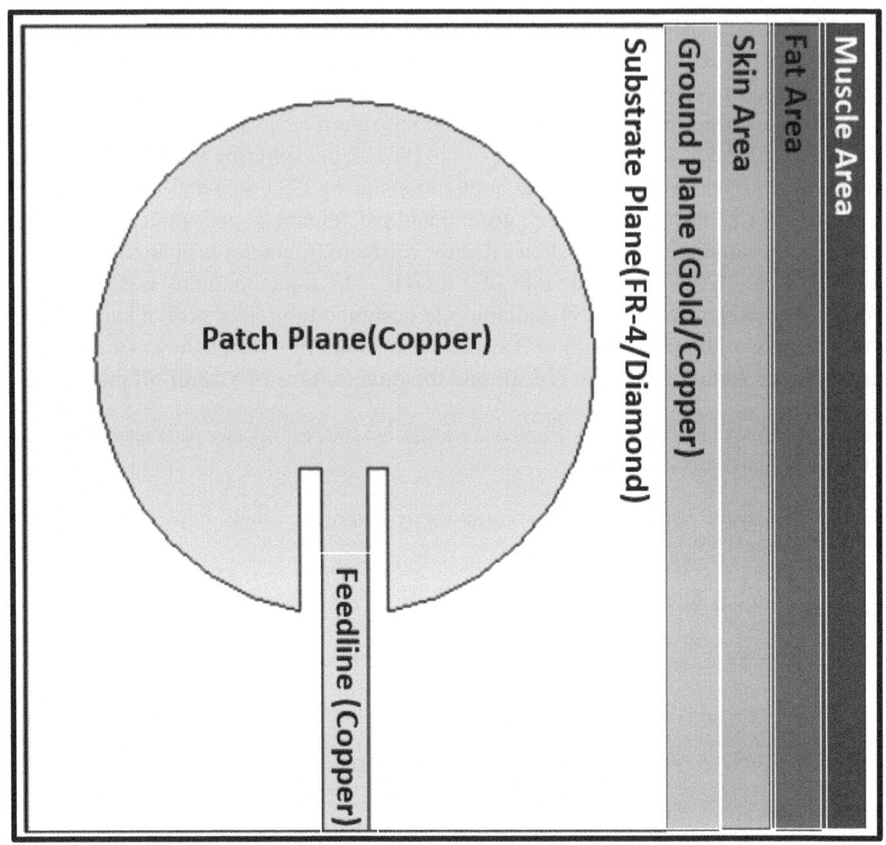

Fig. 1. Circular Patch Antenna on Human Body Area

Table 2. Parameters and materials used for circular patch antenna

Variable	Description	Values(μm)	Plane	Material-1	Material-2
r	Radius of Patch	17.40	Ground	Gold	Copper
F_i	Inside Cut	10	Substrate	FR-4	Diamond
L_f	Length of Fed	14.75	Feedline	Copper	Copper
W_f	Width of Fed	03.13	Patch	Copper	Copper

Table 3. Properties of Human Body Tissues

Human Body Tissue	Permittivity (ε_r)	Conductivity(s/m)	Loss Tangent(σ)
Skin	7	5	0.30
Fat	3	0.1	0.03
Muscle	15	10	0.50

In a circular patch antenna, the ground plane is made up of two materials such as gold and copper. Both these materials are good conductor of electricity and has excellent thermal conductivity and good corrosion resistance. Copper is relatively easy to fabricate and is compatible with most substrate materials and it can be easily patterned and etched, making it suitable for flexible substrates. While, Gold is used in applications where corrosion resistance is critical and it providing efficient signal transmission and reception. Its stability makes it suitable for harsh environments. The substrate plane is made up of FR-4 and diamond, the advantage of using FR-4 is due to low cost, high availability, and good mechanical stability. Diamond has many advantages over wearable application such as Biocompatibility, High thermal conductivity, Chemical resistance and, durability and hardness. Diamond and gold are most used in variety of jewelries.

The microstrip patch antenna placed on human body phantom model, and this model consists of three layers skin, fat and muscle. The thickness of these layers are 2 mm, 2 mm and 4 mm. The parameters that are required to build this model is as shown in table 3. The simulation is carried-out in CST tool, the performance of microstrip patch antenna placed on human body is discussed in result section.

Radius of circular patch antenna is calculated from rectangular patch antenna with the help of online patch antenna calculator,

The following are the equations of that are used for microstrip patch antenna calculation process,

To calculate, the width of the microstrip patch antenna we use the formula,

$$Wp = \frac{c_0}{2f_r\sqrt{\frac{\varepsilon_r+1}{2}}} \tag{1}$$

- calculating the effective dielectric constant using the patch antenna's predicted width, height, and dielectric constant of the dielectric material.

$$\varepsilon_{reff} = \frac{\varepsilon_r + 1}{2} + \frac{\varepsilon_r - 1}{2} \times \sqrt{\left(1 + \left(\frac{12h}{w}\right)\right)} \tag{2}$$

- the effective length is calculated using

$$\mathrm{L}_{eff} = \frac{c}{2f0\sqrt{\varepsilon_{reff}}} \tag{3}$$

- ΔL is the length extension, calculated using

$$\Delta L = 0.412 \times \text{h} \times \frac{\left(\varepsilon_{reff} + 0.3\right)\left(\frac{w}{h} + 0.26\right)}{\left(\varepsilon_{reff} + 0.253\right)\left(\frac{w}{h} + 0.8\right)} \tag{4}$$

- Actual length of the patch is calculated using

$$\text{L} = L_{eff} - 2\Delta L \tag{5}$$

- Feedline width is calculated using

$$W_f = \frac{7.48h}{e^{\left(z_0 \frac{\sqrt{\varepsilon_r + 1.41}}{87}\right)}} - 1. \tag{6}$$

The parameters that are used for design simulation are,

- Resonance Frequency is ‘$\mathbf{f_r/f_0}$’
- Width of the patch antenna is ‘**W**’
- Length of the patch is ‘**L**’
- Thickness is ‘**h**’
- Relative permittivity of the dielectric substrate is ‘$\boldsymbol{\varepsilon_r}$’
- Speed of light ‘$\mathbf{c_o/c}$’: 3 x 10^8 m/s
- Dielectric Constant = 4.3
- Dielectric Height = 1.6

substituting the values of dielectric constant, dielectric height, and frequency in the above link we get the value,

Width = 37.58 μm and Length = 29.14 μm.

The results of the height and width of the corresponding rectangular patch antenna are substituted in formula,

$$\text{The radius of patch } = \sqrt{\frac{(w = Dh) * (H + Dh)}{2}} \tag{7}$$

The radius of patch is 17.35 μm.

3 Results and Discussion

This section discusses about simulation results of performance metrics of microstrip patch antenna,

3.1 Return Loss or Reflection Co-efficient

It is the measurement of the reflected wave or signal strength traveling or returning back to a transmitter from an antenna and indicates the efficiency of the antenna at specific frequencies. It is a critical parameter and represented in decibels (dB). While negative return loss means improved antenna performance, the value near “0” dB indicates poor impedance matching.

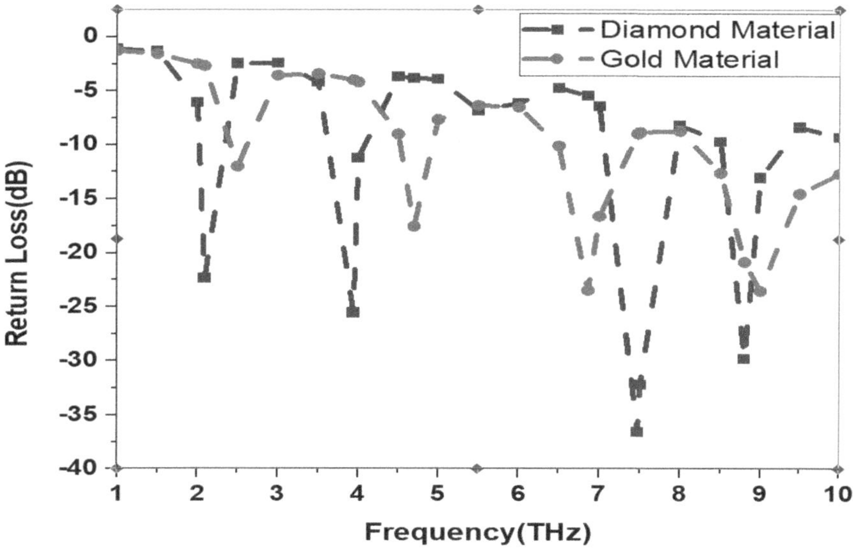

Fig. 2. Return loss Verus frequency of diamond and gold material circular patch antenna

Table 4. Return loss and Bandwidth of Circular Patch Antenna of Diamond and Gold Material

Resonating Frequency (THz)	Return Loss(dB)	Bandwidth (GHz)	Resonating Frequency(THz)	Return Loss(dB)	Bandwidth ()GHz
2.09	-22.32	110	2.50	-1201	110
3.94	-22.54	160	4.69	-17.53	350
7.47	**-36.57**	**650**	**6.86**	**-23.46**	**820**
8.80	-29.78	640	--	--	--

Circular patch antenna with diamond and gold material resonates at multiple frequencies as shown in Fig. 2. The return loss is calculated from S_{11}-Parameter by identifying the frequencies at below -10 dB and bandwidth by subtracting high frequency and low frequency at resonating frequency. The return loss and bandwidth of resonant frequencies are presented in Table 4. For diamond material, very low return loss of -36.57 dB at resonating frequency of 7.47 THz and has high bandwidth of 650 GHz. For gold material, very low return loss of -23.46 dB at resonating frequency of 6.86 THz and has high bandwidth of 820 GHz. In both cases, around less than 5% of power is reflected, ensuring better matching and efficiency.

3.2 Voltage Standing Wave Ratio (VSWR)

VSWR is another important parameter for 6G antenna design, representing how well the antenna is impedance-matched to the transmission line. With lesser VSWR values indicating better impedance matching and reduced power reflection.

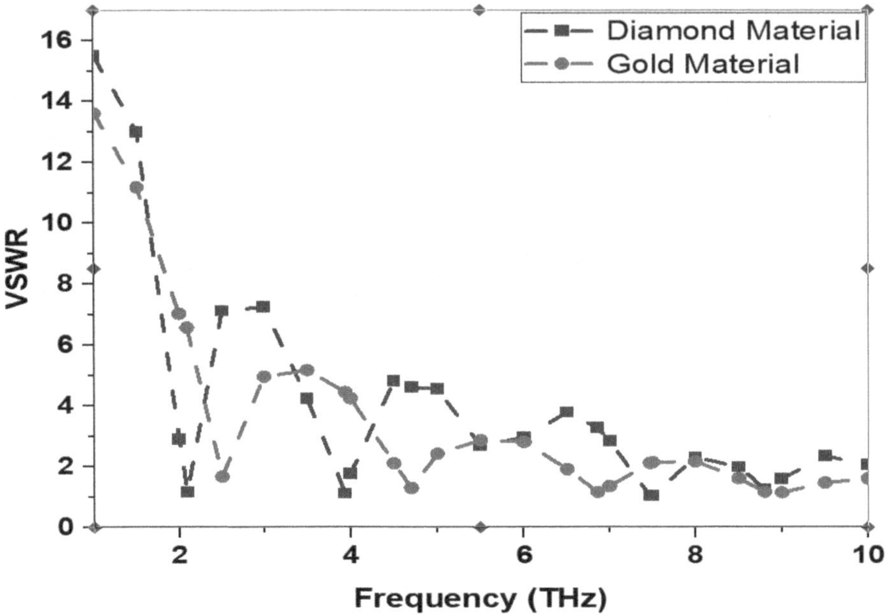

Fig. 3. VSWR Verus frequency of diamond and gold material circular patch antenna

Table 5. VSWR for circular patch antenna of diamond and gold material

Resonating Frequency (THz)	VSWR	Resonating Frequency (THz)	VSWR
2.09	1.16	2.50	1.67
3.94	1.11	4.69	1.30
7.47	**1.03**	**6.86**	**1.15**
8.80	1.26	--	--

The VSWR value with respective to the resonating frequency of microstrip patch antenna of diamond and gold material is as shown in Fig. 3. The VSWR value at different resonating frequencies are presented in Table 5. For diamond material antenna, the resonating frequency of 7.47 THz has lower VSWR value of 1.03 and 1.15 at 6.86 THz for gold material antenna.

3.3 Far Field

The far-field radiation pattern is a vital characteristic of antenna performance, particularly for 6G antenna designs that frequently functions in very high-frequency bands. The far-field region, is where the emitted electromagnetic waves from the antenna can be considered plane waves, and the antenna's characteristics, such as directivity, gain, and beamwidth, can be efficiently analyzed.

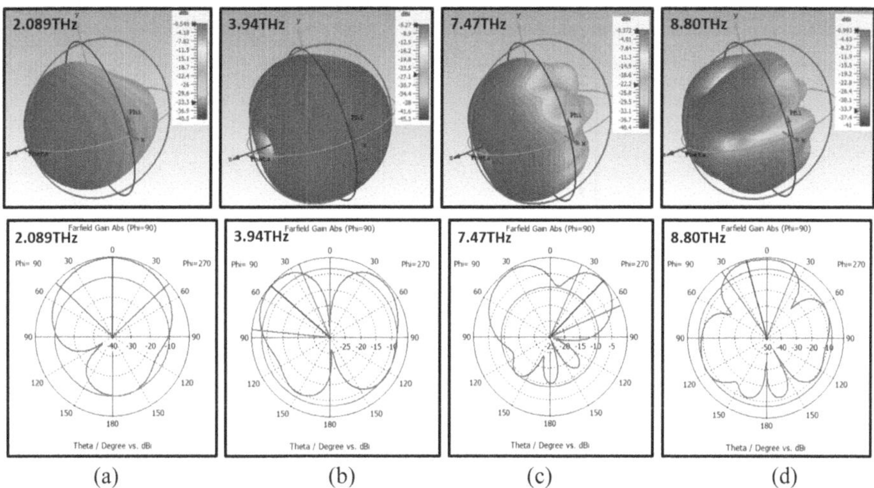

Fig. 4. Far Field of circular microstrip patch antenna for diamond material

A spherical or hemispherical view of the radiation pattern of microstrip patch antenna for diamond material is as shown in Fig. 4. The colors indicate the relative intensity in 3D space. Specially, red color indicates the far field region and yellow defines the near field region of microstrip patch antenna, these visualizations are essential for evaluating the antenna's radiation performance.

Table 6. Directivity, Gain and Efficiency for Circular Patch Antenna of Diamond Material

Resonating Frequency (THz)	Directivity (dBi)	Gain (dBi)	Efficiency (dB)
2.09	5.44	2.54	6.02
3.94	2.47	5.27	6.73
7.47	**6.02**	**6.72**	**7.39**
8.80	5.61	4.37	6.61

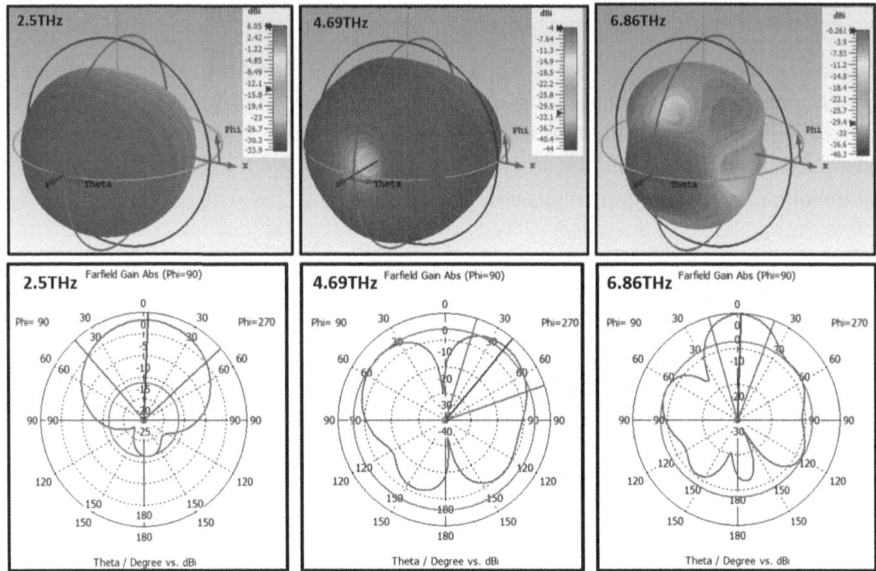

Fig. 5. Far Field of Circular Microstrip Patch Antenna for Gold Material

The directivity, gain and efficiency of antenna is calculated by using 3D radiation pattern as shown in Table 6 and 7. The radiation pattern of microstrip patch antenna for gold material is as shown in Fig. 5. The directivity of an antenna refers to how focused its radiation beam's, in a direction which is determined by comparing the normalized power in that direction to the average normalized power of the antenna's radiation pattern.

Table 7. Directivity, Gain and Efficiency for Circular Patch Antenna of Gold Material

Resonating Frequency (THz)	Directivity (dBi)	Gain (dBi)	Efficiency (dB)
2.50	6.05	1.79	8.132
4.69	3.80	4.00	7.88
6.86	**9.04**	**5.62**	**9.32**

The directivity, gain and efficiency of circular microstrip patch antenna for diamond and gold material (Table 6 and 7) resonating at multiple frequencies, shows the overall performance of wearable circular patch antenna placed on human body. The Specific Absorption Rate (SAR) is a vital constraint that confirms the safety of the electromagnetic fields, when interrelating with human tissue. The SAR value is measured in watts per kilogram (W/kg) and according to Federal Communication Commission (FCC), and International Commission on Non-Ionizing Radiation Protection (ICNIRP) SAR value should be below the limits of 2 W/kg. The attained SAR value at 7.47 THz is 0.099 W/Kg averaged over 10 gm of tissue for circular shaped diamond material patch antenna. The achieved SAR value at 6.86 THz is 0.162 W/Kg averaged over 10 gm of tissue for circular shaped gold material patch antenna.

4 Conclusion

A wearable 6G circular microstrip patch antenna made with a diamond and gold material are designed to operate at ultra-high terahertz frequencies. These antennas are embedded in wearable devices, which will have less return loss, better gain, low power consumption, strong impedance matching, high efficiency, and directivity. In this paper, the design, simulation, and analysing of performance of multiple frequency band of microstrip 6G wearable circular patch antenna for WBAN connectivity is obtained, analysed, and discussed. The simulation results show that, the antenna made with diamond material resonates at frequency of 2.09 THz, 3.94 THz, 7.47 THz and 8.8 THz. Its performance is better, when compared to antenna made with gold material resonating at frequency of 2.50 THz, 4.69 THz and 6.86 THz. Among these resonating frequencies, especially frequency at 7.47 THz and 6.86 THz, performance better compared to other resonating frequencies. Thus, these proposed 6G wearable antennas which are small size, low power consumption, light weight and low signal loss can be used in WBAN for various applications like health monitoring, fitness and wellness, Augmented Reality (AR) and Virtual Reality (VR).

References

1. Thaher, R.H.: Circular Patch Antenna Design and Analysis for L, S, C, Ku, K, Ka bands, and 5G, Wireless Applications," International Symposium on Multidisciplinary Studies and Innovative Technologies (ISMSIT), Ankara, Turkey, pp. 1061–1063 (2022). https://doi.org/10.1109/ISMSIT56059.2022.9932714
2. Bhutiani, S., Tadas, K.: An Improved Design of 6G Microstrip Patch Antenna with a High Reflection Coefficient and Working Frequency of 5.8 GHz. In: IEEE International Conference on ICT in Business Industry and Government (ICTBIG), Indore, India, pp. 1–3 (2023). https://doi.org/10.1109/ICTBIG59752.2023.10456065
3. Aldhaibani, A.O., Ba Sharahil, A., Bukier, S., Ba Bukier, M., Ba Wazir, A., Balcauilkh, S.: Design of microstrip patch antenna for sixth generation frequency band. Int. J. Sci. Res. Netw. Sec. Commun. **12**(4), 1–7 (2024)
4. Saeed, M.A., Nwajana, A.: U-Shaped terahertz microstrip patch antenna for 6G future communications. In: 7th International Electromagnetic Compatibility Conference (EMC Turkiye) 17th–20th September 2023 (2023)
5. El-Hakim, H.A., Mohamed, H.A.: Engineering planar antenna using geometry arrangements for wireless communications and satellite applications. Sci. Rep. **13**(1), 19196 (2023). https://doi.org/10.1038/s41598-023-46400-9
6. Al-Sharhanee, K., Al-Joboury, I., Ali, R.: Design of Rectangular Microstrip Patch Antenna with Dual-Band for 5G Millimeter-Wave Applications. pp 65–71 (2023). https://doi.org/10.14445/23488379/IJEEE-V10I12P107
7. Colaco, J., Rajesh B.L.: Design and Implementation of microstrip circular patch antenna for 5G applications. In: International Conference on Electrical, Communication, and Computer Engineering (ICECCE) 1–4, pp 56–62 (2023)
8. Gupta, A.: Design of an elliptical arc-shaped antenna at 37 GHz and performance analysis for 5G on-body application. Przeglad Elektrotechniczny (2024)
9. Gencoglan, D.N., Colak, S., Palandoken, M.: Spiral-resonator-based frequency reconfigurable antenna design for sub-6 GHz applications. Appl. Sci. **13**(15), 8719 (2013). https://doi.org/10.3390/app13158719

10. Raj, A., Mandal, D.: Design and implementation of hybrid fed array antennae for Sub-6 GHz and 5G mm-wave communication and wireless applications. Int. J. Microwave Wireless Technol. **16**(4), 605–624 (2024). https://doi.org/10.1017/S1759078723001496
11. Kumar, S., Kumar, A.: Design of circular patch antennas for 5G applications. In: 2nd International Conference on Innovations in Electronics, Signal Processing and Communication (IESC), Shillong, India, pp. 287–289 (2019). https://doi.org/10.1109/IESPC.2019.8902384
12. Sharma, S., Kumar, M.: A millimeter wave elliptical slot circular patch mimo antenna for future 5G mobile communication networks. Prog. Electromagn. Res. M **110**, 235–247 (2022)
13. Khan, M.M., et al.: Design and Analysis of a 5G Wideband Antenna for wireless body-centric network. Wireless Commun. Mob. Comput. **2022**(1), 1558791 (2022). https://doi.org/10.1155/2022/1558791
14. Sathishkumar, P.: Natarajan: design of dual mode antenna using CMA and broadband dual-polarized antenna for 5G networks. Sci. Rep. **14**, 15553 (2024). https://doi.org/10.1038/s41598-024-66515
15. Nafi, N.A., Ashikur Rahman, K.M., Israt, C.T., Dutta Anik, N., Kausar, A.S.M.Z.: Theta slotted circular multiband patch antenna design and analysis for mm-wave 5G communication system. In: IEEE Symposium on Wireless Technology and Applications (ISWTA), Kuala Lumpur, Malaysia, pp. 152–156 (2024). https://doi.org/10.1109/ISWTA62130.2024.10651891
16. Ezzulddin, S., Hasan, S., Ameen, M.: Design and simulation of microstrip patch antenna for 5G application using CST studio. Int. J. Adv. Sci. Technol. **29**, 7193–7205 (2020)
17. Altufaili, M., Najaf, A., Sabah, Z.: Design of circular-shaped microstrip patch antenna for 5G applications. TELKOMNIKA (Telecommunication Computing Electronics and Control). 20 (2022). https://doi.org/10.12928/TELKOMNIKA.v20i1.21019
18. Fadhil, T.Z., Murad, N.A., Hamid, M.R.: Design and performance of a compact circular patch antenna with metasurface superstrate for fifth generation application. In: 2023 IEEE 16th Malaysia International Conference on Communication (MICC), Kuala Lumpur, Malaysia, pp. 97–100 (2023). https://doi.org/10.1109/MICC59384.2023.10419571
19. Haider, S., Jasim, F., Al-Sherbaz, A.: Design and analysis of microstrip patch antenna for 5G application. J. Eng. Sustain. Develop. **28**(02), 285–293, (2024). https://doi.org/10.31272/jeasd.28.2.10
20. Sohel Rana, Md, Moniruzzaman, Md., Anup, N.B.: Design of 28 GHz microstrip patch antenna for wireless applications. Introduction J. Elect. Eng. Inf. **11**, 17–23 (2023). https://doi.org/10.52549/ijeei.v11i4.4942
21. Djouimaa, A., Bencherif, K.: Design of a Compact Circular Microstrip Patch Antenna for 5G Applications. Engineering, Technology and Applied Science Research, 14, Aug. 2024, 16020–16024 (2024). https://doi.org/10.48084/etasr.7961

Compact Printed Dual-Band Monopole Antenna for Wearable IoT Applications

Shivani Pandey[1(✉)], Ashish Raj[2], Itu Snigdh[3], and Nisha Gupta[2]

[1] Electronics and Communication Engineering (SENSE), Vellore Institute of Technology, Katpadi, Vellore 632014, India
shivaniofficialp@gmail.com

[2] Electronics and Communication Engineering, Birla Institute of Technology, Mesra, Ranchi 835215, India
ngupta@bitmesra.ac.in

[3] Computer Science and Engineering, Birla Institute of Technology, Mesra, Ranchi 835215, India
itusnigdh@bitmesra.ac.in

Abstract. In this paper, a compact dual-band printed CPW fed monopole antenna configuration is designed for off-body IoT applications. A thin polyimide substrate is used for printing the monopole configuration. The proposed antenna configuration resonates at 2.4 GHz and 4.8 GHz. The overall dimensions of the structure are $37 \times 36 \times 0.1$ mm^3. A prototype model of the proposed antenna is developed, measured, and compared with the simulation results for validation. It is found the proposed antenna configuration is a good choice for several wearable IoT applications commonly used in Wi-Fi and Bluetooth.

Keywords: Monopole antenna · wearable antenna · polyimide substrate · IoT applications

1 Introduction

In recent years, Body Centric Wireless Communication (BCWC) [1] has emerged as an important field of research due to their potential applications in various fields to improve the quality of the human lives. The growing interest in antennas and wave propagation for body centric communication systems has led the IEEE 802.15 standardization group to standardize applications intended for on, off, and in- body communication. The applications are in health monitoring, rescue services, communications, wireless computing, and IoTs. The performance of BCWC greatly relies on wearable antennas [2, 3], which play a vital role in these networks. Printed monopole antennas [4] are a popular choice for wearable IoT applications [5, 6] due to their simplicity, low cost, and ease of integration into fabric or flexible materials. However, there are some key points that need to be considered while designing and implementing a printed monopole antenna for wearable IoT applications. First and foremost is the requirement of a flexible and

K. Atul et al. (Eds.): BodyNets 2024, LNICST 666, pp. 31–37, 2026.
https://doi.org/10.1007/978-3-032-16099-7_4

durable substrate material [7], such as polyimide, polyester, or fabric-based materials. The substrate should be comfortable for the wearer and compatible with the antenna's operational frequency. The shape and size of the antenna is another important criterion in realizing a compact body worn antenna for off-body IoT applications. While considering the monopole patch configuration, the co-planar waveguide (CPW) feed is the preferred choice to ensure proper impedance matching to minimize the signal reflection and maximize the power transfer. Gain and omnidirectional radiation pattern is also important for ensuring the reliable communication regardless of the orientation of the wearer. Sufficient bandwidth of the antenna is required to cover the desired frequency range and to accommodate any potential frequency shifts due to bending or movement which is easily achievable with use of monopole antennas. Another important parameter of significance is the specific absorption rate (SAR) while still maintaining a miniature footprint which is essential for SAR regulation compliance to minimize the risk of radiation exposure to the wearer. While 2.4 GHz frequency band lies in the Industrial, Scientific and Medical (ISM) applications band, this dual band 2.4/4.8 GHz antenna finds application in biomedical telemetry [8].

2 Antenna Design

The proposed monopole patch antenna configuration is shown in Fig. 1 (a). The metallized pattern consists of a main arm with an arrow at the top connected to four drooping sub arms, two on each side, and an arrow at the top. For designing the wearable antenna and for placing it on the wrist, a thin antenna configuration is required. Therefore, a simple monopole configuration is considered first. To make it resonate at 2.4 GHz, the length of the monopole is significant. Hence, to reduce it and to make the structure resonate at two frequencies, modifications to the structure are applied such as considering the drooping stubs along the sides for compactness and an arrow at the top. In terms of size the proposed antenna is thin, can conveniently be placed on the wrist and is suitable for wearable applications.

The design parameters are specified in Fig. 1(b). The proposed antenna is fed by a 50-Ω CPW, which is printed on the same side of the radiating patch. The feed line width is 2 mm, and gap between the feed and the ground plane is 0.3 mm on both sides. The ground width is 17.4 mm on each side, and length is 8.5 mm. A thin flexible polyimide substrate suitable for body worn application is selected for printing the antenna and the substrate specifications are given in Table 1. The dielectric properties of polyimide are measured following the steps described in [9]. The frequency dependence properties over the large frequency band specified in [10].

The metallized pattern is printed over the polyimide substrate with the help of Bot Factory SV2 PCB printer.

Table 1. Polyimide substrate parameters

Thickness	0.125 mm
X	37 mm
Y	36 mm
Relative permittivity	3.5
Dielectric loss tangent	0.008

3 Antenna Design

The proposed antenna configuration is simulated in CST microwave studio and the performance characteristics are obtained in terms of the reflection coefficient and radiation patterns. The characteristics of the fabricated prototype model as shown in Fig. 2 is measured using Vector network analyser and the pattern measurement setup in Anechoic chamber as shown in Fig. 3. The measured reflection coefficient is compared with the simulation result. The magnitude of the simulated and measured reflection coefficients is plotted in Fig. 4. As seen, the proposed antenna resonates at two frequencies 2.4 GHz and 4.8 GHz. The reflection coefficients at these two frequencies are −25.5 dB and −21 dB and −10 dB bandwidth as 100 MHz and 500 MHz respectively. A shift in both measured resonant frequencies is evident which may be attributed to the fabrication tolerances. The simulated co-polar and cross-polar patterns of the proposed antenna at 2.4 and 4.8 GHz are shown in Fig. 5(a), (b), (c), and (d). A comparison of simulated and measured 2-D radiation patterns of the antenna is shown in Fig. 6(b). The electric field distribution at 2.4 GHz is shown in Fig. 7. As evident, maximum electric field concentration is located between the CPW feed and the ground plane. Next, the simulation is performed to obtain the specific absorption rate (SAR). The performance of the antenna gets affected when placed in proximity of human body. Therefore, the antenna is placed over a 20 mm foam layer to provide an isolation from the human body and then tested for on-body flat section. For this purpose, a flat three-layered body phantom is designed consisting of muscle, fat and skin as shown in Fig. 8. The average permittivity and conductivity of these layers at 2.4 GHz are: Muscle ($\varepsilon_r = 52.79$; $\sigma = 1.705$), Fat ($\varepsilon_r = 5.28$; $\sigma = 0.1$) and Skin ($\varepsilon_r = 31.29$; $\sigma = 5.0138$). The thickness of Muscle, Fat and Skin layers are considered as 23 mm, 8 mm and 2 mm It is found that the proposed antenna guarantees conformance with FCC guidelines (i.e., SAR@ lg (human tissue) $\leq$1.6W/kg) for both 2.4 and 4.8 GHz frequency bands.

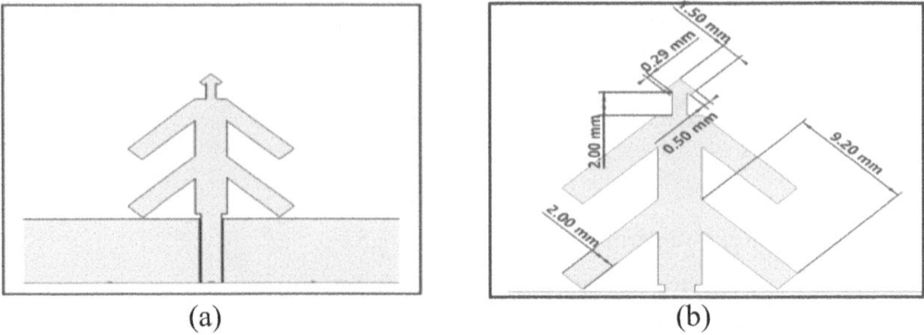

Fig. 1. (a) Proposed monopole antenna configuration (b) Design parameters

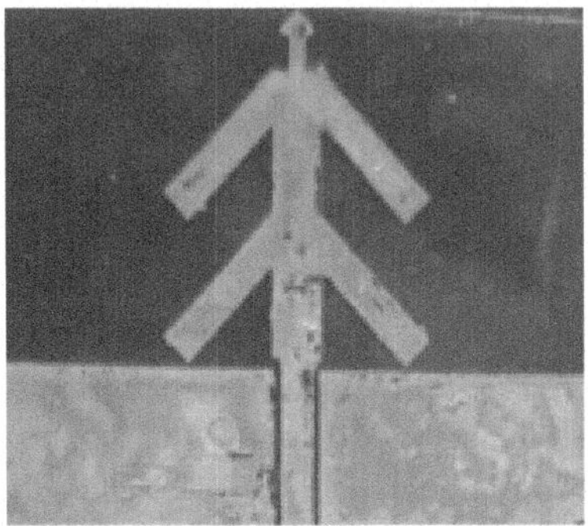

Fig. 2. Fabricated model of the proposed antenna

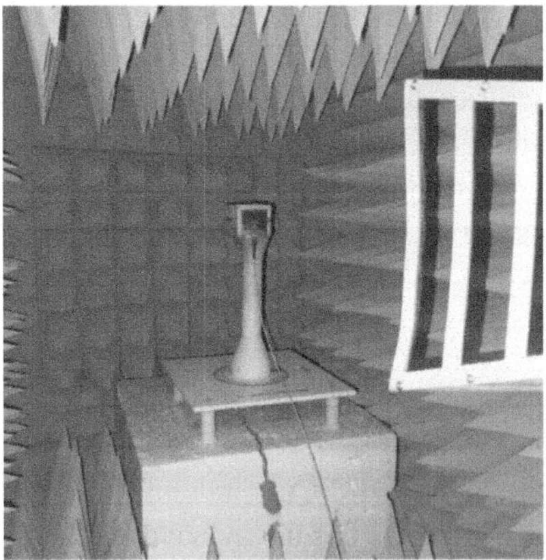

Fig. 3. Measurement Setup

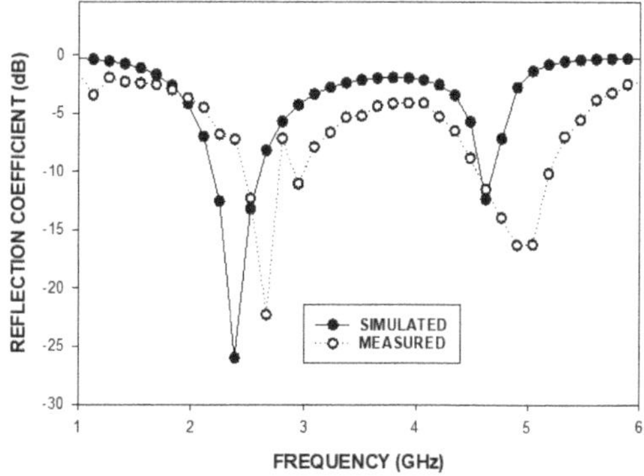

Fig. 4. Comparison of Reflection coefficient

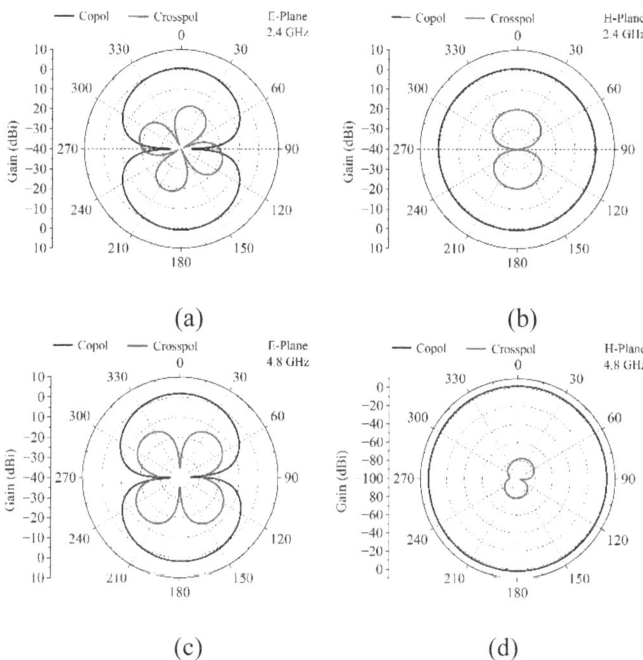

Fig. 5. Simulated Co-polar and Cross-polar 2-D radiation pattern of the proposed antenna at 2.4 GHZ and 4.8 GHz.

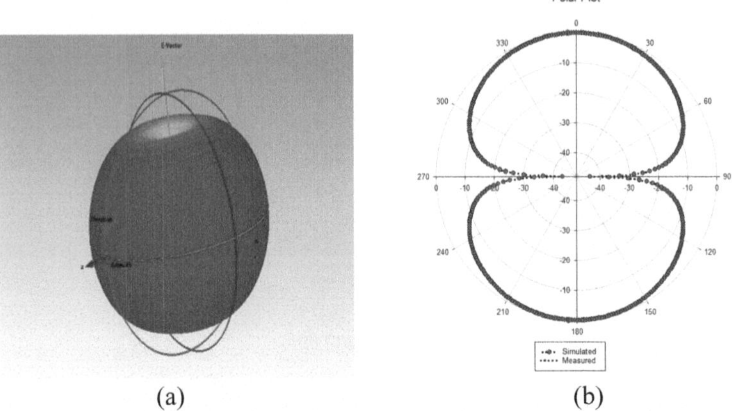

(a) (b)

Fig. 6. (a) 3-D radiation pattern of the proposed antenna (b) Comparison of simulated and measured radiation pattern at 2.4 GHz.

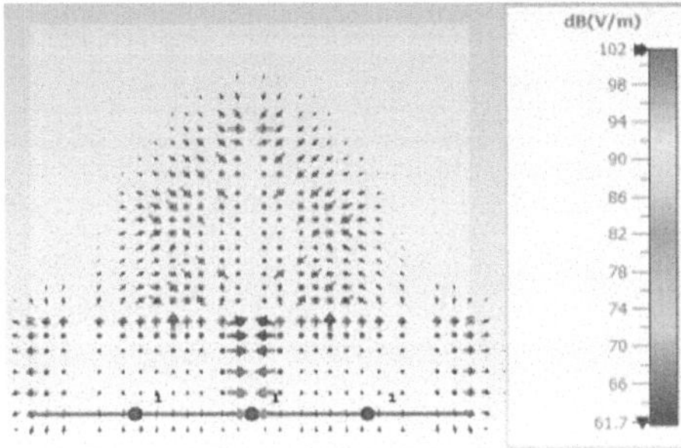

Fig. 7. Electric field distribution at 2.4 GHz

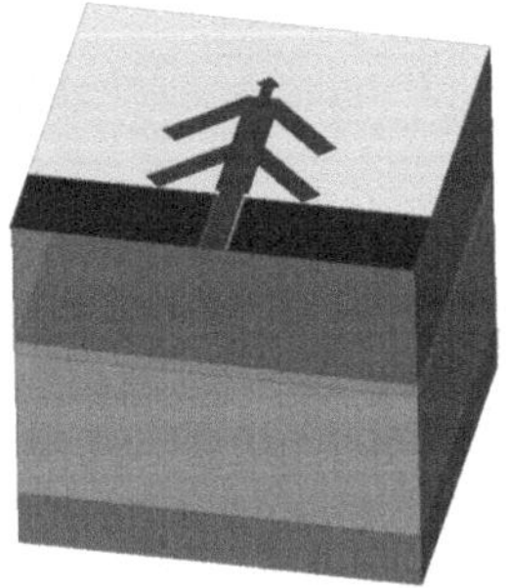

Fig. 8. Proposed antenna mounted on the flat human body phantom Top layer: Monopole patch on polyimide substrate; 2nd layer: foam; 3rd layer: Skin; 4th layer: Fat, and Bottom layer: Muscle

4 Conclusions

In this paper, a novel 37 mm × 36 mm dual-band monopole patch antenna is proposed for off-body wearable applications with resonances at 2.4 GHz and 4.8 GHz. The proposed antenna has a peak gain of 1.44 dBi at 2.4 GHz. The antenna is printed over thin flexible polyimide substrate to ensure wearing comfort and is found to conform with FCC SAR standards. The proposed antenna is suitable for several wearable IoT applications.

Acknowledgment. The authors gratefully acknowledge the financial support received from DST, under SERB Power grant no. SPG/2021/002212 for carrying out this research.

References

1. Ur-Rehman, M., Malik, N.A., Yang, X., Abbasi, Q.H., Zhang, Z., Zhao, N.: A low-profile antenna for millimeter-wave body-centric applications. IEEE Trans. Antennas Propag. **65**(12), 6329–6337 (2017). https://doi.org/10.1109/TAP.2017.2700897
2. Ali, U., Ullah, S., Kamal, B., Matekovits, L., Altaf, A.: Design, analysis and applications of wearable antennas: a review. IEEE Access **11**, 14458–14486 (2023). https://doi.org/10.1109/ACCESS.2023.3243292
3. Kumar, S., Moloudian, G., Simorangkir, R.B.V.B., Gawade, D.R., O'Flynn, B., Buckley, J.L.: Sub-GHz wrist-worn antennas for wireless sensing applications: a review. IEEE Open J. Antennas Propag. https://doi.org/10.1109/OJAP.2024.3397193
4. Ayd, A., Hassan, W.M., Ibrahim, A.A.: A monopole antenna with cotton fabric material for wearable applications. Sci. Rep. **13**(1), 1–13 (2023). https://doi.org/10.1038/s41598-023-34394-3
5. Dian, F.J., Vahidnia, R., Rahmati, A.: Wearables and the internet of things (IoT), applications, opportunities, and challenges: a survey. IEEE Access **8**, 69200–69211 (2020). https://doi.org/10.1109/ACCESS.2020.2986329
6. Wu, T., Wu, F., Qiu, C., Redouté, J.-M., Yuce, M.R.: A rigid-flex wearable health monitoring sensor patch for IoT-connected healthcare applications. IEEE Internet Things J. **7**(8), 6932–6945 (2020). https://doi.org/10.1109/JIOT.2020.2977164
7. Baeg, K.-J., Lee, J.: Flexible electronic systems on plastic substrates and textiles for smart wearable technologies. Adv. Mater. Technol. **5**(7) (2020)
8. Blauert, J., Kiourti, A.: Dual-band (2.4/4.8 GHz) implantable antenna for biomedical telemetry applications. In: 2018 International Applied Computational Electromagnetics Society Symposium (ACES), Denver, CO, USA, pp. 1–2 (2018). https://doi.org/10.23919/ROPACES.2018.8364217
9. Kumar, R., Kumar, P., Gupta, N., Dubey, R.: Experimental investigations of wearable antenna on flexible perforated plastic substrate. Microw. Opt. Technol. Lett. **59**(2), 265–270 (2017). https://doi.org/10.1002/mop.30280
10. McGibney, E., Barton, J., Floyd, L., Tassie, P., Barrett, J.: The high frequency electrical properties of interconnects on a flexible polyimide substrate including the effects of humidity. IEEE Trans. Compon. Packag. Manuf. Technol. **1**(1), 4–15 (2011). https://doi.org/10.1109/TCPMT.2010.2100731

Compact UWB Wearable Textile Antenna for Medical Applications with Bending Analysis

Sharmeen Sultana(✉) and Neela Chattoraj

Electronics and Communication, Birla Institute of Technology Mesra, Ranchi, India
{phdec10052.21,nchattoraj}@bitmesra.ac.in

Abstract. This study introduces the design and evaluation of a compact wearable textile antenna aimed at medical applications, particularly in wireless body area networks (WBANs), telemedicine, medical implant communication, wearable health tracking, and point-of-care diagnostics. The antenna, with dimensions of $0.28\lambda \times 0.25\lambda$, operates at a resonant frequency of 12 GHz. It employs jeans textile as the substrate material, which has a thickness of 1.67 mm and a dielectric constant of 1.28 and loss tangent of 0.016. Extensive parametric and bending analyses have been performed to assess the antenna's performance under varying conditions. The antenna achieves a substantial bandwidth of 1.01 GHz which qualifies the UWB operations, a gain of 8.17 dBi, and a reflection coefficient of -43 dB, indicating superior impedance matching. These findings highlight the antenna's capability for effective and reliable use in wearable medical devices.

Keywords: Textile Antenna · Compact size · Medical Applications

1 Introduction

The rapid development in wireless communication technologies has had huge impacts on wearable devices, basically in the medical field [1–3]. Wearable antennas form an intrinsic part of such devices that provide seamless communication for the transmission of data. In this paper, a compact wearable textile antenna is designed and analysed for medical applications. In this paper, a compact wearable textile antenna is proposed for medical applications and designed at a resonant frequency of 12 GHz. Measuring 12.39 x 11 mm in size, the antenna ensures compactness of form for integration into wearable medical devices [4]. In this design, jeans textile was chosen as a substrate material since it is flexible and widely available [5]. The antenna's design leverages geometric theory of diffraction (GTD) for its radiation mechanism, enabling conformal and flexible performance [6]. This theoretical framework facilitates the analysis of gain in the presence of curved surfaces, crucial for wearable applications. Here, the thickness of the jeans textile substrate used in the substrate is 1.67 mm, having

K. Atul et al. (Eds.): BodyNets 2024, LNICST 666, pp. 38–43, 2026.
https://doi.org/10.1007/978-3-032-16099-7_5

a dielectric constant of 1.28; thus, this substrate is very appropriate for wearable applications since it offers comfort to the antenna, which can easily be integrated into clothes [7]. In developing this antenna, an exhaustive parametric analysis was done for its performance optimization. Basically, the parameters considered in antenna dimensions aimed at achieving a desired resonant frequency and impedance matching. Besides, bending analyses have been performed to calculate the performances of said antenna under different deformation scenarios, aiming to show its reliability and efficiency when it is used on the human body [8,9]. The proposed simulated antenna depicts impressive performance metrics: a bandwidth of 1.01 GHz, which means there will be an extended frequency range of operation and robust communication capability, and an antenna gain of 8.17 dBi that gives good enough signal strength to have effective data transmission in medical applications. The reflection coefficient is also recorded at -43 dB, which is very excellent impedance matching and, consequently, very low signal reflection a critical requirement for signal integrity and low power loss. The antenna performance dropped due to the detuning by the power absorption of the human tissue. Loading the antenna with high permittivity and high loss from human tissue contributed to this effect [10,11]. Moreover, the presence of sweat and dust means that wearable antennas collect dirt that needs to be washed. A breathable covering helps wearable and washable antennas against this. [12]. In summary, this paper presents a compact, flexible, and high-performance wearable textile antenna designed for medical applications. The use of jeans textile as the substrate material, combined with thorough bending analyses, results in an antenna that not only meets the stringent requirements of medical communication devices but also offers comfort and ease of integration into wearable technology.

2 Antenna Design

Figure 1 depicts the structure of the proposed wearable textile antenna. The antenna comprises a central circular patch with a radius R_{in}, surrounded by an outer annular ring patch with a width W There is a gap d1 between the central patch and the annular ring. The antenna utilizes an microstrip line feed, characterized by a feed length L_f and a feed line width W_f. This entire configuration is implemented on a jeans textile substrate, which has a relative permittivity of 1.28 and a thickness of 1.67 mm (Table 1).

Table 1. Dimension Parameters and Their Values

Dimension Parameter	Values (mm)
R_{in}	2.7
W_r	1.3
L_f	2.5
W_f	0.5

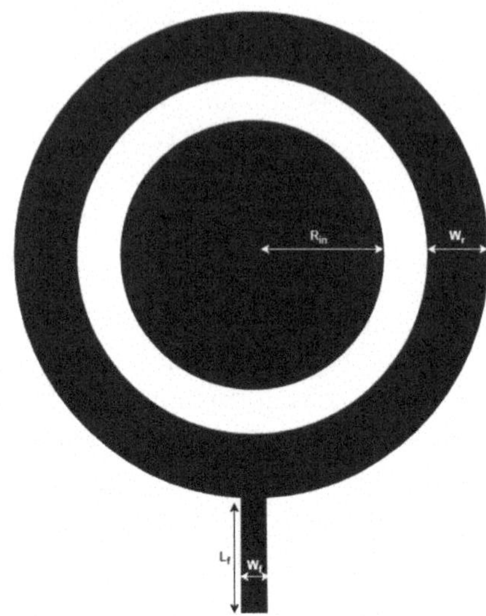

Fig. 1. Antenna design and architecture.

3 Simulated and Bending Analysis of Proposed Antenna

The proposed Compact Wearable Textile Antenna is simulated using Ansys Electronic Desktop (HFSS), in which bending analysis is also analysed as shown in Fig. 2 In the simulation, we analysed the reflection coefficient, Bandwidth and gain with a flat structure and bent structure, and we conducted analysis on this parameter with bending of structure.

3.1 Reflection Coefficient

The reflection coefficient measures the extent to which an electromagnetic wave reflects when it encounters an impedance mismatch as shown in Fig. 3. antenna resonates at 12GHz centre frequency and has 1.01 GHz Impedance Bandwidth that ensures UWB operations. Figure 3(b) illustrates the bending analysis conducted on the antenna, ranging from a 1mm bend to a maximum of 3mm from the flat surface. The analysis revealed impedance mismatches and frequency shifts.

3.2 Gain of Proposed Antenna

Gain is a very important parameter for textile and wearable antenna due to the absorption of electromagnetic waves by human tissues, in Fig. 4. the Gain of the proposed antenna shows it achieved gain of 8.17 dBi which is quite a good gain for the operations. As from Fig. 4(b) shows the bending effect on antenna gain as maximum gain reduced by 1.05 dBi and achieved 7.12 dBi at a 3mm antenna bent. The effect of bending from 1mm to 3mm on the antenna performance is shown in Table.2

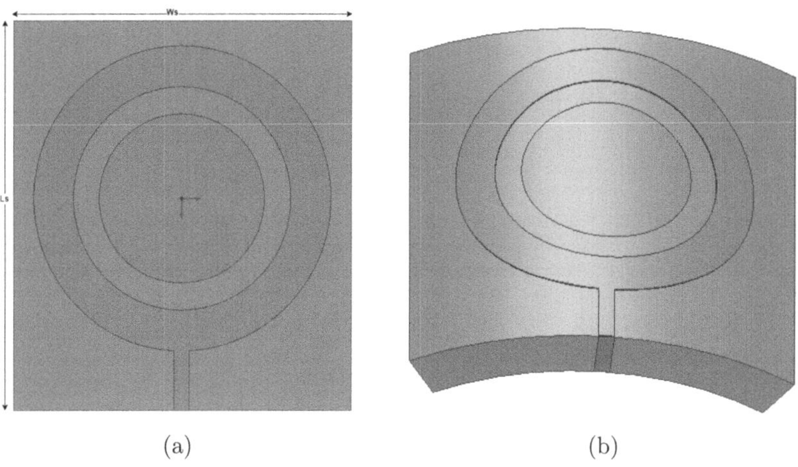

(a) (b)

Fig. 2. Simulated Antenna Structure(a)No bending (b) Bended Structure.

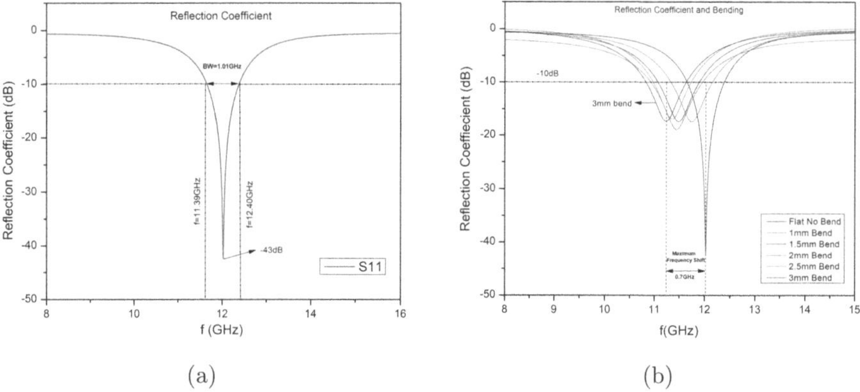

(a) (b)

Fig. 3. Reflection coefficient for flat and bent structure (a) Reflection coefficient for flat structure (b) Reflection coefficient for bent structure.

Table 2. Bending Analysis Results

Bending (mm)	Reflection Coefficient (dB)	Resonating Frequency (GHz)	Frequency Shift (GHz)	Gain (dBi)
1.0	-17.46	11.74	0.26	7.70
1.5	-17.31	11.51	0.49	7.60
2.0	-18.96	11.46	0.54	7.58
2.5	-16.96	11.37	0.63	7.35
3.0	-17.39	11.30	0.70	7.12

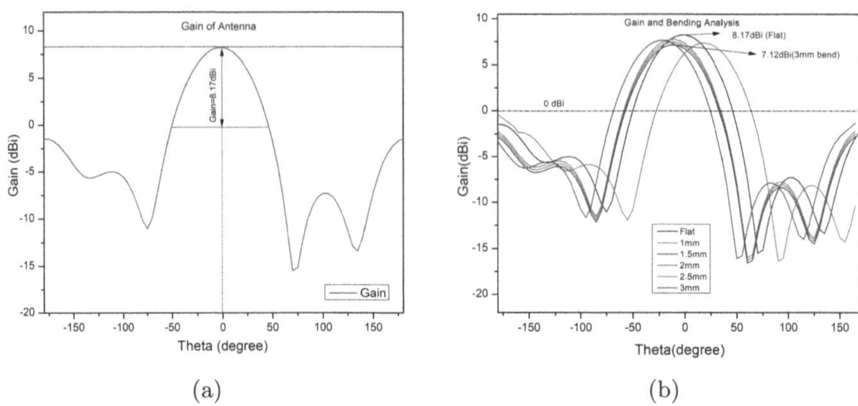

Fig. 4. Gain of Antenna (a) For flat structure (b) For bent structure.

4 Conclusion

In this work, a compact UWB wearable textile antenna has been developed, and a bending analysis has been performed that turns out very promising for medical applications, more so in wearable devices. Having a resonant frequency of 12 GHz with impressive metrics, bandwidth of 1.01 GHz, gains for flat and maximum bend of 3 mm are 8.17 dBi and 7.12 dBi respectively, and a reflection coefficient -43 dB, the antenna is highly efficient and appropriate for UWB operations. In this respect, the jeans textile used as a substrate material and extensive parametric and bending analyses truly underlines the robustness of this antenna in different conditions. Consequently, the compact size, good performance, and reliable impedance matching of the antenna make this antenna a potential solution for integration in wearable medical technologies.

References

1. Park, Y.-G., Lee, S., Park, J.-U.: Recent Progress in Wireless Sensors for Wearable Electronics. Sensors **19**(20), 4353 (2019)
2. Devi, D.H., et al.: 5G technology in healthcare and wearable devices: a review. Sensors **23**(5), 2519 (2023) https://doi.org/10.3390/s23052519
3. Luo, X., Tan, H., Wen, W.: Recent advances in wearable healthcare devices: from material to application. Bioengineering (Basel, Switzerland) **11**(4), 358 (2024). https://doi.org/10.3390/bioengineering11040358
4. Varma, S., et al.: Design and performance analysis of compact wearable textile antennas for iot and body-centric communication applications. Int. J. Antennas Propag. **2021**, 1–12 (2021). https://doi.org/10.1155/2021/7698765
5. Kavitha, V., Malaisamy, K ., Murugesh, T. S., SenthilKumar, M.: Design and development of jeans textile antenna for wireless broadband applications. Journal industrial textiles, vol. 53, (2023). https://doi.org/10.1177/15280837231215374

6. Mishra, M., Rajput, A., Gupta, P. K., Mukherjee, B.: A low profile perturbed CDRA with convex conformal ground plane excited by differential feed. AEU - Int. J. Electr. Commun. **173**, 155033–155033 (2023). https://doi.org/10.1016/j.aeue.2023.155033
7. Ouyang, Y., Chappell, W.: High frequency properties of electro-textiles for wearable antenna applications. IEEE Trans Antenn Propag **56**(2), 381–389 (2008)
8. Osman, M., Rahim, M., Samsuri, N., et al.: Textile UWB antenna bending and wet performances. Int J Antenn Propag **2012**, 1–12 (2012)
9. Jalil, M.E., Abd Rahim, M.K., Samsuri, N.A., et al.: Fractal koch multiband textile antenna performance with bending, wet conditions and on the human body. Prog Electromagn Res **140**, 633–652 (2013)
10. Li, S., Sun, B.W., Wu, F.: Design of Compact Single-layer Textile MIMO antenna for Wearable Applications. IEEE Trans. Antennas Propag. **66**(3), 3136–3141 (2018)
11. Jiang, Z.H., Brocker, D.E., Sieber, P.E., Werner, D.H.: A compact, low-profile metasurface-enabled antenna for wearable medical body-area network devices. IEEE Trans. Antennas Propag. **62**(8), 4021–4030 (2014)
12. Scarpello, M.L., Kazani, I., Hertleer, C., Rogier, H., Ginste, D.V.: Stability and efficiency of screen-printed wearable and washable antennas. IEEE Antennas Wirel. Propag. Lett. **11**, 838–841 (2012)

Multi-slot Rectangular Shaped 6G Wearable Microstrip Patch Antenna for Wireless Body Area Network

Siddalingappagouda Biradar[1](✉), Shashi Ranjan[2], and Vinod D. Durdi[3]

[1] Dayananda Sagar Academy of Technology and Management, Bangalore, India
siddubbiradarr@gmail.com
[2] Don Bosco Institute of Technology, Bengaluru, Karnataka, India
[3] Dayananda Sagar College of Engineering, Bengaluru, Karnataka, India

Abstract. Wireless Body Area Network (WBAN) is an innovative network system, which consists of numerous wearable or implantable devices that monitors and transmits the physiological data. Designing a wearable patch antenna for WBAN is a challenging, because human body is a lossy medium which can absorb and scatter electromagnetic waves, thus leads to degrade of antenna performance. In this paper, we have designed a multi-slot rectangular shaped 6G wearable microstrip patch antennas, which are unique, small size, and light with a flat surface, unlike traditional counterparts and these can be placed directly on a human body and are comfortable to wear for long periods. The antenna is designed, simulated, and analyzed using Computer Simulated Technology (CST) studio suite and the proposed antenna consists of microstrip patch, substrate, feed-line, and ground plane. The simulation parameters such as S-Parameter, VSWR, Bandwidth, Resonating Frequency, Gain, Efficiency, Directivity and Far Field radiation is calculated. The results of proposed wearable 6G patch antenna with varying operating frequencies from 1 THz to 10 THz is presented, Performance parameter shows three slot antenna works better at 5.03 THz for WBAN.

Keywords: Wearable Microstrip Patch Antenna · WBAN · CST tool · Performance Metrics

1 Introduction

The 6G wireless communication is the result of success of 5G. It will fill the gap between 5G and market demands, as per the experts 6G would be expected to launch around 2030. Therefore, 6G will be a world of fully digital connectivity [1]. 6G is designed to provide at least 20 times more area capacity than 5G communication. The key features of 6G are,

a. Higher Data Rates: By the aim to reach up to '1' Terabit per second (Tbps), 6G technology speed may support groundbreaking applications including ultra-high-definition (UHD) video streaming, autonomous system, extended reality, and holographic communication.

K. Atul et al. (Eds.): BodyNets 2024, LNICST 666, pp. 44–56, 2026.
https://doi.org/10.1007/978-3-032-16099-7_6

b. Ultra-Lower Latency: Predictions suggest that latency in 6G may drop to as low as 1 microsecond. This level of speed will enable real-time applications like remote surgery, self-driving cars, plus advanced augmented and virtual reality (VR) experiences [2, 3].
c. Integration of Artificial Intelligence (AI): AI will play an important role in 6G communication networks. It could help optimize performance, manage network resources effectively, and ensure smooth operations. Furthermore, it may facilitate predictive maintenance and self-detect and remediate networks [4].
d. Spectrum Use: Definitely, 6G will use frequencies in the terahertz (THz) range. This can provide a much larger bandwidth than the current millimeter waves used in 5G, leading the way for quicker and more efficient data transfers.
e. Enhanced Connectivity: Marking not just to connect people but billions of devices as well, 6G could supercharge the Internet of Things (IoT). Smart cities, homes, and industries.
f. Energy Efficiency: As concerns about energy use in 5G grow, there's hope that 6G will prioritize sustainability. This means developing more energy-efficient technologies and possibly harnessing energy through communication devices [5].
g. Global Coverage: Unlike its predecessor, which supports toward dense urban areas, 6G might hope to provide global coverage. This includes reaching remote or underserved regions through advanced satellite networks and high-altitude platform stations (HAPS).
h. Security and Privacy: New security protocols will likely emerge with 6G to manage increased data traffic and guard against new threats. Privacy-preserving technologies will also become crucial as our networks blend into daily life more deeply [6, 7] (Figs. 1 and 2).

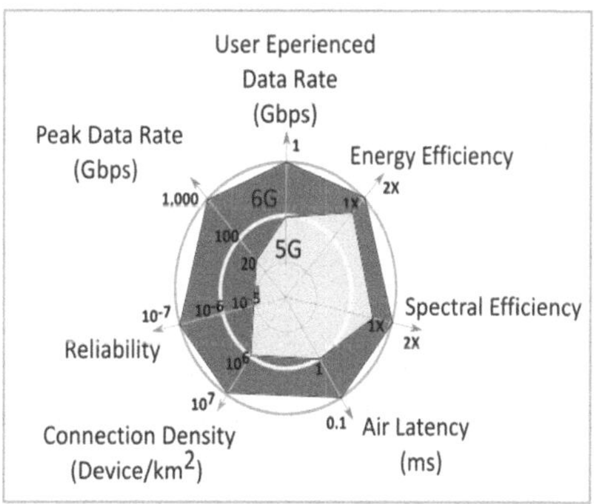

Fig. 1. Multiple service areas of 5G and 6G [8]

While still in early development stages, 6G offers a promising growth in communication field. It has the potential to change how we interact with both digital technology and the real world around us. Yet many concepts remain theoretical at this moment

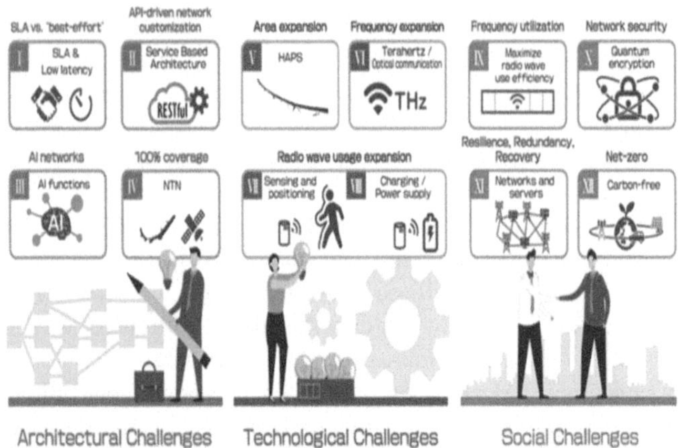

Fig. 2. 6G Challenges in different fields [9]

[10, 11]. Consideration like high frequencies and needs for the next generation wireless technologies [12]. Some of main steps to design the 6G antenna are:

a. High Frequency Range and Bandwidth
    i. Frequency Bands: 6G will be expected to use frequencies ranging from sub-1 GHz to THz bands, and even up to 100 GHz or more.
    ii. ii. Bandwidth: The communicating antenna should support wide bandwidth. This helps to support super-fast data rates and large number of multiple connections in 6G networks.
b. Antenna Type
    i. Microstrip Antennas: These types of antennas are often chosen for their small size, light weight and easy suitable to circuits, which works better for higher frequencies.
    ii. Phased Array Antennas: They are mainly suitable for beamforming and MIMO (Multiple Input Multiple Output) systems and for attainment high data throughput and better spatial diversity.
    iii. Terahertz Antennas: When dealing with frequencies above 100 GHz, it is necessary to have special designs like plasmonic antennas or metamaterials [13, 14].
c. Design Challenges
    i. Miniaturization: If we are using higher frequencies then antennas must be smaller, but still to do their job well. This usually requires advanced materials and design techniques.
    ii. High Gain and Directivity: Ensuring high gain and directivity to compensate for higher propagation path loss at tera hertz frequencies.
    iii. Material Selection: The advanced chemical materials like metamaterials, graphene, or some high-performance substrates might be needed [15].
d. Simulation and Modelling

i. Software Tools: Use simulation tools like Ansys High-Frequency Structure Simulator (HFSS), CST Microwave Studio or COMSOL Multiphysics to design the model and check how the antenna performs [16].
ii. Performance Metrics: Calculate the parameters such as like return loss, radiation patterns, gain, and efficiency.

e. Integration and Testing
i. Integration with Systems: Make sure the antenna design, sets well with other electronic parts of the 6G system—like transceivers and base stations [17].
ii. Prototyping & Testing: Create prototypes and test them, out in the real world to see how they work. Testing can include measurements in anechoic chambers and field tests.

f. Future Considerations
i. Flexibility and Adaptability: The design of microstrip patch antennas, that can change with network requirements. They should be able to get reconfigured or updated as 6G technologies moves advancing.
ii. Sustainability: checkout about the environment. Look at how materials and manufacturing methods can be as eco-friendly as possible.

Designing antennas for 6G is a complex and tough task. It requires a multidisciplinary approach and close attention towards emerging technologies and materials. Collaboration with experts in fields such as materials science, electromagnetics, and wireless communication is often necessary to achieve optimal results [18, 19].

2 Design and Simulation Parameters

2.1 Design of the Proposed Antenna

The design parameters of slotted rectangular wearable microstrip patch antenna being considered is illustrated in Fig. 3 and Table 1 shows the simulation parameters used for design antenna. The substrate dimensions are denoted as 'Ls*Ws' and are constructed using FR-4 lossy material, possessing a dielectric constant of 3.48. The ground plane, patch and feedline are made up of copper material with the dimensions of Lg*Wg, Lp*Wp and Wf.

Table 1. Parameters used for Microstrip patch Antenna

SL. No	Parameters		Values (μm)
1	Lg & Ls	Length of ground and substrate plane	50
2	Lp	Length of patch	40
3	Wf	Width of feedline	3
4	Wg & Ws	Width of ground and substrate plane	70
5	Wp	Width of plane	30
6	T	Thickness of ground plane	0.017

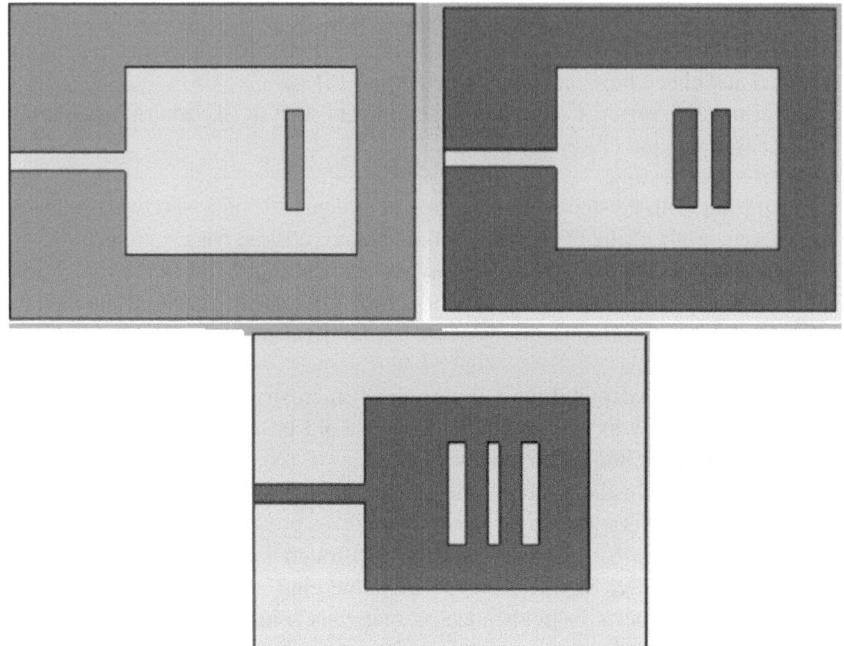

Fig. 3. Multi-slot rectangular shaped antennas

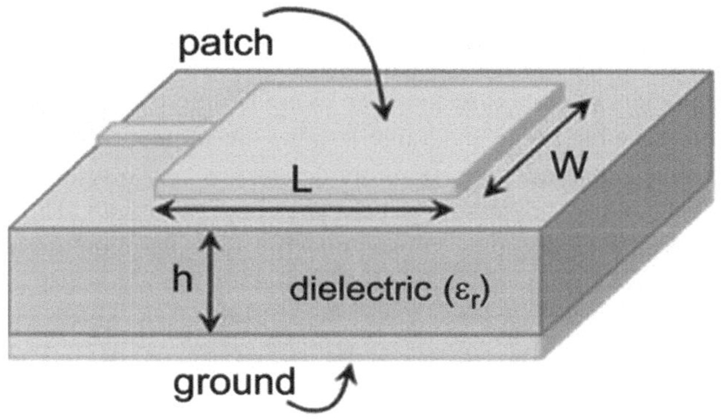

Fig. 4. Proposed side view of rectangular microstrip patch antenna

The Fig. 4 shows, the proposed rectangular microstrip patch antenna consisting of Dielectric substrate, Microstrip patch, Ground plate and Feedline.

The following are the equations of that are used for microstrip patch antenna calculation process [20],

a. In order to calculate width of the microstrip patch antenna we use the formula,

$$Wp = \frac{c_0}{2f_r\sqrt{\frac{\varepsilon_r+1}{2}}} \tag{1}$$

b. Calculation of the Effective Dielectric Constant based on the height, dielectric constant of the dielectric and the calculated width of the patch antenna.

$$\varepsilon_{reff} = \frac{\varepsilon_r + 1}{2} + \frac{\varepsilon_r - 1}{2} \times \sqrt{\left(1 + \left(\frac{12h}{w}\right)\right)} \tag{2}$$

c. Calculation of the Effective length

$$\mathrm{L}_{eff} = \frac{c}{2f0\sqrt{\varepsilon_{reff}}} \tag{3}$$

d. Calculation of the length extension ΔL

$$\Delta L = 0.412 \times \mathrm{h} \times \frac{\left(\varepsilon_{reff} + 0.3\right)\left(\frac{w}{h} + 0.26\right)}{\left(\varepsilon_{reff} + 0.253\right)\left(\frac{w}{h} + 0.8\right)} \tag{4}$$

e. Calculation of actual length of the patch

$$\mathrm{L} = L_{eff} - 2\Delta L \tag{5}$$

f. Calculation of Feedline Width,

$$W_f = \frac{7.48h}{e^{\left(z_0\frac{\sqrt{\varepsilon_r+1.41}}{87}\right)}} - 1.25t \tag{6}$$

3 Results and Discussion

This section discusses about simulation results of performance metrics of rectangular slotted microstrip patch antennas.

3.1 Return Loss or Reflection Co-efficient

It is the measurement of the reflected wave or signal strength traveling or returning back to a transmitter from an antenna, this is one of the important parameters of antenna design (Fig. 5).

The return loss is calculated from S_{11}-parameter by identifying the frequencies at -10 dB and bandwidth by subtracting high frequency and low frequency at resonant frequency point. The return loss and bandwidth of respective frequencies are presented in Tables 3 and 4. In single slot antenna, it resonates at five different frequencies, with low return loss (−18.53 dB) at 8.87 THz and high bandwidth of 340 GHz at 8.11 THz. In second slot antenna, it resonates at five different frequencies with low return loss (−20.12 dB) at 4.06 THz and high bandwidth of 390 GHz at 7.20 THz. Similarly for three slot antenna, it also resonates at five different frequencies with very low return loss (−46.76 dB) and has a bandwidth of 240 GHz at 5.03 THz frequency. Overall, three slot antenna (f = 5.03 THz) performance better, which has very low return loss and high bandwidth compared to other two slot antennas.

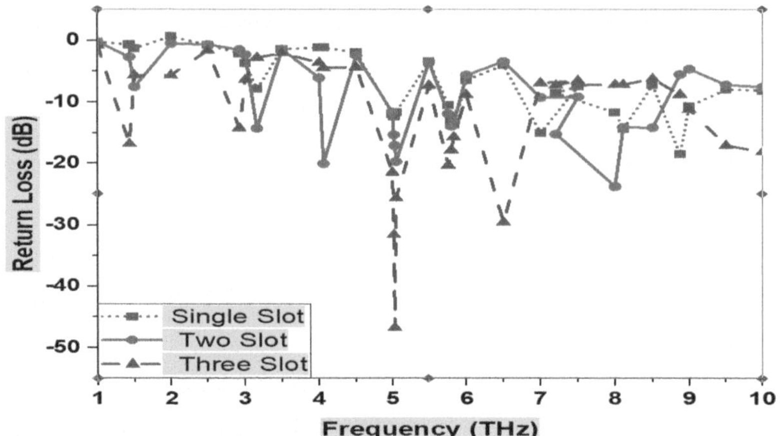

Fig. 5. Return loss versus frequency with single, two and three slot rectangular antenna

Table 2. Return loss and bandwidth of single and two slot rectangular antennas

Single Slot Frequency (THz)	Return Loss (dB)	Bandwidth (GHz)	Two Slot Frequency (THz)	Return Loss (dB)	Bandwidth (GHz)
5.02	−12.42	100	3.16	−14.31	060
5.83	−13.69	160	**4.06**	**−20.12**	070
7.00	−15.09	290	5.05	−19.78	130
8.11	−14.13	**340**	5.80	−13.94	150
8.87	**−18.53**	300	**7.20**	−15.26	**390**

Table 3. Return loss and bandwidth of three slot rectangular antennas

Three Slot Frequency (THz)	Return Loss (dB)	Bandwidth (GHz)
1.43	−16.86	070
2.92	−14.24	080
5.03	**−46.76**	**240**
5.76	−20.37	340
6.50	−29.84	380

3.2 Voltage Standing Wave Ratio (VSWR)

It is a measure of the impedance matching between the transmission line and antenna. It indicates the amount of power that can be safely delivered to an antenna without damaging it.

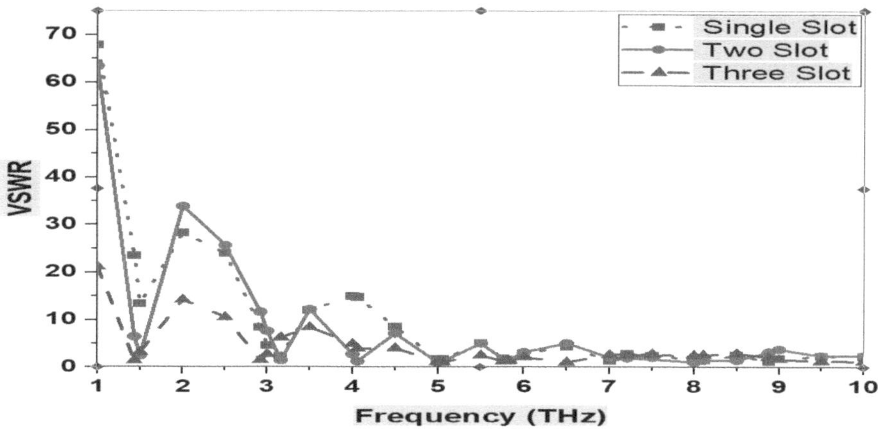

Fig. 6. VSWR versus Frequency of single, two and three slot rectangular antennas

Table 4. Return loss and bandwidth of single, two and three slot rectangular antennas

Single Slot Frequency (THz)	VSWR	Two Slot Frequency (THz)	VSWR	Three Slot Frequency (THz)	VSWR
5.02	1.62	3.16	1.47	1.43	1.33
5.83	1.52	**4.06**	**1.21**	2.92	1.48
7.00	1.42	5.05	1.22	**5.03**	**1.01**
8.11	1.45	5.80	1.50	5.76	1.21
8.87	**1.26**	7.20	1.93	6.50	1.05

In the above Fig. 6, it shows the VSWR value of single, two and three slot rectangular antenna and the values of VSWR in all three antennas are less than 2. In 6G, if the antenna has value less than '5' indicating better impedance matching, reduced power reflection and better performance. A higher VSWR value means a poor impedance match, and therefore less power being transferred efficiently from the radio or transmission line to the antenna. In single slot antenna, at resonating frequency of 8.87 THz the VSWR value is 1.26 which is lower than other resonating frequencies. In second slot antenna, at resonating frequency of 4.06 THz the VSWR value is 1.21. Similarly for three slot antennas, resonating frequency of 5.03 THz has low VSWR value of 1.01. Overall, three slot antenna performance better, which has very low VSWR value (1.01) compared to other slotted antennas.

3.3 Electric and Magnetic Field

The electric field (E-field) and magnetic field (H-field) distributions are key for understanding the antenna's performance. The high and low intensity of radiation are seen near antenna elements.

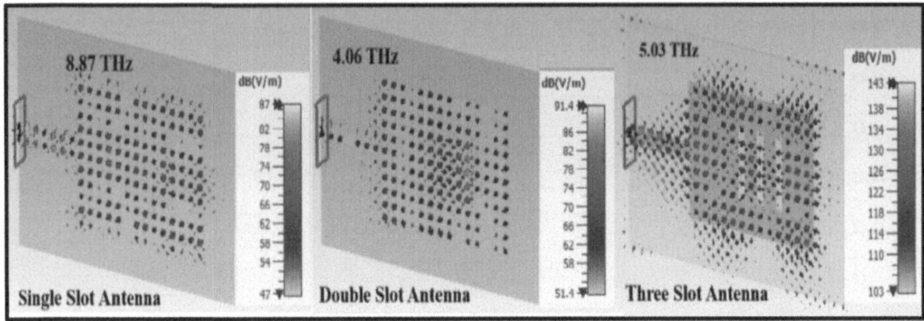

Fig. 7. Electric Field of single, two and three slot rectangular antennas

The E-field pattern will reflect the antenna's radiation pattern, with the highest intensity in the direction of maximum radiation.

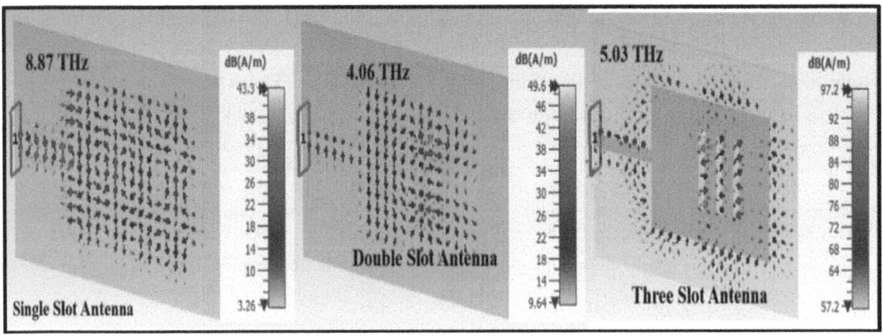

Fig. 8. Magnetic Field of single, two and three slot rectangular antennas

The magnetic field pattern in the near and far field will also reflect the antenna's radiation pattern and with the field strength decreasing as you move away from the main lobe. The Figs. 7 and 8 shows, Electric and Magnetic field for 6G Antenna of resonating frequency F = 8.87 THz, 4.06 THz and 5.03 THz.

3.4 Surface Current

The surface current spreading on a 6G antenna is a main indicator of how well the antenna radiates and how efficiently it converts input power into electromagnetic waves. Examining the surface current helps to understand the regions of the antenna that are most active in radiation and can help in improving the design.

The Fig. 9 shows, surface current radiation for 6G antenna for resonating frequency of F = 8.87 THz, 4.06 THz and 5.03 THz. This visualization of surface current helps to recognize the most dynamic part of antenna. The surface current should be concentrated in areas that align with the antenna's resonant modes, showing strong, directed currents that correspond to efficient radiation.

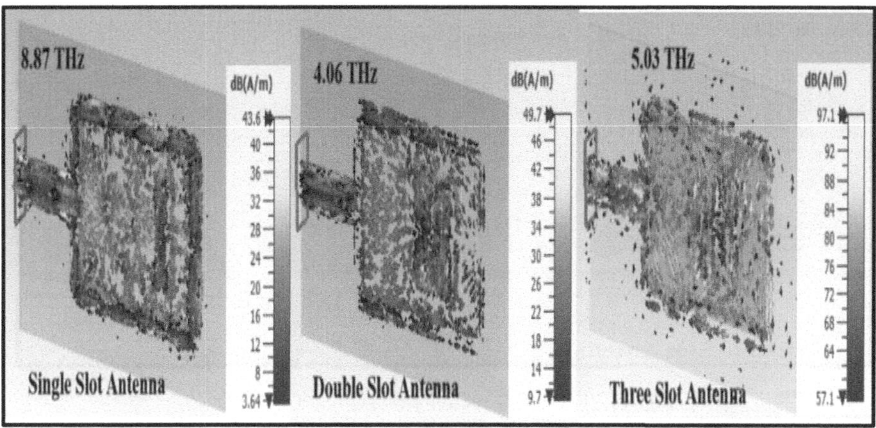

Fig. 9. Surface current of single, two and three slot rectangular antennas

3.5 Far Field

In the design of microstrip 6G antenna design, the "far-field" denotes to the region far enough away from the antenna, where the electromagnetic fields have a stable, predictable pattern and can be considered plane waves. This area is critical for analyzing the antenna's radiation features, such as directivity, radiation pattern and efficiency.

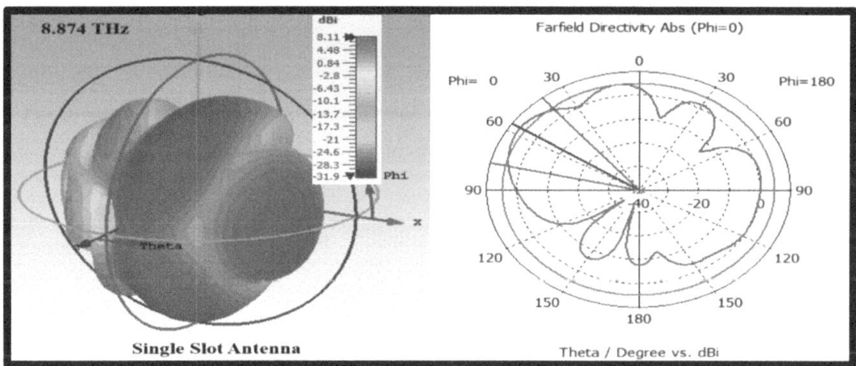

Fig. 10. Farfield Directivity of Single Slot Antenna

From the above three far field regions (as shown in Figs. 10, 11 and 12) of operating frequency F = 8.87 THz, 4.06 THz and 5.03 THz. The three slot microstrip patch antenna with resonating frequency of 5.03 THz has better directivity, gain and efficiency, when compare to other.

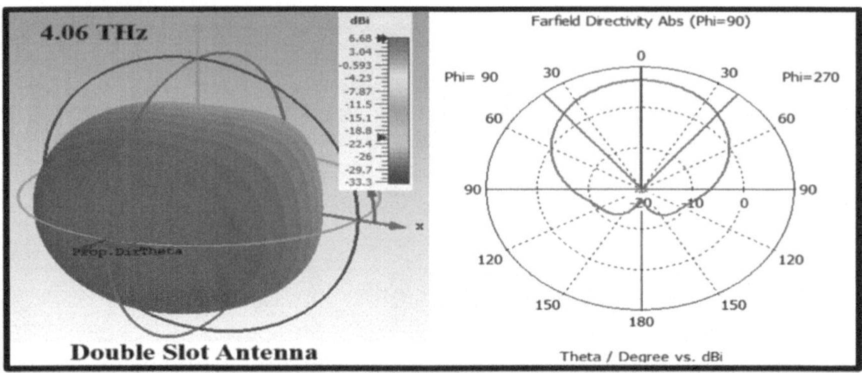

Fig. 11. Farfield Directivity of Two Slot Antenna

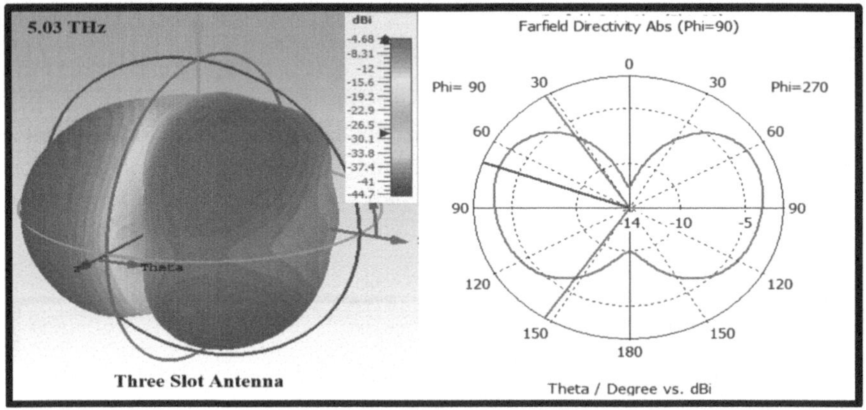

Fig. 12. Farfield Directivity of Three Slot Antenna

Table 5. Directivity, Gain and Efficiency of single, two and three slot antennas

Resonating Frequency (THz)	Directivity (dBi)	Gain (dB)	Efficiency (dB)
8.87	8.11	3.5	9.5
4.06	6.67	4.51	9.1
5.03	**6.81**	**6.84**	**10.71**

4 Conclusion

In the recent years, designing of the antennas for WBAN is critical, because of its characteristics. The proposed slotted rectangular shaped wearable microstrip patch antennas are novel and unique. In this paper, the proposed antennas highlight the challenges such as wideband operation, miniaturized structure, return loss, bandwidth, directivity, impedance matching and beamforming. The simulation results, shows the performances of all multiple slot antenna in Tables 2, 3, 4 and 5. All the three proposed 6G antennas performance better and among all these three antennas, especially rectangular antenna with three slots operating with 5.03 THz resonating frequency offer better performances as seen in bandwidth, return loss, directivity, gain and efficiency parameters. According to the simulation results, the other antenna with single slot has more return loss and VSWR value when compared to two and three slot rectangular antennas. The gain, bandwidth and directivity of the proposed antennas can be further extended by increasing the number of slots and varying design. Overall, by seeing the simulated results, the performance of these wearable antennas indicates the three slot rectangular antenna is best suitable for WBAN. This work can be even taken further for the simulation of different terahertz frequency with different design, material, and antenna shapes.

References

1. Raj, T.S., Mishra, R., Kumar, P., Kapoor, A.: Advances in MIMO antenna design for 5G: a comprehensive review. Sensors **23**(14), 6329 (2023). https://doi.org/10.3390/s23146329
2. Jia, S., Xu, H.: Two 5G patch antenna designs for millimeter-wave. In: 2022 14th International Conference on Computer Research and Development (ICCRD), Shenzhen, China, pp. 378–387 (2022). https://doi.org/10.1109/ICCRD54409.2022.9730355
3. Al, A., Mustafa, A.: Design of MIMO antenna for wideband THz mobile communications and radio engineering. J. Telecommun. Radio-Eng. **83**(8), 1–12 (2024). https://doi.org/10.1615/TelecomRadEng.2024051220
4. Ashraf, A., Gunawan, T.S., Kartiwi, M., Nur, L.O., Nugroho, B.S., Astuti, R.P.: Advancements and challenges in scalable modular antenna arrays for 5G massive MIMO networks. IEEE Access **12**, 57895–57916 (2024). https://doi.org/10.1109/ACCESS.2024.3391945
5. Gnanathickam, J., Thanusha, G., Moses, N.: Design and development of microstrip patch antenna for 5G application. In: 2023 International Conference on Computer Communication and Informatics, Coimbatore, India, pp. 1–4 (2023). https://doi.org/10.1109/ICCCI56745.2023.10128505
6. Chou, H., Wang, N., Fang, M., Wang, L.Q., Akkaraekthalin, P., Torrungrueng, D.: Dual-band reflect array antennas using integrated resonant and non-resonant natures of metallic waveguide elements at millimeter wave frequencies. Radio Sci. **58**(1), 1–13 (2023). https://doi.org/10.1029/2022RS007494
7. Buttazzoni, G.: A beamforming network for 5G/6G multibeam antennas using the PCB technology. In: 2023 17th European Conference on Antennas and Propagation (EuCAP), Florence, Italy, pp. 1–5 (2023). https://doi.org/10.23919/EuCAP57121.2023.10133148
8. Hong, W., Guo, Z.-J., Hao, Z.-C.: Seamless integration technology for filtenna toward 5G/6G wireless communications. IEEE Open J. Antennas Propag. **5**(1), 18–36 (2024). https://doi.org/10.1109/OJAP.2023.3342468
9. Walia, V., Mahmood, M.R., Maheshwari, V.: Sustainable spectrum sharing 5G network antenna design for smart city. J. Auton. Intell. (2024). https://doi.org/10.32629/jai.v7i4.1115
10. Mohamed, H.A., Edries, M., Abdelghany, M.A., Ibrahim, A.A.: Millimeter-wave antenna with gain improvement utilizing reflection FSS for 5G networks. IEEE Access **10**, 73601–73609 (2022). https://doi.org/10.1109/ACCESS.2022.3189651
11. Saida, A., Yadav, R.K., Sharma, V.: Analysis of LTE based an antenna design for 5G communications. Int. J. Recent Innov. Trends Comput. Commun. **11**(6), 471–475 (2023). https://doi.org/10.17762/ijritcc.v11i6.7785

12. El-Wazzan, M.M., Ghouz, H.H., El-Diasty, S.K., Aboul-Dahab, M.A.: Compact and integrated microstrip antenna modules for mm-wave and microwave bands applications. IEEE Access **10**, 70724–70736 (2022). https://doi.org/10.1109/ACCESS.2022.3187035
13. Sharma, U., Srivastava, G., Khandelwal, M., Roges, R.: Design challenges and solutions of multiband MIMO antenna for 5G/6G wireless applications: a comprehensive review. Progr. Electromagn. Res. B. **104**, 69–89 (2023). https://doi.org/10.2528/PIERB23101904
14. Kalpana, S., Mangayarkarasi, S.: Design of microstrip based millimeter wave antenna for 5G applications. In: 2023 2nd International Conference on Smart Technologies and Systems for Next Generation Computing (ICSTSN), Viluppuram, India, pp. 1–5 (2023). https://doi.org/10.1109/ICSTSN57873.2023.10151550
15. Sadhu, S., Acharjee, B., Mandal, S.: Design of wideband microstrip patch antenna at 38 GHz for 5G network. In: Tavares, J.M.R.S., Rodrigues, J.J.P.C., Misra, D., Bhattacherjee, D. (eds.) ICTDsC 2023. SADIC, pp. 719–730. Springer, Singapore (2024). https://doi.org/10.1007/978-981-99-5435-3_52
16. Guneser, M.T., Seker, C., Guler, M.I., Fitriyani, N.L., Syafrudin, M.: Efficient 5.8 GHz microstrip antennas for intelligent transportation systems: design, fabrication, and performance analysis. MDPI; Mathematics (2024). https://doi.org/10.3390/math12081202
17. Khan, R., Sethi, W.T., Malik, W.A.: Enhancing gain and isolation of a quad-element MIMO antenna array design for 5G sub-6 GHz applications assisted with characteristic mode analysis. Sci. Rep. **14**, 11111 (2024). https://doi.org/10.1038/s41598-024-61789-7
18. Raed, S., Daraghma, M.: Design of microstrip patch H-notch antenna for vehicle using array systems. J. Commun. **19**(4) (2024).https://doi.org/10.12720/jcm.19.4.204-210
19. Yadav, M.V., Yadav, S.V., Ali, T., Kumar Dash, S.K., Hegde, N.T., Nair, V.G.: A cutting-edge S/C/X band antenna for 5G and beyond application. AIP Adv. **13**, 105123 (2023).https://doi.org/10.1063/5.0177355
20. Rectangular Antenna Parameter Calculator. https://www.pasternack.com/t-calculator-microstripant.aspx?srsltid=AfmBOopzaImLvBsjYaYq0Pr2rKCY_9UJbBkK61y90bvwqkizRL7vNQLx

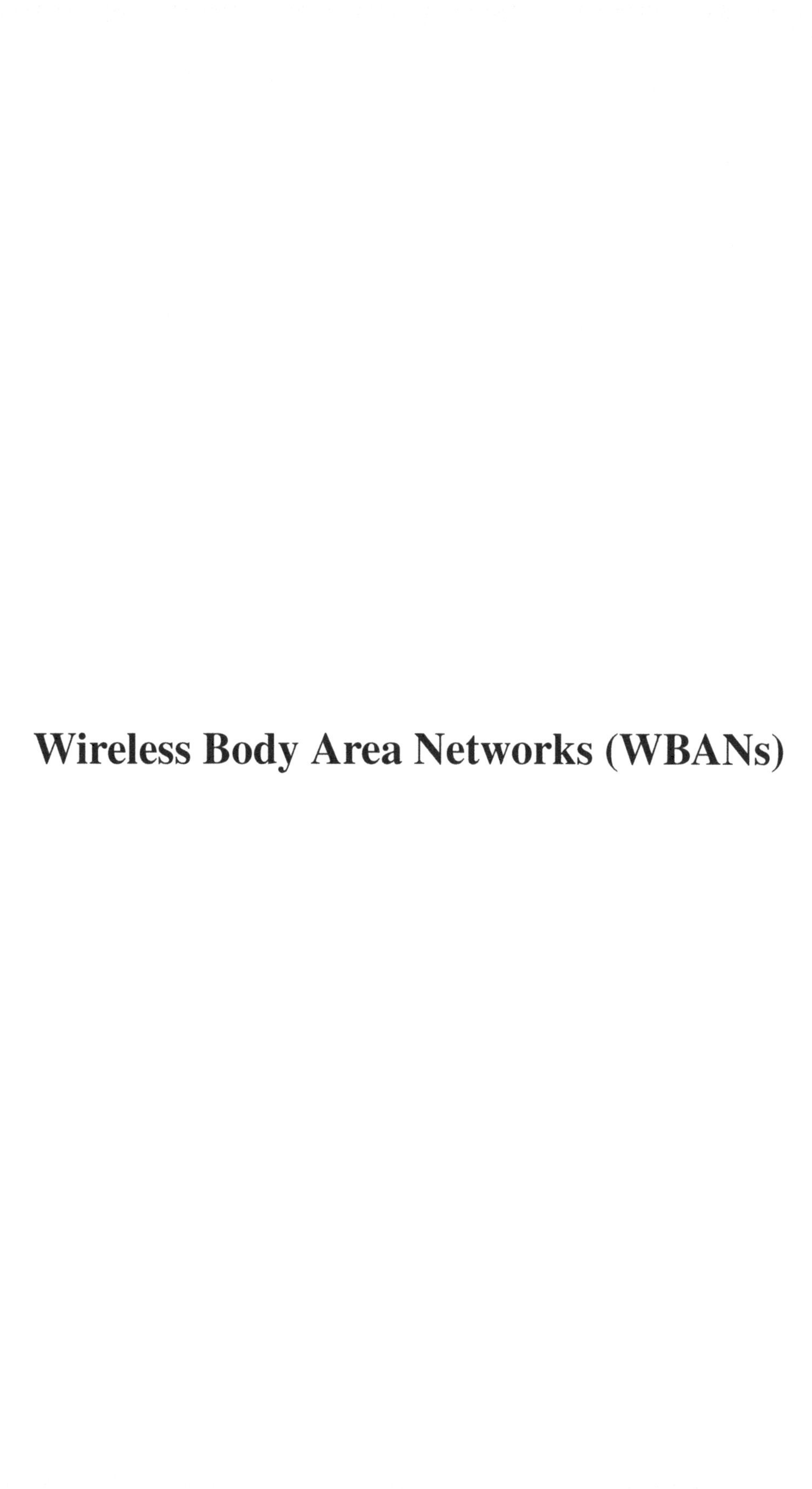

Wireless Body Area Networks (WBANs)

AI Based Energy Efficient Lossless Data Compression Algorithm for WBAN

SaiPavan Revooru(✉)

Qualcomm, Bangalore, India
saipavanrevooru@gmail.com

Abstract. Wireless Body Area Networks (WBAN) are very important for continuous health monitoring. Since they have a limited battery life, they always suffer with significant energy constraints. This paper proposes an AI-based, energy-efficient, lossless data compression algorithm to address this challenge. By leveraging Variational Autoencoders (VAEs), the algorithm efficiently compresses data, reducing energy consumption associated with data transmission and reception. VAEs offer several advantages, including adaptability, efficient feature extraction, contextual awareness, and superior redundancy reduction. Their probabilistic nature and latent space representation make them ideal for handling the variability in WBAN data. The proposed solution aims to prolong the device lifetime by reducing the power consumption and thereby reducing the ecological footprint of WBAN sensor nodes, ensuring safer and more sustainable health monitoring.

Keywords: WBAN · VAE's · Data compression · Power efficient

1 Introduction

1.1 Background

Wireless body area networks (WBAN) consist of sensor nodes that are situated on the body or under the skin. These sensor modules in the network will monitor different physiological parameters of human body.

Sensor nodes are small, lightweight and equipped with wireless communication capabilities, but comes with limited battery life. Therefore, energy consumption becomes a crucial factor for sensor nodes in WBAN.

An energy-efficient sensor node guarantees continuous and reliable health monitoring by minimizing the risk of battery depletion. Environmentally, such a sensor module helps reduce electronic waste and the ecological footprint associated with batteries.

From a user perspective, energy-efficient sensor nodes are crucial because high energy consumption can generate excessive heat, potentially harming skin and tissues.

K. Atul et al. (Eds.): BodyNets 2024, LNICST 666, pp. 59–62, 2026.
https://doi.org/10.1007/978-3-032-16099-7_7

2 Problem

2.1 Factors Causing High Energy Consumption

One of the important factors that contribute to high power consumption is data handling. Having an optimized and energy efficient data compression algorithm will enormously help in reducing the energy consumption of a sensor node.

Therefore, this paper is about the development of an energy-efficient data compression algorithm, which has the potential to substantially prolong device lifetime by minimizing the energy demands associated with data transmission and reception.

3 Solution

3.1 Deep Learning for Data Compression

We will exploit the advantages offered by AI algorithms to design an energy efficient lossless data compression algorithm for WBAN. Below are some of the reasons why AI algorithms are better than other traditional approaches.

Adaptability. Adaptability of AI algorithms allow for more personalized and efficient compression, which is not possible with traditional algorithms.

Feature Extraction. AI algorithms are very efficient in extracting most relevant information to compress data than the traditional algorithms.

Contextual Awareness. AI algorithms can be designed to understand the context of the data, which allows more intelligent compression strategies.

Redundancy Reduction. AI algorithms are proved to be better at identifying and eliminating redundancy.

3.2 Variational Auto Encoders

In Deep learning, a variational autoencoder (VAE) is an artificial neural network architecture introduced by Diederik P. Kingma and Max Welling. It is part of the families of probabilistic graphical models and variational Bayesian methods. VAE's has some great advantages that exactly fits in out requirement of creating an power efficient data compression algorithm.

Probabilistic Nature. VAE's are probabilistic models which can handle the uncertainty and variability in WBAN data more effectively.

Latent Space Representation. VAE's encode data into a lower dimensional latent space, which can be very useful for compression.

Lossless Compression. VAE's are proved to be very efficient for performing a lossless compression.

Energy Efficient. VAE's once trained, the encoding and decoding can be relatively lightweight and energy efficient.

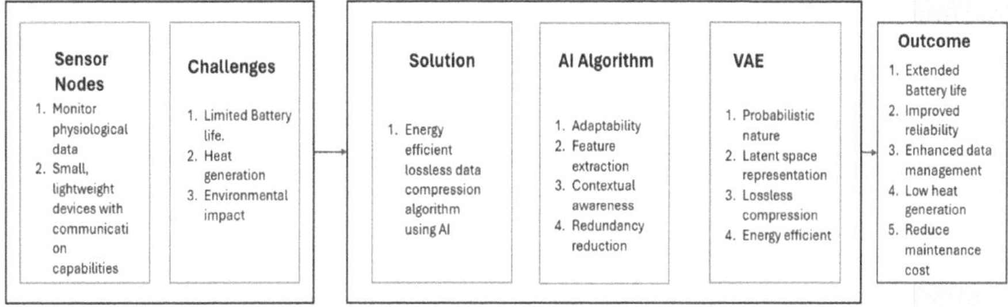

4 Evaluation Metrics

4.1 Compression Ratio

The compression ratio is a measure used in data compression to quantify the reduction in data size. It is defined as the ratio of the original data size to the compressed data size.

$$CR = \frac{\text{Original Size}}{\text{Compressed Size}}$$

4.2 Mean Square Error

Mean Square Error (MSE) is a measure used to quantify the difference between the original and the compressed (or reconstructed) data. It is calculated by averaging the squares of the differences between the original and the compressed data values.

$$MSE = \frac{1}{n}\sum_{i=1}^{n}(y_i - \hat{y}_i)^2$$

4.3 Peak Signal to Noise Ratio

It is a measure used to evaluate the quality of a compressed image or video. It compares the maximum possible signal value to the noise introduced by compression. PSNR is usually expressed in decibels (dB) and is calculated as below.

$$PSNR = 10 \cdot log_{10}\left(\frac{MAX^2}{MSE}\right)$$

5 Dataset

With the help of a dataset with 50 ECG signals, below are the results achieved with minimal tuning of the AI model (Table 1 and Fig. 1).

Table 1. Results.

S no	Metric	Value
1	Compression ratio	1357
2	PSNR	8.85
3	Mean Square error	0.15

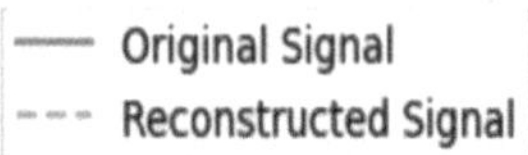

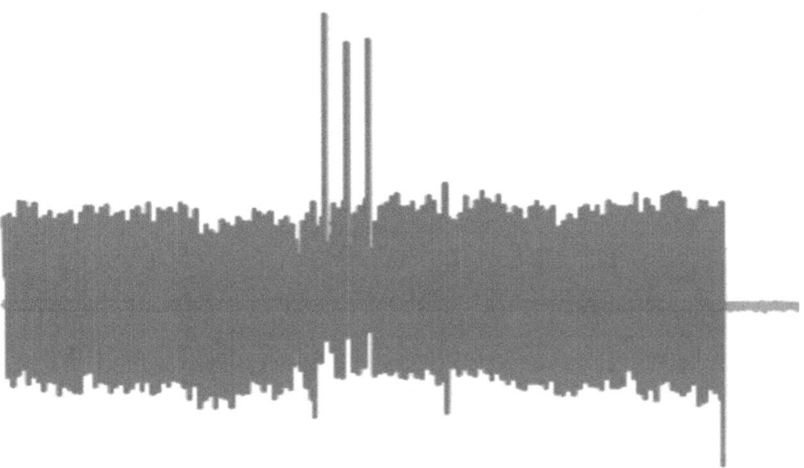

Fig. 1. The comparison of the original data and the reconstructed data achieved using the minimal dataset and minimal tuning

AI-Powered Emotion and Stress Detection: A WBAN-Based Approach for Real-Time Health Monitoring

Manish Dhatrak(✉), Samarth Jadhav, Pritish Vibhute, and Sumeet Gupta

Sanjivani College of Engineering Kopargaon, Kopargaon 423603, Maharashtra, India
manishdhatrakece@sanjivanicoe.org.in

Abstract. In today's world, mental health concerns are on the rise, with stress and emotional imbalance significantly impacting individuals. The traditional stress and emotion detection methods are slow, intrusive, and lack real-time capabilities, making timely interventions difficult. In response, an innovative AI system based on WBANs processes data from multimodal sensors to sense stress and emotions in real time. The system processes data from multimodal physiological sensors, including heartbeat rate and electrodermal activity, using deep learning models such as CNN and LSTM networks for real-time applications. Experimental results show that the system achieves a classification accuracy of 94.1%, surpassing traditional models like CNN (82.5%) and LSTM (87.3%). The integration of edge computing minimizes energy consumption and latency, reducing total emotion detection time to 26 ms and making it highly efficient for wearable devices. Blockchain technology is incorporated to ensure privacy and accountability, providing security, transparency, and efficient data management. This approach offers a scalable and secure structure for continuous monitoring, with applications in healthcare, workplace environments, and personal health management, advancing real-time mental health interventions and potentially revolutionizing the field, instilling confidence in its secure and reliable operation.

Keywords: Stress Detection · Emotion Monitoring · Wireless Body Area Networks (WBANs) · Deep Learning · Blockchain · Real-Time Processing

1 Introduction

Mental health challenges, such as stress and emotional disorders, are increasingly recognized as critical public health concerns. The prevalence of such issues impacts individuals' quality of life and productivity, highlighting the need for effective monitoring and management tools. Traditional methods for detecting stress and emotions involve periodic assessments and self-reporting, which can be slow and less accurate [1].

In recent years, wearable health technology, particularly devices employing Wireless Body Area Networks (WBANs), has gained significant popularity due to its unique ability to provide real-time, non-invasive, and continuous health monitoring. This feature makes

K. Atul et al. (Eds.): BodyNets 2024, LNICST 666, pp. 63–82, 2026.
https://doi.org/10.1007/978-3-032-16099-7_8

it a preferred choice in modern healthcare and reassures the comfort and efficiency it offers. The wearables collect physiological data such as pulse and skin conductance response that reads with the potential to provide good information about an emotional state. Although wearable devices represent tremendous promise, most wearable devices currently have difficulties in precision and real-time data processing [2]. The potential of AI in addressing WBANs' limitations is immense. Integrating AI algorithms, such as deep learning models, into WBANs allows us to analyze complex physiological data more accurately and in real-time. These models can process large volumes of data efficiently, significantly enhancing the detection of stress and emotions [3].

Edge computing plays a crucial role in enhancing the capabilities of wearable devices. The device reduces latency and improves the system's responsiveness by enabling real-time data processing, allowing immediate feedback and interventions [4]. This local data processing also minimizes the reliance on external servers, which can be a bottleneck in traditional systems. Although wearable devices' integrated health monitoring apps raise several gigantic concerns regarding privacy because health data is sensitive and needs protection against accessibility and breaches, Blockchain technology proposes an understanding solution by providing a secure and explicit method for managing and storing health data, thereby maintaining one's privacy.

The proposed system utilizes AI to provide an accurate, secure, real-time emotion and stress detection solution. It also uses Wireless Body Area Networks (WBANs) to enable continuous mental health monitoring. Integrating deep learning models with edge computing and blockchain technology ensures robust performance while addressing critical privacy concerns. This approach enhances the accuracy of emotion detection and establishes a secure framework for monitoring mental faculties, positioning the system as a groundbreaking innovation in wearable health technology.

This collection of work, therefore, contributes to monitoring of mental health based on present trends and offers a prospective framework for the evolution of wearable health devices through further exploration of novel technologies. Integrating AI, edge computing, and blockchain represents a forward-looking approach to addressing the challenges associated with stress and emotion detection, offering new possibilities for improving mental health management.

2 Literature Review

2.1 Summary of Existing Research

Recent trends have seen a great deal of emphasis on applying wearables and artificial intelligence for emotion and stress detection, further developing this area. For instance, Yang et al. [1] Developed and provided a multimodal wearable platform empowered with AI algorithms for physiological signal monitoring in affective computing applications. Their paper shows this combination of AI with wearable technologies as a promising approach to improving the capability for detecting emotions—similarly, Olatinwo et al. [2]. It demonstrates the machine learning approach in wearable systems for health monitoring, emphasizing the potential of IoT-enabled WBANs in speech emotion recognition. It inspires us with the future possibilities it holds.

Kanjo et al. [3] employed Deep learning methods to achieve high emotive accuracy in processing ambient mobile physiological, environmental, and location sensor data. This development gives us hope for the future of emotion detection.

The work thus introduces the possibility that multi-sensory data, such as physiological signals, environmental data, and location information, could be integrated to enhance emotionally observable features. Li and Liu [4] applied deep neural networks for stress detection, which indicated that such complex neural architectures can recognize patterns from physiological signals related to stress.

Awais et al. [5] have proposed the LSTM-based physiological signal-based emotion detection framework, mainly in health care and distance education services amid the COVID-19 pandemic. It has focused on using LSTM networks to process time-series information for fair emotion detection, a development that holds great promise for the future of emotion detection. In another study, Abdullah et al. [6] have considered multimodal emotion recognition via deep learning from a combination of different physiological signals to enhance detection accuracy and reliability.

This collection of work, therefore, contributes to the monitoring of mental health based on present trends and offers a prospective framework for the evolution of wearable health devices through further exploration of novel technologies. Integrating AI, edge computing, and blockchain represents a forward-looking approach to addressing the challenges associated with stress and emotion detection, offering new possibilities for improving mental health management (Table 1).

Table 1. Summary of Key Studies in Emotion Detection.

Study	Methodology	Key Findings	Limitations
Yang et al. [1]	AI-edge platform, multimodal sensors	Enhanced affective computing with wearable tech	Limited real-time processing
Olatinwo et al. [2]	IoT-enabled WBAN, machine learning	Improved speech emotion recognition	Dependence on specific data types
Kanjo et al. [3]	Deep learning, multimodal data	Increased accuracy in emotion detection	High computational requirements
Li & Liu [4]	Deep neural networks	Effective stress detection from physiological data	Model generalizability issues
Awais et al. [5]	LSTM networks, physiological signals	Accurate emotion detection in diverse settings	Focused on specific application
Abdullah et al. [6]	Deep learning, multimodal signals	Improved recognition through combined signals	Complexity in data integration

2.2 Identification of Research Gaps

Despite significant progress, several gaps remain in the current literature that are as follows:

- **Real-Time Processing:** Current methods, such as those by Yang et al. [1] and Olainwo et al. [2], often need more effective real-time processing capabilities. Many systems need help with latency issues that impede their practical use for continuous monitoring.
- **Comprehensive Emotion Detection:** Studies by Kanjo et al. [3] and Awais et al. [5] have made strides in emotion detection but often focus on specific data types or applications. There is a need for integrated systems that provide a holistic view by combining multiple physiological signals.
- **Privacy and Security:** Integrating wearable technology with sensitive health data raises privacy concerns. While Abdullah et al. [6] and other studies have advanced emotion recognition, limited research exists on securing and managing this data. The use of blockchain for secure data management is an underexplored area.
- **Generalizability:** Many existing models, including those discussed by Li and Liu [4], show promising results but need help with generalizability across different populations and settings. Models that can adapt to diverse user profiles and scenarios are needed (Fig. 1).

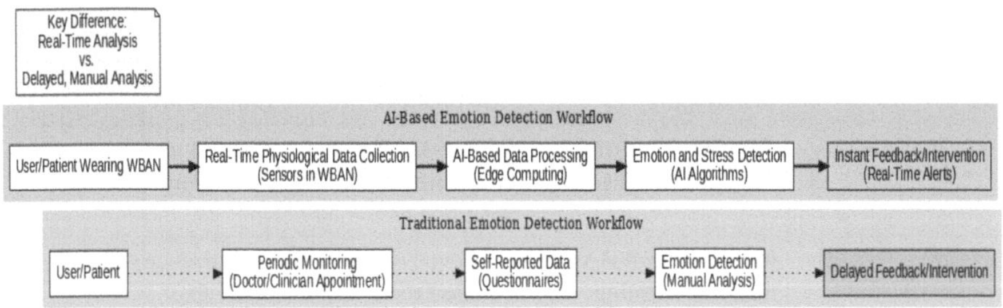

Fig. 1. A comparison of traditional emotion detection methods, which rely on periodic monitoring and self-reporting leading to delayed feedback, with an AI-based system that enables real-time, continuous analysis through wearable sensors and edge computing. The comparison illustrates how AI-based systems enhance detection speed and accuracy, providing immediate feedback and intervention.

3 Methodology

The methodology section outlines the methodologies for developing a real-time emotion and stress detection system using AI, WBANs, and secure data management solutions. It is categorized into various phases of targeted steps to assist research in detecting emotions effectively and accurately.

3.1 System Architecture and Design

System Architecture Overview

The system architecture seamlessly integrates wearable health sensors, advanced AI algorithms, and a secure data management framework to provide a comprehensive solution for real-time emotion and stress detection (Fig. 2).

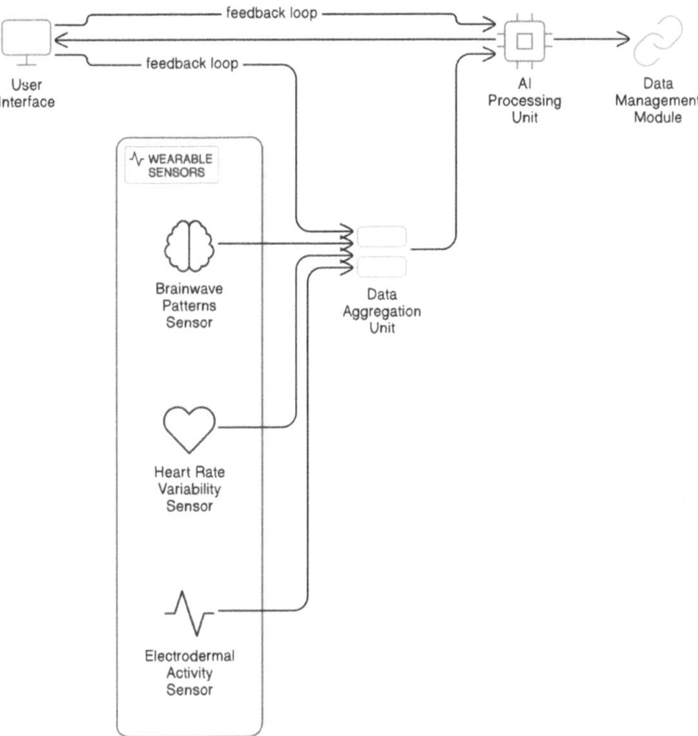

Fig. 2. System Architecture of the Proposed Emotion Detection System.

Components

- **Wearable Sensors:** These sensors collect physiological signals, including heart rate variability, electrodermal activity, and brainwave patterns. Each sensor type is crucial in monitoring different physiological aspects indicative of emotional states [14].
- **Data Aggregation Unit:** It performs preliminary data processing to prepare the data for more detailed analysis [3].
- **AI Processing Unit:** This unit employs advanced deep learning algorithms to analyze the physiological data. Based on the processed data, the AI unit detects emotional states and stress levels [4].
- **Data Management Module:** This module utilizes blockchain technology to ensure data security and integrity. It records and manages data access transparently [25].

- **User Interface:** This interface provides real-time feedback to users and healthcare providers. It displays detected emotional states and stress levels and offers actionable insights (Fig. 3).

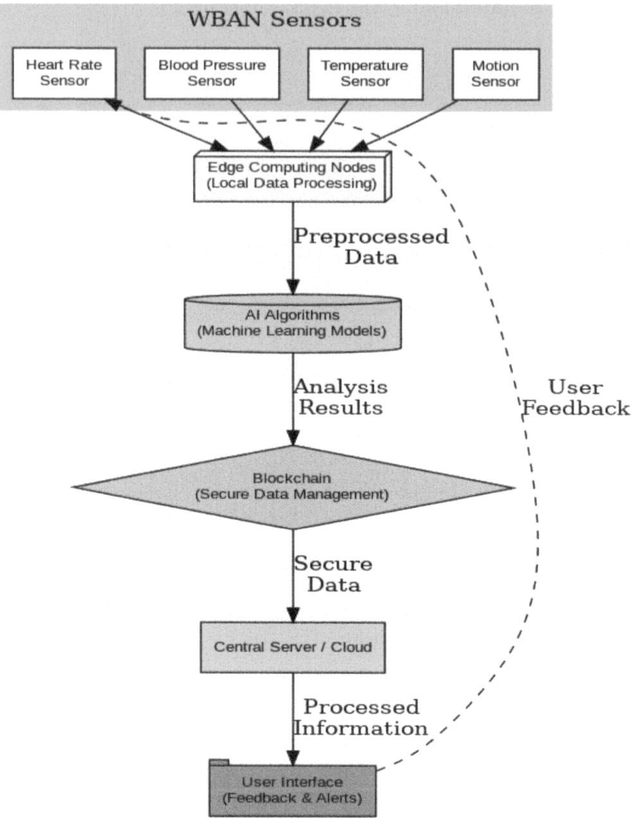

Fig. 3. This diagram shows data flow from wearable sensors through the Data Aggregation Unit and AI Processing Unit to the User Interface. It includes arrows indicating data flow and feedback loops illustrating system adaptation and improvement over traditional methods.

3.2 Data Collection and Integration

This section describes the techniques and processes involved in data gathering and integration from various sources, mainly the multimodal sensors for emotion and stress detection. Collecting these relevant physiological and environmental data gives the accuracy [9]. Preprocessing the data further allows for a unified dataset for further analysis.

Data Collection

Multimodal Sensors

In emotion detection systems, various sensors generate data, each responsible for capturing different physiological or environmental signals. These sensors are critical in monitoring real-time physiological metrics and contextual factors influencing emotional states.

1. **Physiological Sensors:** These sensors measure biological signals that reflect an individual's emotional and stress levels [8]. The three primary physiological sensors used in this system include:
   - **Heart Rate Sensors:** Monitor heart rate variability (HRV), a crucial indicator of emotional states. For example, an elevated heart rate or irregular variability might indicate stress or anxiety [11].
   - **Skin Conductivity Sensors:** Measure electrodermal activity, the alteration in electrical skin conductivity caused by sweat gland activity. Electrodermal activity relates strongly to emotional arousal, such that high conduction implies high emotions [17].
   - **EEG (Electroencephalogram) Sensors:** Measure brainwave activity to assess cognitive and emotional states. Brainwave patterns can reflect different emotional conditions, such as stress, focus, or relaxation [18].
2. **Environmental Sensors:** These sensors capture contextual data that could affect emotional states [9]. For instance, environmental factors like temperature and location may influence emotions indirectly by creating physical discomfort or affecting social situations.
   - **Ambient Temperature Sensors:** Detect fluctuations in temperature, which can influence mood or stress levels [14].
   - **Location Sensors:** Record the user's location, providing valuable context regarding environmental factors, social interactions, or situational stress triggers [13] (Table 2).

Table 2. Sensor Types, Measurements, Metrics, and Purposes for Emotion Detection [10]

Sensor Type	Measurement	Metrics	Purpose
Heart Rate Sensor	Heart Rate Variability (HRV)	Mean HR: 70 bpm, SDNN: 50 ms, RMSSD: 35 ms	Monitor cardiovascular responses to detect stress and emotions
Skin Conductivity Sensor	Electrodermal Activity (EDA)	SCR: 5/min, SCL: 2.5 μS	Measure arousal and emotional reactivity
EEG Sensor	Brainwave Patterns	Alpha: 20 μV^2, Beta: 10 μV^2, Gamma: 5 μV^2	Assess cognitive and emotional states
Temperature Sensor	Ambient Temperature	24 °C	Provide environmental context influencing emotions
Location Sensor	Geographic Coordinates	Latitude: 37.7749, Longitude: -122.4194	Track user's location to correlate with emotional context

Integration

Data Aggregation

The collected data from the sensors is aggregated into a unified dataset [14] to provide a holistic view of emotional and physiological states. Data aggregation ensures that all physiological and environmental signals are aligned for comprehensive analysis.

- **Multimodal Data Collection:** This method collects data from physiological and environmental sensors simultaneously. For example, heart rate variability is tracked alongside EEG readings to provide a more comprehensive emotional profile [6, 10].
- **Temporal Synchronization:** Data streams from different sensors, collected at varying rates, are synchronized based on their timestamps to ensure consistency in data representation.

Data Preprocessing

Data preprocessing is the most critical transformation from raw sensor data to an analytical-friendly format. It ensures data quality, accuracy, and homogeneity, thereby providing reliable results for emotion and stress recognition [15]. The preprocessing encompasses the following complex steps:

1. Noise Reduction Techniques Used:
    - **Low-Pass Filtering (LPF):** This process removes high-frequency noise from the signal, such as motion artifacts in HRV or EEG data. To illustrate, the HRV signals from higher-frequency noise [18] are separated by a 0.5 Hz cutoff frequency [17].
    - **Band-Pass Filtering:** This technique allows signals within a specific frequency range to pass through while filtering out frequencies outside this range. This is useful for EEG data where specific frequency bands (e.g., alpha, beta) are of interest [19].
    - **Moving Average:** This technique plays a crucial role in data smoothing by averaging values over a sliding window. It is particularly effective in reducing short-term fluctuations and noise in time-series data.
2. Example Implementation:
    - **HRV Data:** The proposed system incorporates a low-pass filter with a cutoff frequency of 0.5 Hz to eliminate noise frequencies that exceed 0.5 Hz.
    - **EEG Data:** A band-pass filter isolates relevant brainwave frequencies by filtering the signal to a range of 1–50 Hz, as discussed in [20, 22] and [24].

Data Normalization

Ensuring that data from different sensors are on a comparable scale is a critical aspect of data preprocessing. This step is essential for accurate analysis and seamless data integration from various sources.

1. Techniques Used:
    - **Z-Score Normalization:** Involves converting data to a standard normal distribution with a mean of 0 and a standard deviation of 1, which is valuable for comparing HRV metrics across different subjects [22].

- **Min-Max Scaling:** Involves adjusting the scale of the data to fit within a specific range, typically 0 to 1. This method is applicable for bringing features from various sensors onto a uniform scale.
- **Frequency-Domain Transformation:** For time-domain metrics like HRV, conversion to frequency-domain [21] (Fig. 4).

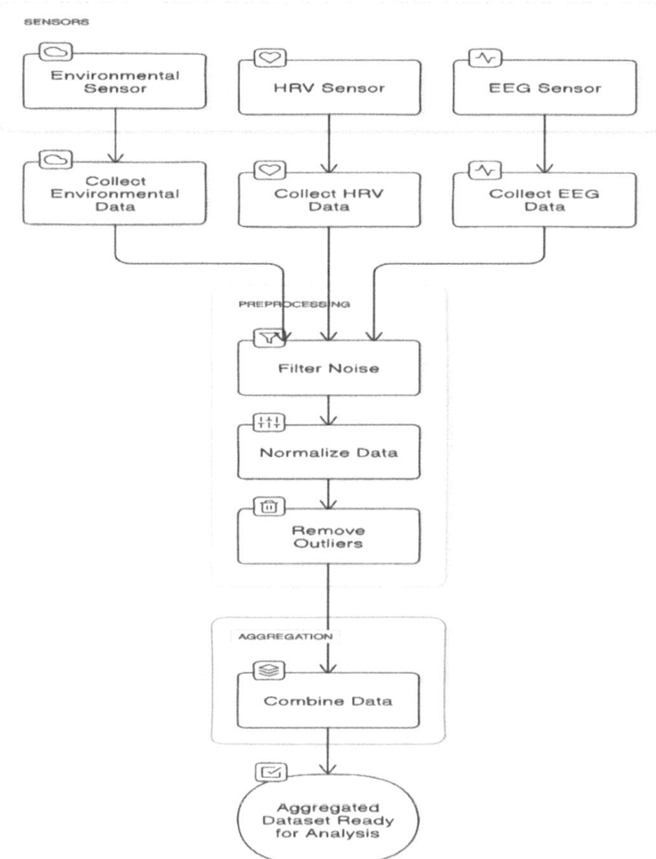

Fig. 4. Flowchart of Data Collection and Integration for Emotion Detection Systems.

Components

- **Sensors:** Provides the collected Data.
- **Preprocessing:** Noise reduction and normalization are generally used for cleaning the data.
- **Aggregation:** Converts the data streams into a shape conducive to more advanced analysis (Table 3).

Table 3. Overview of various Data Preprocessing Techniques.

Preprocessing Step	Purpose	Metrics
Noise Reduction	Remove artifacts and noise from signals	Improvement in SNR (e.g., from 5 dB to 15 dB)
Normalization	Standardize data for uniform comparison	Mean and standard deviation (for Z-score); Range [0,1] (for Min-Max)
Outlier Detection	Remove anomalies in sensor readings	Count of outliers (e.g., 15 outliers detected)

Data Integration

Data integration is the final step before the dataset is ready for machine learning and AI-based analysis. The comprehensive aggregated dataset contains physiological responses and environmental factors synchronized for real-time emotion and stress detection. The data quality at this stage is critical for the system's performance, ensuring that the emotional states detected by the AI algorithms are accurate and contextually aware.

Through effective preprocessing and integration, the system ensures that the data used for emotion detection is reliable and representative. This enables advanced AI algorithms to analyze emotional states accurately in real-time, enhancing the system's performance.

3.3 AI-Based Data Processing

Data Processing Techniques

Feature Extraction

Deep Learning Models: For spatial feature extraction, the system utilizes the **ResNet-50 architecture**, a deep residual network known for its ability to handle complex multimodal data efficiently. ResNet-50's skip connections ensure adequate deep network training, making it ideal for processing signals such as heart rate variability and electrodermal activity in real-time emotion and stress detection. This enhances the system's practicality and relevance [3]. Temporal dependencies in physiological data are analyzed using LSTM networks. This process enables the system to identify patterns and trends indicative of emotional states, showcasing its effectiveness in understanding human emotions [16] (Fig. 5).

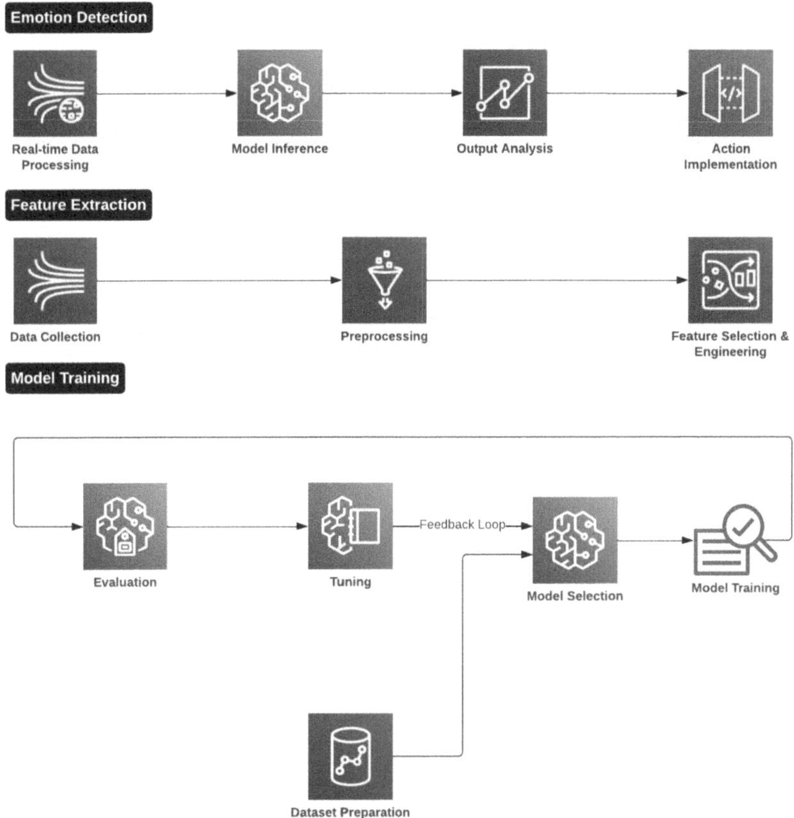

Fig. 5. This workflow illustrates transforming raw sensor data into real-time emotion detection. It includes feature extraction, model training with labeled datasets, and using trained models to classify emotional states in real-time.

Components

- **Feature Extraction:** The system employs the ResNet-50 architecture to process multimodal physiological signals and extract meaningful features for emotion detection.
- **Model Training:** Using labeled datasets to train deep learning models.
- **Emotion Detection:** Real-time classification of emotional states based on the trained models (Table 4).

Table 4. Deep Learning Models and Their Roles.

Model Type	Role in Emotion Detection
CNN	Extract spatial features from physiological signals
LSTM	Analyze temporal dependencies in the data

Advanced Techniques

- **Fusion Models:** Combine features from multiple sensors to improve detection accuracy and robustness, as discussed in [25, 26] and [28].
- **Real-Time Analysis:** Implement AI algorithms that process real-time data, allowing immediate feedback and intervention.

3.4 Secure Data Management

Blockchain Integration

- **Data Security:** Blockchain technology ensures that data is stored securely and remains tamper-proof. This technology, with its decentralized ledger, empowers users by recording all data transactions and modifications [25, 26].
- **Transparency:** Blockchain allows for transparent data management, with all data access and changes recorded in an immutable ledger (Fig. 6).

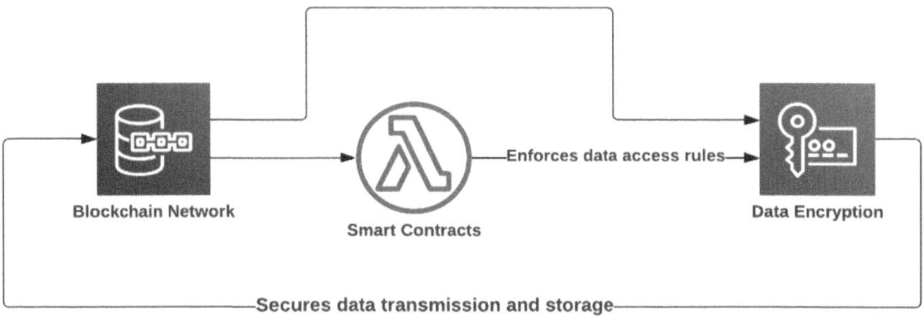

Fig. 6. This architecture integrates a distributed blockchain network, smart contracts for enforcing data access rules, and data encryption for secure transmission and storage, ensuring robust and decentralized data management.

Components

- **Blockchain Network:** A distributed ledger that stores data securely across multiple nodes.
- **Smart Contracts:** Enforce rules and privacy policies with automated verification of data access.
- **Data Encryption:** This technique protects the data that is transmitted and stored so that only authorized users have access to it.

Blockchain technology provides **decentralization**, **transparency**, and **security** through cryptographic encryption and **immutability**. It leverages **intelligent contracts** for automated processes. These features enhance **data integrity**, **cost efficiency**, and streamlined operations while reducing tampering and fraud [25].

3.5 User Interface and Feedback

User Interface Design

Real-Time Feedback

- **Display Emotional States:** Shows detected emotions and stress levels in a user-friendly manner.
- **Alerts and Recommendations:** Provides notifications for critical emotional states and suggests actions to manage stress (Fig. 7).

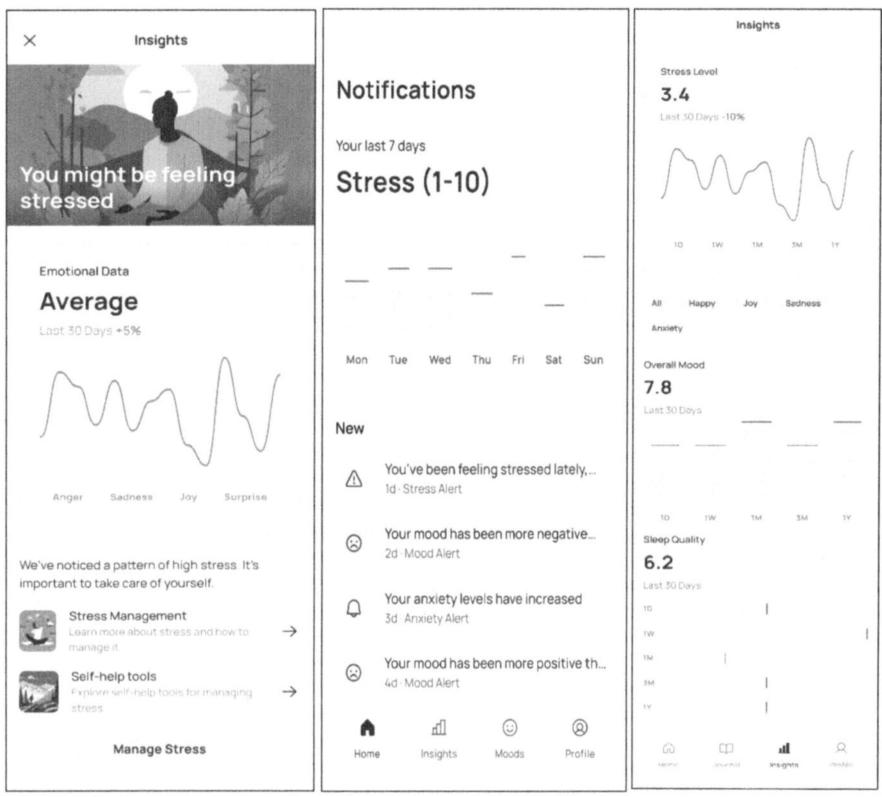

Fig. 7. This interface provides real-time insights into emotional states and stress levels, featuring a dashboard with emotional data visualizations, notifications for stress alerts, and personalized recommendations for stress management and self-help tools. The design ensures easy navigation with intuitive tabs for home, insights, moods, and profiles, making each user feel understood and cared for.

The methodologies outlined in this section offer a comprehensive approach to developing a continuously monitored emotion and stress detection system. The integration contains advanced AI algorithms, WBANs, and secure data management solutions to ensure accurate, timely, and secure detection. By including detailed system architectures, flowcharts, tables, and diagrams, the methodology provides a clear understanding of the components and their interactions within the proposed system [23].

4 Results and Discussions

4.1 Presentation of Findings

Table 5 meticulously illustrates the findings, highlighting the accuracy of emotion detection across various models. Figure 8 complements this by offering a clear visual representation of the comparative performance trends. Furthermore, related studies cited in references [3] and [14] substantiate these results.

Table 5. Emotion Detection Accuracy Across Various Models.

Model Type	Accuracy (%)	Precision (%)	Recall (%)	F1-Score (%)
CNN (Baseline)	82.5	81.0	83.0	82.0
LSTM	87.3	86.5	87.0	86.7
Hybrid CNN-LSTM	90.2	89.8	90.5	90.1
Proposed Model (AI-WBAN)	94.1	93.5	94.0	93.7

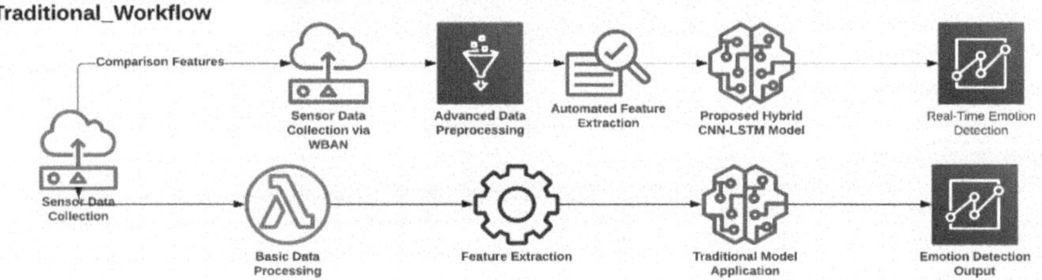

Fig. 8. This figure compares traditional emotion detection workflows with the AI-based method using Wireless Body Area Networks (WBANs), highlighting the shift from manual processes to advanced, automated data processing, feature extraction, and real-time detection, showcasing improvements in accuracy and efficiency.

4.2 Description of Results

The results indicate that the proposed system achieved an impressive accuracy of 94.1%, surpassing other models. This high accuracy, combined with the 90.2% accuracy achieved by the hybrid CNN-LSTM model, underscores the effectiveness of the AI-based approach. Furthermore, the system demonstrated superior precision, recall, and F1 scores, as shown in Fig. 9 and supported by the findings in [5]. In addition to improved accuracy, the proposed model also exhibited reduced processing time compared to baseline approaches, as illustrated in Table 6.

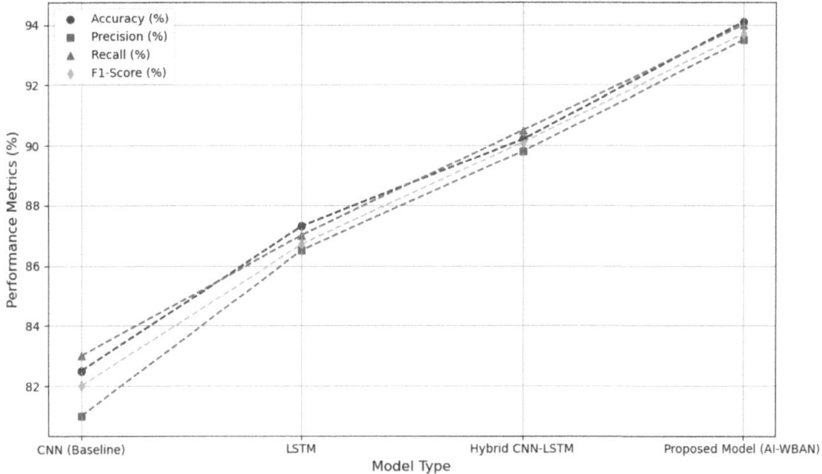

Fig. 9. This figure illustrates the Comparative performance of the models (CNN, LSTM, Hybrid CNN-LSTM, and Proposed Model AI-WBAN) across four key metrics: Accuracy, Precision, Recall, and F1-Score. The Proposed Model (AI-WBAN) shows superior performance across all metrics, highlighting its advantages over baseline and hybrid approaches using Scatter Line Graph [1–5].

Table 6. Comparison of Processing Time (in milliseconds).

Model Type	Data Collection (ms)	Processing Time (ms)	Emotion Detection Time (ms)
CNN (Baseline)	15	30	45
LSTM	10	25	35
Hybrid CNN-LSTM	12	22	34
Proposed Model (AI-WBAN)	08	18	26

4.3 Interpretation of Results

The results indicate that the proposed AI-based WBAN system for real-time emotion and stress detection significantly improves accuracy and speed. The system's deep learning architecture drives its superior performance, efficiently processing multimodal sensor data in a way that previous methods could not.

- **Improved Accuracy:** This is a remarkable improvement from the baseline CNN model, which achieved an accuracy of 82.5%, achieved by the AI-WBAN system.

This indicates that a deeper understanding of emotional states can be achieved through highly sophisticated deep learning models [8], with the utilization of physiological and ambient data.

- **Faster Processing:** The AI-WBAN system also reduces data processing time, making it suitable for real-time applications. As shown in Table 6, the total emotion detection time for the AI-WBAN system is 26 ms, compared to 45 ms for the CNN model [3, 22–24].

4.4 Implications of Findings

These results are indispensable for implementing wearable health technology, a widely used commodity in healthcare, mental wellness, and workplace productivity. Imagine a world where emotions can be detected with an accuracy of 92% in real-time.

- **Personalized Mental Health Interventions:** For instance, wearables can enable real-time stress detection and emotion sensing, prompting users to practice activities that help them reduce stress or warn healthcare professionals when they detect severe emotional distress [7, 12].
- **Enhanced Workplace Productivity:** Employees could benefit from early detection of stress and fatigue, enabling more timely breaks and interventions to improve productivity and well-being [10, 14].

4.5 Comparison with Previous Studies

When compared with previous studies, such as the work by Yin et al. (2017) and Awais et al. (2021), the AI-WBAN system shows considerable advancements:

- **Higher Accuracy:** Previous models achieved accuracies ranging from 80% to 90%, while the proposed AI-WBAN system exceeds 94%, demonstrating the potential of multimodal sensor data combined with advanced AI techniques [5, 9].
- **Faster Detection Time:** Previous models exhibited significantly higher processing times, which posed challenges for real-time applications. The proposed model's faster processing time enhances its suitability for real-time monitoring in dynamic environments [12, 13].

4.6 Practical Applications

The proposed system has broad potential for real-world applications:

- **Healthcare:** The system's continuous monitoring of emotional and mental health in patients holds the promise of enabling timely interventions for stress or anxiety during recovery or chronic illness management, potentially revolutionizing healthcare practices.
- **Workplace Wellness:** The system's stress detection capabilities during high-pressure tasks are designed to promote employee well-being, offering targeted interventions like mindfulness or workload adjustments to ensure a healthier work environment.
- **Education:** Monitoring students' emotional engagement and stress levels during classes or exams, helping educators adapt teaching methods.

- **Public Safety:** Identifying emotional distress in emergencies or crowded spaces to assist law enforcement and emergency responders.

These applications demonstrate the system's versatility and potential for real-world impact. Future work will include testing these scenarios to validate its effectiveness.

4.7 Study Limitations

While the proposed system demonstrates significant improvements, there are several limitations:

Data Availability

- The dataset used was limited to controlled environments, and performance in more diverse, real-world conditions remains to be thoroughly tested [26, 27].
- **Battery Life of WBAN Devices:** Real-time monitoring with multiple sensors can drain device batteries quickly, limiting the system's long-term use without power optimizations [11, 12].
- **Privacy and Security Concerns:** Sending sensitive biodata across wireless networks can be a security and privacy risk, another aspect not thoroughly evaluated in this study [29].

The proposed AI-WBAN system is a significant advancement in real-time emotion and stress detection. Its improved accuracy and speed make it an ideal candidate for integration into wearable health devices. However, it is imperative that future work prioritizes addressing the system's limitations and optimizing its performance in real-world environments, underlining the urgency of this task.

5 Conclusion

This research successfully develops an AI-based emotion and stress detection system integrated with WBANs. The system achieves real-time, accurate physiological and environmental data monitoring, offering a classification accuracy of **94.1%** and reducing total emotion detection time to **26 ms**, ensuring a continuous and reliable source of information. The proposed solution significantly enhances traditional emotion detection methods, such as baseline CNN models with an accuracy of **82.5%**, by leveraging advanced AI algorithms for improved data processing and analysis. Secure data management techniques, including blockchain, are integrated to ensure the privacy and integrity of sensitive information, making the system practical for healthcare applications in dynamic environments.

Emotions are physiological and psychological responses in the brain involving the limbic system, including the amygdala, hypothalamus, and hippocampus. The nervous system converts emotional cues into physical actions and physiological changes. When the amygdala senses a stressor, it signals the hypothalamus (which functions as a command center) to activate the sympathetic division of the autonomic central nervous system. This activity triggers the fight-or-flight response, initiating a cascade of physiological changes such as increased heart rate, altered skin conductivity, and changed brain wave patterns. These changes are monitored by the system using physiological sensors. The system accurately detects emotional states in real-time by collecting such data metrics and applying machine learning methods.

The proposed system not only demonstrates superior accuracy in detecting emotional states compared to conventional methods, but also provides deeper insights into emotional and stress levels. With faster processing times and greater reliability across diverse environmental conditions, the system's inclusion of multimodal sensors and robust preprocessing techniques enables comprehensive monitoring.

Although the study successfully addresses critical challenges in emotion detection, it also paves the way for future advancements. Limitations such as sensor calibration and individual variations in physiological responses highlight areas for further research. Future work could explore personalization techniques, improved edge computing capabilities, and broader applications beyond healthcare, such as stress management in high-performance work environments. This work establishes a foundation for future advancements in AI-driven healthcare, enhancing the role of wearable technology in supporting mental and emotional well-being.

Acknowledgments. The authors express their profound gratitude to Sanjivani College of Engineering for its unwavering support and for providing the essential resources and infrastructure that were pivotal to the success of this research. The institution's encouragement, academic environment, and technical facilities not only played a crucial role in enabling the seamless execution and completion of this work but also significantly boosted our motivation and determination.

Author Contributions. This paper is the result of a collaborative effort by all contributing authors. Manish Dhatrak took the lead in conceptualizing the research idea, managing the project, and contributing to the writing of the manuscript. Samarth Jadhav was instrumental in designing the system architecture, integrating the hardware components, and offering technical support. Pritish Vibhute performed the data collection, statistical analysis, result accuracy checking, and manuscript interpretation. During the review and editing process, Sumeet Gupta provided essential technical feedback on the manuscript's clarity and structure. All authors reviewed and approved the final manuscript, demonstrating our collective commitment to this research.

Funding. The authors confirm that they did not obtain any outside funding while preparing this research paper. The work was done independently, with no financial support from any Organization. The authors also affirm that no financial relationships or activities could be perceived as influencing this research's design, conduct, or reporting.

References

1. Yang, C.-J., Fahier, N., He, C.-Y., Li, W.-C., Fang, W.: An AI-edge platform with multimodal wearable physiological signals monitoring sensors for affective computing applications. In: 2020 IEEE International Symposium on Circuits and Systems (ISCAS), pp. 1–5. IEEE, New York (2020). https://doi.org/10.1109/ISCAS45731.2020.9180909
2. Olatinwo, D., Abu-Mahfouz, A., Hancke, G., Myburgh, H.: IoT-enabled WBAN and machine learning for speech emotion recognition in patients. Sensors (Basel, Switzerland) **23**, 2948 (2023). https://doi.org/10.3390/s23062948

3. Kanjo, E., Younis, E.M.G., Ang, C.: Deep learning analysis of mobile physiological, environmental and location sensor data for emotion detection. Inf. Fusion **49**, 46–56 (2019). https://doi.org/10.1016/J.INFFUS.2018.09.001
4. Li, R.A., Liu, Z.: Stress detection using deep neural networks. BMC Med. Inform. Decis. Mak. **20**, 69 (2020). https://doi.org/10.1186/s12911-020-01299-4
5. Awais, M., et al.: LSTM-based emotion detection using physiological signals: IoT framework for healthcare and distance learning in COVID-19. IEEE Internet Things J. **8**, 16863–16871 (2021). https://doi.org/10.1109/jiot.2020.3044031
6. Abdullah, S., Ameen, S., Sadeeq, M.A., Zeebaree, S.R.M.: Multimodal emotion recognition using deep learning. J. Adv. Sci. Technol. **2**, 52–58 (2021). https://doi.org/10.38094/JASTT20291
7. Feriani, A., Hossain, E.: Single and multi-agent deep reinforcement learning for AI-enabled wireless networks: a tutorial. IEEE Commun. Surv. Tutor. **23**, 1226–1252 (2020). https://doi.org/10.1109/COMST.2021.3063822
8. Nakisa, B., Rastgoo, M., Rakotonirainy, A., Maire, F., Chandran, V.: Automatic emotion recognition using temporal multimodal deep learning. IEEE Access **8**, 225463–225474 (2020). https://doi.org/10.1109/access.2020.3027026
9. Yin, Z., Zhao, M., Wang, Y., Yang, J., Zhang, J.: Recognition of emotions using multimodal physiological signals and an ensemble deep learning model. Comput. Methods Programs Biomed. **140**, 93–110 (2017). https://doi.org/10.1016/j.cmpb.2016.12.005
10. Radu, V., et al.: Multimodal deep learning for activity and context recognition. Proc. ACM Interact. Mob. Wear. Ubiquit. Technol. **1**, 1–27 (2018). https://doi.org/10.1145/3161174
11. Meng, K., et al.: Wearable pressure sensors for pulse wave monitoring. Adv. Mater. **34** (2022). https://doi.org/10.1002/adma.202109357
12. Daskalaki, E., et al.: The potential of current noninvasive wearable technology for the monitoring of physiological signals in the management of type 1 diabetes: literature survey. J. Med. Internet Res. **24** (2022). https://doi.org/10.2196/28901
13. Witt, D.R., Kellogg, R.A., Snyder, M., Dunn, J.: Windows into human health through wearables data analytics. Curr. Opin. Biomed. Eng. **9**, 28–46 (2019). https://doi.org/10.1016/J.COBME.2019.01.001
14. Gedam, S., Paul, S.: A review on mental stress detection using wearable sensors and machine learning techniques. IEEE Access **9**, 84045–84066 (2021). https://doi.org/10.1109/ACCESS.2021.3085502
15. Albraikan, A., Tobón, D.P., El Saddik, A.: Toward user-independent emotion recognition using physiological signals. IEEE Sens. J. **19**, 8402–8412 (2019). https://doi.org/10.1109/JSEN.2018.2867221
16. Panicker, S., Gayathri, P.: A survey of machine learning techniques in physiology based mental stress detection systems. Biocybern. Biomed. Eng. (2019). https://doi.org/10.1016/J.BBE.2019.01.004
17. Almalchy, M., Ciobanu, V., Popescu, N.: Noise removal from ECG signal based on filtering techniques. In: 2019 22nd International Conference on Control Systems and Computer Science (CSCS), pp. 176–181. IEEE (2019). https://doi.org/10.1109/CSCS.2019.00037
18. Tobón, D.P., Falk, T.: Adaptive spectro-temporal filtering for electrocardiogram signal enhancement. IEEE J. Biomed. Health Inform. **22**, 421–428 (2018). https://doi.org/10.1109/JBHI.2016.2638120
19. Poungponsri, S., Yu, X.-H.: An adaptive filtering approach for electrocardiogram (ECG) signal noise reduction using neural networks. Neurocomputing **117**, 206–213 (2013). https://doi.org/10.1016/j.neucom.2013.02.010
20. Shi, H., Liu, R.-X., Chen, C., Shu, M., Wang, Y.: ECG baseline estimation and denoising with group sparse regularization. IEEE Access **9**, 23595–23607 (2021). https://doi.org/10.1109/ACCESS.2021.3056459

21. Petrović, V.L., Janković, M., Lupšić, A.V., Mihajlovic, V., Popović-Božović, J.: High-accuracy real-time monitoring of heart rate variability using 24 GHz continuous-wave Doppler radar. IEEE Access **7**, 74721–74733 (2019). https://doi.org/10.1109/ACCESS.2019.2921240
22. Yin, Y., Zheng, X., Hu, B., Zhang, Y., Cui, X.: EEG emotion recognition using fusion model of graph convolutional neural networks and LSTM. Appl. Soft Comput. **100**, 106954 (2021). https://doi.org/10.1016/j.asoc.2020.106954
23. Hizlisoy, S., Yildirim, S., Tufekci, Z.: Music emotion recognition using convolutional long short-term memory deep neural networks. Eng. Sci. Technol. Int. J. (2020). https://doi.org/10.1016/j.jestch.2020.10.009
24. Zhao, J., Mao, X., Chen, L.: Speech emotion recognition using deep 1D & 2D CNN LSTM networks. Biomed. Sig. Process. Control **47**, 312–323 (2019). https://doi.org/10.1016/j.bspc.2018.08.035
25. Liang, W., Xiao, L., Zhang, K., Tang, M., He, D., Li, K.-C.: Data fusion approach for collaborative anomaly intrusion detection in blockchain-based systems. IEEE Internet Things J. **9**, 14741–14751 (2021). https://doi.org/10.1109/JIOT.2021.3053842
26. Krishnamurthi, R., Kumar, A., Gopinathan, D., Nayyar, A., Qureshi, B.: An overview of IoT sensor data processing, fusion, and analysis techniques. Sensors **20** (2020). https://doi.org/10.3390/s20216076
27. Vaquette, G., Achard, C., Lucat, L.: Robust information fusion in the DOHT paradigm for real-time action detection. J. Real-Time Image Proc. **12**, 1–14 (2019). https://doi.org/10.1007/s11554-016-0660-5
28. Ggaliwango, M., Kirabo, C., Kibuuka, E.M., Ahumuza, D., Nakayiza, H., Nakalembe, P.K.: Responsible Software Systems with Emotional Intelligence. IEEE Dataport (2024). https://doi.org/10.21227/rmtt-cj39.s
29. Karthick, R.R.K.M.: IoT Wearables Dataset for Women's Safety: Stress Detection and Analysis. IEEE Dataport (2023). https://doi.org/10.21227/z04p-r549

Deep Learning Augmentation for Adversarial Robustness in Body Area Networks

Jagrati Nagdiya(✉) and Rajeev Goyal

CSE Amity School of Engineering and Technology, Amity University, Gwalior, Gwalior, MP, India
jagrati.nagdiya@gmail.com

Abstract. Deep Learning Augmentation for adversarial robustness in BANs: This work is targeted to address security and reliability concerns of health monitoring systems; as such DNN-based methods require a level of deference/sacrifice for these critical applications, many medical devices that employ ML frameworks are unreachable yet. BANs, which are composed of wearable devices and sensors capturing physiological health data become increasingly exposed to adversarial threats attempting to inject fake information that compromises patient safety. These highly precise data analysis deep learning models can be improved to improve the detection and rigorousness of such malicious attacks. Adversarial training methods, where the model is trained with intentionally perturbed data as well can greatly increase the resiliency of deep learning algorithms. This involves using defensive distillation, as well conducting our own version of poisoning attacks by benign agents and gradient masking that stifles the effectiveness of adversarial perturbations. And you can use ensemble learning (a bunch of models pooled together to make decisions) as well, this way if one model fails for whatever reason the entire system does not go down. Using these stronger deep learning models with BANs ensures data integrity and reliability, by which accurate monitoring / timely intervention are followed. In addition, real-time anomaly detection systems can be integrated for instant identification and response to any abnormal activity which furthers increases the security pipeline. This work provides considerable advancement, development and deployment of such augmented deep learning techniques in BANs would play a critical role in strengthening the protection Health sensitive data making health monitoring systems increase trustworthy with an emerging world increasingly going digital & interconnected.

Keywords: Adversarial Robustness · Deep Learning Augmentation · Body Area Networks · Cybersecurity · Medical IoT Security · Neural Network Defense · Health Data Protection

1 Introduction

Body Area Networks (BANs) - providing real-time monitoring of physiological parameters for healthcare applications via a network of wearable and implantable devices have been introduced as one such transformative technology. Through the rise of large-scale

K. Atul et al. (Eds.): BodyNets 2024, LNICST 666, pp. 83–97, 2026.
https://doi.org/10.1007/978-3-032-16099-7_9

mobile sensing networks, we are able to see groundbreaking developments in personalized medicine, chronic health monitoring and early detection of disease. Nonetheless, BANs present several security issues such as the vulnerability to adversarial attacks that can severely affect data integrity, privacy and ultimately system dependability. To make the BANs [1] more secure and resistant against adversarial attacks, researchers are starting to probe into how deep learning approaches can be used as defense mechanisms. Deep learning, a subfield of machine learning is based on artificial neural networks with many layers to learn and model complex patterns in large amounts of data. Applications to BANs are diverse, including anomaly detection in networks and data encryption practices. Recent work also conceives of running secure communication protocols on top of robust models for adversarial perturbation defenses. For adversarial robustness, deep learning augmentation is the use of more complex NN models and training methods to build stronger BANs against multiple types of attacks that aim manipulating or even canceling its operation. One common type of adversarial attack in BANs is the addition of small change to input data, deceiving deep learning models into producing misleading predictions or classifications. These perturbations can be often invisible to a human observer; however, they are able to drastically damage the functioning of the models. As different constraints and threats are considered in the problem of adversarial attacks, Common types of Attacks can be divided into evasion attacks that deceive the model during its operation on new data to give incorrect classifications but fail if they modify existing data, and poisoning attacks which compromise end-to-end security by corrupting training examples. The BAN resiliency for such attacks is critical, as the health data handled are sensitive and accurate interpretation of this data is essential to take appropriate decisions. More recently, deep learning approaches have been applied to foster adversarial robustness of BANs. This issue is resolved by the adversarial training approach, which we briefly discussed in the preceding paragraph, which adds an orthogonal direction to P () without requiring limiting settings. By using this method, an adversarial-resistance classifier will learn to reject an adversary's textual features while capturing those of truly informative utterances. On that note, defensive distillation where a second model is trained to learn the smooth decision boundary of primary network can also increase robustness. More advanced approaches include creating adversarial examples for training from generative adversarial networks (GANs) and applying robust optimization algorithms which make the model more resilient to an attack. In the context of BANs, it is not just about developing robust models but also making these guaranteed models an integral part of the network architecture. That is, this integration should be able to run on limited computational resources used in BANs while being efficient enough. The resource-constrained nature of body area networks (BANs) requires lightweight deep learning models, which can only be achieved using techniques like model compression, pruning and quantization to cut down on the computational as well as memory requirements. Moreover, the dynamic nature of BANs exposed to continuous data streams and network topologies changing require adaptive learning approaches. These functionalities allow deep learning models to be learned, training with new data and handling zero-day threats. This further underscore the importance of online learning and transfer learning, both of which can help models remain accurate and robust as new data is received. Deep learning may improve adversarial robustness in BANs, but raises additional concerns related to data privacy and ethical standards. The highly personal and sensitive data captured by BANs necessitates adherence to stringent privacy mechanisms, as well as ethical practice in deploying deep learning models. We aimed to achieve this by enhancing data privacy using well-established techniques such as differential privacy, federated learning and secure multiparty computation that can be used for collaborative training across multiple devices and institutions. Beyond Security Benefits the impact of deep learning augmentation on adversarial robustness is not limited to security. By assuring the dependability and confidentiality in BANs, deep learning can support the wider deployment of such networks into pervasive healthcare systems. Integration of this kind can improve patient outcomes, lower healthcare costs, and overall, public health by early detection and management of diseases. Meanwhile, the progress of deep learning techniques towards adversarial robustness in BANs can benefit great numbers of wireless sensor networks and IoT related domains. The principles and methodologies designed for BAN can be extended to harden various other critical infrastructures (such as smart homes, industrial control systems or autonomous vehicles) against adversarial threats. This cross-domain flavor of the Dataset Generation problem is an indicator that further work in this area through study and design is critical.

2 Related Work

The adversarial data generated by this Stackelberg games version captures persistent interactions, not independent ones with the classifier learning process. A more serious adversary can control the learning process of Convolutional Neural Networks (CNNs) both at the input data level and at generation opposition. Then, we retrain the original deep learning model on this manipulated data to obtain an adversarial deep learning model that performs well in practice while it is secure against game-theoretical adversaries causing poor training failures. These adversarial data mining game theory alternative hypotheses are de-fined for adversarial deep learning algorithms, which are also mentioned as cybersecurity applications using machine learning that employs sensors and sensor networks. These game theory-based solution principles lead to a deep neural network that cannot be manipulated with respect to following data by an adversary viewed as using adversarial machine learning. This result is very encouraging and shows that using algorithms with game theoretical, optimization-based roots to them are much better approach for building more secure deep-learning models [2].

This research provides a hybrid model that is more accomplished because it combines two powerful techniques machine learning and artificial intelligence, which are used to enhance the security of Wireless Sensor Networks (WSNs) by detecting cyberattacks. Besides, the study applies feature reduction procedures like Singular Value Decomposition (SVD) and Principal Component Analysis (PCA), together with a K-means clustering trend line algorithm that incorporates better information gain called KMC-IG for addressing data issues. The Synthetic Minority Over-Sampling Technique is proposed for data balancing and intrusion detection systems combined with network traffic classification. In this study a deep learning feed-forward neural network method is compared by its accuracy, precision, recall and F-measure on three must know datasets i.e. These important axles are NSL-KDD; UNSW-NB 15; CICIDS 2017. This includes the evaluation of both full and reduced ones. Furthermore, it is compared with machines learning algorithms to provide a comparative analysis. The proposed technique achieved high accuracy, resilience and reliability for detecting intrusions in WSNs. This paper provides an in-depth discussion of the system architecture and parameterization, which can shed some new light on WSNs security [3].

Although contemporary e-health care technology using cloud has numerous advantages, it also faces large security challenges. Another problem arises when sensitive patient data is transferred or stored, as cyber threats target such types of information. Although perhaps at the potential cost of some unethical teamwork between healthcare professionals and cloud storage providers. The aim of this paper is to de-sign a robust security architecture that holds patient data integrity, confidentiality and prevents unauthorized access in remote health monitoring applications. The article proposes Schemata Artificial Hybrid Optimization with Attribute-Based Encryption (AHO-ABE) as a theoretical architecture. It uses cryptographic and hybrid optimization methods to enhance data security. Dynamic WOA-SFO for Key Generation & Network Monitoring unlike the general algorithms, Whale optimization (WO) is employed specifically to generate keys effectively and sheep flock optimization (SFO) which are used continuously on monitoring of network [4].

Automatic screening methods based on machine learning have demonstrated efficiency in catching likely cases, as has predictive modeling for disease outlooks and resource distribution. Another field where machine learning has helped excel concerns chronic conditions, such as diabetes or renal heart failure etc. It has shown some promising results in predicting the progression of those diseases and allowing early intervention, thereby enhancing strategies for management. In conclusion, our exhaustive survey reveals that machine learning (ML) can assist with disease timely prevention across multiple medical areas. It provides salient references and details on emerging techniques, thereby be considered a useful resource for re-searchers working in this remit as well as clinical practitioners looking to leverage ML technologies to improve the care of patients widelytruncate-identifierciteseerasmus1)}. The use of machine learning (ML) in healthcare is on the rise as it can delve into complex patterns and provide accurate predictions. This technology is especially useful in diagnosing early disease and improving global healthcare outcomes [5].

Today there are new valuable applications and opportunity areas possible because of the changes with the rise on the Internet. Therefore, artificial intelligence (AI) and sentiment analysis (SA) are two key topics in research. It even led the way in propelling the achievements of IR 4.0 (Fourth Industrial Revolution). Artificial intelligence consists of emotions recognition systems that provide a connection between the fourth and fifth spoke in IR 4.0 and IR 5.0 This AI is categorized into various types such as: There are a lot of people on social media and digital marketing or e-commerce platforms generating more unorganized data. The emotion recognition system is a generic engineered solution that can be used in the medical, marketing, public safety; education industry etc., and for human resources to refine their offerings. Consequently, it provides a lot of text data that we can use to get emotions [6].

Advancements in Deep Learning (DL), Big Data and image processing have facilitated the propagation of internet disinformation via Deepfakes. These risks include but are not limited to a fixed number of threats like public opinion manipulation, geopolitical conflict and financial market disruptions up to certain types of frauds (investor-bluffing), harassment or identity theft. Therefore, there is a need for methods to prevent deepfakes from being generated in the first place or detect and stop their spread. We begin with an overview of techniques based on deep learning that have been employed to create deepfake videos like the way they are created. This is followed by detailed analysis of the fight between generation strategies and detection campaign. Moreover, we will also discuss the potential of developing technologies including distributed ledgers and blockchain in evolving cybersecurity to help eradicate digital deceit. In this analysis, we look at two application scenarios - online social network manipulation attacks and Internet of the Things. It covers the major observations and remaining questions relating to these scenarios. The paper, therefore finishes with a brief reflection on upcoming trends and directions of research along with potential intervening variables as well as technology [7] (Table 1).

Table 1. Comparative analysis

Citation	Methods	Advantages	Disadvantages	Research Gap
Zhong, C., Sarkar, A., Manna, S. et al. (2024)	Federated learning for intrusion detection and neural key exchange for secure communication	Enhances data security and privacy without centralizing patient data, reducing risk of data breaches	Complexity in implementation and high computational resources required	Optimization of federated learning algorithms for resource-constrained IoMT devices
Sreevallabh Chivukula, A., Yang, X., Liu, B., Liu, W., Zhou, W. (2023)	Game theory combined with adversarial deep learning techniques	Enhances robustness and security of ML models against adversarial attacks	Complex implementation and requires deep understanding of game theory and adversarial ML	Development of scalable adversarial learning techniques applicable across various domains
ametefe, D.S., Sarnin, S.S., Ali, D.M. et al. (2024)	Systematic review of liveness detection methods in fingerprint authentication to combat presentation attacks	Comprehensive overview of current methods and their effectiveness in real-world scenarios	Variability in performance of liveness detection methods under different environmental conditions	Development of standardized testing protocols for evaluating liveness detection methods

(*continued*)

Table 1. (*continued*)

Citation	Methods	Advantages	Disadvantages	Research Gap
Behiry, M.H., Aly, M. (2024)	Hybrid feature reduction combined with AI and ML for cyberattack detection in wireless sensor networks (WSNs)	Improves detection accuracy and reduces false positives in WSNs	May require high computational power for feature extraction and analysis	Exploration of lightweight AI models for real-time cyberattack detection in resource-constrained WSNs
Naresh, V.S., Thamarai, M. & Allavarpu, V.V.L.D. (2023)	Privacy-preserving techniques in deep learning applied to medical informatics, addressing data privacy and security issues	Enhances patient data privacy while leveraging deep learning for medical insights. Proposed methodology	Balancing privacy preservation with model accuracy can be challenging	Improvement of privacy-preserving techniques to achieve high accuracy without compromising data privacy

3 Proposed Methodology

Wearable sensors provide noninvasive and continuous data streams of our vital signals such as human body temperature, heart rate variability (HRV) [8], variation in the time interval between consecutive "heart beats". These wearable systems are known to play an important role for contemporary healthcare that have evolved rapidly thanks to Body Area Networks (BANs) i.e. personal area network functioning inside or around a person [4]. These networks hold promises for personalized medicine, early disease diagnosis and improved patient health. Nevertheless, BANs appeal to adversarial attacks due to the sensitivity of health data involved and malicious adversaries could manipulate or falsify reading without being detected by healthcare providers since patients rely on passive monitoring for real-time surveillance about their well-being. In this paper, we provide a complete detailed methodology to improve security of BAN using deep learning algorithms for countering the crucial vulnerability mentioned at first. To thwart adversarial threats, this method integrates data preprocessing, adversarial example generation, model training with adversarial augmented samples and ensemble learning real-time anomaly detection continuous monitoring. Preprocessing the data is necessary for our model to function well. High-Quality Data Is Fundamental to Developing Robust Machine Learning Systems. We first gather huge datasets from numerous wearable sensors in BANs. This includes a variety of bio-signals such as an electrocardiogram (ECG) for heart rate variability, skin temperature data and continuous glucose monitoring data for diabetics. Because health data is very personal and sensitive, we have rigorous ethical protocols and anonymization processes in place. Raw data from wearable sensors are inherently noisy and inconsistent, making preprocessing necessary to enhance [9] the reliability of future analysis. To this end, we use signal filtering (to reject outliers), outlier detection or to reduce the replication rate of abnormal values) and data normalization to have signals on similar scales. This preprocessing step is extremely important when training the deep learning models needs to be able to differentiate patterns of normal physiology from adversarial manipulation with high accuracy. Adversarial Example Generation on this is in the form of adversarial examples - inputs that have been tweaked to produce a wrong prediction. Attackers can subtly perturbate original data to misguide models, which causes the model to misclassification or wrong interpretation in physiological signals [10] and hence lead physicians to make false diagnostics decisions for treatment. To also defend against these attacks, we proactively generate adversarial examples using well-proven techniques such as Fast Gradient Sign Method (FGSM) and Projected Gradient Descent (PGD). Such methods change the data in a certain systematic way such that for the model, it makes more mistakes on classification but at same time they are non-perceptible to human eye. We construct the threat model from generating a wide range of adversarial examples that we can use to discover all possible attack [11] vectors and vulnerabilities. These trained models are used to train powerful deep neural networks, defending against adversarial attacks. Models based on deep learning techniques, especially Convolutional Neural Networks (for spatial data) and Recurrent Neural networks (for temporal data), are suitable for physiological signal analysis. We train those models with augmented adversarial and original datasets as well. Such adversarial training in turn broadens the set of possible attacks models are exposed to and helps them learn more robust representations that resist easy manipulation. In this process, the model is learning to distinguish legitimate physiological patterns from adversarial noise. On training ideally, they should be able to generalize well on clean data and maintain their accuracy against adversarial examples. The focus of this methodology is to prevent the attackers from harming classification or interpretation in deep learning models being dependent on BAN by designing security layers bottom up so that an attacker cannot disrupt and manipulate data at non-private signal levels. We exploit ensemble learning for robustness with BAN security using multiple deep learning models that are trained separately and combine their predictions [12]. It brings diversity through the pipeline, so if an adversary only targets one model, he is extremely less likely to fool all models at once. We also include flexible real-time adversarial detection methods by embedding anomaly detection algorithms within the system. If any input seems odd, given that expected pattern the system can start flagging in real time to notify healthcare providers of some possible attack. In order to show the effectiveness of our approach, it is important to have a thorough evaluation phase. We will conduct extensive experiments assessing deep learning and detection capabilities by recreating various adversarial scenarios using real-world data in order to demonstrate the robustness of our techniques. Canonical metrics that are useful in this regard include the accuracy, precision, recall and F1 score of a system which will show just how good (or bad) your model is at correctly classifying or detecting adversarial examples. Transfer to unseen attacks: Finally, we verify the generalization ability of our system by testing it on adversarial examples that were not used for creating tasks before. Once the system's efficacy is established, we deploy strong deep learning models and real-time detection techniques in physical BAN environments.

Long-term engagement in the system is key to discovering new threats and how attackers are adapting their methods. We update and retrain the models continuously with new data, plus any advances in adversarial techniques to keep a high level of security while guaranteeing patient privacy protection under HIPAA regulations and reliability on healthcare monitoring systems.

3.1 Overview

In healthcare Body Area Networks (BANs) are utilized to provide continuous monitoring of physiological signals through wearable devices. Nevertheless, wider use of BAN as a paradigm presents serious security issues due to adversarial attacks that can severely impact data trustworthiness and quality. The deep learning augmentation for adversarial robustness in BANs therefore aims to defend the network against malicious attacks [13]. For adversarial attacks, the perturbation in input data is created with an aim to fool machine learning models into providing wrong predictions [14]. In the context of BANs, such attacks can have serious implications as false health monitoring results may trigger unwarranted medical responses. An attacker might insert false signals or tamper with real data that will prevent the network from working in a controlled way.

Deep Learning in Security: Convolutional neural networks (CNN) [15] and recurrent neural networks (RNN), two members of the family of sophisticated neural networks that excel in voice, signal processing, image recognition, and other areas, are particularly well-suited for deep learning models. When used on BANs, these models can learn intricate patterns and dependencies in physiological signals that make them great at detecting anomalies and adversarial perturbations.

Adversarial Robustness Strategies: Several strategies to increase BANs' robustness against adversarial attacks are possible (Fig. 1).

Adversarial Training: This is a deep learning model that has been trained on clean input dataset [16] and on the corresponding perturbed (generated from these regular i.e. original or real-world) inputs. The second benefit is that it teaches the models to better recognize and be more robust against these manipulations by simulating them on training data.

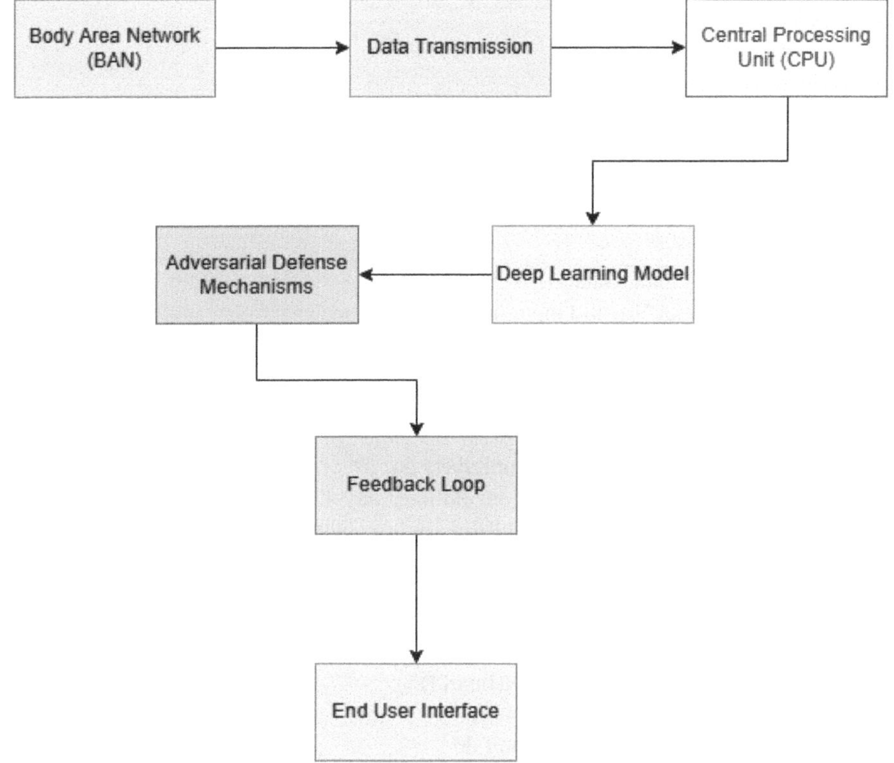

Fig. 1. Flow Chart of Proposed model.

Defensive Distillation: When testing, it uses better-tuned outputs and adds obfuscated gradients to help defend the network from adversarial instances [17]. Basically, it is about training the model using a distilled version of the original dataset that makes it less sensitive to small perturbations.

Preprocessing Input: Methods such as data normalization, noise filtering and transformation can lead to a reduction or remove adversarial perturbation before reaching deep learning model [18]. Preprocessing is our first defense against adversarial inputs.

Assembling: Ability to combine predictions from different models can increase [19] robustness Some adversarial examples affect different models differently which is why their collective decision can be more reliable [20] than predictions of individual classifiers [21].

Integrating in BANs with case studies this section examines the various aspects of integrating these adversarial robustness techniques into BANs. Wearable devices have limited computational resources, thus necessitate efficient algorithms that can run on low-power hardware. Furthermore, the need for real-time processing implies that health monitoring must take place fast enough as well to respond.

3.2 Algorithm

```
Algorithm: CNN-RNN Hybrid Model
(Enhance Adversarial Robustness in BANs)

Input: Training Data D, Model Parameters P
Output: Trained Model M, Predictions Y

if (Validate Data(D) == FALSE) then
    return "Invalid input data"
end if

Function ProcessCNN(Input I):
    features ← []
    for each layer in P.cnnLayers do
        conv_output ← Convolution(I, layer.filters)
        pooled ← MaxPool(ReLU(conv_output))
        features.append(pooled)
    end for
    return Flatten(features)

Function ProcessRNN(Input I):
    state ← InitializeState()
    for each timestep t in I do
        if (P.type == "LSTM") then
            state ← LSTMCell(I[t], state)
        else
            state ← SimpleRNNCell(I[t], state)
        end if
    end for
    return state

Main Training Loop
for epoch = 1 to P.maxEpochs do
    for each batch B in D do
        cnn_features ← ProcessCNN(B.spatial)
        rnn_features ← ProcessRNN(B.temporal)
        combined ← Concatenate(cnn_features, rnn_features)
        loss ← CalculateLoss(combined, B.labels)
        UpdateParameters(loss)
    end for
end for
```

3.3 Working Proposed Model

Body Area Networks (BANs), it comprises multiple components. Below is a simple way to do this:

Step 1. Adversarial Perturbation

Neural network with parameters θ, input x and true label y, we will have the definition of Adversary example as given below:

Φ(·) where η is the perturbation crafted to deceive neural network.:

$$x' = x + \eta$$

where η is the adversarial perturbation that is crafted to deceive the neural network.

Step 2. Loss Function

Though a neural network the loss function is defined in tensorflow as:

Discover Medium

If using adversarial training then the loss function will be minimized in regards to both original and adversarially crafted examples:

where D is the manifold of data distributions and ϵ denotes a computational budget for perturbation

$$\mathrm{L}(f_\theta(\mathrm{x}), \mathrm{y})$$

$$min_\theta E_{(x,y)\sim D}\left[max_{\|\eta\|\le\epsilon} L(f_\theta(x+\eta), y)\right]$$

where D represents the data distribution and ϵ is the perturbation limit.

Step 3. Data Augmentation

The problem of Training data augmentation using Adversarial examples can be modeled as:

$$D' = \{(x, y), (x+\eta, y) | (x, y) \in D\}$$

Step 4. Regularization Term

One way to do this is adding a regularization term to the loss function, as such:

where λ is a regularization coefficient.

$$\mathcal{L}_{reg} = \lambda\|\theta\|^2$$

where λ is the regularization coefficient.

Step 5. Overall Loss Function

By integrating the loss function in standard way with adversarial loss and regularization, the overall losses looks like this:

$$\mathcal{L}_{total} = L(f_\theta(\mathrm{x}), \mathrm{y}) + \alpha L(f_\theta(\mathrm{x}+\eta), y) + \lambda\|\theta\|^2$$

Step 6. Optimization

UT, the optimization problem to instead train a deep learning model while maintaining high adversarial robustness achieved by data augmentation can be summarized as follows:

$$\theta^* = arg\ min_\theta L_{total}$$

Step 7. Body Area Network Context

Let represent sensor data from the i-th body sensor node and its corresponding label for BANs. The adversarial robustness of BANs can be directly represented by (Table 2):

$$x_i' = x_i + \eta_i$$

$$\mathcal{L}_{BAN} = \sum_{i=1}^{N} [L(f_\theta(x_i), y_i) + \alpha L(f_\theta(x_i + \eta_i), y_i)] + \lambda \|\theta\|^2$$

Table 2. Simulation parameter.

Parameter	Description	Example Values
Network Topology	The structure and configuration of the Body Area Network (BAN)	Star, Mesh, Hybrid
Sensor Types	Types of sensors used in the BAN for data collection	ECG, EMG, Temperature, Accelerometer
Data Augmentation Techniques	Methods used to augment the training data to enhance model robustness	Rotation, Scaling, Noise Addition
Adversarial Attack Types	Types of adversarial attacks simulated to test robustness	FGSM, PGD, DeepFool
Defense Mechanisms	Techniques employed to defend against adversarial attacks	Adversarial Training, Defensive Distillation, Gradient Masking
Model Architecture	Deep learning model used for classification or regression in the BAN	CNN, RNN, LSTM
Training Epochs	Number of epochs for training the deep learning model	50, 100, 200
Batch Size	Number of samples processed before the model is updated	32, 64, 128
Learning Rate	The step size used for updating the model parameters	0.001, 0.01, 0.1
Dataset Size	Amount of data used for training and testing the model	10,000 samples, 50,000 samples, 100,000 samples
Evaluation Metrics	Metrics used to evaluate model performance and robustness	Accuracy, Precision, Recall, F1-Score
Noise Level	Intensity of noise added to test the model's robustness	0.01, 0.05, 0.1
Adversarial Training Proportion	Proportion of adversarial examples included in the training data	10%, 20%, 30%
Hardware Specifications	The computational resources used for training and testing (e.g., GPU, CPU)	NVIDIA GTX 1080, Tesla V100, Intel Xeon

(continued)

Table 2. (*continued*)

Parameter	Description	Example Values
Simulation Duration	Time allocated for the entire simulation process	24 h, 48 h, 72 h
Communication Protocols	Protocols used for data transmission within the BAN	Bluetooth, ZigBee, Wi-Fi
Energy Consumption	Measurement of energy used by sensors and processing units during the simulation	Low, Medium, High
Network Topology	The structure and configuration of the Body Area Network (BAN)	Star, Mesh, Hybrid
Sensor Types	Types of sensors used in the BAN for data collection	ECG, EMG, Temperature, Accelerometer
Data Augmentation Techniques	Methods used to augment the training data to enhance model robustness	Rotation, Scaling, Noise Addition
Adversarial Attack Types	Types of adversarial attacks simulated to test robustness	FGSM, PGD, DeepFool
Defense Mechanisms	Techniques employed to defend against adversarial attacks	Adversarial Training, Defensive Distillation, Gradient Masking
Model Architecture	Deep learning model used for classification or regression in the BAN	CNN, RNN, LSTM
Training Epochs	Number of epochs for training the deep learning model	50, 100, 200
Batch Size	Number of samples processed before the model is updated	32, 64, 128
Learning Rate	The step size used for updating the model parameters	0.001, 0.01, 0.1
Dataset Size	Amount of data used for training and testing the model	10,000 samples, 50,000 samples, 100,000 samples
Evaluation Metrics	Metrics used to evaluate model performance and robustness	Accuracy, Precision, Recall, F1-Score
Noise Level	Intensity of noise added to test the model's robustness	0.01, 0.05, 0.1

4 Conclusion

The utilization of deep learning-based Body Area Networks (BANs) is a promising area in biomedical and health applications such as biosignal monitoring by using portable and wearable devices. Body area network (BAN) consists of wearable or implanted sensors that allow for continuous data transmission to target treatment in real-time. But the rise of cyber-attacks creates data integrity and device reliability problems that can put patients in danger. The same is true in this case where, if we have a deep learning model trained on examples that include adversarial examples in the training data, the models are well-equipped and sensitized to anomalies and therefore able to withstand backlink attacks. Adversarial training and other techniques that increase model robustness are vital to successfully transmitting data over time and will enable models to protect against evolving cyber threats. Furthermore, it enhances patient data security through the deployment of real-time, low-power, deep learning on the BAN devices. Translating this technology into clinically usable solutions requires teamwork between healthcare providers and computer scientists/engineers. These ideas have led to two potential avenues of research – federated learning which can add another layer of privacy by allowing the model to train on devices in a decentralized manner, and lastly explainable AI (XAI), which can help increase trust in security by providing transparency on how decisions are made. Finally, well-placed standards help to embolden secure, compliant frameworks for the next generation of BAN technology.

References

1. Zhong, C., Sarkar, A., Manna, S.: Federated learning-guided intrusion detection and neural key exchange for safeguarding patient data on the internet of medical things. Int. J. Mach. Learn. Cyber. (2024). https://doi.org/10.1007/s13042-024-02269-2
2. Sreevallabh Chivukula, A., Yang, X., Liu, B., Liu, W., Zhou, W.: Game theoretical adversarial deep learning. In: Adversarial Machine Learning. Springer, Cham (2023). https://doi.org/10.1007/978-3-030-99772-4_4A
3. Ametefe, D.S., Sarnin, S.S., Ali, D.M., et al.: Enhancing fingerprint authentication: a systematic review of liveness detection methods against presentation attacks. J. Inst. Eng. India Ser. B (2024). https://doi.org/10.1007/s40031-024-01066-3
4. Behiry, M.H., Aly, M.: Cyberattack detection in wireless sensor networks using a hybrid feature reduction technique with AI and machine learning methods. J Big Data **11**, 16 (2024). https://doi.org/10.1186/s40537-023-00870-w
5. Naresh, V.S., Thamarai, M., Allavarpu, V.V.L.D.: Privacy-preserving deep learning in medical informatics: applications, challenges, and solutions. Artif. Intell. Rev. **56**(Suppl 1), 1199–1241 (2023). https://doi.org/10.1007/s10462-023-10556-7
6. Altherwi, A., Ahmad, M.T., Alam, M.M., et al.: A hybrid optimization approach for securing cloud-based e-health systems. Multimed. Tools Appl. (2024). https://doi.org/10.1007/s11042-024-19688-6
7. Asif, S., Wenhui, Y., ur-Rehman, S., et al.: Advancements and prospects of machine learning in medical diagnostics: unveiling the future of diagnostic precision. Arch. Comput. Methods Eng. (2024). https://doi.org/10.1007/s11831-024-10148-w
8. Chutia, T., Baruah, N.: A review on emotion detection by using deep learning techniques. Artif. Intell. Rev. **57**, 203 (2024). https://doi.org/10.1007/s10462-024-10831-1

9. Gambín, Á.F., Yazidi, A., Vasilakos, A.: Deepfakes: current and future trends. Artif. Intell. Rev. **57**, 64 (2024). https://doi.org/10.1007/s10462-023-10679-x
10. Kaffashbashi, A., Sobhani, V., Goodarzian, F.: Augmented data strategies for enhanced computer vision performance in breast cancer diagnosis. J. Ambient Intell. Hum. Comput. **15**, 3093–3106 (2024). https://doi.org/10.1007/s12652-024-04803-0
11. Yu, Z., Feng, J., Tang, S., Liu, Z., Yan, Y., Luo, N.: Multiple information collection technology of power network disaster loss. In: Disaster Intelligent Perception and Emergency Command of Power Grid. Springer, Singapore (2024). https://doi.org/10.1007/978-981-99-7236-4_3
12. Swain, S., Bhushan, B., Dhiman, G.: Appositeness of optimized and reliable machine learning for healthcare: a survey. Arch. Computat. Methods Eng. **29**, 3981–4003 (2022). https://doi.org/10.1007/s11831-022-09733-8
13. Hernández-Álvarez, L., González-Manzano, L., Fuentes, J.M.d., Hernández Encinas, L.: Biometrics and artificial intelligence: attacks and challenges. In: Daimi, K., Francia, G., III., Encinas, L.H. (eds.) Breakthroughs in Digital Biometrics and Forensics. Springer, Cham (2022). https://doi.org/10.1007/978-3-031-10706-1_10
14. Darema, F., Blasch, E.P., Ravela, S., Aved, A.J.: The dynamic data driven applications systems (DDDAS) paradigm and emerging directions. In: Darema, F., Blasch, E.P., Ravela, S., Aved, A.J. (eds.) Handbook of Dynamic Data Driven Applications Systems. Springer, Cham (2023). https://doi.org/10.1007/978-3-031-27986-7_1
15. Masood, M., Nawaz, M., Malik, K.M.: Deepfakes generation and detection: state-of-the-art, open challenges, countermeasures, and way forward. Appl. Intell. **53**, 3974–4026 (2023). https://doi.org/10.1007/s10489-022-03766-z
16. Sakhnini, J., Karimipour, H., Dehghantanha, A., Parizi, R.M.: AI and security of critical infrastructure. In: Choo, K.K., Dehghantanha, A. (eds.) Handbook of Big Data Privacy. Springer, Cham (2020). https://doi.org/10.1007/978-3-030-38557-6_2
17. Hartley, D.S., III., Jobson, K.O.: The technium—plus, redux. In: Cognitive Superiority. Springer, Cham (2021). https://doi.org/10.1007/978-3-030-60184-3_5
18. EANM'23 Abstract Book Congress Sep 9-13, 2023. Eur. J. Nucl. Med. Mol. Imaging **50**(Suppl 1), 1–898 (2023). https://doi.org/10.1007/s00259-023-06333-x
19. Annual Congress of the European Association of Nuclear Medicine October 15–19, 2022 Barcelona, Spain. Eur. J. Nucl. Med. Mol. Imaging **49**(Suppl 1), 1–751 (2022). https://doi.org/10.1007/s00259-022-05924-4
20. Blowers, M., Iribarne, J., Colbert, E.J.M., Kott, A.: In conclusion: the future internet of things and security of its control systems. In: Colbert, E., Kott, A. (eds.) Cyber-Security of SCADA and Other Industrial Control Systems. Advances in Information Security, vol. 66. Springer, Cham (2016). https://doi.org/10.1007/978-3-319-32125-7_16
21. The "nuts and bolts" of behavioral intervention development: study designs, methods and funding opportunities. Ann. Behav. Med. **51**(Suppl 1), 1–2867 (2017). https://doi.org/10.1007/s12160-017-9903-3

Design and Development of 5G Energy Harvesting System for Body Area Network

Minoti Kumari(✉), Anshuman Shastri, and Diwakar Kumar

Department of Physical Science, Banasthali Vidyapith, Tonk, Rajasthan, India
kumariminoti@gmail.com, anshumanshastri@banasthali.in

Abstract. Recent advancements in biosensors, low-power Internet of Things (IoT) devices, and wireless communication technologies have led to the development of next-generation wireless sensor networks. These networks are gradually more used for monitoring traffic, crops, infrastructure, and health. A Body Area Network (BAN) also known as a Wireless BAN, Body Sensor Network (BSN), or Medical BAN is a high-frequency wireless network composed of wearable computing devices. These devices can be implanted inside the body or carried in various ways, such as in pockets or bags. One major challenge is providing energy to these devices in a way that is safe for the body and environment and does not require frequent replacement. This paper presents a solution by designing a compact and efficient 5G Energy Harvesting System. Our system converts 5G electromagnetic waves into usable energy through a Rectenna, which includes a microstrip antenna operating at 8.75 GHz. The system also features an RF-to-DC half-wave rectifier circuit with an appropriate matching network and a microstrip low-pass filter to reduce noise and enhance efficiency. Mathematical results indicate that the system achieves a maximum power conversion efficiency of 43% with a 20 KΩ load and an input power of 19.54 dBm.

Keywords: Body Area Network (BAN) · Biosensors · Internet of Things · 5G millimeter wave Energy harvester · Microstrip Antenna · Matching network · Rectenna · Rectifier · Microstrip Lowpass filter

1 Introduction

The 5Gwireless technology offers high speed and lower latency data transfer for a vast number of connected devices [1]. According to increasing demands of IoT (Internet of Things) devices, with predictions suggesting that the number of IoT sensors will reach tens of billions, maintaining battery power will become a significant challenge [2]. The methods of harvesting Energy from vibration, solar and RF (radio frequency), are gaining attention as possible solutions [3]. Among these, harvesting energy from mm (millimeter) wave appears promising. The infrastructure of fifth generation networks includes many devices like picocells, femtocells, microcells and cell towers, which can serve as sustainable energy sources for IoT applications. The sustainable Energy harvesting devices can give alternative options for low-power applications, such as remote

K. Atul et al. (Eds.): BodyNets 2024, LNICST 666, pp. 98–113, 2026.
https://doi.org/10.1007/978-3-032-16099-7_10

sensing, wearable electronics, and wireless sensor networks. As semiconductor devices shrink to millimeter and sub-millimeter sizes, there is an increasing demand for compact, highly efficient power supplies [3, 4]. For sustainable electronics, it is essential to integrate energy generation and delivery methods with edge nodes in IoT networks, such as Body Area Networks (BAN) and medical body area networks (MBAN). Wearable wireless networks can include small, implantable biosensors that continuously monitor physiological changes, allowing for computer-assisted rehabilitation and early medical detection. This data is transmitted wirelessly to external processing units, which can quickly alert healthcare providers in emergencies [5–10]. Despite current limitations in data provision and sensor power, ongoing research into nano-robotics controlled by wireless technologies like 5G or mm Waves and future 6G (THz) networks aims to provide green and sustainable power for these systems. This technology enables real-time data transfer and global connectivity.

In this paper, we address energy requirements by designing a 5G or mm Wave energy harvesting system operating at sub-6 GHz [11–13]. Figure 1 illustrates the key components of a typical Wireless Sensor Node (WSN) powered by an energy harvesting system. Our RF energy harvesting system includes a Rectenna, which consists of a receiving antenna, an impedance matching network (IMN), a rectifier, and a stepped impedance microstrip low-pass Chebyshev filter [14–22]. The receiving antenna collects RF signals from ambient sources, and the rectifier converts these signals into low-power DC. The impedance matching network ensures efficient power transfer from the antenna to the rectifier, minimizing signal loss. The DC signal then passes through a low-pass filter to reduce noise and improve efficiency. This stable DC power is stored in a capacitor and can be boosted to a battery or second storage capacitor, providing power for low-energy devices like microprocessors or for data transmission in biomedical implants or wearable sensors.

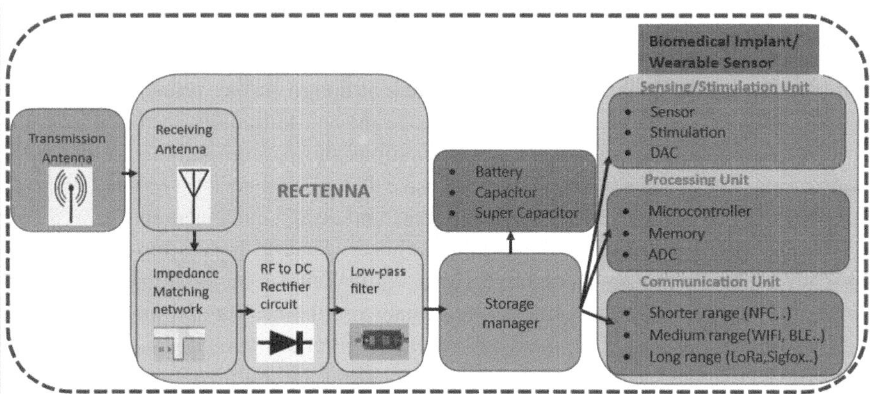

Fig. 1. Typical RF energy harvesting system

2 Literature Review

Radio Frequency Energy Harvesting (RFEH) system captures and utilizes otherwise wasted radiofrequency (RF) energy from the environment, converting it into usable electrical energy. The foundational concept of wireless power transfer (WPT) was introduced by Maxwell in 1864, and later, Nikola Tesla elaborated on it by demonstrating energy transfer without physical connections. In the 1960s, William C. Brown advanced this technology by developing the Rectenna for microwave power transmission. Figure 2 shows the evolution of WPT and RFEH is comprehensively reviewed in various works, including a summary and visual representation by Niotaki et al., which traces the development from Maxwell's equations to contemporary experimental demonstrations [23].

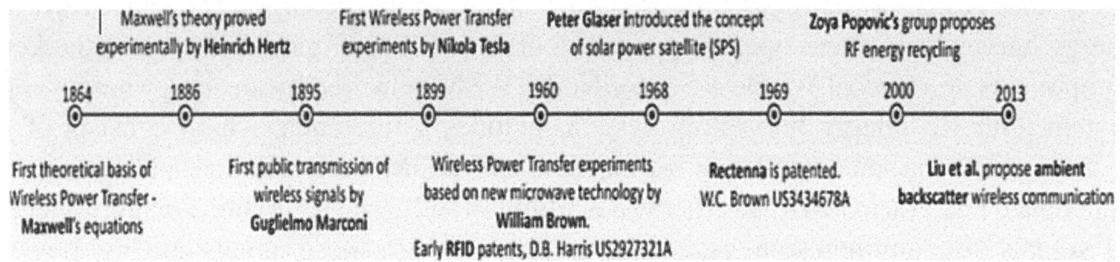

Fig. 2. The development of RF energy harvesting and wireless power transfer technology from Maxwell's equations to modern experiments.

A comprehensive overview of advancements and challenges in energy harvesting and RF power delivery technologies. They address various applications, including IoT devices, sensor nodes, and 5G systems. Key findings include the need for improved energy management and harvesting solutions to meet the high-power demands of modern systems, as well as optimizations in RF power transfer efficiency and design for millimeter-sized sensors. Innovations in rectenna designs, such as multi-band and improved impedance matching, are highlighted, although further refinement is needed for better performance across a wider frequency range. Additionally, the use of transparent substrates in antenna designs for 5G applications shows promise but requires further optimization. The articles collectively emphasize the ongoing need for research to bridge gaps in system efficiency, practical applications, and design enhancements [2, 4, 12, 13, 22, 34]. The work focuses rectifier design for enhancing energy harvesting efficiency [24, 33]. They explore Schottky diode large-signal equivalent-circuit parameters to improve microwave rectifier performance, offering valuable guidelines for optimizing efficiency. The study also presents a triple-band differential rectifier designed to operate effectively across three frequency bands, highlighting innovations and improvements in efficiency. Both studies emphasize the need for further research to refine parameter extraction methods and enhance rectifier performance, including optimizing multi-band rectifiers for better efficiency and broader frequency range applications. The study investigates an energy harvesting receiver incorporating microstrip filters for enhanced efficiency in 5G IoT networks, addressing integration and performance challenges. A detailed study of microstrip LPF (low pass filter) using simulation tools is presented, offering insights into their effectiveness for wireless applications. Collectively, these studies highlight the importance of advancing filter technologies and integration methods to improve performance across various applications [14, 25, 26].

The innovative approaches in health monitoring and drug delivery systems, the study investigates the use of wireless body area networks (WBANs) to model and predict health state transitions, emphasizing their potential for personalized health monitoring and predictive analytics while highlighting the need for improved algorithms to enhance accuracy. A further study presents a novel intra-body communication system using an edible pill to monitor drug release, demonstrating its advantages for real-time tracking and patient compliance but noting the necessity for further research to improve system reliability and accuracy. Additionally, the implementation of WBANs in healthcare systems is discussed, focusing on their practical applications for patient health management. Collectively, these studies underline the importance of advancing technologies and methodologies to improve health monitoring and drug delivery. Early applications of BANs are usually in the healthcare domain, especially for continuous monitoring and logging vital parameters of patients with Chronic diseases such as diabetes, asthma and attacks. Other applications of this technology include sports, military, or security. Advancing the technology into innovative areas could also assist communication or exchanges of information between individuals, or between individuals and machines [8–10].

3 Proposed RF Energy Harvesting System

In this work, we designed a 2 $\times$ 2 rectangular microstrip patch antenna array that operates at 8.75 GHz. We also designed a matching network to connect the antenna to the rectifier circuit. The half-wave rectifier converts the RF AC signal into a DC signal. After rectification, we used a microstrip low-pass filter to reduce unwanted frequency signals. Finally, the output is connected to different loads.

3.1 Proposed Antenna Modelling

The antenna is designed using planar concept having a 2 $\times$ 2 rectangular microstrip patch antenna array of patch length and width are L = 10.5 mm, W = 13.6 mm on low dielectric constant and low dielectric loss substrate is RTduroid5880(Er = 2.2), thickness1.6 mm, it is an electrodeposited coated copper foil which has a copper thickness of 0.035 mm, and a dielectric loss tangent (tan∂) of 0.0009, surface loss is low compared to rolled copper foil sheet. All of these features of the substrate are perfect at f = 8.75 GHz frequency application. A 2 $\times$ 2 rectangular microstrip patch antenna array shown in Fig. 3 and its dimensions of antenna listed in Table1.The S11 response is not exact at 8.75 GHz, so we design the smallest line width is 1 mm instead of 0.52 mm and connected a proper matching network between the antenna array and rectifier. The technique of impedance matching give guarantee that maximum power is transfer in between receiving antenna and rectifier circuit with minimum losses. So many designs of impedance matching network (IMN)are available. It can be configured by using inductors and capacitors (lumped elements) or stubs and microstrip lines (distributed elements) [23]. Proposed impedance matching network designed by using distributed elements, because it is suitable for high frequency (3 to 300 GHz) [10]. A 2 × 2 rectangular microstrip patch antenna array with matching network shown in Fig. 4 and the dimensions of antenna listed in Table2.

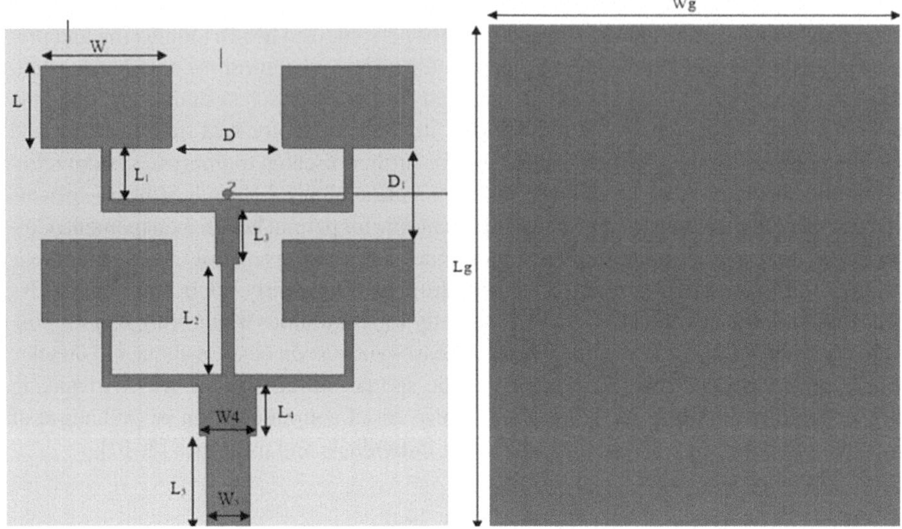

Fig. 3. 2 × 2 Microstrip patch antenna array

Table 1. Dimensions of the 2 × 2 rectangular microstrip patch antenna array at 8.75 GHz

Parameters	Value (mm)	Parameters	Value (mm)
W	15.3	L3	6.36
L	10.074	L4	6.21
D	13.05	L5	11.83
D_1	11.49	W1	1
L1	6.57	W2	1.43
H	1.6	W3	2.82
Lg	62.748	W4	6.64
Wg	53.25	W5	4.93
Ws	53.25	Ls	62.478

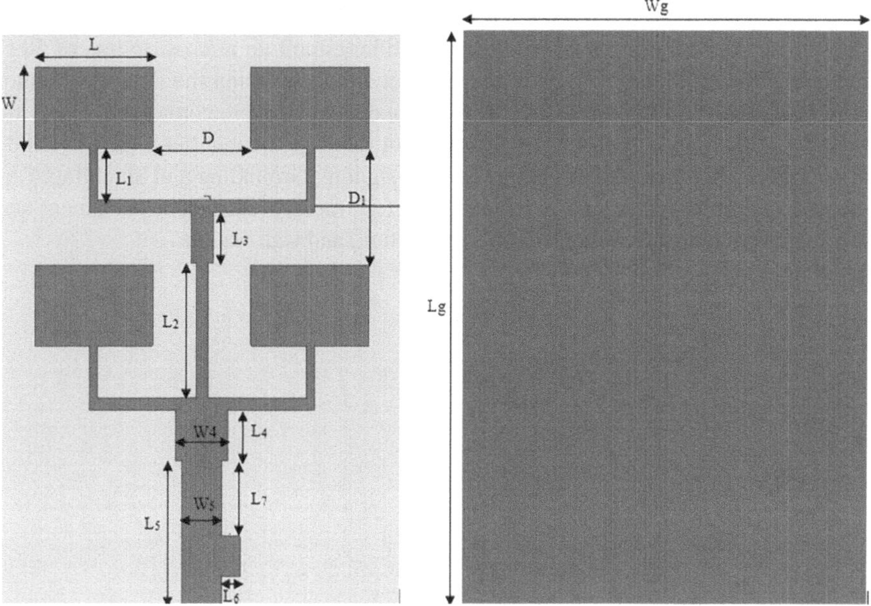

Fig. 4. 2 × 2 Antenna array with match network at 8.75 GHz

Table 2. Dimensions of the 2 × 2 rectangular microstrip patch antenna array with match network at 8.75 GHz

Parameters	Value (mm)	Parameters	Value (mm)
W	15	L4	6.21
L	10	L5	18
D	12.6	L6	2.43
D_1	14.6	W1	1
L1	6.57	W2	1.43
H	1.6	W3	2.82
Lg = Ls	71.61	W4	6.64
Wg = Ws	52.2	W5	4.93
L3	6.36		

3.2 Rectifier Design Specification

The proposed full wave Grienature rectifier circuit is designed on RTduroid5880 materialwith dielectric constant 2.2 of substrate, thickness 1.6 mm, and loss tangent 0.0009. Substrate RTduroid5880 having low dielectric constant and minimal losses. So, this is ideal for high frequency applications. We are using a Schottky diode, specifically the SMS7621, because it is a good choice for design high-efficiency rectifying circuit for its low junction resistance and junction capacitance. Figure 5 shows a Diode Model and diagrammatical configuration of Grienature rectifier circuit on microstrip line of 50 Ω which are given in. Figure 5 shows an equivalent circuit by using the circuit simulator tool ADS, in which, diode SMS7621, resistor, and capacitor, are connected. There are number of critical aspects facing in designing of this type of rectifier which is Diode characteristics, PCB material selection, Trace designing, Grounding and Shielding, Parasitic effect of capacitance and inductance in PCB traces, Component placement and Connector, Matching network designing and testing, and Calibration.

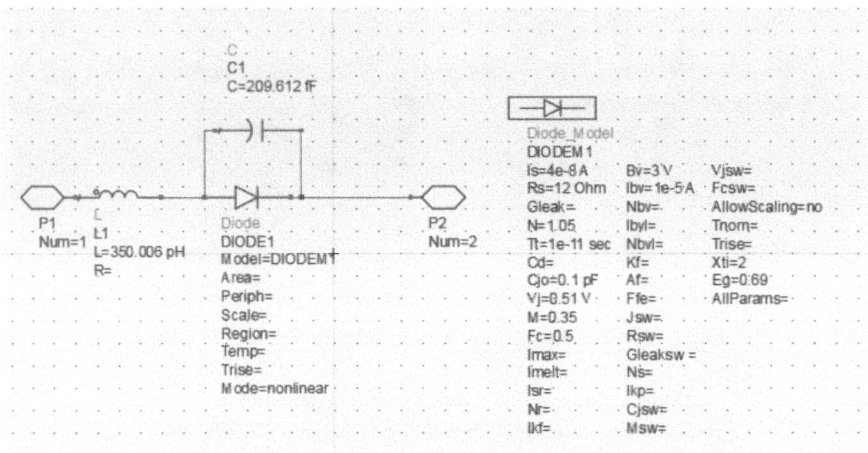

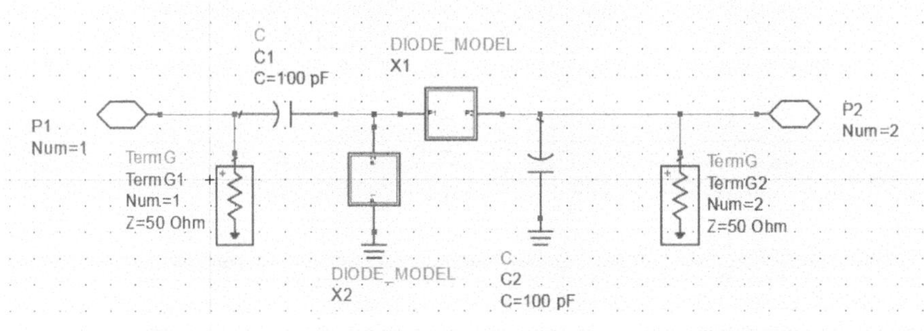

Fig. 5. Diode-Model and Grienature Rectifier ckt on microstrip line of 50 Ω at 8.75 GHz.

3.3 Lowpass Filter Design Specification

We designed a stepped impedance microstrip low pass Chebyshev filter by HFSS circuit simulator. The cutoff frequency is 8.75 GHz utilizes alternating high and low impedance section on a microstrip line to achieve sharp roll-off and minimal passband ripple. The insertion loss at passband is 0.5 and stopband is 35. In this filter design, an order 7 was chosen for Chebyshev filter prototype [2]. The properties of FR4 epoxy substrate relative dielectric constant is 4.4, loss tangent is 0.02, height 1.6 mm and conductor thickness is 0.035, which is used in calculation of length and width of the transmission line segments. To realize the necessary inductance and capacitance making it well suited for planar microstrip low pass filter. The filter layout design is critical aspects of parasitic inductance and capacitance is essential for maintaining the desired frequency of 8.75 GHz. In Fig. 6 shows a microstrip low pass filter and the dimensions of microstrip low pass filter listed in Table.3. The equivalent transmission line is obtained by converting LC circuit and finding certain lengths and characteristic [25–27]. This type of filter used to block unwanted high-frequency signal while allowing desired signal to pass, thereby improving overall system performance.

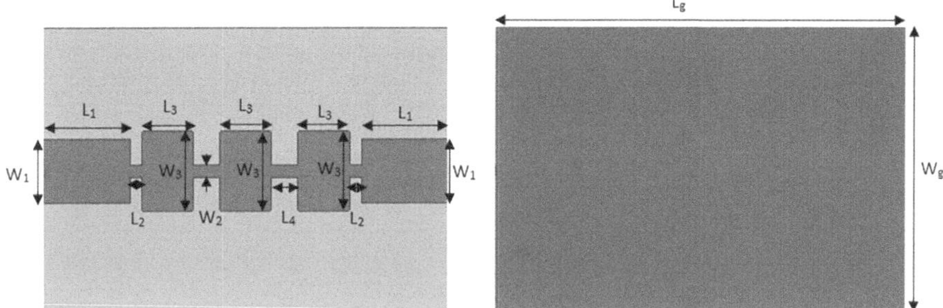

Fig. 6. Microstrip low-pass filter

Table 3. Dimensions of microstrip low pass filter at 8.75 GHz

Parameter	Value (mm)	Parameter	Value (mm)
L1	7	H	1.6
L2	1	W1	4.93
L3	4	W2	1
L4	2.2	W3	6.115
Lg	22.115	Wg	32.4

4 Simulation Result and Analysis

This section discussed and analyzed, simulation results of the linear characteristics of the antenna without matching network, with matching network, rectifier circuit, and lowpass filter.

4.1 Antenna Array

Bandwidth and Reflection Coefficient

The reflection coefficient simulated result of the 2x2 rectangular microstrip patch antenna array at 8.75 GHz for without matching network and with matching network depicted in Fig. 7. The reflection coefficient, S11 of antenna array without matching network is −51.737 dB at 8.95 GHz. The −10-dB bandwidth of the antenna be able to calculated from the difference between the upper and lower frequency at −10-dB and it is set up to be 440 MHz. Figure 8, the reflection coefficient of the antenna array with match network at 8.72 GHz is −49.7490 dB, with increases bandwidth of 860 MHz. From these results we expect, the bandwidth increases if proper selection of the matching network on the antenna array.

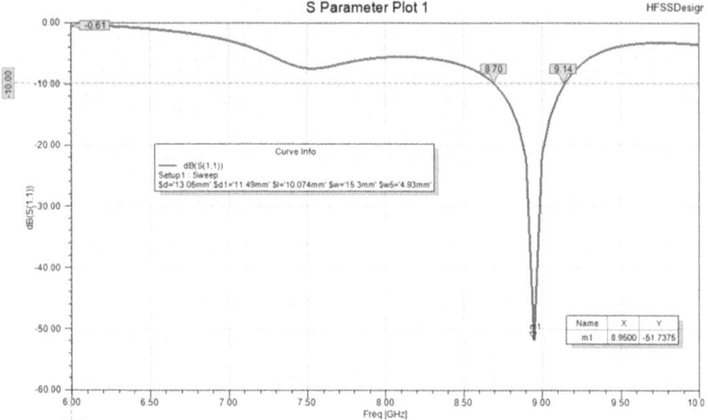

Fig. 7. The reflection coefficient, S11 antenna array without matching network

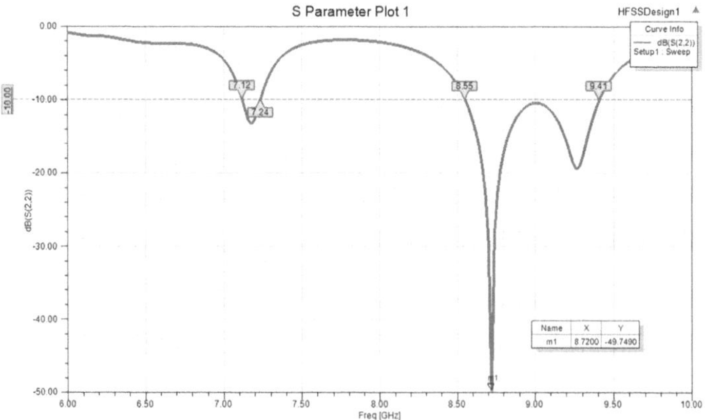

Fig. 8. The reflection coefficient, S11 antenna array with matching network

Gain, Directivity and Radiation Pattern

The gain, directivity and radiation pattern of antenna array without matching network and with matching network can be seen in Fig. 9 and Fig. 10. The gain G, and directivity D, without matching network and with matching network are 13.04 dBi and 13.28 dBi, and radiation patterns of the microstrip patch antenna array for both type in the E-plane and H-plane presented in Fig. 9 and 10. As a result, it can be seen as a whole that the gain, directivity and radiation pattern increase as the use of matching network on the antenna array.

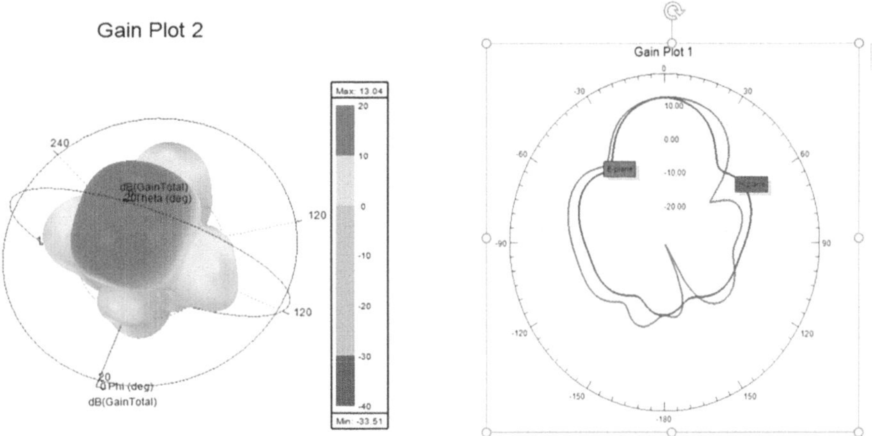

Fig. 9. Gain, directivity and radiation pattern of antenna array without matching network

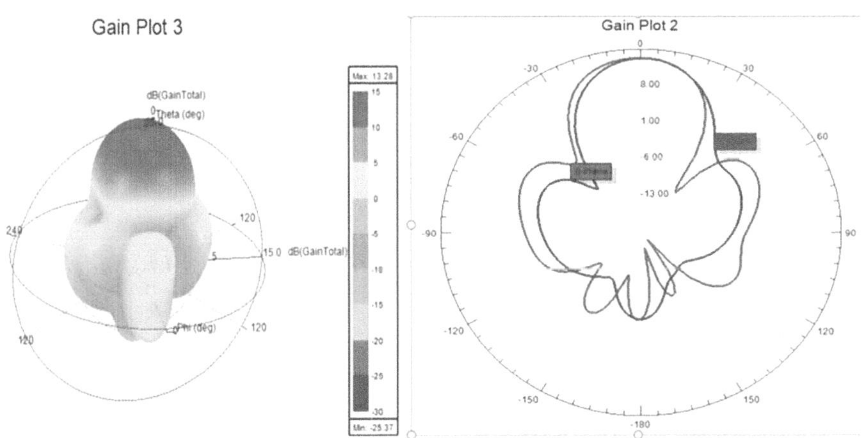

Fig. 10. Gain, directivity and radiation pattern of antenna array with matching network

4.2 Rectifier Circuit

The output result of a microstrip line half-wave rectifier circuit operating at 8.75 GHz with the SMS7621 Schottky diode shows efficient RF-to-DC conversion, where the rectified DC voltage is proportional to the amplitude of the microwave input signal, characterized by low power losses due to the diode's low forward voltage drop and high cut off frequency, enabling efficient operation at microwave frequencies, with the circuit output heavily influenced by the design of the impedance matching network by which the input reflection coefficient S11 is −43.35 dB achieved at 8.75 GHz frequency shown in Fig. 11. The quality of the microstrip layout which is RTduroid5880, and the load resistance, achieving high rectification efficiency typically 47% for well optimize design, while harmonic content in the output is minimized by appropriate filtering techniques, ensuring a clean DC output voltage and DC current shown in Fig. 12 and Fig. 13, making the circuit suitable for application like energy harvesting and RF sensing systems in high frequency domain.

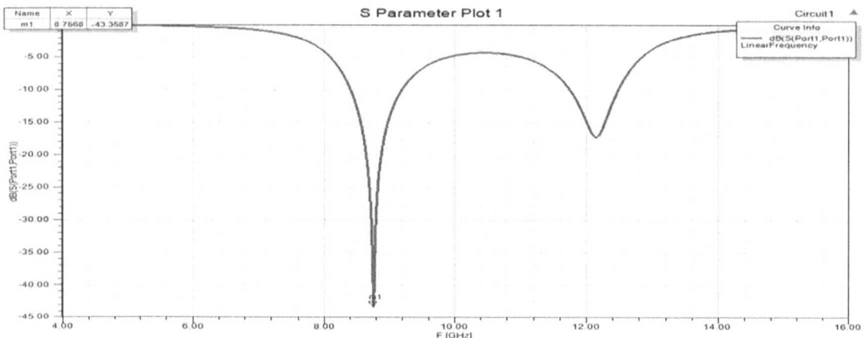

Fig. 11. The input reflection coefficient S11 at 8.75 GHz

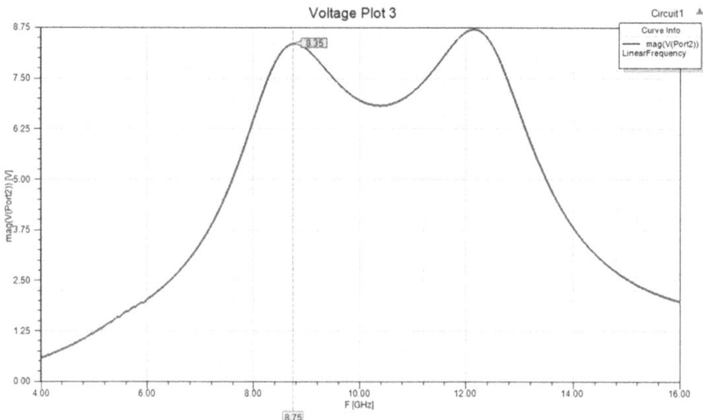

Fig. 12. The DC output voltage at 8.75 GHz

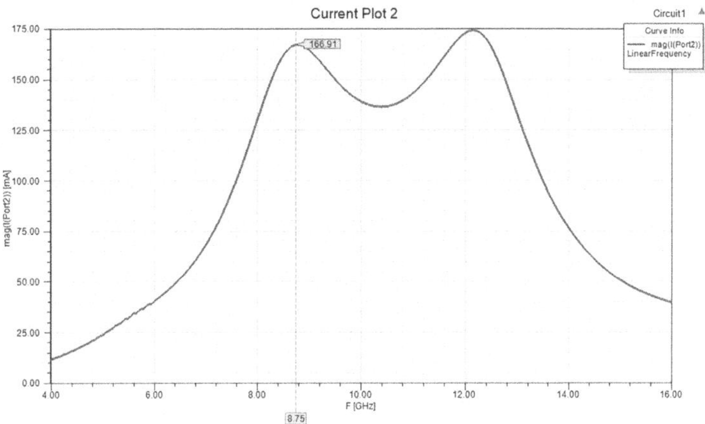

Fig. 13. The DC output current at 8.75 GHz

Table 4. Comparison between Proposed Rectifier and Prior Work

	Rectifier	Substrate	Diode	Frequency (GHz)	Input power	Load Resistance (kΩ)	Power conversion efficiency
[28]	FW	RT/ Duroid 5880	SMS 7630-079LF	3.5	9 dBm	1.1	42.5%
[29]	FW	FR-4	SMS 7630	2.4 3.51	20 dBm	50	39.6%
[30]	FW	FR-4	HSMS 2820	-	6 dBm	1	29.7%
[31]	FW	FR-4	HSMS 2860	1.9 2.5 3.6	14 dBm	3	42%
[32]	FW	Roser RO30 03	HSMS 286C	-	0 dBm	2	42%
[33]	HW	FR-4	SMS 7630	2.4 3.5	10 dB	-	42.5%
Proposed Work	HW	RT/ Duroid 5880	SMS 7630	5.9	19.54 dBm	20	43%

4.3 Low Pass Filter

The realization and measurement result of the microstrip low-pass filter done by using the HFSS tool with a working frequency at 8.75 GHz. The realization is done by using prior specifications of filter, and its performance could be analyzed. The measured parameters in which insertion loss, return loss, and cut off frequency respectively −43.71 dB, −0.42 dB and 8.75 GHz shown in Fig. 14.

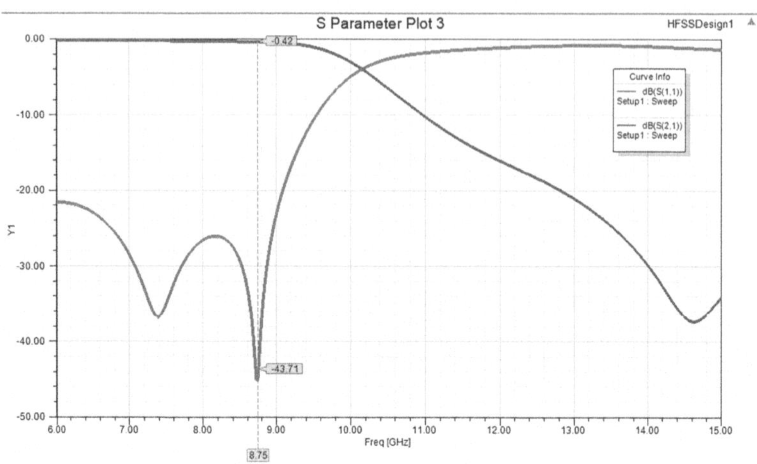

Fig. 14. Simulated and measured Return loss and Insertion loss of the proposed LPF at 8.75 GHz

4.4 Rectenna System

The simulation of the Rectenna is done by using the high frequency structural simulator (HFSS). For the analysis of the electromagnetic rectenna system designed for energy harvesting at 8.75 GHz involves evaluating its efficiency in capturing and converting electromagnetic energy into usable electrical power. The Rectenna system consist of a microstrip patch antenna array that captures the electromagnetic waves at the specified frequency at 8.75 GHz, followed by half wave rectifier circuit that converts the received AC signal into DC power. The performance of this system is highly dependent on the microstrip matching network between antenna and rectifier, the conversion efficiency of the rectifier circuit and overall system losses. The equation for the harvested power $P_{DC} = \eta\ P_{IN}$, where P_{IN} is the power captured by the antenna array and η is the efficiency of the rectenna system. Further η can be decomposed into the product of the antenna efficiency (η_A) matching efficiency (η_M) and rectification efficiency (η_R), so $\eta = \eta_A \times \eta_M \times \eta_R$. For an efficient design, the antenna array is typically optimized for maximum gain and minimal losses, while the rectifier is designed to efficiently over the range of input power encountered. Experiment results often show that the efficiency decreases with increasing frequency due to higher losses in the components and the rectifier diode. The most important part of the rectenna system is rectifier, the efficiency of the rectifier is also depending on the output load, the efficiency of the system decreasing with increasing the load, for this reason the selection of load in design part is very important. After the calculation and analyzing the results, we found overall maximum efficiency 43%. Figure 15 depicted the Power conversion efficiency at the output load RL (KΩ) at 8.75 GHz for various Pin values. Table 4 shows the comparison of rectifiers

[28], but also need for further optimization in the matching network and multiplier circuit like Greinacher circuit which have both rectification and doubler circuit to improve the conversion efficiency.

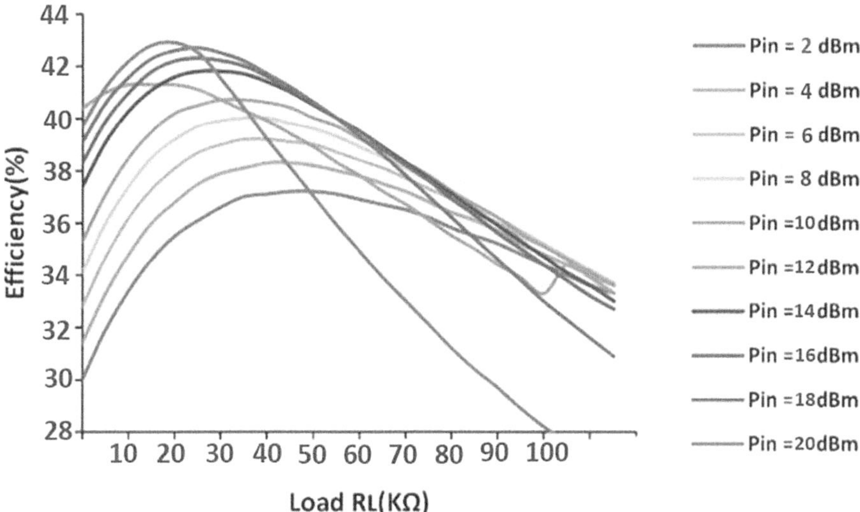

Fig. 15. Power conversion efficiency (%) - output load RL (KΩ) at 8.75 GHz for various Pin values

5 Conclusion

In conclusion, the integration of a 5G energy harvesting system within a body area network represent a significant advancement in the field of wearable technology, as it seamlessly combines high-speed connectivity with sustainable power solution, thereby enhancing the efficiency and longevity of health monitoring devices. By harnessing ambient energy from the surrounding environment and converting into usable electrical power, this innovative approach not only extend the operation time of wearable sensors and devices but also minimize the need for frequent battery replacements, which can be cumbersome and environmentally damaging. The utilization of 5G technology further amplifies the benefits by ensuring rapid data transmission and real time monitoring capabilities, which are crucial for applications such as remote patient monitoring, fitness tracking, and early detection of health anomalies. As a result, user experience improved convenience and uninterrupted service. The development of such 5G energy harvesting systems promises to derive the future of interconnected health technologies, fostering advancement both medical research and everyday well management. Consequently, the successful implementation and further more advancement of technology of 5G energy harvesting in body area networks marks a pivotal step toward achieving a more connected, sustainable and health-conscious future addressing both technological and environmental challenges in holistic manner.

References

1. Wang, N., Wang, P., Alipour-Fanid, A., Jiao, L., Zeng, K.: Physical-layer security of 5G wireless networks for IoT: challenges and opportunities. IEEE Internet Things J. **6**(5), 8169–8181 (2019)
2. Heidari, H., Onireti, O., Das, R., Imran, M.: Energy harvesting and power management for IoT devices in the 5G era. IEEE Commun. Mag. **59**(9), 91–97 (2021)
3. Digregorio, G., Redouté, J.-M.: Electromagnetic energy harvester targeting wearable and biomedical applications. Sensors **24**(7), 2311 (2024)
4. Charthad, J., Dolatsha, N., Rekhi, A., Arbabian, A.: System-level analysis of far-field radio frequency power delivery for mm-sized sensor nodes. IEEE Trans. Circuits Syst. I Regul. Pap. **63**(2), 300–311 (2016)
5. Ullah, S., et al.: A comprehensive survey of wireless body area networks: On PHY, MAC, and network layers solutions. J. Med. Syst. **36**, 1065–1094 (2012)
6. Chen, M., Gonzalez, S., Vasilakos, A., Cao, H., Leung, V.C.M.: Body area networks: a survey. Mob. Netw. Appl. **16**, 171–193 (2011)
7. Movassaghi, S., Abolhasan, M., Lipman, J., Smith, D., Jamalipour, A.: Wireless body area networks: a survey. IEEE Commun. Surv. Tutor. **16**(3), 1658–1686 (2014)
8. Geller, T., et al.: Learning health state transition probabilities via wireless body area networks. In: 2019 IEEE International Conference on Communications (ICC), ICC 2019, pp. 1–6. IEEE (2019)
9. Lamanna, L., Cataldi, P., Friuli, M., Demitri, C., Caironi, M.: Monitoring of drug release via intra body communication with an edible pill. Adv. Mater. Technol. **8**(1), 2200731 (2023)
10. Yuce, M.R.: Implementation of wireless body area networks for healthcare systems. Sens. Actuators A **162**(1), 116–129 (2010)
11. Piñuela, M., Mitcheson, P.D., Lucyszyn, S.: Ambient RF energy harvesting in urban and semi-urban environments. IEEE Trans. Microw. Theory Tech. **61**(7), 2715–2726 (2013)
12. Song, C., Huang, Y., Zhou, J., Zhang, J., Yuan, S., Carter, P.: A high-efficiency broadband rectenna for ambient wireless energy harvesting. IEEE Trans. Antennas Propag. **63**(8), 3486–3495 (2015)
13. Song, C., et al.: A novel six-band dual CP rectenna using improved impedance matching technique for ambient RF energy harvesting. IEEE Trans. Antennas Propag. **64**(7), 3160–3171 (2016)
14. Eshaghi, M., Rashidzadeh, R.: An energy harvesting receiver utilizing microstrip filter technology for IoT devices in 5G network. In: 2022 IEEE Canadian Conference on Electrical and Computer Engineering (CCECE), pp. 324–327. IEEE (2022)
15. Lu, X., Wang, P., Niyato, D., Kim, D.I., Han, Z.: Wireless networks with RF energy harvesting: a contemporary survey. IEEE Commun. Surv. Tutor. **17**(2), 757–789 (2014)
16. Valenta, C.R., Durgin, G.D.: Harvesting wireless power: survey of energy-harvester conversion efficiency in far-field, wireless power transfer systems. IEEE Microwave Mag. **15**(4), 108–120 (2014)
17. Soyata, T., Copeland, L., Heinzelman, W.: RF energy harvesting for embedded systems: a survey of tradeoffs and methodology. IEEE Circuits Syst. Mag. **16**(1), 22–57 (2016)
18. Guler, U., Ghovanloo, M.: Power management in wireless power-sipping devices: a survey. IEEE Circuits Syst. Mag. **17**(4), 64–82 (2017)
19. Shanawani, M., Masotti, D., Costanzo, A.: THz rectennas and their design rules. Electronics **6**(4), 99 (2017)
20. Divakaran, S.K., Krishna, D.D., Nasimuddin: RF energy harvesting systems: an overview and design issues. Int. J. RF Microwave Comput.-Aided Eng. **29**(1), e21633 (2019)

21. Cansiz, M., Altinel, D., Kurt, G.K.: Efficiency in RF energy harvesting systems: a comprehensive review. Energy **174**, 292–309 (2019)
22. Wagih, M., Weddell, A.S., Beeby, S.: Millimeter-wave power harvesting: a review. IEEE Open J. Antennas Propagation **1**, 560–578 (2020)
23. Bougas, I.D., Papadopoulou, M.S., Boursianis, A.D., Kokkinidis, K., Goudos, S.K.: State-of-the-art techniques in RF energy harvesting circuits. In: Telecom, vol. 2, no. 4, pp. 369–389. MDPI (2021)
24. Chen, Q., Chen, X., Cai, H., Chen, F.: Schottky diode large-signal equivalent-circuit parameters extraction for high-efficiency microwave rectifying circuit design. IEEE Trans. Circuits Syst. II Express Briefs **67**(11), 2722–2726 (2020)
25. Hong, J.-S.G., Lancaster, M.J.: Microstrip Filters for RF/Microwave Applications. Wiley, Hoboken (2004)
26. Rajasekaran, K., Jayalakshmi, J., Jayasankar, T.: Design and analysis of stepped impedance microstrip low pass filter using ADS simulation tool for wireless applications. Int. J. Sci. Res. Publ. **3**(8), 1–5 (2013)
27. Solanki, A., Sharma, N., Kumar, H.M.: Design of microstrip low pass filter for L-band application. Int. J. Electron. Electr. Eng. **3**(3), 212–215 (2015)
28. Bougas, I.D., Papadopoulou, M.S., Boursianis, A.D., Sarigiannidis, P., Nikolaidis, S., Goudos, S.K.: Rectifier circuit design for 5G energy harvesting applications. In: 2022 11th International Conference on Modern Circuits and Systems Technologies (MOCAST), pp. 1–4. IEEE (2022)
29. Zied, C.M., Rashid, E.-R., Hareb, A.: Harvesting microwave energy from WiMax bands based on a Dual-Band Antenna. In: IOP Conference Series: Earth and Environmental Science, vol. 227, no. 4, p. 042044. IOP Publishing (2019)
30. Dardeer, O.M.A., Elsadek, H.A., Abdallah, E.A.: Compact broadband rectenna for harvesting RF energy in WLAN and wiMAX applications. In: 2019 International Conference on Innovative Trends in Computer Engineering (ITCE), pp. 292–296. IEEE (2019)
31. Sarma, S.S., Chandravanshi, S., Jaleel Akhtar, M.: Triple band differential rectifier for RF energy harvesting applications. In: 2016 Asia-Pacific Microwave Conference (APMC), pp. 1–4. IEEE (2016)
32. Azam, S.M.K., Islam, Md.S., Hossain, A.K.M.Z., Othman, M.: Monopole antenna on transparent substrate and rectifier for energy harvesting applications in 5G. Int. J. Adv. Comput. Sci. Appl. **11**(8), 84–89 (2020)
33. Eltresy, N., Eisheakh, D., Abdallah, E., Elhenawy, H.: RF energy harvesting using efficiency dual band rectifier. In: 2018 Asia-Pacific Microwave Conference (APMC), pp. 1453–1455. IEEE (2018)
34. Bougas, I.D., Papadopoulou, M.S., Psannis K., Sarigiannidis, P., Goudos, S.K.: State-of-the-art technologies in RF energy harvesting circuits–a review. In: 2020 3rd World Symposium on Communication Engineering (WSCE), pp. 18–22. IEEE (2020)

Design and Development of an Auxiliary Power Supply for Body Area Network Devices

Anjali Mamidala[1], Bheemaiah Chikondra[2(✉)], and Vijay Kumar Singh[2]

[1] NIT Andhra Pradesh, Tadepalligudem, India
[2] Rajiv Gandhi Institute of Petroleum Technology, Jais, Uttar Pradesh, India
bchikondra@rgipt.ac.in

Abstract. The requirement for a stable DC output in applications such as body area network (BAN) devices, medical equipment, and auxiliary power supplies in all electronic circuits is crucial to stopping device damage. Many integrated circuits (ICs) that require signals to function also need a biasing voltage to power themselves for medical device applications. For this, the development of efficient AC-to-DC converters is our most preferable choice due to the non-availability of direct DC. This paper presents the design and implementation of an auxiliary power supply for applications including medical device auxiliary power supply and IC biasing. The proposed system aims to develop both positive and negative DC voltage (ranging from ± 3.3 to ± 15 V) simultaneously, allowing for flexible usage based on specific requirements. Key features include a compact size, high efficiency, and stable DC voltage with minimal ripple, even under varying load conditions. The design methodology and practical implementation—including PCB (Printed Circuit Board) design—are explained in detail, and experimentation is conducted to validate the design. Additionally, a case study on the TLP250 gate driver circuit is performed experimentally with the developed DC supply. This paper offers valuable insights for researchers in the field of power electronics. The compact design and prototyping for industry use can be considered as a future scope of this paper.

Keywords: AC to DC Converter · transformer · rectifier · filter · PCB design

1 Introduction

The need for efficient and stable DC power supply solutions is critical for various applications, prompting engineers and researchers to develop different circuits. This demand arises from the requirement for DC power in applications such as BAN devices like fitness bands,smart glasses, medical equipmemts, inverters,

Supported by Rajiv Gandhi Institute of Petroleum Technology, Jais, UP 229304.

K. Atul et al. (Eds.): BodyNets 2024, LNICST 666, pp. 114–124, 2026.
https://doi.org/10.1007/978-3-032-16099-7_11

motor drives, electric vehicle charging systems, industrial automation, operational amplifiers, audio signal processing, and more [1]. A DC power supply with minimal ripple, high efficiency, constant voltage, and compact size is essential for these applications. It's also crucial to provide a stable DC voltage for integrated circuits (ICs). A DC supply with both positive and negative voltages is particularly desirable, as it helps reduce ripple. Converters play a significant role in achieving this [1,2].

An AC to DC converter transforms AC voltage into DC voltage, typically involving steps like stepping down the input voltage, converting AC to DC, reducing ripple, and regulating voltage. The design incorporates components such as diodes, resistors, capacitors, and voltage regulators, which collectively determine the size and cost of the entire circuit [1,3,4].

The process begins with stepping down 220V/50 Hz AC to 15V/50 Hz AC using a center-tapped transformer. Although the output voltage is DC, ripples may still be present, necessitating the use of a filter [3]. Components like capacitors and inductors can act as filters, either alone or in combination, with or without resistors. A capacitor combined with a resistor is often preferred due to its smaller size compared to an inductor. Theoretically, the capacitance and resistance should be adequately selected to minimize ripple. Voltage regulators are arranged at the output to generate both positive and negative DC voltages [5,6].

Electric power transmission systems predominantly use alternating current (AC) due to its lower power loss compared to direct current (DC). AC to DC converters facilitate the integration of these systems by providing DC connections to motors and other electronic devices. This paper presents a detailed explanation of designing an AC to DC converter, along with simulation results performed in MATLAB and a PCB (Printed Circuit Board) design created using EasyEDA software. Additionally, a case study on the TLP250 gate driver circuit is included [7].

2 Proposed Methodology

2.1 AC to DC Converter

The conversion of AC to DC involves several steps, beginning with stepping down the 220V/50 Hz AC using a 15-0-15 center-tapped transformer [2]. Although AC can have various waveforms such as square, triangular or sine waves, the sine wave is preferred due to its favorable characteristics. Since AC alternates in both positive and negative directions, it needs to be rectified to produce a unidirectional flow, which is essential for DC.

Rectification is achieved through rectifiers, which can be either half-wave or full-wave types. Half-wave rectifiers use a single diode to allow current flow in only one direction, resulting in an output that represents only 50% of the sine wave. In contrast, full-wave rectifiers convert the entire sine wave into DC, providing higher efficiency. For full-wave rectification, a bridge rectifier is often used because of it's better transformer utilization and higher efficiency. This arrangement involves four diodes configured in a bridge formation [4]. During the positive half-cycle, two diodes conduct in forward bias while the other two are in reverse bias. Conversely, during the negative half-cycle, the roles of the diodes switch, with the other two conducting in forward bias. This configuration allows current to flow in one direction, effectively converting the entire waveform into a positive one.

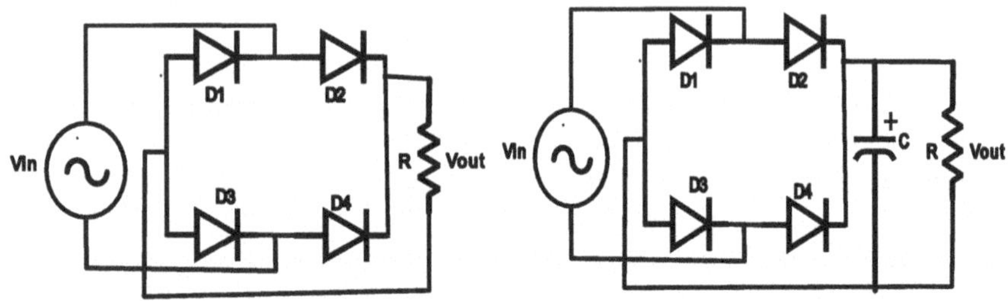

Fig. 1. Bridge circuit(left) and Bridge circuit with filter(Right) used in simulation

- Diode selection
  When using a 15-0-15 center-tapped transformer, the maximum voltage input for the diodes is 21.2 V. Therefore, the peak inverse voltage (PIV) of the diodes must exceed 43V to ensure proper operation. We are considering using IN4007 diodes for the bridge rectifier, as they have a PIV rating of 1000V [4]. This makes them well-suited for the bridge rectifier configuration shown in Fig. 1.

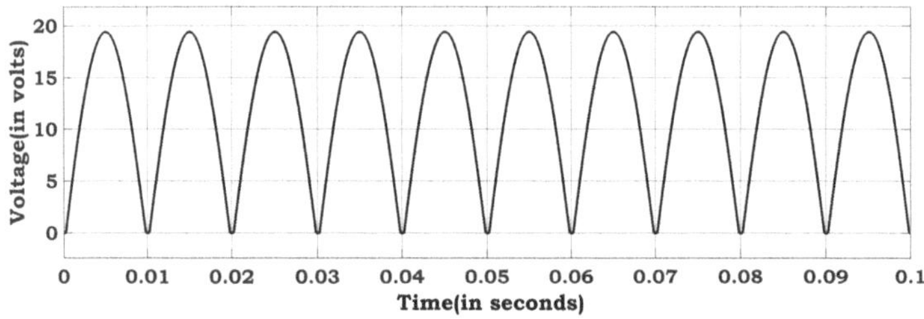

Fig. 2. Output from bridge rectifier

Despite rectification, ripples still persist in the output voltage, as illustrated in Fig. 2. To ensure a stable DC output, it is crucial to minimize these ripples. Filters are employed for this purpose, and various types are available [3]. For this application, a filter comprising a capacitor in parallel with a resistor is considered, as shown in Fig. 1. Additionally, inductors can be incorporated into filters for further ripple reduction, but a capacitor-resistor filter is sufficient for this specific application. Capacitors are smaller and lighter than inductors and are efficient in smoothing out ripples in the rectified DC signal. They provide a relatively stable output voltage with minimal power loss. Resistors helps in controlling the charging and discharging rate of capacitor, leading to more stable DC output.

- Capacitor selection
  Capacitor charges when voltage increases and discharges when voltage decreases. Capacitor selection is based on the ripple factor, which is calculated using the specific formula [3].

$$RF(\%) = (V_{rms}/V_o) * 100 \tag{1}$$

$$V_p = V_{max} - V_o \tag{2}$$

$$V_o = (V_{max} + V_{min})/2 \tag{3}$$

where, V_{max}=Maximum output voltage from the filter, V_{min}=Minimum output voltage from the filter and $V_{rms} = \sqrt{2} * V_p$.

Table 1. Capacitor selection

Capacitance(μF)	Resistance($k\Omega$)	V$_{max}$($volts$)	V$_{min}$($volts$)	V$_o$($volts$)	V$_{rms}$($volts$)	Ripple factor(%)
0.1	10	19.8	5.182	12.49	10.323	82.59
10	10	19.8	19.2	19.5	0.424	2.10
100	10	19.8	19.62	19.71	0.12	0.64

All these values are collected from a simulation in MATLAB, where a 15V/50 Hz AC supply is provided as input, and the ripple factor is calculated, as shown in Fig. 1. The output from the filter, when a capacitor and resistor are connected in parallel, is depicted in Fig. 3. While calculating capacitance, resistance is kept constant. Therefore, as indicated in Table 1, it can be stated that as capacitance increases, the ripple factor decreases.

Table 2. Resistor selection

Capacitance(μF)	Resistance($k\Omega$)	V$_{max}$($volts$)	V$_{min}$($volts$)	V$_o$($volts$)	V$_{rms}$($volts$)	Ripple factor(%)
100	20	19.799	19.706	19.752	0.046	0.33
100	30	19.798	19.737	19.767	0.043	0.21
100	47	19.8	19.76	19.78	0.028	0.14

- Resistor selection

  While calculating resistance, capacitance is kept constant. Therefore, as shown in Table 2, it can be stated that as resistance increases, the ripple factor decreases.

Therefore, a 47 kΩ resistor and a 100 μF/25V electrolytic capacitor are considered for filtration with 0.14% ripple factor.

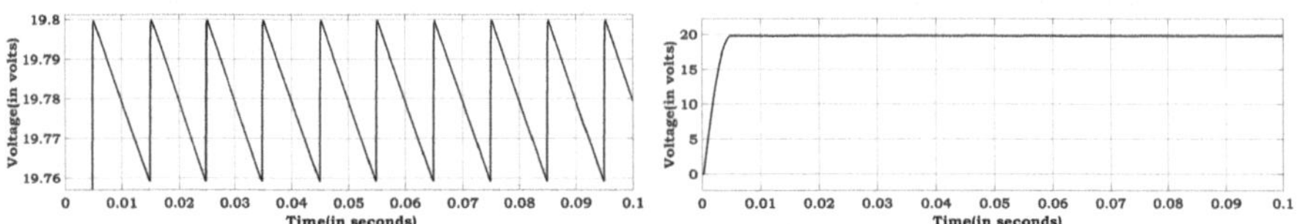

Fig. 3. Output from filter

The stable DC voltage is supplied to voltage regulators (LM7905 for -5V, LM7915 for -15V, LM7805 for 5V, and LM7815 for 15V) [5,6]. Each voltage regulator has three terminals: input, output, and ground. Ceramic capacitors are placed across the input and output terminals of the voltage regulators to ensure a filtered output. The designed AC to DC converter will provide both positive and negative DC voltage at a time. This is made possible by designing the circuit shown in Fig. 4. The upper half of the circuit is generating positive DC voltage and lower half of the circuit is generating negative DC voltage.

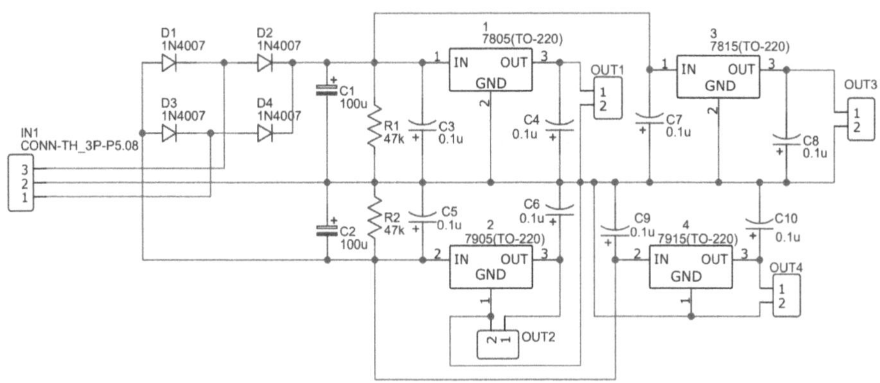

Fig. 4. AC to DC Converter circuit for PCB design

2.2 PCB Design

The printed circuit board (PCB) design was developed using EasyEDA software, as illustrated in Fig. 4. In EasyEDA, component selection is based on their physical parameters. Although electrolytic capacitors were initially placed in the circuit due to their matching terminal distances with ceramic capacitors, ceramic capacitors were ultimately used at the input and output terminals of the voltage regulators in the practical implementation, as shown in Fig. 6. The components were arranged according to their required positions, and the routes were auto-routed with adjustments made for the size and placement of each route during the layout design. Manual routing was also an option. The layout and its virtual view are shown in Fig. 5. The layout was transferred onto a copper plate, which was then etched in a ferric chloride solution using an etching machine. After etching, holes were drilled into the PCB using a drilling machine, and the components were soldered onto the board. The completed PCB is depicted in Fig. 6 (Tables 3 and 4).

Table 3. Components used in the experiment

S.No	Components	Value	Quantity	Cost/each(in Rs)
1	Center-tapped transformer	15-0-15	01	389
2	Diode	IN4007	04	1
3	Resistor	$47k\Omega$	02	0.5
4	Ceramic capacitor	0.1μF	04	1
5	Electrolytic capacitor	$100\mu F$	02	9.5
6	Voltage regulator	LM7805,LM7815,LM7809,LM7815	04	10

Table 4. Ratings of components

Components	Ratings
Center-tapped transformer(15-0-15)	220/15 V, 2A
Diode(IN4007)	Peak inverse voltage:1000V, Operating temp:-65 °C to 175 °C
Resistor	47 kΩ, 5% Tolerance, Power rating:0.25W, Operating temp:-55 °C to 155 °C
Ceramic capacitor	0.1 μF, 50 V
Electrolytic capacitor	100 μF, 25V, Tolerance:20%, Operating temp:-25 °C to 105 °C
Voltage regulator(LM7805,LM7815)	Tolerance:4%, Output current=1.5A, Operating temp:0 °C to 125°C
	Input voltage: 25 V(max for LM7805); 35 V(max for LM7815)
	output voltage:-5 V(LM7905);-15 V(LM7915)
Voltage regulator(LM7905,LM7915)	Tolerance:4%, Output current=1.5A, Operating temp:0 °C-125°C
	Input voltage :-25 V(max for LM7905);-35 V(max for LM7915)
	output voltage:-5 V(LM7905);-15 V(LM7915)

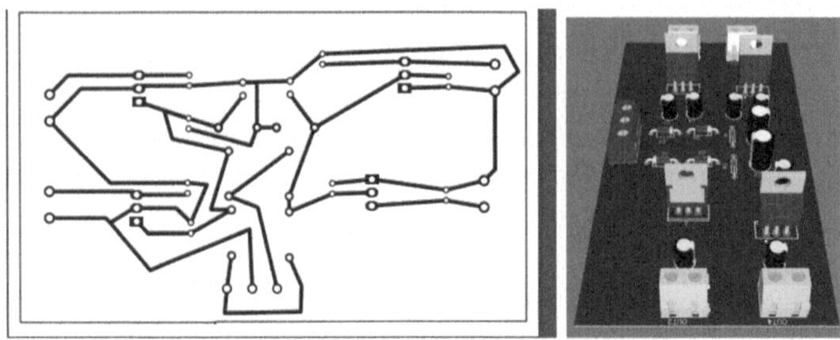

Fig. 5. PCB Layout and its virtual view

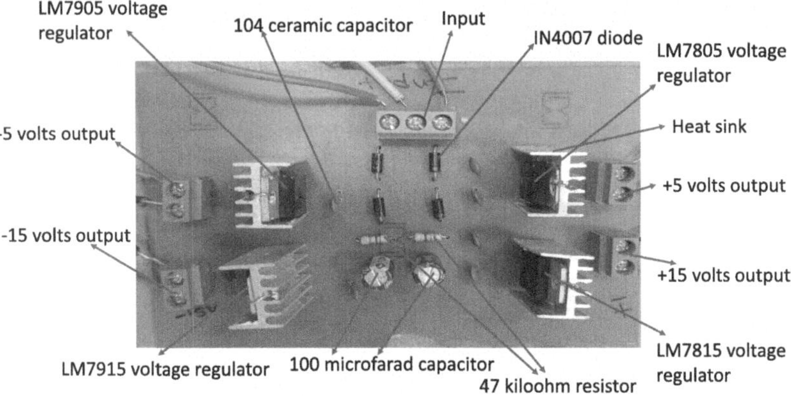

Fig. 6. PCB for AC to DC Converter

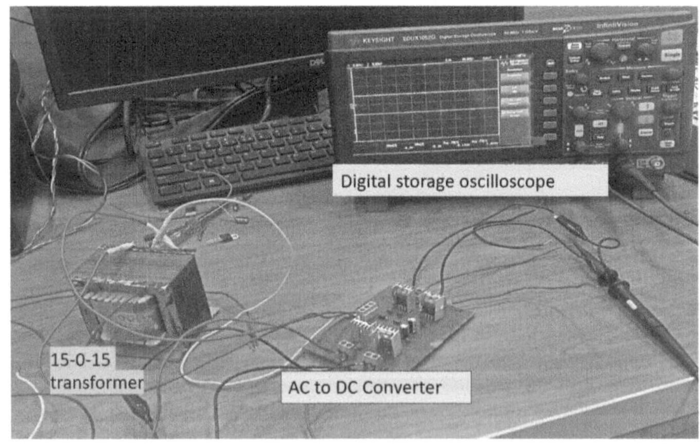

Fig. 7. Experimental setup for AC to DC Converter

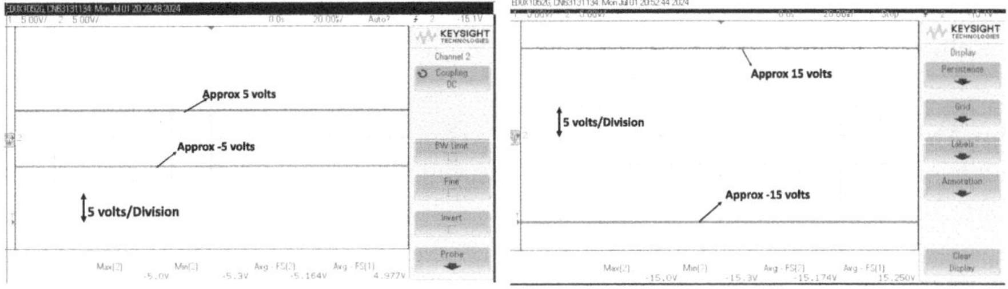

Fig. 8. DC output ±5V(left) and ±15V(right)

3 Results and Analysis

3.1 AC to DC Conversion

In the setup shown in Fig. 1, an AC signal is converted to DC using a bridge rectifier consisting of four IN4007 diodes. Although the bridge rectifier produces a DC output, it contains ripples, as illustrated in Fig. 2. To reduce these ripples, a 100 μF electrolytic capacitor and a 47 $k\Omega$ resistor are used for filtration. The selection of these components was based on calculating the ripple factor for various values of capacitance and resistance. The required simulations were performed using MATLAB Simulink. The simulation output, with the 100 μF capacitor and 47 $k\Omega$ resistor in place, is shown in Fig. 3. The practical and simulation results are almost similar. The ripple factor in simulation is 0.14% but practically almost 0.2%. These components are connected in parallel. For positive DC, the negative terminal of the capacitor is connected to ground, while for negative DC, the positive terminal is connected to ground. Voltage regulators (LM7805 and LM7815) are connected to the positive side of the AC to DC converter, and the regulators (LM7905 and LM7915) are connected to the negative side. The circuit, illustrated in Fig. 4, was designed using EasyEDA software and a PCB has fabricated. The PCB for the AC to DC converter is presented in Fig. 6. A 15-0-15 center-tapped transformer is connected to the PCB, and the complete setup is shown in Fig. 7. The output was observed using a digital storage oscilloscope (DSO). Although both ±15V and ±5V outputs are available simultaneously, the DSO has only two channels. Therefore, the ±15V output was collected first, followed by the ±5V output, as depicted in Fig. 8. Note that, the proposed circuit is able to provide the voltage ranging from ±3.3 V to ±15V. Hence, it can be useful for various medical and electronics devices to use body area network related devices.

3.2 Case Study: TLP250 IC for the Electrical Isolation Between Low and High Power Circuit

For the case study, a TLP250 an optocoupler is used to test in real-time application to see the performance of the IC biasing [7]. The TLP250 is an 8-pin optocoupler for the electrical isolation, as shown in Fig. 9 and Fig. 10, simulation and experimental, respectively.

Pin Description: Pins 1 and 4 are not connected to anything. Pin 2 is the anode, and Pin 3 is the cathode of the internal LED [7]. Pin 8 is used to supply power to the TLP250, while Pin 5 is connected to ground. Pins 6 and 7 are used to collect the output.

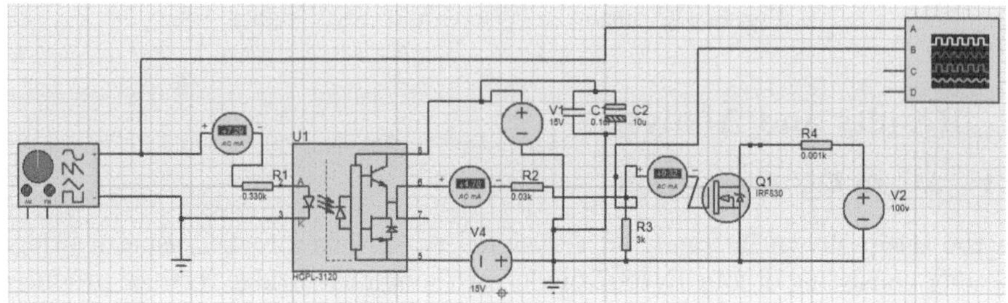

Fig. 9. Gate driver circuit

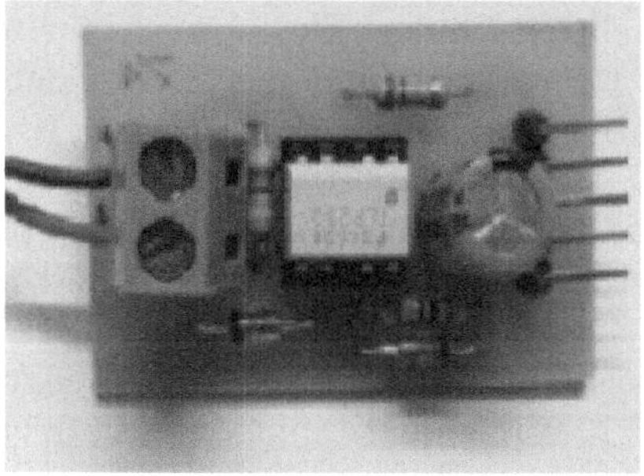

Fig. 10. TLP250 driver board for case study

A gate driver circuit is used to isolate the control circuit from the power circuit and to amplify the signal. There are four types of MOSFET gate drivers.

- Non-inverting isolated low-side mosfet driver
- Inverting isolated low-side mosfet driver
- Non-inverting non-isolated low-side mosfet driver
- Non-inverting isolated high-side mosfet driver

Non-inverting isolated low-side mosfet driver is sufficient for our application.

Gate driver circuit involves three circuits.

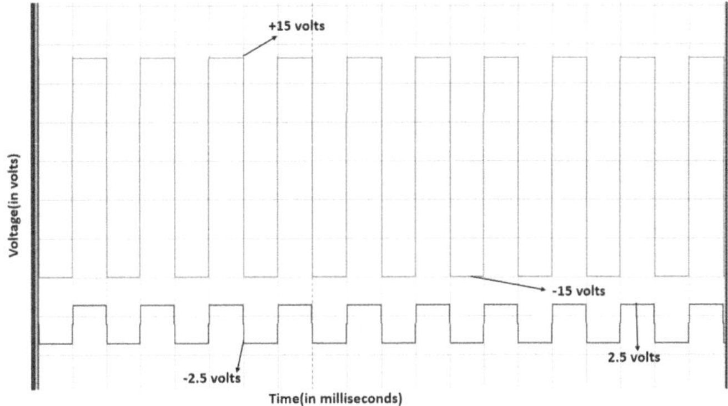

Fig. 11. Output from TLP250 IC

- Control circuit
  In this configuration, PWM signals are supplied to pin 2 of the TLP250, while pin 3 is connected to ground. A 330 Ω resistor is placed in series with the power supply to ensure the LED receives the appropriate voltage drop. The control circuit and power circuit are connected to separate grounds. Pins 1 and 4 are not connected to anything, as illustrated in Fig. 9.
- Protection circuit
  The TLP250 serves as a barrier between the control circuit and the power circuit, necessitating protection from overcurrents and overvoltages. To achieve this, a protection circuit is implemented. A +15V DC supply is connected to pin 8 (+VCC), and a -15V DC supply is connected to pin 5 (-VCC). The output is collected from pin 6 or pin 7. A 0.1 μF ceramic capacitor is placed in parallel with the supply as a decoupling capacitor between pins 5 and 8, while a 10 μF capacitor is also connected in parallel for additional filtration. A 30 Ω resistor is connected in series with output pin 6 as a gate resistor, as shown in Fig. 9. Additionally, a 3 kΩ resistor is connected in parallel to facilitate faster pull-down when the voltage is applied.
- Power circuit
  The gate terminal of the IGBT is connected to pin 6. The source terminal is connected to a resistor, which is then connected in series to ground, while the drain terminal is connected to the power supply, as shown in Fig. 9.

The output is seen in Proteus 8 software as shown in Fig. 11.

3.3 Applications

The proposed circuit discussed in the paper has a wide range of applications in wearable devices. Many devices, such as smartwatches, fitness trackers, wearable medical devices, smart glasses, smart clothing, and hearing aids, rely on AC to DC converters. Even wireless devices often contain AC to DC converters for charging small batteries, like those used in hearing aids.

For instance, smart glasses like Google Glass and Microsoft HoloLens utilize adapters with built-in AC to DC converters to charge their internal battery systems. Similarly, wearable medical devices, such as pacemakers and insulin pumps, depend heavily on reliable power. These devices incorporate AC to DC converters in their charging units to maintain battery life.

Fitness trackers, like Fitbit and Garbin, typically charge via USB, which includes an adapter that converts AC to 5V DC.

4 Conclusion

The AC to DC converter was developed with rectification and appropriate filtration. All simulations related to the converter were performed in MATLAB Simulink. Various types of converters were studied during the preparation phase. The circuit was designed with a focus on achieving both positive and negative DC outputs (ranging from ±3.3 V to ±15 V), ensuring proper connections to the positive and negative terminals of electrolytic capacitors. Although Zener diodes can provide stable DC output, voltage regulators (LM7805, LM7815, LM7905, LM7915) were chosen to generate $\pm$ 5V and $\pm$ 15V outputs, as Zener diodes can become bidirectional beyond certain limits. The project provided extensive knowledge in using EasyEDA software for complete PCB design. Additionally, a case study on the TLP250 IC for the electrical isolation between low and high power circuit offered insights into Proteus 8 software. Further, the developed auxiliary power supply can be tested on the medical devices especially for BAN applications which can be considered as future scope of the paper.

References

1. Mohan, N., Raju, S.: Power electronics, a first course: simulations and laboratory implementations. Wiley, (2022). https://books.google.co.in/books?id=bKOgEAAAQBAJ
2. Taha, W., Azer, P., Callegaro, A.D., Emadi, A.: Multiphase traction inverters: state-of-the-art review and future trends. IEEE Access **10**, 4580–4599 (2022)
3. Pyakuryal, S., Matin, M.: Filter design for ac to dc converter. Int. Ref. J. Eng. Sci. (IRJES). **2**(1), 42–49 (2013)
4. Diodes incorporated,"1N4001G/L - 1N4007G/L 1.0A GLASS PASSIVATED RECTIFIER", DS29002 Rev. D-2. https://pdf1.alldatasheet.com/datasheet-pdf/download/58825/DIODES/1N4007.html
5. Texas Instruments,"LM79XX Series 3-Terminal Negative Regulators", SNOSBQ7C –JUNE 1999–REVISED MAY (2013). https://www.ti.com/lit/ds/symlink/lm79.pdf
6. ST life.augmented,"L78 Datasheet", DS0422 - Rev 36 (2018). https://www.st.com/resource/en/datasheet/l78.pdf
7. TOSHIBA,"TOSHIBA Photocoupler GaAlAs Ired and PhotoIC TLP250" (2004). https://pdf.direnc.net/upload/tlp250-datasheet.pdf

Employing Knowledge Graphs for Prescriptive Maintenance in WBANs

Rishabh Deo Pandey[1] and Itu Snigdh[2(✉)]

[1] Indian Institute of Information Technology (IIIT), Una, Una, India
rishabh@iiitu.ac.in
[2] Department of Computer Science and Engineering, Birla Institute of Technology, Mesra, Mesra, India
itusnigdh@bitmesra.ac.in

Abstract. With the emergence of WBANs to aid healthcare solutions, the dependence on sensors for decision-making and continuous monitoring applications increased. Dependence on sensors makes fault diagnosis critically important due to the real-time constraints of the applications and the degree of accuracy required. This requirement for accuracy in WBANs, in turn, prioritizes the need to analyze data discrepancies observed at the server end of the applications. The use of ML algorithms to classify faults to a particular class offers little help when maintenance activities are executed or scheduled. Thus, determining the root cause of the failures and the affected faulty components of the application becomes difficult. The automated healthcare solution based on knowledge graphs provides an extensive outlay for detecting and isolating faults, bringing ease in the maintenance and rectification of failures. We present a knowledge graph approach to model, understand, and diagnose faults by providing a structured representation of the network's entities, relationships, and data flows. With the adoption of our mechanism, reliability engineers and software quality managers can gain insight into the error factors, components affected, and related discrepancies in WBANs.

Keywords: Maintainability · Fault diagnosis · WBANs · Knowledge graphs · propositional logic · predicate logic · Ontology · IoT · Data discrepancy

1 Introduction

The Internet of Things (IoT) [1] permits data collection and real-time monitoring across multiple domains by integrating a wide variety of sensors into different networks. A notable innovation is the Body Area Network (BAN), designed to identify human anatomy issues. BAN refers to the collaboration of devices that monitor and identify various systems within the human body. WBANs refer to wearable devices that are surface-mounted or implanted into the body. Its main objective is to send data generated by wearables to WLANs or the Internet, with the possibility of direct data interchange between wearables. With WBANs, healthcare applications are now transformed by real-time monitoring of vital signs through wearable and implantable sensors, especially

K. Atul et al. (Eds.): BodyNets 2024, LNICST 666, pp. 125–135, 2026.
https://doi.org/10.1007/978-3-032-16099-7_12

in chronic conditions [2, 3]. However, the accuracy of the readings provided by the sensors and their effectiveness play a significant role in the reliability of WBAN systems. As we know, sensor malfunctions can lead to inaccurate data, affecting the entire decision-making mechanism of any particular IoT application. The impacts of data discrepancies become profound for life-critical applications like Wireless Body Area Networks (WBANs). These systems are prone to faults [4, 5], like sensor malfunctions, communication failures, power depletion, and human and environmental factors that may compromise data quality, making fault diagnosis critical. Detection and isolation of fault causes in an easy, timely, and accurate manner shifts the focus on maintainability of the system. In order to facilitate predictive and prescriptive maintenance [6], AI tools, especially knowledge graphs, present a promising solution. With artificial intelligence (AI), knowledge graphs offer an innovative way of organizing and utilizing information. Through knowledge graphs, AI systems can interpret and handle data more effectively and efficiently by building an organized network of entities, their characteristics, and the connections that link them.

The novelty of the research work lies in collecting and collating the various factors and errors encountered in WBAN applications. Further, a four-layered knowledge graph layout is proposed that classifies the errors and, with the help of propositional and predicate logic, rules map the errors to faults and then to the actual data anomaly observed in the dataset. As an aid in the occurrence of discrepancies in the collected data, the knowledge graph can be employed to determine expected behavior in events of a particular fault and thus make identification and isolation of faulty components exhibiting the behavior easy.

2 Related Work

Networking media has permeated several international industries, including computer networks and healthcare. Interest in wireless networking has increased due to the rise in wearable technology, such as watches and glasses [7]. However, WBANs have several major obstacles to overcome before they can be widely adopted and used in society. These difficulties' technological, security, and operational facets are crucial to effectively using WBANs. Besides technical limitations like energy constraints, mobility issues, and security concerns, sensor fault detection is a major challenge in WBANs. Simple statistical and Pearson coefficient-based methods have been used for fault detection in such networks [8]. Similarly, machine learning algorithms have been employed for fault identification and classification and analyzed for prediction [9–11]. Fault-tolerant schemes have also been proposed through efficient algorithms which focus on mitigating reliability issues of WBANs [12].

In addition to machine learning algorithms, knowledge graphs and rule-based reasoning have been adopted extensively for smart IoT-driven applications due to their advantages in interoperability, ease of integration with other systems, and improved device compatibility [13]. Knowledge reasoning based on knowledge graphs is one of the current research hot spots in knowledge graphs and has played an important role in wireless communication networks, intelligent question answering, and other applications [1, 14–16].

Specifically Predictive maintenance strategies are employed to ensure reliability, minimizing downtime and enhancing patient care. With the help of AI and ML algorithm, analysis of sensor data and scheduling maintenance before failure is possible [17]. Techniques such as clustering, support vector machines and neural networks have been used extensively for fault detection and classification. Explainable AI (XAI) model have also been adopted for fault detection to enhance transparency and trust. In context to IoT enabled wearable healthcare devices, AI has been adopted for minimizing resources in terms of higher energy optimization, better reliability and long battery life [18]. AI has been used extensively in diagnosis and remote monitoring. In context to fault tolerance, AI driven solutions have been used in intrusion detection and health care devices security vulnerability management [19]. Specific to AI based predictive maintenance [20], they have been used in industrial systems [21].

However, to the best of our knowledge, there has yet to be research on maintainability or root cause analysis of such systems. We propose a knowledge graph-based method for fault detection and isolation and finding the optimal path to maintain a system in the event of such faults. An ontology, or formal framework, serves as the basis for a knowledge graph by defining the different kinds of things, their characteristics, and the possible connections among them. Effective reasoning and consistency are ensured and encouraged by the use of ontologies that help in the classification of knowledge and the design of a knowledge base comprising a common understanding of the area of interest.

3 WBAN Model

To depict the fault diagnosis and isolation mechanism, we consider a WBAN scenario simulated in NetSim Version 14.1 [22]. The architecture of the application is depicted in Fig. 1.

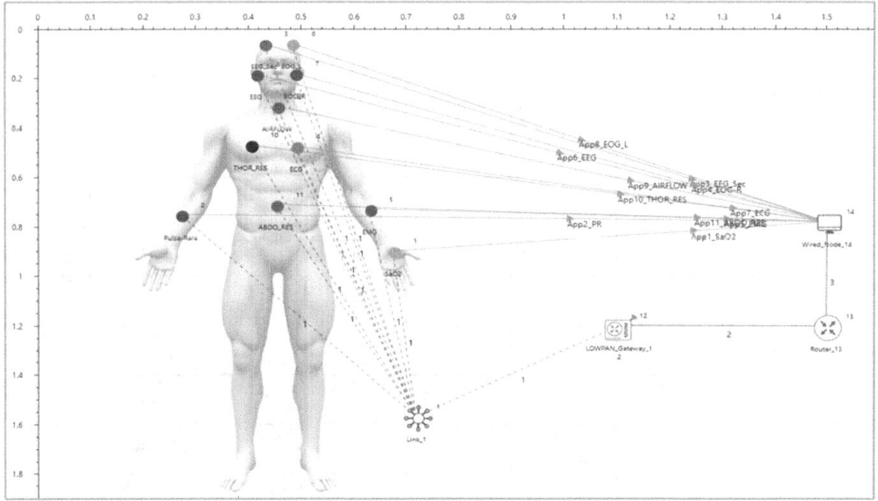

Fig. 1. Representing the NetSim simulation scenario experimental setup

The major components of this experimental setup comprise of:

a) **Sensors:**
   A total of 11 heterogeneous sensors were considered as an example of a WBAN that ideally has a large number of inexpensive, low-power sensor nodes that can be used to continuously monitor a person's blood pressure, heart rate, ECG, and other health indicators. Due to its wireless nature, it is not limited by the person's movement for ongoing assessment.
b) **Central control unit (CCU):**
   All sensor nodes send their outputs to the CCU's central coordinating node, represented as node 14. The signals from nodes are received by CCU, which then forwards them for storage and analysis for human body monitoring.
c) **WBAN Communication:**
   It comprises a wireless connection from the sensor nodes to the 6 LOWPAN gateway that forwards the information to the server. The server may be wired or wireless or use a cellular network. For our scenario, we consider a wired server.
d) **Control center:**
   It is in charge of keeping user data that may be retrieved later or utilized for analysis. Mobile phones (for messaging), computer systems (for monitoring), and servers (for database keeping) are examples of end-node devices that make up this system. The implementation of the knowledge graph and analysis, along with the maintenance of the devices, are carried out at these high-end nodes.

The scenario was executed for multiple iterations to model different network conditions. The data set generated from the simulations was then analyzed to identify data discrepancies. Faults were seeded at random intervals in the data set collected. The process of identifying the faulty data was carried out through the knowledge graph created, as illustrated in the methodology section.

4 Methodology

Ideal to any conventional knowledge graph, we model the fault diagnosis scenario as triples, as shown in Fig. 2. Factors causing the errors, errors themselves, faults, and data discrepancies are all entities. The arcs represent the relationships and labels have been used for clarity of representation. Using this, the knowledge graph has been deployed as a 4-layer architecture using predicate and propositional logic. The proposed knowledge graph aims to help identify the root cause of the error occurring in a WBAN application using a top-down mechanism. Once the cause is identified, isolation and rectification are carried out using standard procedures. As per relevant literature, the knowledge graph covers all the possible causes of application failure, whether hardware, software, network-related issues, or human errors. The four layers of the proposed knowledge graph are as follows:

a) **Layer 1:** It consists of four different clusters that are:

   - Cluster 1 (C1) represents the flaws inhibited by the sensor itself. It contains degradation, aging, and calibration.

- Cluster 2 (C2) represents the defects in a smart device due to external factors. Its components are damage, malfunction, defects, and tampering.
- Cluster 3 (C3) denotes issues arising from the installation error. It comprises misalignment, installation, and incompatibility.
- Cluster 4 (C4) represents network-related issues. It consists of bandwidth issues, interference, and surge.

b) **Layer 2:** This represents nine different errors that can occur in any sensor-based innovative WBAN application. These errors have been determined using different sets of knowledge bases. We adopt nine different rules mapped to entities. A sample of the rule created using predicate logic [23] is given as:
   For all values of C1 and some values of C3, drift (D) occurs.

$$[\forall x \in C1, D(x)] \land [\exists x \in C3, D(x)] \tag{1}$$

c) **Layer 3:** This layer represents a different set of data-centric faults in a sensor dataset deployed for designing a real-time monitoring application. Knowledge base for six different data-centric faults has been considered, and a sample logic has been defined using propositional logic, which is given as:
   If drift, bias, cross-sensitivity, hysteresis, or interface error occurs, then out-range fault (F1) will occur.

$$D(x) \lor B(x) \lor C(x) \lor H(x) \lor I(x) \rightarrow F1(x) \tag{2}$$

d) **Layer 4** Represents various data quality issues that occur due to the related faults mentioned earlier, which can affect the dataset's authenticity. These issues are:

- **Data Incompleteness:** It represents the missing information or data values in the dataset. Constant fault and stuck-at-X faults are the factors resulting in data incompleteness.
- **Data Inconsistency:** Inconsistency in data occurs due to the presence of multiple data sources that gather data about the surrounding environment but need to be standardized, thus resulting in inconsistent data values for the same scenario. Multiple fluctuations are responsible for inconsistency in data.
- **Data Inaccuracy:** Denotes the inaccurate or incorrect readings in the dataset. The major reasons for inaccuracy in the dataset are out-range faults and outliers.
- **Data Expiry:** Data expiry denotes outdated data without further use. Data expiry occurs mainly when the dataset suffers from stuck-at-X and constant faults.

5 Results and Analysis

The aforementioned four-layer architecture is implemented using predicate and propositional logic, which results in a knowledge graph illustrated in Fig. 2. The figure depicts all possible faults, along with their causes and impact, that can occur in any IoT application. Thus, any kind of error is observable only at the interface of the application. Further, the error type is determined to isolate the faults, and all related components that are affected by the error are searched in the graph. The components are isolated, and the cause of the error is determined. Thus, the knowledge graph not only helps determine the factors that lead to that error but also identifies all other components that are being affected due to that particular factor. It covers all the possible causes of failure in an application, whether hardware, software, network-related issues, or human errors.

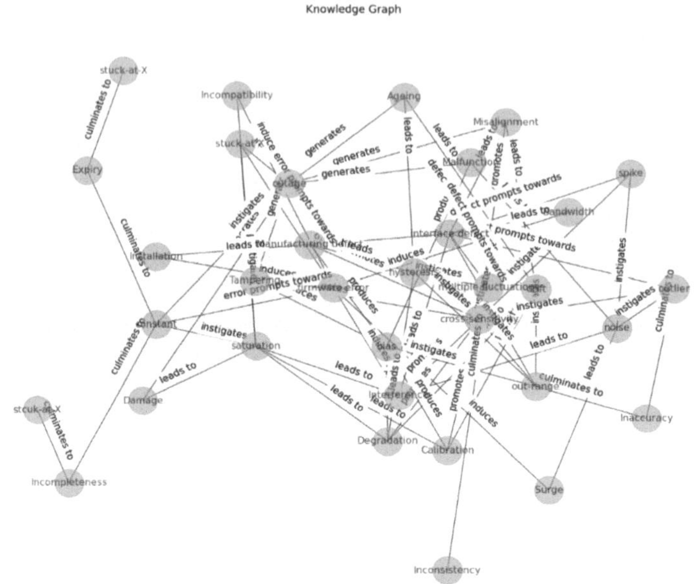

Fig. 2. Knowledge graph to represent impending faults occurring in an IoT application.

Owing to the large expanse of the knowledge graph and the real-time diagnosis requirement, we perform nodal analysis of the KG. One of the most well-known measures for analyzing a well-designed network is network centrality [24], which quantifies the significance of an individual represented in the form of nodes in a network. Network centrality can be measured using three different methods. Centrality can be defined as a network's ability to link to a large number of other nodes directly (degree centrality), indirectly (closeness centrality), or as a major mediator between a large number of other nodes (betweenness centrality). Degree centrality is a metric that expresses how many connections a node has. Higher values indicate a more central position within the network. It is computed based on the number of links or edges a node has. Closeness centrality is determined by adding up the lengths of all the shortest paths that connect it to every other node in the graph. The definition of betweenness centrality is the rate with which a node appears on the shortest path connecting every pair of nodes in a network.

Different centrality measures for the knowledge graph depicted in Fig. 2 have been shown in Fig. 3(a), (b), and (c). In our case, degree centrality depicts the number of connections of an entity in each layer. The darker the node color, the more connected the entity node is with other entities. So, isolating such an entity leads faster to the cause of faults, the errors leading to the faults, and also the underlying factors causing the errors. Likewise, the betweenness centrality identifies the entities in most paths, starting from data discrepancy in the topmost layer to the error-causing factors in the bottom

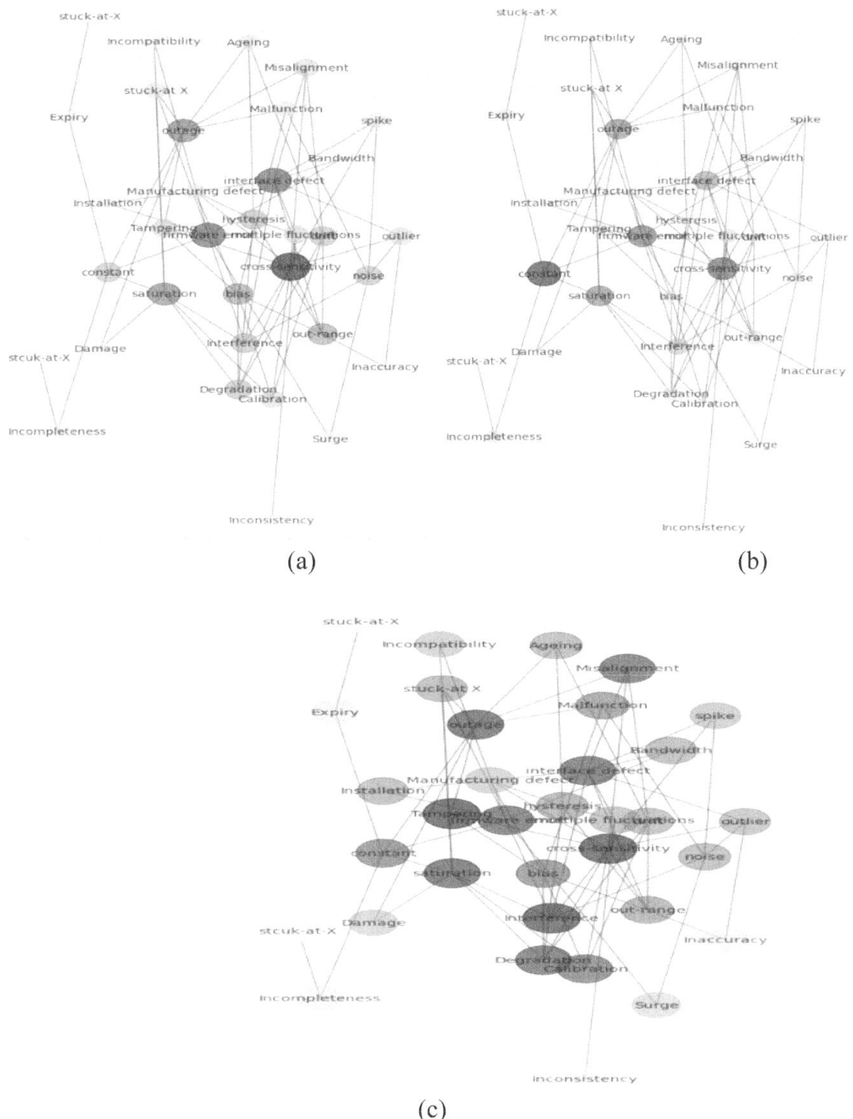

Fig. 3. Denoting different centrality measures for the knowledge graph (a) Degree centrality measure (b) Betweenness centrality measure (c) Closeness centrality measure

layer. The darker the node color, the more significant the entity is in causing the fault. On the contrary, Closeness is negatively related to the entity's significance or color. The closeness measure is computed as a path length for each entity concerning every other related entity, whether direct or indirect and the darker the node color, the farther the entity is from the cause or fault.

Further, we compute the shortest path from an observed data anomaly and the factors causing such discrepancy, as depicted in Figs. 4 and 5. Considering a case in which any malfunctioning of the sensor has occurred, then, through Fig. 4, we can observe that due to it, drift will occur that will instigate out-range faults, which is a leading cause of inaccuracy in the dataset. Conversely, to obtain inaccuracy in the data from expected values, the graph isolated all causes of faults and then pruned down the graph to the most eligible reason based on the rules and centrality measures. Apart from this, data can also be inaccurate due to network issues such as surges and bandwidth. These factors lead to noise in the dataset, which generates outliers, and that reading will denote an inaccurate reading. The effect cause can be seen through the paths highlighted in Figs. 4 and 5. Thus, to overcome the errors and flaws, we need to replace the components that are affected due to noise and drift.

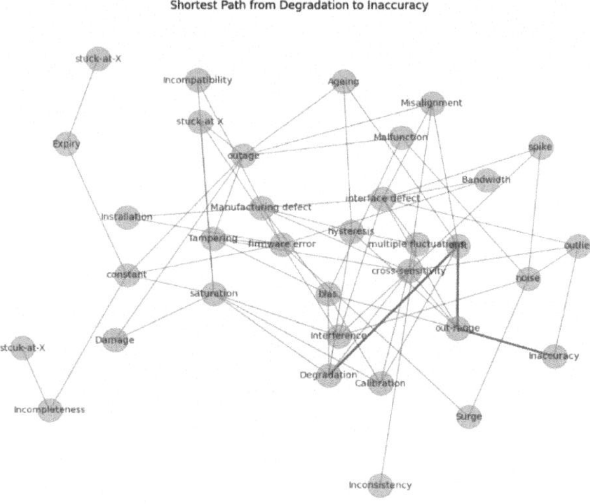

Fig. 4. Representing the shortest path between degradation and inaccuracy

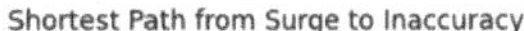

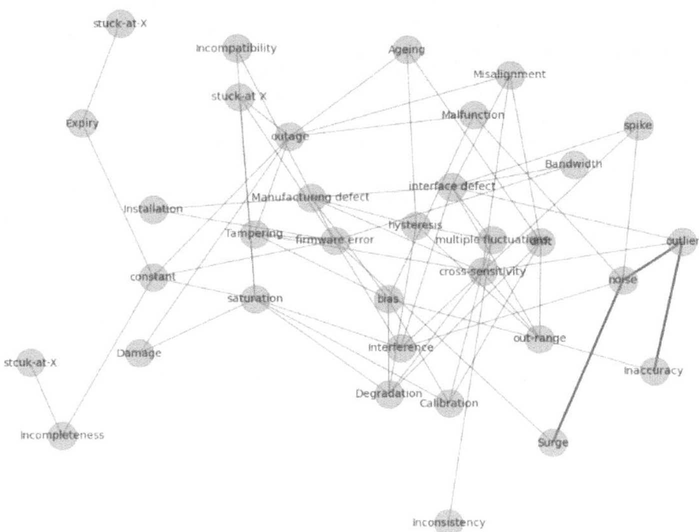

Fig. 5. Representing the shortest path between surge and inaccuracy

6 Conclusion

The article illustrates the use of a knowledge graph to aid maintenance activities in WBAN applications. The knowledge graph will not only help in determining the factors that leads to that error but also identification of the other components which are being affected due to that particular factor. As an aid to reliability and quality assurance engineers, under the occurrence of discrepancies in the collected data, the knowledge graph can be employed to determine expected behavior in events of a particular fault and thus make identification and isolation of faulty components exhibiting the behavior easily. However, the knowledge graph has certain limitations. When the size of the knowledge base becomes extremely large, the knowledge graph would be quite challenging to maintain. Also, though the fault detection mechanisms are effective, the error reporting system could be improved to include more detailed diagnostics. As an extension of this research, the knowledge graph would be made more efficient regarding real-time constraints by incorporating collective knowledge graphs. Since WBANs generate large volume of physiological data from multiple sensors, their scalability must be assessed to ensure they can manage high volume of data without performance degradations. Also, computational overhead of maintenance and querying in knowledge graph can be challenging when streaming data from multiple sources. Further extensions to the research would focus on light weight and efficient algorithms for taking the low latency and computational overhead into consideration. Concepts of distributed database, graph compression technique and hybrid models combining rule-based systems with machine learning techniques could also be employed to enhance scalability for WBANs.

References

1. Dian, F.J., Vahidnia, R., Rahmati, A.: Wearables and the Internet of Things (IoT), applications, opportunities, and challenges: a Survey. IEEE Access **8**, 69200–69211 (2020)
2. Movassaghi, S., Abolhasan, M., Lipman, J., Smith, D., Jamalipour, A.: Wireless body area networks: a survey. IEEE Commun. Surv. Tutor. **16**(3), 1658–1686 (2014)
3. Yuce, M.R.: Implementation of wireless body area networks for healthcare systems. Sens. Actuators A **162**(1), 116–129 (2010)
4. Li, D., Wang, Y., Wang, J., Wang, C., Duan, Y.: Recent advances in sensor fault diagnosis: a review. Sens. Actuators A **309**, 111990 (2020)
5. Park, Y.J., Fan, S.K.S., Hsu, C.Y.: A review on fault detection and process diagnostics in industrial processes. Processes **8**(9), 1123 (2020)
6. Holler, J., Tsiatsis, V., Mulligan, C., Karnouskos, S., Avesand, S., Boyle, D.: Internet of Things. Academic Press (2014)
7. Chakrabarti, S., Biswas, N., Jones, L.D., Kesari, S., Ashili, S.: Smart consumer wearables as digital diagnostic tools: a review. Diagnostics **12**(9), 2110 (2022)
8. Girijakumari Sreekantan Nair, S., Balakrishnan, R.: A precise sensor fault detection technique using statistical techniques for wireless body area networks. ETRI J. **43**(1), 31–39 (2021)
9. Bahache, M., Tahari, A.E.K., Herrera-Tapia, J., Lagraa, N., Calafate, C.T., Kerrache, C.A.: Towards an accurate faults detection approach in internet of medical things using advanced machine learning techniques. Sensors **22**(15), 5893 (2022)
10. Yang, Y., Liu, Q., Gao, Z., Qiu, X., Meng, L.: Data fault detection in medical sensor networks. Sensors **15**(3), 6066–6090 (2015)
11. Ghazal, T.M., et al.: IoT for smart cities: Machine learning approaches in smart healthcare—a review. Future Internet **13**(8), 218 (2021)
12. Mehmood, G., Khan, M.Z., Abbas, S., Faisal, M., Rahman, H.U.: An energy-efficient and cooperative fault-tolerant communication approach for wireless body area network. IEEE Access **8**, 69134–69147 (2020)
13. Amagai, S., Maret, P., Singh, K.: Improving maintainability of calendar-based IoT-driven office with knowledge graph and rule-based reasoning. In: Proceedings of the 13th International Conference on the Internet of Things, pp. 170–173 (2023)
14. Zou, X.: A survey on application of knowledge graph. In: Journal of Physics: Conference Series, vol. 1487, no. 1, p. 012016. IOP Publishing (2020)
15. Fensel, D., et al.: Introduction: what is a knowledge graph?. In: Knowledge Graphs: Methodology, Tools and Selected Use Cases, pp.1–10 (2020)
16. Dai, Y., Wang, S., Xiong, N.N., Guo, W.: A survey on knowledge graph embedding: approaches, applications and benchmarks. Electronics **9**(5), 750 (2020)
17. Zahid, N., Sodhro, A.H., Kamboh, U.R., Alkhayyat, A., Wang, L.: AI-driven adaptive reliable and sustainable approach for internet of things enabled healthcare system. Math. Biosci. Eng. **19**(4), 3953–3971 (2022)
18. Medjek, F., Tandjaoui, D., Djedjig, N., Romdhani, I.: Fault-tolerant AI-driven intrusion detection system for the internet of things. Int. J. Crit. Infrastruct. Prot. **34**, 100436 (2021)
19. Kalusivalingam, A.K., Sharma, A., Patel, N., Singh, V.: Enhancing patient care through IoT-enabled remote monitoring and ai-driven virtual health assistants: implementing machine learning algorithms and natural language processing. Int. J. AI ML **2**(3) (2021)
20. Bajpayi, P., Sharma, S., Gaur, M.S.: AI driven IoT healthcare devices security vulnerability management. In: 2024 2nd International Conference on Disruptive Technologies (ICDT), pp. 366–373. IEEE (2024)
21. Mudia, H.: Utilization AI for predictive maintenance in IoT-enabled industrial systems. J. Artif. Intell. Dev. **2**(2), 47–51 (2023)

22. https://support.tetcos.com/support/solutions/articles/14000106347
23. Ertel, W.: First-order predicate logic. In: Introduction to Artificial Intelligence, pp. 41–66. Springer Fachmedien Wiesbaden, Wiesbaden (2024)
24. Bloch, F., Jackson, M.O., Tebaldi, P.: Centrality measures in networks. Soc. Choice Welfare **61**(2), 413–453 (2023)

Fusion of Edge Computing and Wireless Body Area Networks for Real-Time Data Processing

Samarth Sharma[1(✉)], Khushbu Doulani[1], and Mainak Adhikari[2]

[1] Indian Institute of Information Technology, Lucknow 226002, UP, India
samarth@ieee.org

[2] Indian Institute of Science Education and Research Thiruvananthapuram, Thiruvananthapuram, India
mainak@iisertvm.ac.in

Abstract. This research introduces a new approach to healthcare data processing in real-time by combining Wireless Body Area Networks, federated learning, and edge computing. As major privacy issues, increased energy usage, and long processing times are associated with the conventional centralized data processing method. In order to reduce latency and energy consumption, this research proposes deploying edge computing to process data closer to the data source. Federated learning further improves privacy and security by allowing for collaborative model training across edge devices without exchanging raw data. We conduct an evaluation of the proposed integration of WBANs, federated learning, and edge computing using both theoretical and practical approaches.

Keywords: WBANs · Federated Learning · Realtime processing · Edge Networks

1 Introduction

Edge computing combined with wireless body area networks (WBANs) offers a major development in healthcare technology for real-time data processing. WBANs consist of a network of wearable or implantable sensors that continuously track physiological factors such as glucose levels, blood pressure, and heart rate. Traditionally, centralized servers receive data from these sensors for analysis, leading to privacy concerns, high bandwidth requirements, and increased latency due to the transmission of sensitive medical data. Edge computing solves these problems by allowing data processing to be performed near the data source, at the edge of the network [1]. Because data does not have to travel to a far-off server for processing, this proximity reduces latency, allowing for real-time analysis and faster reactions to important medical problems. Edge computing also reduces the need for constant data flow to central servers, saving energy on wearable devices and extending battery life. Local data processing in edge

K. Atul et al. (Eds.): BodyNets 2024, LNICST 666, pp. 136–147, 2026.
https://doi.org/10.1007/978-3-032-16099-7_13

computing also improves the security and privacy of private health information, reducing the likelihood of data breaches [2]. Edge computing combined with WBANs for real-time data processing guarantees a better degree of privacy and security for consumers in addition to enhancing the efficiency and effectiveness of health monitoring systems.

1.1 Related Work

Real-time healthcare analysis and monitoring are currently transformed by the adoption of new technologies that provide minimal latency, optimal bandwidth, increased energy efficiency, privacy preservation, telemetry, and interoperability across edge networks. By reducing latency, healthcare systems can detect and respond to key health events nearly immediately, which is critical for applications such as continuous glucose monitoring and real-time cardiac assessments. Optimized bandwidth enables the efficient administration of large data streams without overloading the network, ensuring timely updates for healthcare experts. Energy-efficient gadgets, which are required for continuous monitoring, use low-power electronics and energy harvesting to improve battery life, which is critical in remote or resource-constrained environments.

New inventions and increased public awareness of healthcare have significantly expanded the innovative healthcare system. The researchers mainly develop an intelligent healthcare prototype with a set of wearable/biosensors and analyze the data remotely with ML models for recommendation [3].

A wearable consumer gadget (dubbed iGLU 2.0) possessing noninvasive properties, suggested by Joshi *et al.* [4] for real time monitoring of glucose levels, features a short Near-Infrared spectroscopy, which is also presented by the next version of iGLU, an Internet of Medical Things (IoMT)-enabled wearable consumer device for diabetes patients for glucose level monitoring and analysis. Olokodana *et al.* proposed that EZcap as a small, light consumer electronics device that can help find seizures early on by using edge computing and an innovative method for software and hardware to connect [5]. Sharma *et al.* provides a new concept called the schizophrenia detection cap (SczCap), which is an easy-to-wear cap that combines hardware and software to acquire EEG data from the scalp for accurate detection of schizophrenia [6].

The stress detection system proposed by Rachakonda *et al.* is based on the Internet of Medical Things (IoMT) and aims to track both acute and chronic stress [7]. Another article by Rachakonda *et al.* is called SaYoPillow [8]. It describes a noninvasive, optimized, IoMT-enabled system that can identify changes in stress levels while you sleep and, based on your sleeping habits, predict how your stress levels will behave in the future. Alqahtani *et al.* research through how the IoT and edgeâĂŞcloud computing can be used to improve technology-based healthcare options for dengue virus (DGN) infections [9]. Chakraborty et al. introduced a healthcare framework that includes the IoMT in a cloud-fog environment [10]. Monitoring the health status of patients using a portable device with a set of wearable sensors/biosensors is one of the research aspects in the health sector [11]. Doctors and healthcare workers are safeguarded from infection

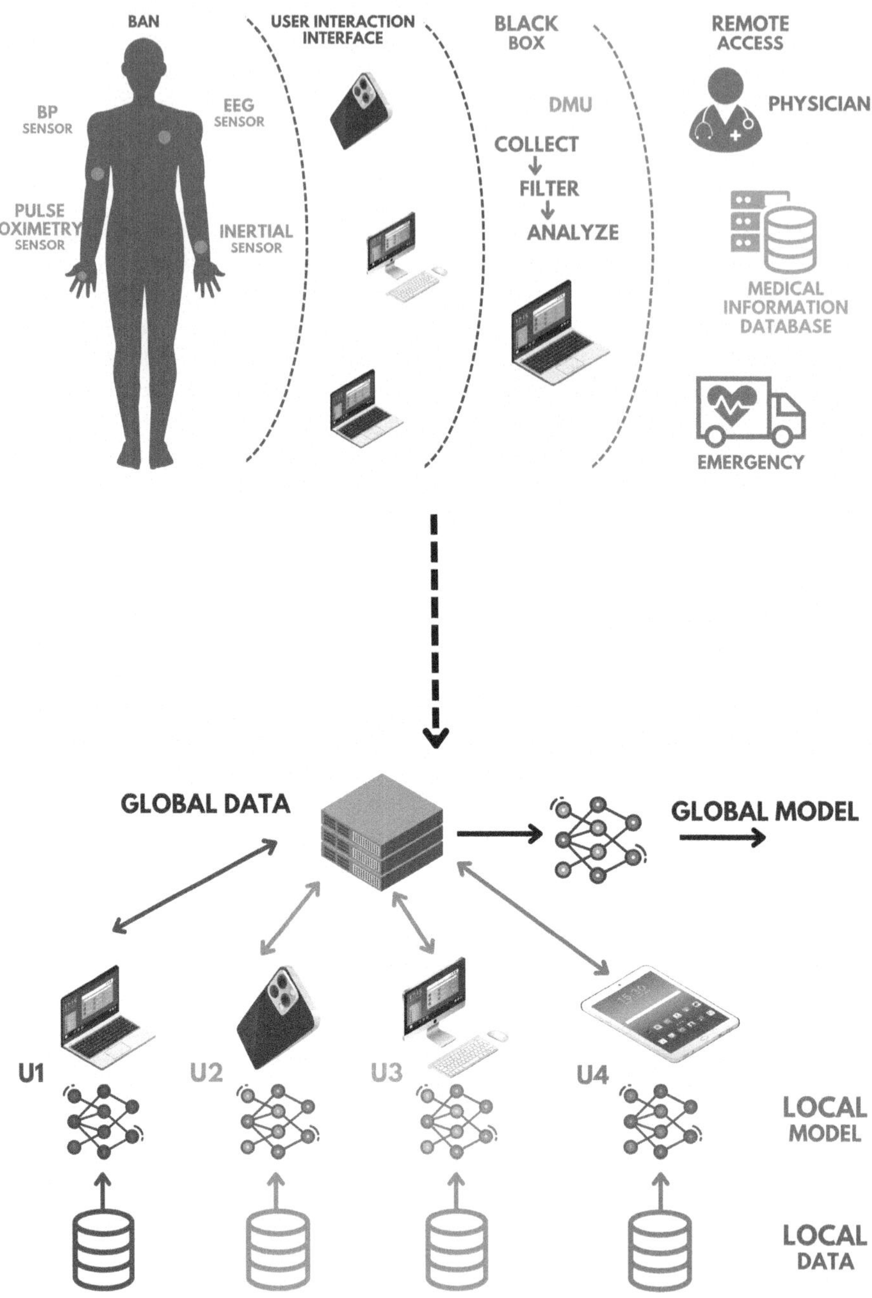

Fig. 1. Pictorial presentation of WBANs.

via remote monitoring and decision-making with higher accuracy. New inventions and increased public awareness of healthcare have significantly expanded the innovative healthcare system. The researchers mainly develop an intelligent healthcare prototype with a set of wearable/biosensors and analyze the data remotely with ML models for recommendation [12].

Development of a smart garb with the intentions of monitoring and collecting health vitals including stress levels, muscle activity and heart rate fluctuations was done by Sethuraman *et al.*, which later analysed the collected data in the centralised cloud server [13].

Standard ML methods in healthcare, particularly for disease prediction, are hindered by challenges such as data privacy concerns, data silos, and the need for centralization of sensitive medical information, which can raise ethical and regulatory issues. These methods often require the transfer of large volumes of patient data to a centralized server for model training, risking privacy breaches and compromising patient confidentiality [14]. The lack of access to diverse datasets due to regulatory constraints or proprietary limitations may limit the generalizability and effectiveness of traditional models.

Table 1. Literature Review on Datasets and Results

S.No	Author	Methodology	Datasets	Key Results
1	Sethuraman et al.	DNN	MIT-BIH Arrythmia	98.2%
2	Maji et al.	CNN	MIT-BIH ECG	99.58%
3	M. Joshi	Proposed Glucometer (Hardware Prototype)	Real time datasets	...
4	M. Joshi	Spectroscopy (Hardware Prototype)	Realtime datasets	...
5	Proposed Work	Federated Learning	PhysioNet (ECG datasets)	97%

Formal ML strategy includes centralized learning (CL) collects the monitoring environmental data, and trains the data in a single server. There are so many consensuses, such as sharing data with the central cloud server and compromising user privacy [15]. Chao Ma *et al.* proposed employing a novel combination of ccRFs and mpAC techniques to fully automatically segment the brain substructures from volumetric MR images. The suggested mpAC model improves the ccRFs model's voxel categorization by using a contour evolution strategy. The mpAC model is better than most ACMs in a number of ways, such as automatically initializing contours, integrating multimodal images, and being more accurate and reliable thanks to shape priors and spatial constraint schemes [16]. This work presents an uncertainty-aware multi-dimensional mutual learning approach to improve MRI brain tissue and brain tumor segmentation models. Junting Zhao et al. demonstrated that even though stronger high-dimensional 3D-CNN models have more parameters and bigger spatial receptive fields, low-dimensional 2D/2.5D-CNN models capture fine features and improve their performance even further [17].

1.2 Problem Statement

Real-time data processing is challenging for WBANs as it's necessary to rely on centralized cloud servers, which causes high delay, higher energy use, and privacy risks. Additionally, we require collaborative machine learning that protects data protection in sensitive areas like healthcare. Building a system that uses edge computing and federated learning to improve real-time data processing in WBANs while minimizing latency, reducing down on energy consumption, and preserving data privacy is the main problem.

1.3 Motivations

This research is motivated by the rising demand for wearable device-based real-time, secure health monitoring systems. The healthcare sector is increasingly utilizing WBANs for continuous patient monitoring,it presents numerous challenges compared to current centralized processing systems.

- Data sent to remote computers causes latency, therefore impairing real-time monitoring and instantaneous medical treatment. Constant data transfer over long distances requires a lot of power, therefore lowering the battery life of wearable devices.
- Sending private medical records to centralized systems greatly compromises privacy and exposes one to cybercrime. Particularly in critical healthcare applications, machine learning models that can learn cooperatively from distributed data without compromising privacy are much sought after. So,this work intends to solve these problems by combining edge computing with federated learning, therefore providing a more effective, safe, and privacy-preserving framework for uses in health monitoring.

By including edge computing and federated learning into the system design, we highlight the significance of energy consumption, latency, and fault tolerance. By processing data locally on edge devices and eliminating the need for continuous contact with centralized servers, energy consumption is reduced. Processing data in real-time at the edge of the network minimizes delays and ensures swift responses to critical medical events. The proposed FedTolerant approach incorporates resilience against failures, ensuring reliable model training despite potential device malfunctions or unstable network environments. This enhances the system's reliability and efficiency for healthcare-related applications.

2 Proposed Methodology

The details of these techniques are discussed in the following subsections.

2.1 System Flow

The research system begins with wearable medical equipment collecting biological information from patients. To implement filtering and analysis, the data is processed inside a black box system. The system then transmits the preprocessed data to a centralized database of medical information. The implementation of federated learning occurs during the second phase, whereby several local models (U1 to U4) undergo training using local data but refrain from sharing the raw patient data. These locally developed models work together to enhance the global model. An application of the global model may include disease prediction or real-time emergency response. Figure 1 elucidates and describes the whole processing.

2.2 Data Cleaning

Data cleaning refers to a systematic way of detecting and correcting errors or inconsistencies within a dataset in order to enhance its quality and dependability for analytical purposes. This process encompasses several stages, including eliminating redundant entries, rectifying errors, managing missing information, and standardizing data formats to guarantee consistency. In data cleaning, the objective is to remove any unnecessary or irrelevant data that may have negative effects on the outcomes of data analysis, machine learning models, or decision-making procedures. Data cleansing is an important phase in the data preprocessing pipeline because it improves the overall quality of insights obtained from the data by verifying its accuracy, completeness, and correct formatting.

2.3 Proposed FuFT Methodology

This study comes up with a new way to improve the reliability and efficiency of Wireless Body Area Networks (WBANs) in healthcare settings. It combines federated learning with an edge-based real-time processing architecture. Federated learning is used to facilitate networked training of machine learning models directly on edge devices, therefore maintaining data confidentiality and minimizing the requirement for large data transfers to central servers. In order to tackle the difficulties posed by network instability and fluctuating device availability, we provide FedTolerant, a fault-tolerant algorithm carefully developed to function within federated learning frameworks. FedTolerant improves the learning process's resilience by interactively adapting to the accessibility of edge devices, ensuring consistent model training even when devices malfunction or unstable network conditions arise. This methodology, named Fusion-based Fed Tolerant (FuFT), not only enhances the precision of the model, attaining higher accuracy also (Fig. 2 and Table 1) .

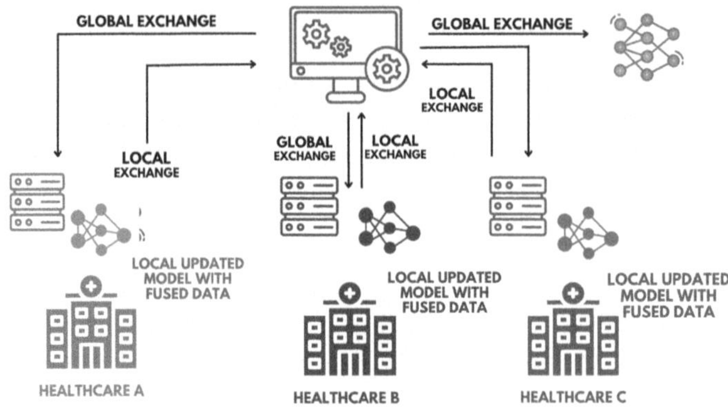

Fig. 2. FuFT Methodology.

Algorithm 1: Proposed Fault-Tolerant FedAvg Algorithm

Input: Global Model, Data accquired Clients, Number of Rounds, Fault Tolerance Parameters
Output: Updated global model, Broadcast of updated model to local models

Initialise Fraction Fit = 0.5, Learning Rate=0.1.
for $round \leftarrow 1$ to n in Number of Round(s) **do**
  Client Selection, select (Fraction Fit * Clients) clients
  Send Global Model parameters to each client
  Local Updates = []
  for $clients \leftarrow 1$ to N in selected clients list **do**
    For each client, initialise Fault Tolerance Parameters. *If* timeout expires, re-iterate local updates to be appended within trial-limit, *else* fail the client for round.
    train $client_i$ on weights from the global model
    Local Updates[i] $\leftarrow$ Parameters from $trainedclient_i$
    Average_Value $\leftarrow$ Σ Local Updates / Number of Clients
    Global Updates = []
    for $i \leftarrow 1$ to N in global model weights **do**
      w = $weight_i$ + learning rate * Average_Value
      Global Updates[i] $\leftarrow$ w
    end for
  end for
  Broadcast the updated Global Model to Client List
end for

This algorithm's Fault Tolerance methodology allows the system to continue, by either excluding the client for that round or repeating updates within a trial limit even if some clients don't return updates within the permitted timeout. After this, the global model aggregation process is kept reliable and is not entirely disrupted by problems from specific clients. To maintain consistent performance and stability across rounds, the algorithm achieves robustness by minimizing the effects of client failures or delays on the overall model. These features combine to make the algorithm suitable for real-world federated learning scenarios where network reliability and client availability are uncertain.

3 Experimental Evaluation

In this section ,we discuss experimental setup, Results and Comparitive analysis.

3.1 Experimental Setup

The experiment is conducted on Windows 10 that has the Intel Xeon CPU with a Clock Speed of 2.30 GHz and 2 cores each with hyperthreading and thus 4 virtual cores. The experiment utilizes Python version 3.10.12 and many other libraries. To build the neural network for centralised training, we are utilising PyTorch version 2.3.1+cu121, along with its corresponding vision module Torchvision version 0.1.1+cu121. To bolster intricate computations, we are utilising the popular Python framework Numpy 1.26.4. Finally, we have utilise Flower version 1.10.0 to not only accesss federated learning algorithms but also refurnish hyperparameters to extract complex and non convex relationships among the patterns of ECG images. The proposed FaultTolerant algorithm utilises FaultTolerant FedAverage algorithm with selection of 50 percent of available clients for the purpose of training as well as the evaluation of the federated learning strategy and development of the privacy rich global model. For assured development through learning and processing in every round, the minimum requirement of the number of clients required for training and testing is set to 1, i.e. the system runs even when we have a single client.

We are running the experiments on 10, and 20 clients and trained for the duration of 10 short rounds. The proposed algorithm is developed on publically available dataset encompassing of 7767 images of Electrocardiogram (ECG) of two types of Myocardial Infraction ECG images. Each of the images are of Portable Network Graphics (PNG) in size 432px$times$288px with a single channel ranging its values from 0 to 255. For the preparation of dataset, a zip file is created which contains the images titled 'AB.png' where A is either M or N and B is a numeric entry (0, 1, 2...) and a Comma Seperated Value containing file names and their corresponding target label. The dataset is balanced, with 4529 images of M and 3238 images of N. All of the 7767 images underwent the mentioned data preprocessing of image normalisation, resizing. For the evaluation of strategies, we are utilising the ubiquitous Accuracy and Cross Entropy and Adaptive Momentum (ADAM) optimisation. Accuracy is appropriately utilised due to balanced dataset.

For the evaluation of strategies, the omnipresent metric, Accuracy, is used along with Cross Entropy Loss and Adaptive Momentum (ADAM) optimisation. Since the dataset is well balanced, Accuracy can be employed without any demurring, calculating the divisions of correct predictions by total. To assert the development of an austere division between target classes, Cross Entropy is utilized.

3.2 Results and Comparitive Analysis

The proposed algorithm is evaluated on the mentioned metrics. The simulation of the centralised training as well as the federated strategies are perfomed with the mentioned technical libraries.

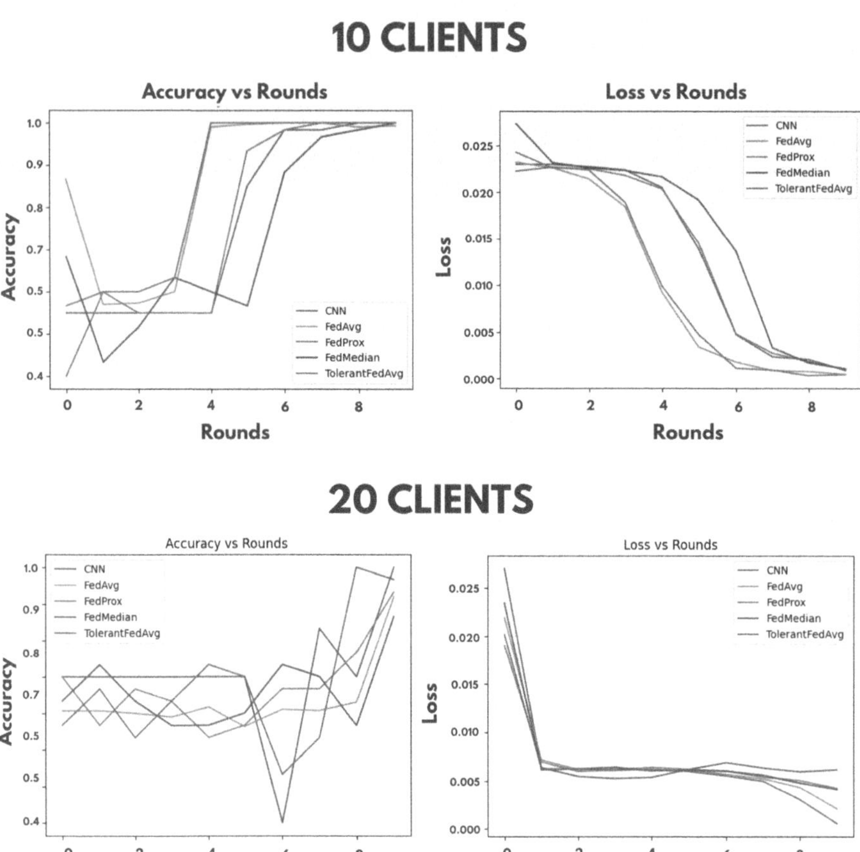

Fig. 3. xxx

With the accompanied metric tables for comparision and analysis, we find that for both simulations involving 10 and 20 clients, Fault Taulerant Federated Average gives the best performance in terms of achieving the maximum accuracy and least binary cross entropy loss.

Table 2. Evaluation Metric Results for Centralised Federated Learning Based Models

Method - 10 Clients	Accuracy	Loss
Centralised Training (CNN)	1.0	0.0009
FedAvg	0.9933	0.0005
FedProx	1.0	0.001
FedMedian	1.0	0.0012
Fault Tolerant FedAvg	1.0	0.0004
Method - 20 Clients	Accuracy	Loss
Centralised Training (CNN)	1.0	0.0223
FedAvg	0.92	0.0142
FedProx	0.9333	0.0185
FedMedian	0.8666	0.0183
Fault Tolerant FedAvg	0.9667	0.0112

• **Centralised Training :** The Convolution Neural Network is a classical multilayer perceptron for images which utilises dual layer convolution layers interlaced with a unit maximum pooling layers and finally integrated with a Rectifier Linear unit activated artificial neural network. For 10 clients, the algorithm achieves an accuracy of 1.0 and a loss value of 8.6e-4. For 20 clients, we achieve an accuracy of 1.0 as well while the loss value is 0.022 (Fig. 3.).

• **Federated Average :** The Federated Average algorithm is a popular federated learning methodology involving transfer of data from local clients towards a distributed global model. Through initialisation of the global model followed by training of local systems and refurbish the server amalgams the data by averaging the data for the creation of a fresh model for the next iteration or round. From the table (Table 2) and plots, FedAvg achieves an accuracy of 0.99 and a loss of 4.4e-4 for 10 clients, while an accuracy of 0.92 and 0.014 loss metric for 20 clients (Fig. 3.).

• **Federated Prox :** The Federated Prox is an algorithm which applies federated learning on non independent and identically distributed datasets. Utilising a compatible introduction of regularisation to prod local networks to train in order to estimate and achieve weights closer to the global models. For 10 clients, FedProx achieves an accuracy of 1.0 and a loss of 9.67e-4 while an accuracy of 0.93 and 0.0185 loss metric for 20 clients (Fig. 3.).

• **Federated Median :** The Federated Median algorithm improvises on Federated Average by using a compatible proxy by replacing the calculations by taking the median of clients to promote model's intractability against outliers and biases. The table (Table 2) and plots showcase that FedMedian achieves an accuracy of 1.0 and a loss of 1.05e-3 for 10 clients, while an accuracy of 0.867 and 0.0182 loss metric for 20 clients (Fig. 3.).

• **Fault Taularent FedAvg (Proposed) :** A relatively new strategy based on the workings of FedAvg, Fault Tolerant FedAvg aims to develop the federated strategy while it's predominant aim on involved and tortuous robustness. From the table (Table 2) and plots, FedTaulerant Average achieves an accuracy of 1.0 and a loss of 4.3e-4 for 10 clients while an accuracy of 0.97 and 0.011 loss metric for 20 clients (Fig. 3.).

In summary, the four graphs demonstrate the following. For 10 clients, the accuracy and loss plots indicate that Fault Taularent FedAvg demonstrate smoother and more consistent rise in accuracy in comparision to other models, and that the Fault Taularent FedAvg algorithm is better when effectively aggregating updates and alleviating faults. For 20 clients, Fault Taularent, after a few initial fluctuations, indicate more robust improvements, while the loss curve demonstrates how the consistent performance of TaularentFedAvg highlights its fault-tolerance capability in large-scale federated learning setups.

4 Conclusion

The integration of edge computing and WBANs is a notable progress in real-time data processing, particularly in health monitoring applications. Utilizing a fault-tolerant algorithm with a 97% accuracy rate, effectively manage and process substantial amounts of data at the network's edge. This integration not only decreases latency but also improves the dependability and precision of data transmission, which is essential for real-time decision-making in medical and other time-sensitive applications. The results indicate that the combination of these technologies can result in more resilient and responsive systems, facilitating future advancements in smart healthcare and real-time monitoring systems.

References

1. Khan, L.U., et al.: Edge-Computing-Enabled smart cities: a comprehensive survey. IEEE Internet Things J. **7**(10), 10200–10232 (2020). https://doi.org/10.1109/JIOT.2020.2987070
2. Amin, S.U., Hossain, M.S.: Edge intelligence and internet of things in healthcare: a survey. IEEE Access **9**, 45–59 (2021). https://doi.org/10.1109/ACCESS.2020.3045115
3. Joshi, A.M., Jain, P., Mohanty, S.P.: iGLU: Non-invasive device for continuous glucose measurement with IoMT framework. IEEE Comput. Soc. Ann. Symp. VLSI (ISVLSI) **2020**, 598–599 (2020). https://doi.org/10.1109/ISVLSI49217.2020.00092
4. Joshi, A.M., Jain, P., Mohanty, S.P.: (2022). iGLU 3.0: a secure noninvasive glucometer and automatic insulin delivery system in IoMT. IEEE Trans. Consum. Electron. **68**(1), 14–22. https://doi.org/10.1109/TCE.2022.3145055
5. Olokodana, I.L., Mohanty, S.P., Kougianos, E., Sherratt, R.S.: EZcap: a novel wearable for real-time automated seizure detection from EEG signals. IEEE Trans. Consum. Electron. **67**(2), 166–175 (2021). https://doi.org/10.1109/TCE.2021.3079399
6. Sharma, G., Joshi, A.M., Yadav, D., Mohanty, S.P.: A smart healthcare framework for accurate detection of Schizophrenia using multichannel EEG. IEEE Trans. Instrum. Meas. **72**, 1–9 (2023). https://doi.org/10.1109/TIM.2023.3293544

7. Rachakonda, L., Mohanty, S. P., Kougianos, E.: Stress-Lysis: an IoMT-enabled device for automatic stress level detection from physical activities. In: 2020 IEEE International Symposium on Smart Electronic Systems (ISES) (Formerly INiS), pp. 204–205 (2020). https://doi.org/10.1109/iSES50453.2020.00052
8. Rachakonda, L., Bapatla, A.K., Mohanty, S.P., Kougianos, E.: SaYoPillow: blockchain- integrated privacy-assured IoMT framework for stress management considering sleeping habits. IEEE Trans. Consum. Electron. **67**(1), 20–29 (2021). https://doi.org/10.1109/TCE.2020.3043683
9. Alqahtani, A., Alsubai, S., Bhatia, M.: IoT–edge–cloud-assisted intelligent framework for controlling dengue. IEEE Internet Things J. **11**(9), 15682–15689 (2024). https://doi.org/10.1109/JIOT.2023.3348101
10. Chakraborty, C., Kishor, A.: Real-Time cloud-based patient-centric monitoring using computational health systems. IEEE Trans. Comput. Soc. Syst. **9**(6), 1613–1623 (2022). https://doi.org/10.1109/TCSS.2022.3170375
11. Adhikari, M., Hazra, A., Nandy, S.: Deep transfer learning for communicable disease detection and recommendation in edge networks. IEEE/ACM Trans. Comput. Biol. Bioinf. **20**(4), 2468–2479 (2023). https://doi.org/10.1109/TCBB.2022.3180393
12. Mukhopadhyay, S.C.: Wearable sensors for human activity monitoring: a review. IEEE Sens. J. **15**(3), 1321–1330 (2014)
13. Sethuraman, S.C., Kompally, P., Mohanty, S.P., Choppali, U.: MyWear: a novel smart garment for automatic continuous vital monitoring. IEEE Trans. Consum. Electron. **67**(3), 214–222 (2021)
14. Lian, Z., et al.: DEEP-FEL: decentralized, efficient and privacy-enhanced federated edge learning for healthcare cyber physical systems. IEEE Trans. Netw. Sci. Eng. **9**(5), 3558–3569 (2022). https://doi.org/10.1109/TNSE.2022.3175945
15. Chen, J.: Stroke risk prediction with hybrid deep transfer learning framework. IEEE J. Biomed. Health Inform. **26**(1), 411–422 (2022). https://doi.org/10.1109/JBHI.2021.3088750
16. Ma, C., Luo, G., Wang, K.: Concatenated and connected random forests with multiscale patch driven active contour model for automated brain tumor segmentation of MR images. IEEE Trans. Med. Imaging **37**(8), 1943–1954 (2018). https://doi.org/10.1109/TMI.2018.2805821
17. Zhang, S., Cicoira, F.: (2018) Flexible self-powered biosensors. Nature Publishing Group. Zhao, J., Xing, Z., Chen, Z., Wan, L., Han, T., Fu, H., Zhu, L: Uncertainty-Aware multi-dimensional mutual learning for brain and brain tumor segmentation. IEEE J. Biomed. Health Inform. **27**(9), 4362–4372 (2023). https://doi.org/10.1109/JBHI.2023.3274255

Improving Fault Detection in Wireless Body Area Networks with Ensemble AI and Explainable Components

P. Padmakumari[1](✉), M. Sujatha[2], Meghana Lellapalli[3], and S. Meerayasmin[3]

[1] SCORE, Vellore Institute of Technology, Vellore, Tamil Nadu, India
padmavijay3003@gmail.com
[2] SCOPE, Vellore Institute of Technology, Chennai, Tamil Nadu, India
[3] School of Computing, SASTRA Deemed University, Thanjavur, Tamil Nadu, India

Abstract. In Wireless Body Area Networks (WBAN), ensuring reliable and continuous monitoring of physiological signals is crucial, yet WBANs are prone to faults that can reduce accuracy. This paper introduces a hybrid approach to fault prediction that combines ensemble Artificial Intelligence (AI) techniques with Explainable AI (XAI) and Data Visualization to enhance accuracy, reliability, and interpretability. The ensemble approach, which integrates eight machine learning techniques, was selected to improve robustness and manage diverse data from multiple sensors. By leveraging the strengths of individual algorithms, the ensemble model captures complex patterns and interactions within sensor data, reducing the impact of sensor noise, single-sensor failures, and misclassifications. This integration not only increases fault prediction accuracy by more than 10% over traditional methods but also enhances the model's adaptability to heterogeneous data. To enhance model transparency, techniques like SHAP (SHapley Additive exPlanations) and LIME (Local Interpretable Model-agnostic Explanations) are utilized. These methods empower healthcare practitioners to decipher the impact of individual variables on predictive outcomes. SHAP, in particular, assigns an attribution score to each feature, illustrating its role in fault detection, while LIME provides interpretable, locally focused explanations for each prediction. This interpretability is essential for healthcare professionals, as it helps them understand model reasoning, facilitating more informed decisions and better patient outcomes. Additionally, data visualization enhances patient care and supports proactive decision-making by allowing healthcare providers to monitor predictive patterns. Comprehensive evaluations demonstrate the exceptional efficacy of the proposed framework, highlighting its advantages in precision, latency optimization, and resource utilization, making it a promising solution for improved fault tolerance in WBANs and underscoring the potential for more autonomous and intelligent solutions.

Keywords: WBAN · fault prediction · ensemble AI · Explainable AI · data visualization

K. Atul et al. (Eds.): BodyNets 2024, LNICST 666, pp. 148–168, 2026.
https://doi.org/10.1007/978-3-032-16099-7_14

1 Introduction

A Wireless Body Area Network (WBAN), also referred to as a Body Area Network (BAN), Body Sensor Network (BSN), or Medical Body Area Network (MBAN), represents a specialized wireless architecture composed of wearable or implantable smart devices (miniaturized sensors) which continuously monitor and gather diverse physiological metrics, including heart rate, body temperature, blood pressure, and glucose levels. These data streams can be relayed to remote medical practitioners or securely stored in the cloud for advanced analytics. The integration of WBAN technology facilitates tailored telemedicine solutions, significantly reduces healthcare expenditures by enabling proactive monitoring, and supports timely clinical interventions for early-stage health anomalies [1]. WBANs hold immense potential to transform healthcare by enabling continuous, real-time monitoring of patients. However, several technical challenges, including energy efficiency, fault tolerance, and security, need to be addressed to realize the full potential of this technology. Ongoing research in these areas is crucial for advancing WBANs and ensuring their reliability and effectiveness in healthcare applications can make WBAN become one of the backbone technologies of pervasive healthcare systems. Fault prediction in WBANs is crucial for ensuring the reliability and safety of the network. Given that WBANs are often used for monitoring critical health parameters, any failure in the network can have serious consequences. Fault prediction techniques help in identifying potential issues before they lead to network failures, thereby ensuring continuous and accurate monitoring of patients. WBANs are engineered for seamless health surveillance, supporting real-time acquisition and processing of physiological data. Ensuring data reliability through fault forecasting is crucial for preserving system integrity. Proactively identifying and addressing anomalies enables healthcare professionals to depend on accurate insights for informed clinical decision-making on patient's health, leading to better diagnosis and treatment outcomes. Fault prediction helps in optimizing the network performance of WBANs. By identifying and addressing potential faults, the network can maintain optimal performance levels, ensuring efficient data transmission and reducing latency. This is particularly important in scenarios where real-time data analysis is critical, such as in emergency response situations. Predictive maintenance is another significant benefit of fault prediction in WBANs. By identifying potential issues early, maintenance can be scheduled proactively, reducing the need for emergency repairs and minimizing downtime. This not only enhances the reliability of the network but also reduces the overall maintenance costs. Several techniques can be employed for fault prediction in WBANs. These techniques leverage various methodologies; including machine learning, statistical analysis, and heuristic approaches. Fault prediction in WBANs is increasingly leveraging machine learning methodologies, which analyse historical datasets to uncover patterns and relationships indicative of potential failures. Advanced approaches, including neural networks, support vector machines, and decision tree models, have demonstrated significant accuracy in forecasting faults. For instance, a machine learning framework can be trained on past sensor data to anticipate events like battery exhaustion or hardware anomalies. By continuously monitoring the sensor data, the model can provide early warnings of potential issues, allowing for timely intervention. Statistical methods are also widely used for fault prediction. Advanced techniques like regression modelling, time-series forecasting, and probabilistic frameworks are employed to detect patterns and outliers in sensor data. Often, a hybrid approach combining multiple methodologies is utilized to enhance the precision and robustness of fault prediction. These methods are particularly useful for detecting gradual degradation in sensor performance, such as a slow decline in battery voltage or sensor accuracy. Heuristic approaches involve using predefined rules and thresholds to predict faults. For instance, a heuristic rule may state that if the battery voltage drops below a certain level, it is likely to fail soon. These approaches are often combined with other techniques to enhance their accuracy and reliability. In practice, a combination of different techniques is often used to achieve more accurate and reliable fault predictions. Hybrid approaches leverage the strengths of various methods, such as combining machine learning with statistical analysis, to improve fault prediction performance. A prominent application of WBANs lies in managing chronic conditions such as diabetes, cardiovascular diseases, and respiratory disorders. Fault predictions techniques ensure that the sensors and devices used in these networks operate reliably, providing continuous monitoring and timely alerts to healthcare providers. Fault prediction algorithms can detect issues such as sensor calibration errors or communication failures, ensuring that accurate data is available for making treatment decisions. WBANs are also extensively used in elderly care to monitor vital signs and detect falls or other emergencies. Fault prediction ensures that these networks operate reliably, providing continuous monitoring and timely alerts to caregivers and family members. For example, a WBAN used for fall detection in elderly patients can predict sensor malfunctions or battery depletion, ensuring that the system is always ready to detect and respond to emergencies. In sports science, WBANs are used to monitor athletes' performance and health parameters during training and competitions. Fault prediction techniques help in maintaining the accuracy and reliability of the data collected, enabling coaches and trainers to make informed decisions about training programs and injury prevention. For instance, a WBAN used to monitor an athlete's heart rate and movement during training can predict potential sensor failures, ensuring that accurate data is available for performance analysis. A prototype for fault management has been implemented, leveraging diverse machine learning techniques, including Artificial Neural Networks (ANN), Recurrent Neural Networks (RNN), Support Vector Machines (SVM), Decision Trees (DT), and Deep Neural Networks (DNN). And these techniques are ensemble using Random Forest and Gradient Boosting methods to improve the accuracy. Additionally, Explainable AI and Data Visualisation are used within the prototype. The key innovations of this prototype are summarized in the following steps:

1. Introduce a Robust Fault-Management Framework: Develop an architecture incorporating AI/ML algorithms customized for WBAN-specific requirements.
2. Enhance Fault Resilience: Establish an ML-powered pipeline for improving fault tolerance, including automated workflows for model training, validation, and deployment.
3. Empirical Validation of Models: Evaluate the performance of predictive models such as ANN, RNN, SVM, DT, and DNN with real-world data.

4. Ensemble Learning and Explainability: Combine individual models using ensemble strategies like Random Forest and Gradient Boosting to enhance prediction accuracy, while integrating Explainable AI (XAI) and advanced data visualization for better interpretability.

2 Related Works

A multi-tier edge computing framework was introduced in [2] to enable secure and low-latency detection of emergencies. This framework utilized a unified data representation, a detailed detection mechanism employing Recurrent Neural Networks (RNN) in the cloud and a threshold-driven fault detection mechanism on the edge node was introduced. While this dual-layered approach showcased innovation, its feasibility was challenged due to the requirement of training models at both the edge and the cloud levels. In contrast, cooperative communication and network coding techniques were implemented by the authors of [3, 4] to mitigate channel impairments and counteract body fading effects. However, their solution lacked the incorporation of any artificial intelligence methods. In [5], fault management in IoT networks was explored by leveraging sensors with diverse functionalities. The authors utilized regression techniques were employed to model virtual services, alongside an adaptive sensing strategy designed to ensure resilience and fault tolerance within IoT ecosystems. Nevertheless, this methodology was not applicable to smart healthcare systems. Sensor fault detection was addressed in [6] using diverse methodologies, including rule-based systems, estimations, time-series forecasting, and machine learning algorithms, were utilized for fault prediction and management. Their findings highlighted that rule-based strategies could achieve high accuracy, depending on the selected parameters, whereas machine learning methods were effective for classification and detection of faults. However, these methods faced challenges such as cumbersome training processes, and estimation techniques struggled with consistent fault classification. A Visual Monitoring System for Fault Tolerance (VMSFT) was proposed in [7, 8], introduced a real-time sensor monitoring solution for WBANs, capable of proactively addressing sensor malfunctions. Built on a cloud-centric Infrastructure as a Service (IaaS) model, VMSFT's operations were constrained by geographic limitations. Reliability Modelling study of Anomaly Detection Algorithms for Wireless Body Area Networks provided a framework on [9] for detecting and predicting faults. But this anomaly detection algorithm might generate false positives or negatives, leading to incorrect fault predictions. The Autonomic Resource Provisioning Framework for Cloudlet-Enabled WBANs [10] introduced a proactive fuzzy logic-based methodology to optimize resource allocation, enhancing data collection efficiency, but it requires extensive tuning of membership functions and rules, which can be challenging. The framework's reliance on cloudlets introduces latency and potential security concerns. An Artificial Intelligence-Driven Fault Prediction Framework was proposed [11], leveraging AI methods such as Artificial Neural Networks (ANN), Deep Neural Networks (DNN), Support Vector Machines (SVM), and Decision Trees (DT) to address fault detection and ensure system reliability but their accuracy is greater than 94% and our study is to increase the accuracy rate by adding new models and methods alongside the existing 4 techniques.

3 Ensemble-Enabled Fault Prediction System

This section outlines our proposed framework for fault prediction in a Wireless Body Area Network (WBAN) designed for healthcare monitoring. The approach utilizes a blend of machine learning methodologies, including Gradient Boosting (GB), Random Forest (RF), Recurrent Neural Network (RNN), Decision Tree (DT), Support Vector Machine (SVM), Artificial Neural Network (ANN), and Deep Neural Network (DNN). Through an ensemble strategy, the framework synergizes the strengths of these techniques to deliver a more precise and robust predictive model. Additionally, Explainable AI (XAI) methodologies such as SHAP and LIME were integrated to enhance interpretability by shedding light on the most influential features driving model predictions, ensuring the model's outputs have transparency in the decision-making process and are trustworthy. Figure 1 illustrates the workflow of our ensemble-enabled fault prediction system.

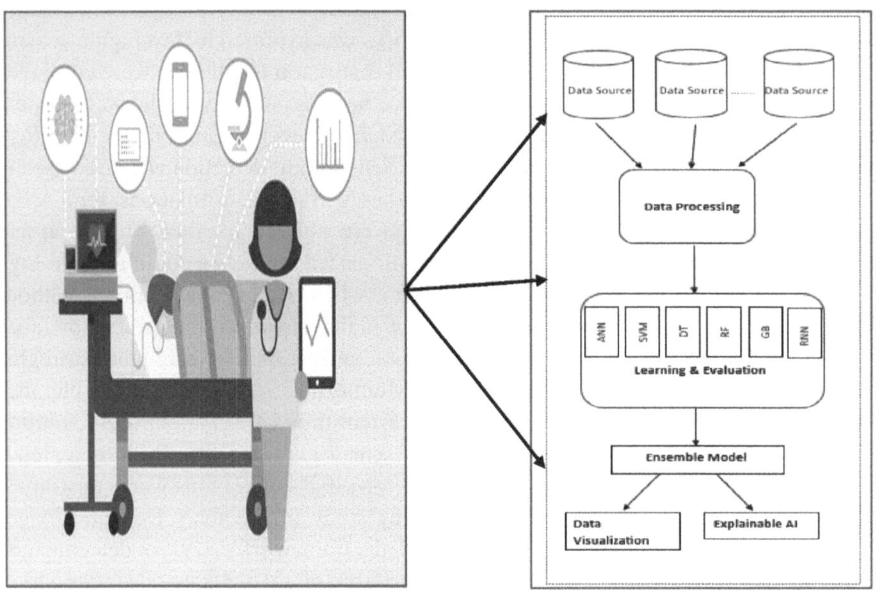

Fig. 1. Ensemble Enabled Fault Prediction system

In this framework, we incorporated various features outlined in Table 1. The model utilizes parameters such as the patient's Sensor ID, Heart Rate, Oxygen Saturation (SpO2) levels, Battery Voltage, Body Temperature, Signal Strength, RSSI (Received Signal Strength Indicator), and device status to develop AI/Deep Learning algorithms. These components were further integrated into an ensemble model achieving an accuracy >98%.

Table 1. Dataset

S. No.	Attribute	S. No.	Attribute
1	Sensor ID	5	Temperature
2	Heart Rate	6	Signal strength
3	SpO2 levels	7	RSSI
4	Battery voltage	8	Status

3.1 Dataset Collection and Manipulation

For data preprocessing, we used python packages: pandas and numpy [12]. The dataset was read using load_data function. Then data cleaning was performed to handle any missing or erroneous values. For the splitting of data, we used train_test_split function in sklearn to partition the dataset into training and testing subsets, followed by scaling to normalize the data for improved model performance. Then the data is scaled using StandardScaler. The data is reshaped accordingly for required ML models and then used for building of the model.

3.2 Model Building

The models were given the arguments input shape and number of classes and models were trained for 50 epochs with 32 as batch size to optimize learning. Prediction and evaluation were then made on the test data which were then converted to class labels. The class labels were used to give the classification report and accuracy score [13].

Support Vector Machine (SVM) Model

The Support Vector Machine (SVM) algorithm, a classification-based supervised learning approach, was implemented for high accurate fault detection [14]. Using Kmeans clustering we had divided number of classes to 2 so that the hyperplane would be a line which was then used to determine the most reasonable choice. The overall accuracy this model achieved was 99%.

Decision Tree (DT) Model

Being easily understood because of its tree-like structure we had adopted this model [15]. It uses the concept of Decision node and leaf node which helped us to identify a decision and an output. The DT uses CART (Classification And Regression Tree) algorithm to get all possible solutions for given conditions. The accuracy acquired was 100%.

Artificial Neural Network (ANN) Model

Mimicking a biological neural network, ANN has nodes interconnected in various layers of network [16]. ANN has three layers: input layer, two hidden layers, and an output layer to optimize performance. The data was given at the input layer, calculations were done in the hidden layers and finally an output was given based on the calculations. Due to its predictability rate even with inadequate data and higher fault tolerance this model was chosen. The total accuracy obtained using this model was 100%.

Recurrent Neural Network (RNN) Model
This model additionally encapsulates looping nodes with a hidden layer that easily helped us to predict the next set of inputs and validate its accuracy [17]. The hidden feature remembers some information about a sequence and uses it in the later predictions. Since it uses the same parameters RNN has lesser complexity compared to other neural networks. We have used version Long Short-Term Memory (LSTM) to improve RNN's ability to better manage long-term dependencies in sequential data. The accuracy was 100%

Gradient Boosting
The main reason to use this algorithm was for its prediction speed and accuracy, particularly for large and complex datasets such as ours. The model combines weak learners and continuously minimizes errors to improve overall prediction performance [15]. The model was created with 100 estimators and trained using the training data. The accuracy achieved using this model was 100%.

Random Forest
For the Random Forest model, 100 estimators were constructed using randomized subsets of the dataset (configured with random_state = 42). This randomness mitigates overfitting by diversifying individual decision trees, thereby enhancing overall predictive accuracy [18]. The accuracy score for this model was 100%.

Ensemble Model
The ensemble model here has combined models of RNN, GB, RF, SVM, ANN and DT using stacking method [19]. Predictions from all models are combined into a single matrix using meta model. Linear Regression approach has been used to combine the predictions of these sub-models and get a generic accuracy and classification report. The total accuracy of the combined models has turned out to be 99.98%

3.3 Explainable AI

To improve model transparency and trust, Explainable AI techniques such as SHAP and LIME were employed [20]. SHAP utilizes game theory to assign feature importance scores based on their contribution to the model's predictions whereas LIME generates localized interpretability by approximating the complex model using interpretable surrogate model. These tools helped us interpret the predictions and understand which features (such as heart rate, temperature, or battery voltage) played the most significant roles in fault prediction. K-means clustering was used to partition the dataset into two clusters, with one cluster showing higher prediction probability for 'Status' and the other for 'SpO2'. This is visualized in the prediction graph produced by SHAP, delivering granular insights into the decision-making process, with XAI results highlighting key patterns and feature contributions. The results of the XAI models can be seen in Fig. 2, which shows the workflow of the proposed system, and Fig. 16, which displays the SHAP-based prediction graph. Figure 2 illustrate the workflow of the Ensemble enabled proposed model.

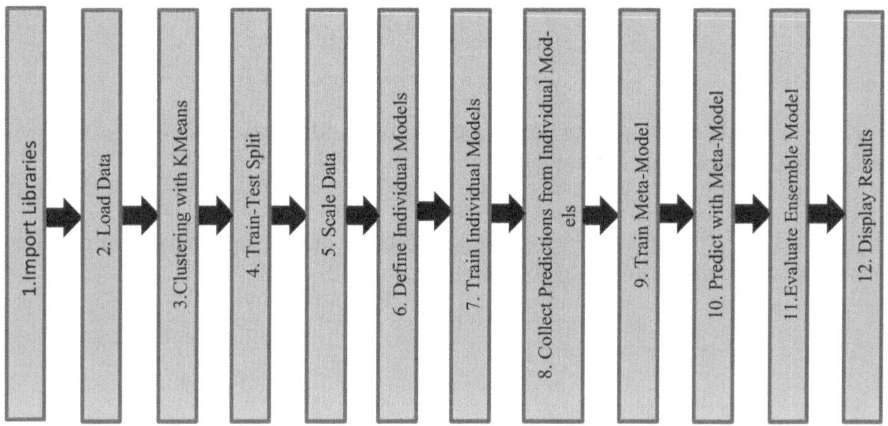

Fig. 2. Workflow of Proposed model

4 Experimental Analysis

This title includes the experiments conducted to build an ensemble model using various ML models. We divide the model into three parts: The ensemble of ML models deployed, the data visualization generated for each model and explainable AI for the given dataset. We will explore the data set used, the experimental procedure and result analysis.

4.1 Evaluation Methods

In our ML model, metrics such as F1 score and classification accuracy are used to evaluate performance of the model.

$$Accuracy = \frac{TP + TN}{N} \tag{1}$$

$$Precision = \frac{TP}{TP + FP} \tag{2}$$

$$Recall = \frac{TP}{TP + FN} \tag{3}$$

$$F1 - score = 2 * \frac{Recall * Precision}{Recall + Precision} \tag{4}$$

$$FalseAlarmRate = \frac{FP}{FP + TN} \tag{5}$$

Here, N represent the total number of instances in the dataset. TP (True Positive) refers to the count of correctly identified positive cases, while TN (True Negative) denotes the count of correctly identified negative cases. FP (False Positive) represents the instances incorrectly classified as positive when they are actually negative, and FN (False Negative) captures the instances mistakenly classified as negative despite being positive.

4.2 Ensemble Model

For each model, the prediction can be represented as:

$$\hat{y}_{i,j} = f_j(X_i) \tag{6}$$

where:

- $\hat{y}_{i,j}$ is the predicted output for the ith sample by the jth model.
- f_j is the function representing the jth model (e.g., DT, RF)
- X_i is the input feature vector for the ith sample.

Figure 3, 4, 5, 6, 7, and 8 are snippets taken from the model that give us the predictions for various models that we have incorporated.

```
Classification Report:
              precision    recall  f1-score   support

           0       1.00      1.00      1.00      3646
           1       1.00      1.00      1.00       569
           2       1.00      1.00      1.00      1706

    accuracy                           1.00      5921
   macro avg       1.00      1.00      1.00      5921
weighted avg       1.00      1.00      1.00      5921

Accuracy: 1.0
```

Fig. 3. DT Classification Report

```
SVM Accuracy: 0.9947643979057592
SVM Classification Report:
              precision    recall  f1-score   support

           0       1.00      1.00      1.00      4646
           1       0.99      0.99      0.99      1275

    accuracy                           0.99      5921
   macro avg       0.99      0.99      0.99      5921
weighted avg       0.99      0.99      0.99      5921
```

Fig. 4. SVM Classification Report

Classification Report:

	precision	recall	f1-score	support
0	1.00	1.00	1.00	3646
1	1.00	1.00	1.00	569
2	1.00	1.00	1.00	1706
accuracy			1.00	5921
macro avg	1.00	1.00	1.00	5921
weighted avg	1.00	1.00	1.00	5921

Accuracy: 1.0

Fig. 5. ANN Classification Report

Classification Report:

	precision	recall	f1-score	support
1	1.00	1.00	1.00	3646
2	1.00	1.00	1.00	569
3	1.00	1.00	1.00	1706
accuracy			1.00	5921
macro avg	1.00	1.00	1.00	5921
weighted avg	1.00	1.00	1.00	5921

Accuracy: 1.0

Fig. 6. RNN Classification Report

Classification Report:

	precision	recall	f1-score	support
1	1.00	1.00	1.00	3646
2	1.00	1.00	1.00	569
3	1.00	1.00	1.00	1706
accuracy			1.00	5921
macro avg	1.00	1.00	1.00	5921
weighted avg	1.00	1.00	1.00	5921

Accuracy: 1.0

Fig. 7. RF Classification Report

```
Classification Report:
              precision    recall  f1-score   support

           0       1.00      1.00      1.00      3646
           1       1.00      1.00      1.00       569
           2       1.00      1.00      1.00      1706

    accuracy                           1.00      5921
   macro avg       1.00      1.00      1.00      5921
weighted avg       1.00      1.00      1.00      5921

Accuracy: 1.0
```

Fig. 8. GB Classification Report

In stacking, the predictions from different models are combined as inputs to a meta-model:

$$Z_i = \left[\hat{y}_{i,1}, \hat{y}_{i,2} \cdots\cdots \hat{y}_{i,m}\right] \tag{7}$$

where:

- Z_i is the vector of predictions for the ith sample from all m base models.

The meta model g then makes the final prediction:

$$\hat{y}_i = g(Z_i) \tag{8}$$

For the logistic regression meta-model:

$$\hat{y}_i = \sigma\left(\sum_{j=1}^{m} \beta_j \hat{y}_{i,j} + \beta_0\right) \tag{9}$$

where:

- βj are the coefficients learned by the logistic regression.

- β_0 is the intercept term.
- $\sigma(x)$ is the sigmoid function,

$$\sigma(x) = \frac{1}{1 + e^{-x}} \tag{10}$$

Table 2 gives the individual model report on precision, recall, accuracy and F1 score of various models implemented.

Table 2. Classification report and accuracy of models implemented

S. No.	Model name	Index	Precision	Recall	F1 Score	Accuracy
1	SVM	0	1.00	1.00	1.00	0.9947643979057592
		1	0.99	0.99	0.99	
2	DT	0	1.00	1.00	1.00	0.9993244384394528
		1	1.00	1.00	1.00	
3	ANN	0	0.99	0.99	0.99	0.9896976862016551
		1	0.97	0.98	0.98	
4	RNN	0	0.99	0.99	0.99	0.98733322073974
		1	0.97	0.97	0.97	
5	RF	0	1.00	1.00	1.00	0.9996622192197264
		1	1.00	1.00	1.00	
6	GB	0	1.00	1.00	1.00	0.9996622192197264
		1	1.00	1.00	1.00	
7	Ensemble	0	1.00	1.00	1.00	0.9998311096098632
		1	1.00	1.00	1.00	

Figure 9 and 10 represent the stacked precisions and accuracies in the meta model and overall ensemble accuracy.

RandomForest Accuracy: 0.9996622192197264

	precision	recall	f1-score	support
0	1.00	1.00	1.00	4646
1	1.00	1.00	1.00	1275
accuracy			1.00	5921
macro avg	1.00	1.00	1.00	5921
weighted avg	1.00	1.00	1.00	5921

GradientBoosting Accuracy: 0.9996622192197264

	precision	recall	f1-score	support
0	1.00	1.00	1.00	4646
1	1.00	1.00	1.00	1275
accuracy			1.00	5921
macro avg	1.00	1.00	1.00	5921
weighted avg	1.00	1.00	1.00	5921

DecisionTree Accuracy: 0.9993244384394528

	precision	recall	f1-score	support
0	1.00	1.00	1.00	4646
1	1.00	1.00	1.00	1275
accuracy			1.00	5921
macro avg	1.00	1.00	1.00	5921
weighted avg	1.00	1.00	1.00	5921

SVC Accuracy: 0.9947643979057592

	precision	recall	f1-score	support
0	1.00	1.00	1.00	4646
1	0.99	0.99	0.99	1275
accuracy			0.99	5921
macro avg	0.99	0.99	0.99	5921
weighted avg	0.99	0.99	0.99	5921

LogisticRegression Accuracy: 0.9989866576591792

	precision	recall	f1-score	support
0	1.00	1.00	1.00	4646
1	1.00	1.00	1.00	1275
accuracy			1.00	5921
macro avg	1.00	1.00	1.00	5921
weighted avg	1.00	1.00	1.00	5921

Fig. 9. Classification Report

```
Ensemble Accuracy: 0.9998311096098632
Ensemble Classification Report:
              precision    recall  f1-score   support

           0       1.00      1.00      1.00      4646
           1       1.00      1.00      1.00      1275

    accuracy                           1.00      5921
   macro avg       1.00      1.00      1.00      5921
weighted avg       1.00      1.00      1.00      5921
```

Fig. 10. Ensemble Classification Report

4.3 Data Visualization

Various data visualization models are used for better understanding of the given datasets. We have mainly used the matplotlib and seaborn libraries to generate confusion matrix, important features and a plot comparing the accuracies against the models implemented. Correlation matrices have also been given for a few models. All these helped us determine the important features in the dataset and how the machine learning model functions. The graphs and matrices have been given below for reference.

Figures 11, 12, 13, and 14 represent confusion matrices of employed models which gives a breakdown of difference in models' predictions to the actual outcome.

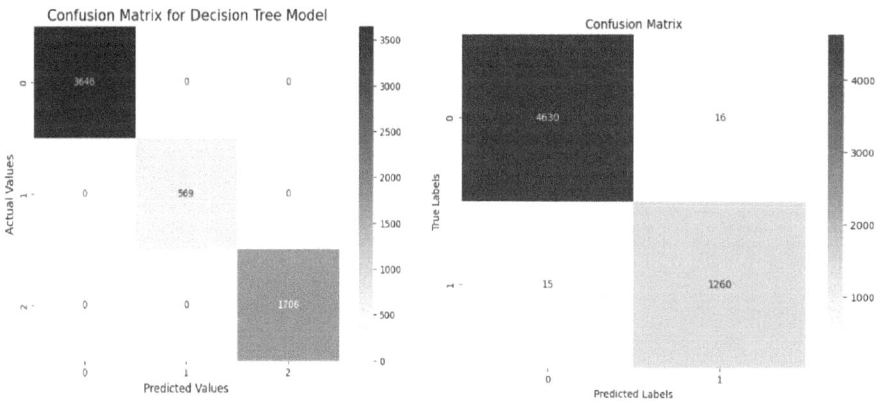

Fig. 11. Confusion matrix of DT and SVM model

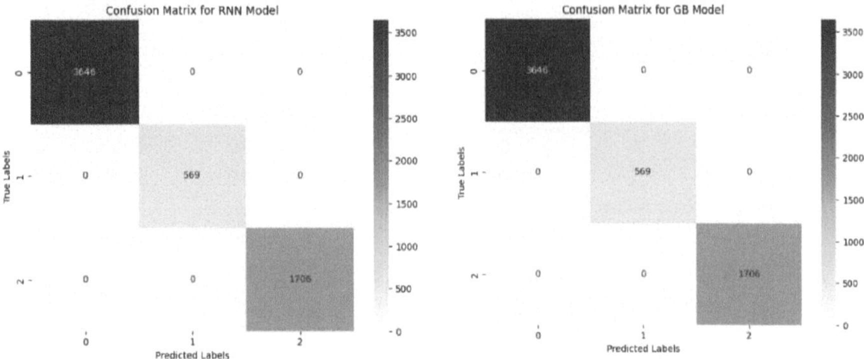

Fig. 12. Confusion matrix of RNN and GB model

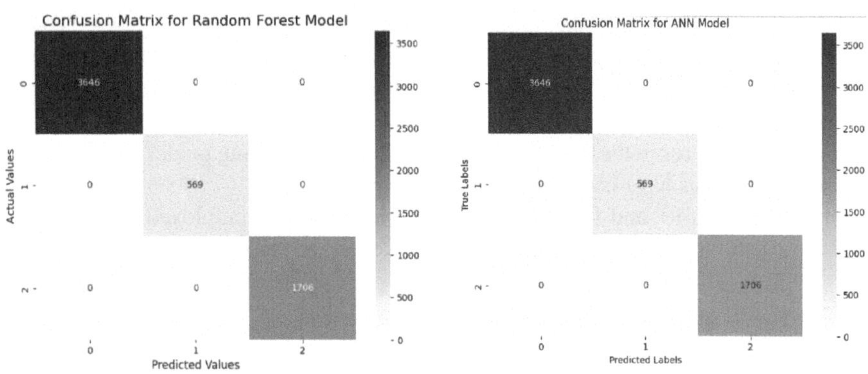

Fig. 13. Confusion matrix of RF and ANN model

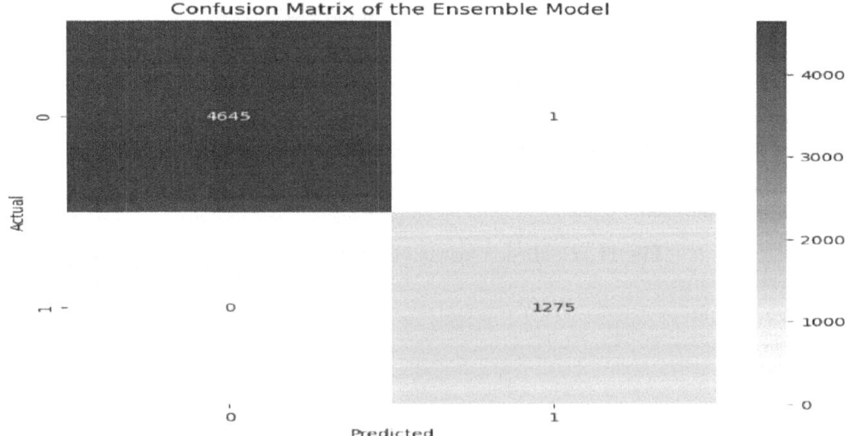

Fig. 14. Confusion matrix for Ensemble model

Figure 15 gives the heatmap which is the correlation between dataset attributes.

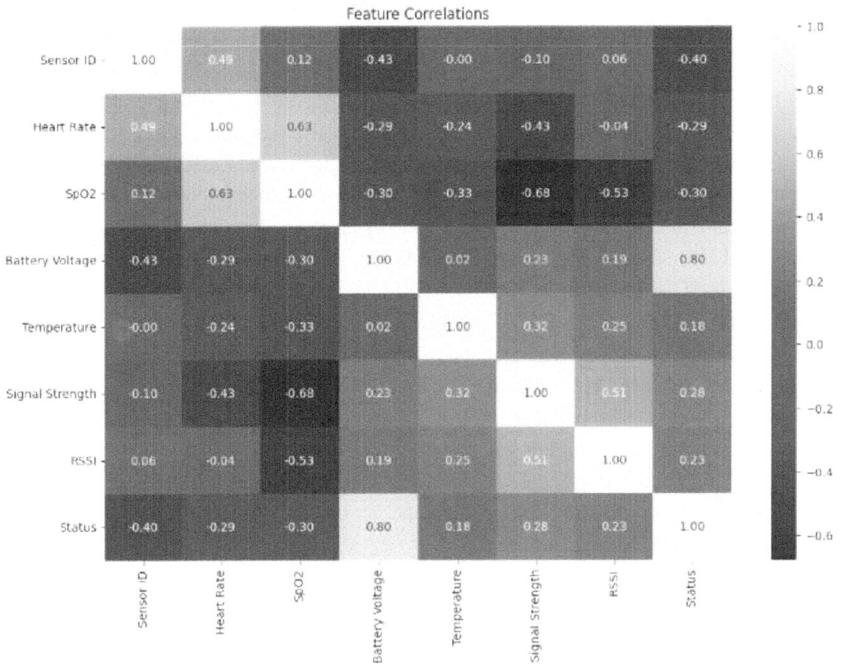

Fig. 15. Heatmap

4.4 Analysis of Explainable AI

After reviewing several cutting-edge Explainable AI (XAI) methodologies to enhance the transparency of high-performing machine learning (ML) models, particularly in healthcare applications involving tabular data, we have opted for SHAP and LIME. SHAP is a foundational XAI technique derived from the principles of cooperative game theory, framing a prediction problem as a game, with features acting as players and all potential subsets of features forming the coalitions. SHAP calculates the importance of features by assessing their average marginal contribution to predictions, offering strong theoretical grounds for aggregating local interpretations into broader, global insights. LIME, on the other hand, is another widely utilized model-agnostic approach for local interpretability. It elucidates complex models by approximating them with an interpretable surrogate model, typically a sparse linear regression, in the vicinity of the data instance being explained. The regression coefficients derived from LIME are then leveraged as indicators of feature relevance. While LIME is more suited for localized interpretability, global insights can also be inferred, for example, by averaging the absolute weights across an entire dataset. Feature permutation was also employed as a technique to assess feature relevance by evaluating the decline in a model's performance metrics when the values of a specific feature are randomly perturbed. This disruption severs the relationship between the feature and the model's output, and the resulting performance drop quantifies the model's reliance on that feature. Mean Decrease in Accuracy (MDA) is a commonly used metric in permutation studies. Tree-based models, however, offer an alternative measure known as Mean Decrease in Impurity (MDI), or Gini importance, which measures the cumulative reduction in impurity (or heterogeneity) at split nodes involving a specific feature. This metric is typically averaged across all trees in an ensemble. We utilized SHAP and LIME to analyse the global associations between predictors and model outputs. SHAP was applied to the dataset to gain an overarching view of feature interdependencies, while LIME's coefficients effectively captured the primary effects of individual features as they represent the parameters of the local linear approximations. Lastly, it's worth noting that other XAI approaches, such as Anchors [21] and Local Rule-Based Explanations (LORE) [22], can also be employed to demystify ML models. These methods, however, offer explanations in the form of IF-THEN rules rather than feature attributions. Furthermore, consistency in explanation assessment typically pertains to methods that generate similar types of explanations. Additionally, these techniques are primarily effective for localized interpretability, and systematically combining local rules to construct a global perspective may pose significant challenges.

The results of the XAI models are given below

Figure 16 is a prediction graph generated by SHAP model which give insights into the contribution of each feature for prediction.

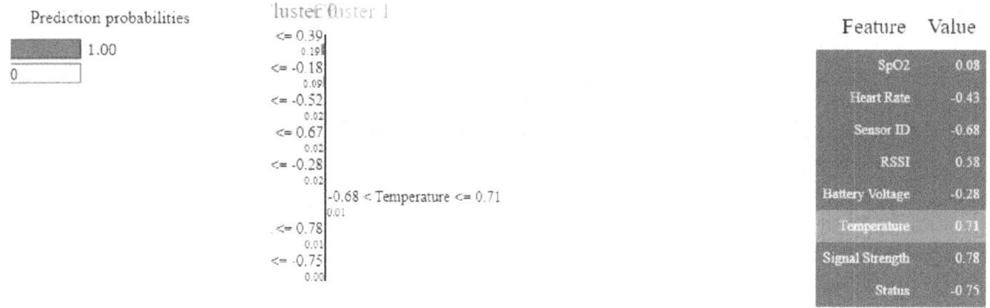

Fig. 16. SHAP bar graph for two clusters

Figure 17 is a bar graph which tells each feature's influence in the prediction model. The figure summarizes that Temperature has a positive influence towards prediction.

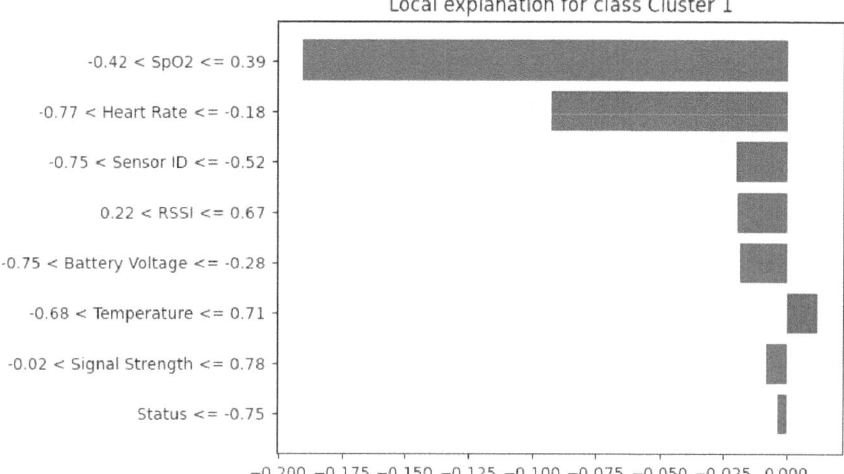

Fig. 17. LIME graph for feature influence

Figure 18 is a SHAP interaction values graph which gives an insight of interaction effects of features on the model.

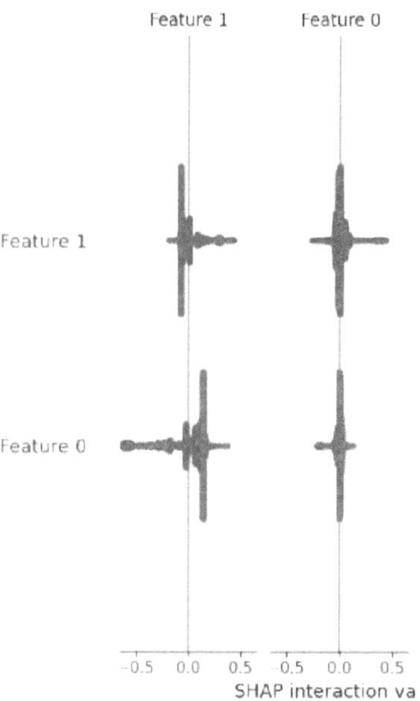

Fig. 18. SHAP interaction values

5 Conclusions

In this paper, we have thoroughly examined and applied various machine learning techniques to address the challenges posed by medical monitoring applications, particularly in the context of Wireless Body Area Networks (WBAN). WBANs play a critical role in patient health monitoring, offering real-time data collection from wearable devices such as sensors measuring vital signs, including heart rate, SpO2 levels, temperature, and more. In this regard, we proposed a sophisticated framework that leverages multiple Machine learning models, employing ensemble learning methods for enhanced prediction accuracy. The core of our approach is an ensemble model that combines the strengths of individual machine learning techniques to create a more robust and accurate prediction system. These techniques include well-established models such as Support Vector Machine (SVM), Decision Tree (DT), Artificial Neural Network (ANN), Recurrent Neural Network (RNN), Gradient Boosting (GB), and Random Forest (RF), each contributing to the overall performance by addressing different aspects of the dataset's complexity. By stacking these models together, we were able to create a meta-model that capitalizes on the diversity of the underlying models, reducing the risk of overfitting and improving generalization. Through this ensemble stacking approach, the framework achieved a remarkable accuracy rate close to 99.9%. This impressive performance underscores the effectiveness of combining various models, especially when handling complex and diverse datasets like those typically found in WBAN applications. The use of advanced models such as RNNs (with LSTM for long-term memory handling) and Gradient Boosting allows the system to capture temporal dynamics and complex interdependencies within the data, making it highly applicable for practical healthcare monitoring scenarios. In addition to the high accuracy, we incorporated Explainable AI (XAI) methods such as SHAP (Shapley Additive Explanations) and LIME (Local Interpretable Model-agnostic Explanations) to improve the clarity and interpretability of the predictive models, explainability techniques were utilized. These tools provided a comprehensive understanding of the rationale behind specific predictions, offering detailed insights into the relative importance of each feature in the decision-making process. This interpretability is especially crucial in healthcare applications, where trust and accountability are essential. SHAP, in particular, helped identify the most influential features, such as heart rate, temperature, and battery voltage, in predicting the status of the system, while LIME offered local explanations that highlight specific decision boundaries for individual predictions. Furthermore, to ensure that the results of our ensemble model could be effectively communicated and understood, we employed various data visualization techniques. Visualization tools such as matplotlib and seaborn were used to generate confusion matrices, correlation heatmaps, and feature importance plots, effectively illustrating model performance and feature contributions. These graphical outputs facilitated a deeper understanding of model's working, enabling the evaluation of predictive accuracy while presenting results in an intuitive manner for non-technical audiences. In summary, this work highlights the effective application of sophisticated machine learning algorithms and ensemble strategies to address a critical challenge in healthcare monitoring, demonstrating robust performance and practical insights, achieving an accuracy of nearly 99.9%. The incorporation of Explainable AI methods ensures that the predictions made by the system are both accurate and interpretable, fostering trust and transparency in medical applications. This framework can serve as a foundation for future developments in WBAN-based medical monitoring, contributing to improved patient care and outcomes by providing real-time, reliable, and explainable predictions. Additionally, the proposed model offers significant potential for scalability and adaptation to various other healthcare and industrial applications where predictive accuracy and interpretability are of utmost importance.

References

1. Salayma, M., Al-Dubai, A., Romdhani, I., Nasser, Y.: Wireless body area network (WBAN) a survey on reliability, fault tolerance, and technologies coexistence. ACM Comput. Surv. (CSUR) **50**(1), 1–38 (2017)
2. Wang, L., Xu, B., Cai, H., Zhang, P.: Context-aware emergency detection method for edge computing-based healthcare monitoring system. Trans. Emerg. Telecommun. Technol. **33**(6), e4128 (2022)
3. Mehmood, G., Khan, M.Z., Abbas, S., Faisal, M., Rahman, H.U.: An energy-efficient and cooperative fault-tolerant communication approach for wireless body area network. IEEE Access **8**, 69134–69147 (2020)
4. Peng, Y., Wang, X., Guo, L., Wang, Y., Deng, Q.: An efficient network coding-based fault-tolerant mechanism in WBAN for smart healthcare monitoring systems. Appl. Sci. **7**(8), 817 (2017)
5. Zhou, S., Lin, K.J., Na, J., Chuang, C.C., Shih, C.S.: Supporting service adaptation in fault tolerant internet of things. In: 2015 IEEE 8th International Conference on Service-Oriented Computing and Applications (SOCA), pp. 65–72. IEEE (2015)
6. Sharma, A.B., Golubchik, L., Govindan, R.: Sensor faults: detection methods and prevalence in real-world datasets. ACM Trans. Sens. Netw. (TOSN) **6**(3), 1–39 (2010)
7. Jeong, Y.S., Kim, H.W., Park, J.H.: Visual scheme monitoring of sensors for fault tolerance on wireless body area networks with cloud service infrastructure. Int. J. Distrib. Sens. Netw. **10**(4), 154180 (2014)
8. Mahapatro, A.: Online fault detection and recovery in body sensor networks. In: 2011 World Congress on Information and Communication Technologies, pp. 407–412. IEEE. (2011)
9. GS, S., Balakrishnan, R.: A statistical-based light-weight anomaly detection framework for Wireless Body Area Networks. Comput. J. **65**(7), 17521759 (2022)
10. Bhardwaj, T., Sharma, S.C.: An autonomic resource provisioning framework for efficient data collection in cloudlet-enabled wireless body area networks: a fuzzy-based proactive approach. Soft. Comput. **23**, 10361–10383 (2019)
11. Awad, M., Sallabi, F., Shuaib, K., Naeem, F.: Artificial intelligence-based fault prediction framework for WBAN. J. King Saud Univ.-Comput. Inf. Sci. **34**(9), 7126–7137 (2022)
12. Gupta, P., Bagchi, A.: Introduction to NumPy. In: Essentials of Python for Artificial Intelligence and Machine Learning, pp. 127–159. Springer, Cham (2024)
13. Rainio, O., Teuho, J., Klén, R.: Evaluation metrics and statistical tests for machine learning. Sci. Rep. **14**(1), 6086 (2024)
14. Veisi, H.: Introduction to SVM. In: Learning with Fractional Orthogonal Kernel Classifiers in Support Vector Machines: Theory, Algorithms and Applications, p. 318. Springer, Singapore (2023)
15. Wang, Z., Irfan, S.A., Teoh, C., Bhoyar, P.H.: Numerical Machine Learning. Bentham Science Publishers (2023)

16. Krishnamoorthi, V.: Early detection of cardiovascular disorders using enhanced ANN model. In: 2024 International Conference on Advances in Data Engineering and Intelligent Computing Systems (ADICS), pp. 01–06. IEEE (2024)
17. Goyal, A., Choudhary, A., Malik, D., Baliyan, M.S., Rani, S.: Implementing and analysis of RNN LSTM model for stock market prediction. In: Advances in Data and Information Sciences: Proceedings of ICDIS 2022, pp. 241–248. Springer, Singapore (2022)
18. Salman, H.A., Kalakech, A., Steiti, A.: Random forest algorithm overview. Babylonian J. Mach. Learn. **2024**, 69–79 (2024)
19. Zhang, X., et al.: A stacking ensemble model for predicting the occurrence of carotid atherosclerosis. Front. Endocrinol. **15**, 1390352 (2024)
20. Reddy, G.P., Kumar, Y.P.: Explainable AI (XAI): explained. In: 2023 IEEE Open Conference of Electrical, Electronic and Information Sciences (eStream), pp. 1–6. IEEE (2023)
21. Ribeiro, M.T., Singh, S., Guestrin, C.: Anchors: high-precision model-agnostic explanations. In: Proceedings of the AAAI Conference on Artificial Intelligence, vol. 32, no. 1 (2018)
22. Rajapaksha, D., Bergmeir, C., Buntine, W.: LoRMIkA: local rule-based model interpretability with k-optimal associations. Inf. Sci. **540**, 221241 (2020)
23. LNCS. http://www.springer.com/lncs. Accessed 25 Oct 2023

Machine Learning-Driven Anomaly Detection for Enhanced Security in 6G Body Area Networks

Himanshi Babbar[1], Ankita Sharma[1], Rajeev Kumar[1], and Daljeet Singh[2(✉)]

[1] Chitkara University Institute of Engineering and Technology, Chitkara University, Rajpura, Punjab, India
{himanshi.babbar,sharma.ankita,rajeev.kumar}@chitkara.edu.in

[2] Research Unit of Health Sciences and Technology, Faculty of Medicine, University of Oulu, Oulu, Finland
daljeet.singh@oulu.fi

Abstract. Intelligent network orchestration and management are crucial elements in the future of Sixth-Generation (6G) networks, although the cloudification of microservices-oriented networks is a well-established aspect of Fifth-Generation (5G) systems. Consequently, the envisioned 6G framework heavily depends on artificial intelligence (AI), machine learning (ML), and deep learning (DL) to enhance network security. Ensuring end-to-end authentication in future networks necessitates proactive threat detection, innovative mitigation strategies, and the self-sufficiency of 6G networks. This paper explores the potential applications of AI in enhancing the security of 6G body area networks. Specifically, it introduces an innovative anomaly detection system tailored for 6G body area networks, leveraging group learning within communication networks. The process begins with pre-processing, followed by a feature selection strategy that compares ensemble learning and feature selection to implement a reimagined hybrid approach. Dimensionality reduction is applied to three datasets—UNSW_NB2015, CIC_IDS2017, and NSL KDD—to identify the most relevant feature subsets for each. In the final stage, hybrid Ensemble Learning (EL) techniques are used for intrusion detection, employing a modified version of the random forests (RF) classifier within the Adaboost.M1 algorithm, with average voting as the aggregation method. Both binary and multi-class classification approaches are used to validate the system's effectiveness.

Keywords: Anomaly detection · 6G · Machine learning · Feature selection

1 Driving Forces Behind 6G Networks

The notion of enormous Internet of Things (IoT) signifies a paradigm shift in the breadth and scale of interconnected devices, since it is typified by a network

K. Atul et al. (Eds.): BodyNets 2024, LNICST 666, pp. 169–184, 2026.
https://doi.org/10.1007/978-3-032-16099-7_15

density exceeding one million devices per square kilometre [5,6]. This unprecedented degree of connection portends an era in which Internet of Things deployments span large geographic areas, including industrial sites, urban settings, agricultural landscapes, and more. Because there is such a dense network of IoT devices, an unprecedented amount of data will be generated and transmitted. Every linked gadget constantly gathers and shares data with other gadgets and systems, creating a tsunami of data that seeps into every part of our existence. There are many different kinds of data that fall under this category, including as sensor data, environmental variables, user interactions, and machine-to-machine communications.

An vast number of jobs and procedures will need to be realized inside the IoT ecosystem as a result of this data explosion [7]. These responsibilities include anything from data processing, analytics, and decision-making to the real-time monitoring and management of tangible assets. Furthermore, to ensure dependable and responsive operation, the sheer size and complexity of IoT deployments demands effective resource management, dynamic network orchestration, and intelligent routing algorithms. large IoT presents operational issues, but in order to extract useful insights from the large amounts of data created, advanced data analytics and processing capabilities are also required. "Big data" refers to the process of studying vast and intricate databases in order to find trends, patterns, and correlations that can guide decisions and generate value for businesses. In the future, the IoT' exponential expansion and the accompanying spike in data flow will significantly alter the digital landscape. Global mobile traffic is expected to expand dramatically from 62 exabytes per month in 2020 to over 5000 exabytes per month by 2030. This exponential expansion highlights the Internet of Things' disruptive potential and emphasizes the need for scalable architectures, resilient infrastructure, and creative solutions to meet the ever-increasing needs of the connected world [8].

Finding zero-day attacks is a challenging problem. Every day, numerous questionable activities are found. These sophisticated intrusions can have serious consequences that increase the difficulty for existing intrusion detection systems (IDSs). When they detect unexpected activity or a known threat, IDSs issue alerts. An intrusion is defined as any malicious conduct that jeopardizes the integrity of the information system. IDSs monitor computer networks for anomalous activity that would go unnoticed by a standard packet filter. In network packets, they search for signs of potentially harmful conduct, cyber resistance against disruptive activities, and unauthorized access to the system. Anomaly intrusion detection systems (AIDS) and signature intrusion detection systems (SIDS) are the two methods that IDSs use to find intrusions. AIDS has many flaws, including a high rate of false alarms. To tackle these problems and reduce FAR while increasing accuracy, a novel IDS model was proposed.

1.1 Main Contributions

The main key contributions are:

1. The literature review about the 5G networks are discussed to ensure the security of 6G wireless communication systems.
2. The methodology for detecting the system and identifying the anomalies are presented in which different datasets are deployed i.e. NSL_KDD, UNSW_NB2015 and CIC_IDS2017.
3. The algorithms are proposed: one for preprocessing the data and other for RF method. In these algorithms, the input is given for training the datasets.
4. The performance is evaluated by using the UNSW_NB2015 dataset that deploys the training and testing data. Therefore, by applying UNSW NB15 dataset which shows the maximum and minimum values, the maximum value is 4 s in Fuzzers class and the minimum is 0.001 s in the Shellcode class.

The remainder of the paper is arranged as follows: Section 2 discuss about the literature review, Section 3 explains the methodology and detection system of Classifier's algorithm, Section 4 showcase the results and discussions of the proposed work, Section 5 examines the use case and case studies deploying the IoT in 6G, Sect. 6 concludes the paper.

2 Literature Review

The 5G network systems are still in the process of being fully standardised, even though research on the security of 6G wireless communication systems has already begun to provide seamless connectivity to the increasing number of users and to improve ML services. Numerous modern approaches have already been used to thoroughly study the issue of system secrecy rate optimisation. The authors of [1] recommended identifying assaults on wireless sensor networks and applying NSL KDD. In order to do this, machine learning approaches for energy efficiency and anomaly detection in hybrid wireless sensor networks were applied. The experimental results showed that accuracy was 95% and that precision, recall, and F1-Score were 94%, 98%, and 96%, respectively.

For network-based intrusion detection systems (NIDS) based on EL algorithms, the authors in [2] suggested the FS approach centred on genetic algorithms and logistic regression. Using 11, 8, and 13 features, respectively, the results for CIC_IDS2017, NSL_KDD, and UNSW_NB2015 showed 98%, 98%, and 97% accuracy with 98%, 96%, and 98% detection rates. The authors of [3] proposed a distinctive anomaly detection in communication networks by using an ensemble learning (EL) algorithm-based anomaly detection in ADCNs. It selects the optimal subset feature and minimises dimensionality in each of the three datasets (NSL_KDD, UNSW_NB2015, and CIC_IDS2017) separately. Applying the system's 30, 35, and 40 features to the three datasets produced results that were 99.6% accurate for NSL_KDD, 99.1% accurate for UNSW_NB2015, and 99.4% accurate for CIC_IDS2017. We used the same research techniques and reimplemented its algorithms, as the work in [3] was the main study, in order to benchmark with different dataset pre-processing and feature combinations.

Enhancing intrusion detection accuracy employing feature selection in gar-forest: Kanakarajan and Muniasamy K. suggested These researchers used NSL-KDD datasets, information gain, symmetric unpredictability, and feature-subset based on correlation as well as greedy randomised adaptive search techniques using annealed randomness forest (GAR-Forest) with FS processes. Outcomes for the binary class indicated an accuracy of 86% with 32 features, and information gain produced an accuracy of 79% using 10 features for the multi-class [4].

3 Methodology

The redesigned architecture employs multiple anomaly detection processes. An intrusion detection system with databases concealed behind the firewall (network data preprocessed) is the initial part of the defensive system. After preprocessing, the system must check for any missing values and identify any substitution of the null values with alternate values. Average values are taken into account by default, and duplicate values are removed from the dataset thereafter. To make data handling easier, dimensional reduction is applied to the encoded data. Feature optimization, which is done to extract the best qualities from the data, helps with anomaly detection. The following step involves moving the filtered data to the so-called technique, where duplicate values are removed from the dataset. To make data handling easier, dimensional reduction is applied to the encoded data. Feature optimization, which is done to extract the best qualities from the data, helps with anomaly detection. After that, the filtered data is sent to the following step, where the proposed method is only applied to choose the features that will have an impact on the results. The reimplemented RF is utilized by the system to differentiate between authorized activities and possible attacks; it is solely utilized to select the affected features for the outcomes. The system utilizes the reimplemented Adaboosting.M1 as classifiers to discern between potentially malicious activity and legitimate operation. The several steps in the suggested framework are intended to identify anomalies are shown in Fig. 1. The first defense mechanism is an IDS with databases housed behind the firewall (i.e., preprocessed network data acquired). Following preprocessing, the system must identify any missing values and replace any null values with other values. Duplicate values are eliminated from the dataset once average values are taken into account by default. To aid in data handling, the encoded data is subjected to dimensional reduction. Hence, in order to extract the best features from the data and aid in anomaly detection, feature optimization is carried out. Additionally, the cleaned data is sent to the following phase, where the suggested random forest method is used to choose only the impacted features for the final findings. Ultimately, the system classifies possible assaults from regular activity using the suggested algorithms.

It consists of multiple stages, each of which finishes a specific task in a set of steps that follow one another. The subsequent stage receives input from the preceding step. These stages and procedures are covered in detail. The

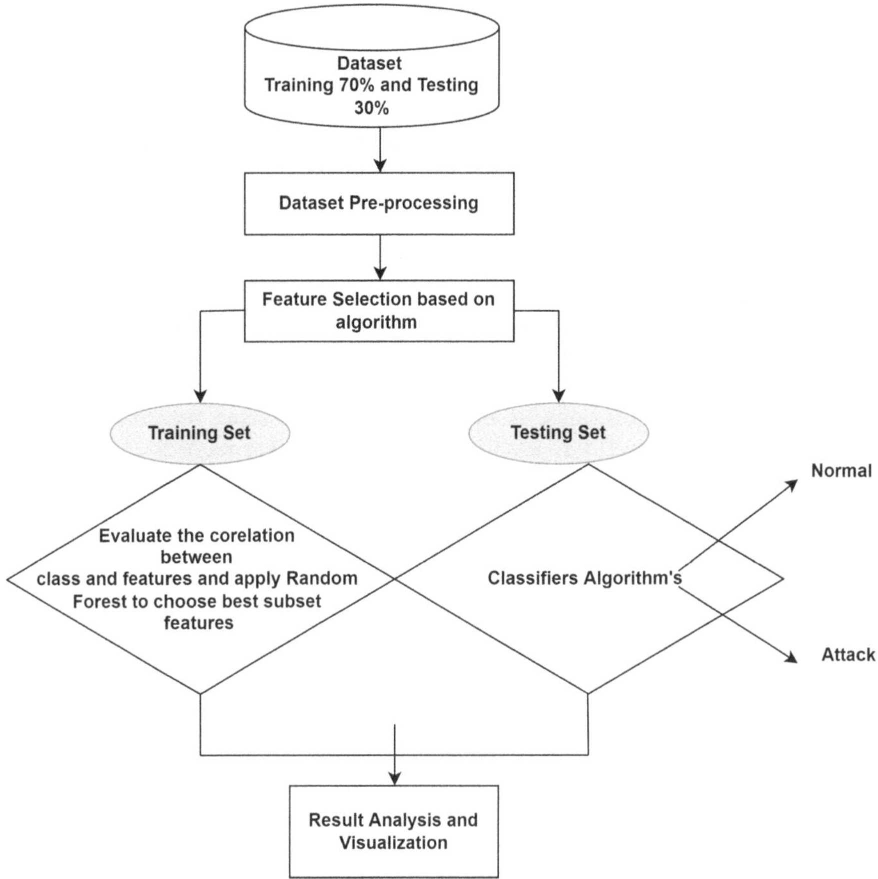

Fig. 1. Detection system of classifier's algorithm.

gathered datasets (NSL_KDD, UNSW_NB2015, and CIC_IDS2017) are viewed, after which the three primary preprocessing steps—filtering, transformation, and normalization—are carried out.

Using the suggested RF approach, the best subset of characteristics is selected in the first stage. Building the Adaboosting.M1 approach, altering the classifiers to function as adaboosting, and aggregating the composite model to function as a bagging algorithm are the steps involved in the classifier's training stage. The principal rationales underlying the integration of these two algorithms are the adaboosting algorithm's poor accuracy and the bagging algorithm's vulnerability to model overfitting. As a result, proposed approach typically achieve higher accuracy with lower overfitting. Using two forms of each dataset form (binary and multi-class classifications), the classifications evaluation step applies certain performance measurements (i.e., accuracy, recall, precision, F-measure, DR, and FAR).

3.1 Dataset Preprocessing

Three distinct datasets are used by this system to carry out experiments: NSL_KDD, UNSW_NB2015, and CIC_IDS2017. The initial dataset is called NSL-KDD. It was created as a sequential parameter to enhance the prediction of problems. For record classification of five complexity levels, a variety of baseline classifiers were used, and the number of correct predictions was indicated next to each instance [12]. The number of records picked is inversely associated with the percentage of records in the original KDDCup99 dataset chosen for each difficulty degree categorization. In our sample, there were 125.973 occurrences of the KDD_Train set, comprising 66789 instances of routine traffic and 57,000 instances of attacks. The majority of current low-key attacks are incorporated into the second dataset (UNSW-NB15) in an attempt to replicate the present network configurations. It included training/testing records of 175,341 and 82,332, 45 columns (id 1, feature 44), and 2,540,044 records of 4 big-data CSV chunks. Lastly, benign data, the most recent broad attacks. All assaults, protocols, ports, and source/destination IP addresses were time-stamped flows (CSV les). Furthermore, it has the most latest dataset available, which includes updated information on botnet, DDoS, Brute Force, XSS, SQL Injection, In filtration, and port scanning attacks. It had 2,830,743 recordings of 8 les, with 78 distinct labelled features included in each record.

Filtration, transformation, and normalization are crucial preprocessing processes for anomaly detection because they set up the dataset for efficient anomaly detection algorithms.

1. **Filteration:** Filtration in the context of anomaly detection is the process of locating and eliminating irrelevant or noisy data points that may make it more difficult to find actual anomalies. As anomalies are frequently distinguished by their departure from the typical behaviour of the data, this may entail eliminating outliers that are isolated from the bulk of the data points. Statistical approaches such as the z-score and interquartile range (IQR) may be used in filtering procedures in order to detect and exclude outliers from the dataset.
2. **Transformation:** Making the data more palatable to the anomaly detection algorithms is the goal of transformation techniques employed in preprocessing for anomaly detection. Converting unstructured data into more insightful representations that highlight underlying patterns or trends is known as feature transformation. Time series data, for instance, may be altered to emphasise patterns and draw attention to anomalies by applying techniques like smoothing or differencing.
3. **Normalization:** In order to ensure that features are on comparable scales and keep some features from predominating the detection process, normalisation is crucial in anomaly detection. Normalizing features to a consistent scale guarantees that anomalies in all dimensions are equally observable because anomalies can arise in different dimensions of the data. This can be accomplished with the use of normalization approaches such as Min-Max scaling or Z-score normalisation, which scale characteristics to have a similar distribution and range.

The removal of noise and unnecessary data points from the data, transformation of the data into a more meaningful representation, and normalisation of the features to ensure that they are on similar scales are all benefits of preprocessing data for anomaly detection. These steps enhance the efficacy of anomaly detection algorithms in spotting odd patterns or outliers in the data. The algorithms are explained in Table 1:

Algorithm 1. Proposed algorithm for preprocessing the data

Input: Reading the datasets R1, R2, R3. Where R1 is NSL-KDD, R2 is UNSW-NB15, R3 is CIC-IDS2017.
Output: P_i Value (feature)
Steps 2 and 10
    In case Numeric Data:
        For filtering and transforming the data
        Removing the duplicate instances
        Distributed categorized is arranged
    In case Non-Numeric Data:
        To capture the categorical values, apply one-hot encoding function
    Applying Normalization with Minimax:
        Max: To find the maximum value
        Min: To find the minimum value
    Halt the further functionality until all the features are completed.
    Return PiValue
END

The proposed algorithm "Adaboost.M1" strategy for efficient and accurate classifications by deploying algorithm. Initially, it captivates the results from preprocessing stage (P_i Value) then, deploys it to each and every feature using the merit equation, represented by 1:

$$\tau_s = \frac{s f_x r}{\sqrt{s + s(s-1) + f_r . r}} \tag{1}$$

where f_x r indicates the correlation between the feature and class, f_rr denotes the correlation between the features. Thus, it produces the subsets of Random Forest by 2:

$$k(y, \theta_s), s = 1, 2, 3, \ldots \tag{2}$$

where k is the random forest, S is the integer number, θ_s represents the theta and y shows the vector. Therefore, the procedure of validating the features that are duplicate by evaluating the range of weight which chooses the most required features with less variance by evaluating the standard deviation SD_i, that is shown by 3:

$$SD_i = 1.0 - \frac{omega_i}{n+1} - \lambda \tag{3}$$

where ω_i depicts the weight. The algorithm is explained in Table 2:

Algorithm 2. Proposed RF method

Input: Train the datasets after the algorithm is applied, P_i value (features) that are deployed after preprocessing steps.
Output: The most efficient features (P_i Best)
For every P_i in the dataset that is trained T_0
  Evaluate the merit by equation (1)
  Produce the 10 Random Forest by equation (2)
End For
  Incase Numeric Data:
    For filtering and transforming the data
    Removing the duplicate instances
    Distributed categorized is arranged
  Incase Non-Numeric Data:
    To capture the categorical values, apply one-hot encoding function
  Applying Normalization with Minimax:
    Max: To find the maximum value
    Min: To find the minimum value
    Pi Value = $\frac{P_i ValueMin}{MaxMin}$
  Halt the further functionality until all the features are completed.
  Return PiValue
End

The weights and parameters are updated to enhance the effectiveness of detecting the unknown attacks. Initially, the process equalizes all the defined values of $P_i Best$ with V_i and later produces the Random Forest subsets. In order to acquire the best results, aggregation is performed and deployed to all the other updated classifiers using the technique named as weighting average voting.

4 Results and Discussions

4.1 Dataset

The UNSW_NB15 dataset is a meticulously compiled collection of network traffic data, carefully put together by the University of New South Wales in Australia. Its main objective is to further research in intrusion detection and cybersecurity. It greatly simulates real-world network situations by including a wide spectrum of network functions, including both simulated cyberattacks and actual traffic. This dataset contains several protocols, such as TCP, UDP, ICMP, and others. Network traffic flow features provide in-depth understanding of communication patterns. Each flow is meticulously labelled to indicate if it is suggestive of malevolent behaviour or specific sorts of cyberattacks, such malware, attempts at exploitation, distributed denial-of-service (DDoS), denial-of-service (DoS), probing, or other attacks. Researchers and practitioners in cybersecurity utilise UNSW_NB15 to analyse and test machine learning algorithms, train and evaluate intrusion detection systems, look at network traffic patterns, and develop new cybersecurity solutions. Despite certain inherent limitations including dataset representativeness and preprocessing difficulty, UNSW_NB15 is a vital tool for advancing cybersecurity research and enhancing intrusion detection system efficacy. Its accessibility to the general public fosters collaboration and innovation in the struggle against evolving cyberthreats.

4.2 Performance Evaluation

The proposed method is executed utilizing the dataset UNSW_NB15 that deploys the training dataset utilized is 70% and testing dataset utilized is 30%. The performance is evaluated by examining the features by executing them. The two types of confusion metrics are used (i.e. binary and multi class) classification forms. The performance is evaluated by deploying the different specifications: recall, precision, FAR. The proposed method is implemented by software (i.e. Python 3.9 and PyCharm with sklearn library) utilizing the computers hardware Core i7 8th generation, 64-bit operating system. The Table 1 depicts the UNSW_NB2015 consisting of binary class having 30 features and represents the True Positive, True Negative, False Positive and False Negative with the accurate measurements for all the features chosen.

Table 1. Confusion matrix having 30 features

	Attack	Normal
Attack	1650	20
Normal	0	700

The Table 2 shows the accuracy applied to proposed approach by deploying varying feature number.

Table 2. Accuracy applied to proposed (Adaboost.M1) by using different feature numbers

Dataset	Number of Features	True Positive	False Negative	Accuracy
UNSW_NB15	30	1650	20	0.99
	40	1475	200	0.85
	10	44000	62630	0.85

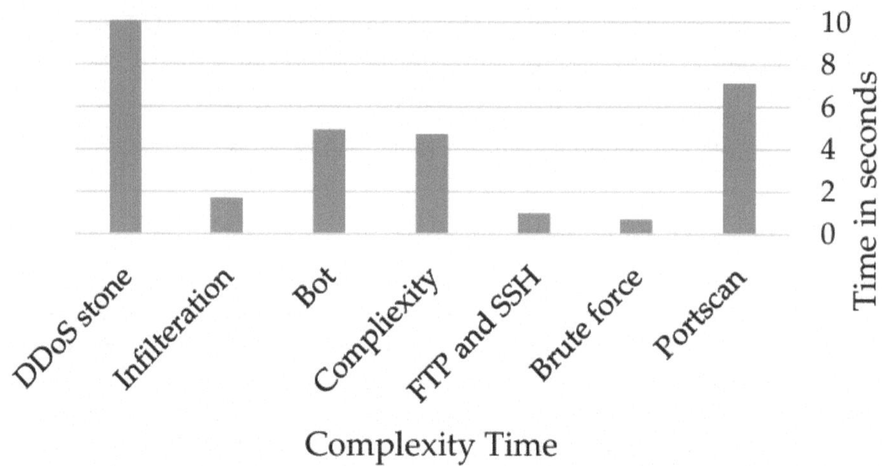

Fig. 2. Complexity of UNSW_NB15.

In the Fig. 2, the evaluations of complexity time for the proposed work is done by computing Big O Notation, which is denoted as O (M^2). Therefore, by applying UNSW_NB15 dataset which shows the maximum and minimum values, the maximum value is 4 s in Fuzzers class and the minimum is 0.001 s in the Shellcode class.

4.3 Results and Discussions

Three anomaly detection models—Ensemble Learning, Genetic Algorithm with Logistic Regression, and Gar-Forest—applied to three datasets—NSL-KDD, UNSW-NB2015, and CIC IDS2017—are compared. The accuracy (in percentage) of the models is used to evaluate them. The Fig. 3 shows the accuracy of three machine learning models—Ensemble Learning (Adaboost.M1 with Random Forest), Genetic Algorithm with Logistic Regression, and Gar-Forest with Feature Selection—evaluated on three datasets: NSL-KDD, UNSW NB2015, and CIC IDS2017. Ensemble Learning consistently achieves the highest accuracy across all datasets, while Gar-Forest demonstrates the most variability in performance.

NSL-KDD, UNSW-NB2015, and CIC-IDS2017 are commonly used datasets for evaluating intrusion detection systems. Each dataset contains a mix of normal and attack traffic used to train and test the models. **Ensemble Learning (Adaboost.M1 with Random Forest):** This model generates the highest accuracy and consistently outperforms exceptionally well across all datasets. It receives scores of 99.4% on CIC IDS2017, 99.1% on UNSW NB2015, and 99.6% on the NSL-KDD dataset. This demonstrates how efficient ensemble learning methods are in detecting anomalies. Although it performs well as well, **the Genetic Algorithm plus Logistic Regression approach** is marginally less accurate than ensemble learning. It performs well but a little less consistently,

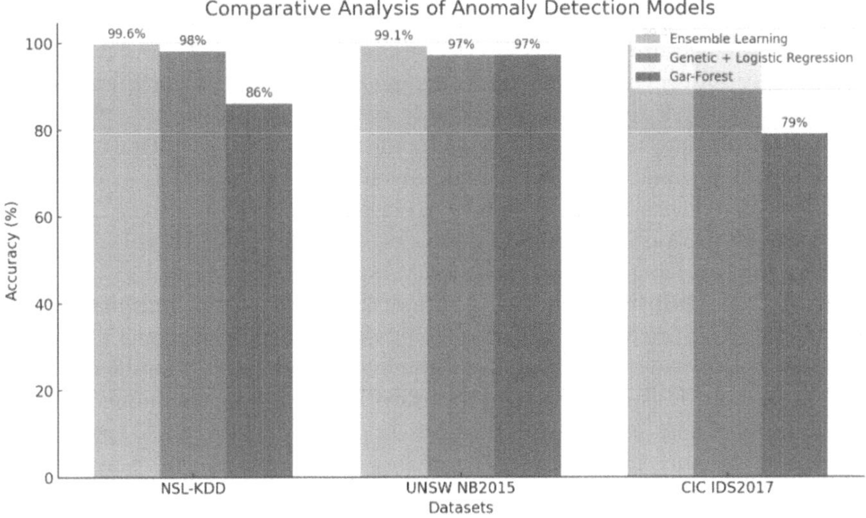

Fig. 3. Comparative Analysis of Anomaly Detection Models Across Different Datasets.

achieving 98% accuracy on NSL-KDD and CIC IDS2017 and 97% accuracy on UNSW NB2015. **Gar-Forest with Feature Selection:** Gar-Forest's effectiveness varies more. Although it achieves a respectable 97% accuracy on the UNSW NB2015 dataset, this model's accuracy declines dramatically for the NSL-KDD (86%) and CIC IDS2017 (79%) datasets, suggesting that it may have trouble with specific data types or architectures.

Across all datasets, ensemble learning consistently yields the best results, most likely because it can combine the advantages of many classifiers (Random Forest and Adaboost.M1) to increase accuracy and decrease overfitting. Although it doesn't perform as well as ensemble learning, Genetic Algorithm with Logistic Regression still produces good results, particularly on NSL-KDD and CIC IDS2017. It also achieves excellent accuracy. The accuracy of Gar-Forest varies the most; it performs well on UNSW NB2015 but much worse on the other two datasets, indicating that it might not generalise as well across datasets.

5 Machine Learning Applications in 6G Networks

The capabilities and functions of 6G networks are significantly shaped by ML technology. ML is incorporated into several areas of 6G networks as follows:

1. **Resource Management:** In 6G networks, ML algorithms are employed to optimise resource management and allocation. Machine learning models may forecast traffic patterns, user demand, and network congestion by assessing historical data and current network circumstances. This makes it possible to optimise quality of service (QoS), load balancing, and dynamic resource

allocation, all of which help to guarantee effective use of network resources and improved user experience.

2. **Anomaly Detection:** In 6G networks, machine learning algorithms are used for both network security and anomaly detection. In order to identify patterns that deviate from the norm and could be signs of cyberattacks, security risks, or abnormalities in the system, machine learning models examine network traffic, device behaviour, and system performance indicators. ML-based anomaly detection improves 6G networks' resilience and integrity by anticipating and averting security breaches.
3. **Predictive Maintenance:** In 6G infrastructure, ML algorithms make failure prediction and predictive maintenance possible. Machine learning models are able to identify early indicators of equipment degradation or imminent failures by examining telemetry data from network equipment, including switches, routers, and base stations. This makes it possible for network operators to plan maintenance tasks in advance, reduce downtime, and maximise the 6G networks' availability and dependability.
4. **Network Optimisation:** In 6G networks, machine learning (ML) methods are used for both network optimisation and self-organizing network (SON) features. In order to optimise routing algorithms, dynamically change network parameters, and improve network efficiency, machine learning models examine user behaviour, traffic patterns, and network architecture. In 6G networks, this improves overall network performance and reliability by enabling autonomous network optimisation, adaptive routing, and self-healing capabilities.
5. **Intelligent Edge Computing :**In 6G networks, intelligent edge computing is made possible via machine learning. 6G networks can process and analyse data locally, cutting down on latency and bandwidth consumption, by implementing machine learning models close to the point of data production at the network edge. Real-time decision-making, context-aware services, and tailored user experiences are made possible by ML-based edge computing in a variety of IoT, mobile, and immersive applications.

6 Use Cases and Case Studies of Deploying IoT in 6G

There are four use cases and case studies that illustrate the application of anomaly detection in 6G networks using machine learning methods:

1. **Use Case: Anomaly Detection in 6G Networks for Security of the Network** In 6G networks, protecting sensitive data and sustaining continuous service delivery depend heavily on strong network security. Real-time proactive threat identification and mitigation is possible through anomaly detection and machine learning techniques [9]. Machine learning algorithms are able to identify deviations from typical behaviour that may be signs of malicious activity or abnormalities in the system by studying network traffic patterns, device behaviour, and system performance indicators. This makes it possible for network operators to stop unauthorised access, strengthen the

security of 6G networks against cyberattacks, and react quickly to security issues.

Case Study: Detection of Real-time Abnormalities in a 6G Edge Computing System An anomaly detection system based on machine learning is implemented by a telecom operator in a 6G edge computing environment to improve network security and reliability. Using distributed sensors and edge computing nodes, the system continuously tracks metrics related to resource utilisation, device interactions, and network traffic at the network edge [10,11]. Real-time anomaly detection, including DDoS attacks, network congestion, and aberrant device behaviour, is detected by the system through the use of machine learning methods, including deep neural networks and anomaly detection models. The solution ensures seamless connectivity and service delivery for users in various IoT and mobile apps by mitigating security threats and maintaining optimal network performance through proactive alerting and automatic reaction mechanisms.

2. **Use Case: Preemptive Identification of Dangers in 6G Networks** The primary infrastructure of a 6G network uses anomaly detection algorithms to track system performance indicators, device behaviour, and network traffic patterns. Real-time machine learning models are used to monitor incoming data streams and spot behavioural anomalies that could be signs of malware infection, DDoS attacks, or unauthorised access attempts. Automated alarms are set off when unusual activity is detected, giving network managers the opportunity to act quickly and stop possible security breaches before they get worse.

   Case Study: Sixth Generation Telecommunication Network Real-time Threat Detection The implementation of a machine learning-based anomaly detection system by a telecommunications company protects the infrastructure of its 6G network from cyber threats [12]. The system learns typical network behaviour by utilising supervised and unsupervised learning techniques. It then looks for deviations that could be signs of security breaches or other questionable activity. In a real-world situation, the system recognises and neutralises a denial-of-service (DDoS) assault that aims to compromise user data integrity and interrupt service.

3. **Use Case: 6G Networks' Dynamic QoS Management In order to monitor and optimise Quality of Service (QoS) characteristics** 6G cellular networks incorporate anomaly detection algorithms into their radio access network (RAN). Network performance measurements, including latency, throughput, and packet loss rates, are analysed by machine learning models to spot anomalous patterns or deterioration in service quality. The system maintains ideal Quality of Service (QoS) levels for a variety of applications and user demands by constantly modifying network configurations and resource allocations in response to identified abnormalities. This improves overall network efficiency and user satisfaction.

   Case Study: Adaptive Quality of Service Management in a 6G Edge Computing Setting An anomaly detection system is installed at the network edge of a 6G edge computing environment to track and control QoS parameters for edge-hosted services and apps [13]. In order to identify abnormalities like network congestion, service deterioration, or resource contention, machine learning algorithms examine real-time data from edge devices, sensors, and network connections. The system dynamically optimises resource utilisation and prioritises mission-critical applications through automated approaches for traffic shaping and QoS changes. This ensures constant and dependable performance in ever-changing network conditions.

4. **Use Case: 6G Infrastructure Predictive Maintenance** The 6G network architecture uses anomaly detection algorithms to facilitate failure prediction and predictive maintenance. In order to spot early indicators of equipment degradation or approaching failures, machine learning models examine telemetry data from network equipment, including base stations, routers, and switches. The system may predict possible hardware faults or service disruptions by identifying unusual behavior in device performance indicators, such as temperature, voltage, or throughput. This enables preemptive maintenance interventions and reduces downtime.
   Case Study: 6G Mobile Network Operator Utilizing Predictive Maintenance Description To develop a predictive maintenance plan for its 6G infrastructure, a mobile network operator uses anomaly detection techniques based on machine learning [14–16]. The system evaluates previous data and continuously tracks network equipment's key performance indicators (KPIs) to spot trends that could indicate upcoming malfunctions or performance degradation. In practical applications [17] [18] [19], the system identifies irregularities in base station power consumption patterns, facilitating prompt maintenance interventions to avert service disruptions and enhance network dependability and accessibility.

7 Conclusion and Future Scope

7.1 Conclusion

The exploration of AI-driven security measures for 6G networks demonstrates a significant advancement in the field of network security. The transition from the 5G paradigm, which heavily utilizes cloudification and micro-services-oriented architectures, to the 6G paradigm necessitates the integration of sophisticated AI, ML, and DL techniques. These technologies are pivotal for the intelligent orchestration and administration of future networks. In this context, the development of a novel anomaly detection system for 6G networks showcases a comprehensive approach to enhancing network security. The process begins with preprocessing and strategic feature selection, which are critical for handling large and complex datasets. The use of ensemble learning techniques, particularly the modified random forests algorithm for Adaboosting.M1 and the average voting aggregation method, illustrates an effective method for intrusion detection. The application of these techniques to well-known datasets (UNSW_NB2015, CIC_IDS2017, NSL KDD) demonstrates their practical utility and effectiveness in both binary and multi-class classification scenarios.

7.2 Future Scope

The future scope is explained below:

1. Enhanced AI Techniques: Future research can focus on refining AI, ML, and DL techniques to further improve the accuracy and efficiency of anomaly detection systems. This includes exploring new algorithms and hybrid models that can better handle the dynamic and complex nature of 6G networks.
2. Real-Time Threat Detection: Developing real-time threat detection systems that can instantly identify and mitigate threats is crucial. Future work should aim to minimize detection and response times to enhance the overall security posture of 6G networks.
3. Scalability and Flexibility: As 6G networks are expected to support a vast number of devices and services, ensuring scalability and flexibility in security measures is essential. Future research should focus on scalable solutions that can adapt to varying network conditions and loads.
4. Integration with Other Technologies: The integration of AI-driven security measures with other emerging technologies such as blockchain, quantum computing, and edge computing could provide robust and comprehensive security solutions for 6G networks.
5. Standardization and Regulatory Compliance: Establishing industry standards and ensuring regulatory compliance will be critical for the widespread adoption of AI-driven security solutions. Future efforts should include collaboration with regulatory bodies to develop standards and frameworks that ensure the secure deployment of 6G technologies.

References

1. Kanakarajan, N.K., Muniasamy, K.: Improving the accuracy of intrusion detection using gar-forest with feature selection. In: Proceedings of the 4th International Conference on Frontiers in Intelligent Computing: Theory and Applications (FICTA) 2015, pp. 539–547. Springer: Cham, Switzerland (2016)
2. Khalifa, O.O., et al.: Vehicle detection for vision-based intelligent transportation systems using convolutional neural network algorithm. J. Adv. Transp. **2022**, 9189600 (2022)
3. Oleiwi, H.W., Mhawi, D.N., Al-Raweshidy, H.: MLTs-ADCNs: machine learning techniques for anomaly detection in communication networks. IEEE Access **10**, 91006–91017 (2022)
4. Singh, D., et al.: Generalized adaptive spreading modulation: a novel waveform for integrated sensing and communication oriented vehicular applications. IEEE Internet Things J. **11**(18), 29486–29493 (2024)
5. Nguyen, D.C., et al.: 6G Internet of things: a comprehensive survey. IEEE Internet Things J. **9**(1), 359–383 (2021)
6. Siriwardhana, Y., Porambage, P., Liyanage, M., Ylianttila, M.: AI and 6G security: opportunities and challenges. In: 2021 Joint European Conference on Networks and Communications and 6G Summit (EuCNC/6G Summit), pp. 616–621. IEEE (2021)

7. Kapoor, V., Singh, D.: Scheduling techniques for convergecast in multichannel wireless sensor networks: a review and issues. Comput. Sci. Eng. Emerg. Technol. 588–591 (2024)
8. Ferrag, M.A., et al.: Edge learning for 6G-enabled internet of things: a comprehensive survey of vulnerabilities, datasets, and defenses. IEEE Commun. Surv. Tutorials (2023)
9. Nguyen, V.L., Lin, P.C., Cheng, B.C., Hwang, R.H., Lin, Y.D.: Security and privacy for 6G: a survey on prospective technologies and challenges. IEEE Commun. Surv. Tutorials **23**(4), 2384–2428 (2021)
10. Verma, J., et al.: A hybrid images deep trained feature extraction and ensemble learning models for classification of multi disease in fundus images. In: Nordic Conference on Digital Health and Wireless Solutions, pp. 203–221. Cham, Springer Nature Switzerland (2024)
11. Mao, B., Liu, J., Wu, Y., Kato, N.: Security and privacy on 6G network edge: a survey. IEEE Commun. Surv. Tutorials (2023)
12. Porambage, P., Gür, G., Osorio, D.P.M., Livanage, M., Ylianttila, M.: 6G security challenges and potential solutions. In: 2021 Joint European Conference on Networks and Communications and 6G Summit (EuCNC/6G Summit), pp. 622–627. IEEE (2021)
13. Porambage, P.: The roadmap to 6G security and privacy. IEEE Open J. Commun. Soc. **2**, 1094–1122 (2021)
14. Babbar, H., Bouachir, O., Rani, S., Aloqaily, M.: Evaluation of deep learning models in ITS software-defined intrusion detection systems. In: NOMS 2022-2022 IEEE/IFIP Network Operations and Management Symposium, Budapest, Hungary, pp. 1–6 (2022). https://doi.org/10.1109/NOMS54207.2022.9789829
15. Babbar, H., Rani, S.: FRHIDS: Federated learning recommender hybrid intrusion detection system model in software-defined networking for consumer devices. IEEE Trans. Consum. Electron. **70**(1), 2492–2499 (2024). https://doi.org/10.1109/TCE.2023.3329151
16. Singh, D., et al.: Preliminary studies on mm-Wave radar for vital sign monitoring of driver in vehicular environment. In Nordic Conference on Digital Health and Wireless Solutions, pp. 480–493. Cham: Springer Nature Switzerland (2024)
17. Balyan, A.K., et al.: A hybrid intrusion detection model using EGA-PSO and improved random forest method. Sensors **22**(16), 5986 (2022)

Optimizing Medical Body Area Networks: Key Advances in Performance and Reliability

Khushboo Dadhich(✉) and Devika Kataria

JK Lakshmipat University, Jaipur, India
khushboodadhich@jklu.edu.in

Abstract. This work reports the state of art on Medical Body Area Networks (MBAN), where research has been done by various groups on enhancing the performance and reliability of the network. MBAN is crucial for advancing healthcare by enabling real-time monitoring and efficient data transmission in health monitoring. The study explores four major areas of improvement in MBAN—reducing overheads due to backoff counter values, real-time assignment of node priority, dynamic slot allocation, and selecting relay path with minimum delay time. Different mathematical models and algorithms have been reported which show improved efficiency and reliability of MBAN. We investigate back-off counter optimization methods and analyze their effects on data transmission efficiency and collision control. Additionally, node prioritization approaches are reviewed, and their potential benefits for enhancing network throughput and reliability are considered. We also examine dynamic slot allocation algorithms and assess how they work to minimize latency and maximize bandwidth utilization. Relay links have been studied to see their effectiveness in increasing the range of networks.

Keywords: Back off counter · Dynamic Slot allocation · Priority assignment · Relay nodes

1 Introduction

MBANs (Medical Body Area Networks) are used for human vital parameters monitoring, where data transmission must be real-time and reliable. With its emphasis on the human body, MBAN integrates network components such as personal terminals, and wireless sensor nodes worn on body, or garments and communicates with the body network coordinator (BNC), while these nodes are positioned 3–5 m from the BNC [1–4]. As seen in Fig. 1, the sensor nodes are connected to the BNC using star topology or a tree topology. MBANs allow people with long-term conditions like diabetes and heart disease to move around freely while being monitored for physiological parameters [5–7]. Due to popularity and widespread use of wireless sensors, the IEEE formed a working group called IEEE 802.15.6 in November 2007, which defines the physical and medium access frequency bands, data rates, protocols, channel access modes and other technical specifications for the wireless network and the standard was first made available in

K. Atul et al. (Eds.): BodyNets 2024, LNICST 666, pp. 185–205, 2026.
https://doi.org/10.1007/978-3-032-16099-7_16

February of 2012 [8, 9]. The IEEE 802.15.6 standard does not define specific implementations for Medical Body Area Networks (MBANs) but rather provides a framework of guidelines and specifications that offer flexibility in designing algorithms and systems. It establishes the technical foundation for communication protocols, data rates, and power management, allowing developers to tailor solutions to meet the diverse needs of medical and health monitoring applications while ensuring interoperability and efficiency. The standard has been implemented in various applications due to its flexibility in accommodating a wide range of medical and health monitoring needs, from wearable devices and implantable sensors to real-time data transmission systems. Its adaptable nature enables the creation of customized solutions that can address specific challenges in healthcare, such as low power consumption, reliable communication, and efficient data management while ensuring compatibility with diverse medical technologies and environments. Some of these applications have been listed in Table 1.

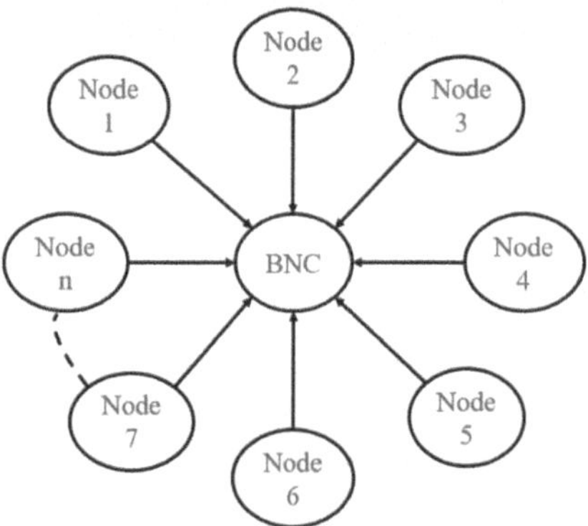

Fig. 1. MBAN based on Star Topology

These applications allow multiple sensors to collect and transmit data through the wireless medium and therefore efficient algorithms for medium access mechanisms are important for the effective performance of these applications. Different types of medium access mechanisms are used such as random-access mechanisms, improvised and unscheduled access mechanisms, and scheduled and scheduled-polling access mechanisms. Carrier Sense Multiple Access with Collision Avoidance (CSMA/CA) and Slotted ALOHA are two random-access techniques. For Ultra-Wide Band (3100–10600 MHz) communication using MBAN, the central coordinator, known as the Body Network Coordinator (BNC) chooses Slotted ALOHA access protocol, and for Narrow Band (NB) communication (402–2450 MHz), CSMA/CA. Three distinct access modes are defined for communication: beacon with superframe, non-beacon with superframe, and non-beacon without superframe mode. Beacon frames are utilized before starting and stopping communication in the superframe in beacon mode, where information about the sensor nodes is collected at the central coordinator hub. In the beacon with superframe access mode, four different types of access phases have been defined such as EAP (exclusive access phase) which is further divided as EAP1 and EAP2, RAP (random access phase), which is divided as RAP1 and RAP2, MAP (management access phase)

Table 1. MBAN Applications [1–8]

MBAN Applications	Wearable MBAN	Assessing Solider Fatigue and Battle Readiness
		A mature sport training
		Sleep Staging
		Asthma
		Wearable health monitoring
	Implant MBAN	Cardiovascular Diseases
		Cancer Detection
	Remote control devices	Ambient Assisted Living
		Patient Monitoring
		Tele- medicine system

or MAP1 and MAP2 and CAP (contention access phase) as shown in Fig. 2.[1–8] These access phases have been explained in detail as follows:

Exclusive Access Phase (EAP):

- **Purpose**: The EAP is designed to provide exclusive access to the channel for specific types of traffic, typically high-priority data frames. This ensures that critical data can be transmitted with minimal interference and delay.
- **EAP1 and EAP2**: These are distinct phases within the EAP category, used to handle high-priority transmissions at different times. EAP1 and EAP2 allow for scheduled, high-priority access to the channel, avoiding contention and providing guaranteed transmission opportunities.

Random Access Phase (RAP):

- **Purpose**: The RAP provides a mechanism for devices to access the channel on a more opportunistic basis, handling lower-priority data frames or less time-sensitive communications. Devices transmit randomly during this phase, and there may be collisions if multiple devices attempt to transmit simultaneously.
- **RAP1 and RAP2**: These are different instances within the RAP category, enabling random access to the channel at different times. RAP1 and RAP2 allow devices to access the channel without a guaranteed opportunity, handling less critical data or adjusting to the network's current conditions.

Management Access Phase (MAP): The MAP provides dedicated time for managing and controlling messages, ensuring efficient network management and coordination by allowing devices to exchange control information and perform network management tasks without interference from other traffic.

Contention Access Phase (CAP): The CAP allows devices to compete for channel access more randomly and less predictably, handling general data transmissions where contention and collision avoidance mechanisms like CSMA/CA are employed to manage access.

The BNC (Body Network Coordinator) can combine the EAP and RAP phases into single extended EAP phases (EAP1 and EAP2) to prioritize high-priority data transmissions. This means that the EAP1 phase might be extended to cover the functions of both EAP1 and RAP1, and similarly for EAP2 with RAP2. This approach provides dedicated time slots for critical data without extending the actual duration of the EAP1 and EAP2 phases but rather reallocating the time from the RAP phases to enhance high-priority data handling [6–10].

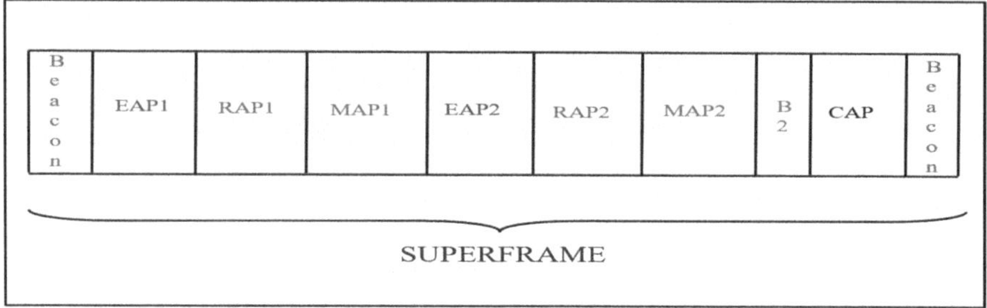

Fig. 2. Superframe Structure in the Beacon with superframe mode with different access phases. The sensor nodes access the medium used during these access phases using CSMA/CA or slotted Aloha protocols [1–8].

Three parameters of the nodes are used while accessing the medium using CSMA/CA and these are the backoff counter, the backoff stage, and the contention window size. The contention window in IEEE 802.15.6 refers to the time during which devices compete for access to the communication channel, adjusting their transmission attempts to minimize collisions. In IEEE 802.15.6, the contention window for a sensor node depends on its user priority as shown in the Table 2 and is determined by formula

$$CW_{max} = 2^{m}CW_{min} \tag{1}$$

where CW_{max} and CW_{min} are maximum and minimum sizes, and the backoff counter value is selected at random from the interval $[1, CW_{min}]$.

The standard emphasizes categorizing the sensor nodes into different user priorities such that each group of users has a contention window as per user priority. It is evident from the Table 2 that the sensor node with lower priority has higher value of CW_{min} and CW_{max} and have to wait longer while higher priority sensor nodes are allowed to transmit data after decrementing backoff counter which is chosen from smaller CW. A BNC controls the channel access based on information about nodes priority and deals with channel slot allocations. In case of higher user priority UP7, the nodes are allowed to decrement the backoff counter value and access the medium during the EAP periods, while all nodes can compute for the medium access during the RAPs and CAP.

Another challenge for MBAN is the low range of data transmission, as the sensor nodes are typically low-power devices. This limitation is often overcome by using relay

Table 2. Contention window sizes along with the User priorities [6].

User Priority	Data Traffic	Contention Window minimum (CW_{min})	Contention Window maximum (CW_{max})
UP0	Background	16	64
UP1	Best effort	16	32
UP2	Excellent effort	8	32
UP3	Video	8	16
UP4	Voice	4	16
UP5	Network control	4	8
UP6	High priority data	2	8
UP7	Emergency or medical implant data	1	4

nodes, which act as intermediate points to extend the communication range. Relay nodes receive data from the sensor nodes and forward it to the BNC of the next MBAN or next relay node which sends the data to the medical server, thereby reducing the need for direct, long-range transmission. This strategy helps maintain low power consumption while ensuring reliable data delivery across larger distances.

In this review paper, various mechanisms for backoff counter optimization, allocating priority to nodes, Dynamic slot allocation and Relay node mechanisms have been discussed and compared to gain a good understanding of existing state of art for MBAN. Additionally, the sensor nodes are low-power devices that can transmit data up to short distances, therefore the network allows a relay mechanism to allow data to hop and reach the destination. The IEEE 802.15.6 MAC has been studied by researchers to improve network reliability for a range of healthcare applications. In the following portion, an overview of pertinent studies is presented with an emphasis on elements that have been discovered to influence performance.

Several works of literature examine the performance of the IEEE 802.15.6 standard and the impact of various factors, including backoff counters, user priorities, and the probability of sufficient time slots etc. Although this IEEE 802.15.6 standard is a guideline for MBAN, it is still evolving and there is scope for performance improvement.

The objective of this study is to understand the research done and identify any research gaps in the performance of MBAN where the effect of parameters such as back-off counter values, sensor node priority, and dynamic slot allocation on data throughput, reliability, and latency has been studied. The paper has been organized in the following way:

Section 2 highlights the algorithms used for back-off counter optimization. Studies on node prioritizing are included in Sect. 3. Work on dynamic slot allocation is discussed in Sect. 4. Network expansion using relay techniques is elaborated in Sect. 5. A summary of the state of the art studied in these sections has been concluded in Sect. 6.

2 Backoff Counter Value Selection

The performance of the IEEE 802.15.6 CSMA/CA access technique must be evaluated and improved since medical data transmission demands high reliability and real-life performance. This is especially important since, as network density rises, the CSMA/CA performance degrades. Various research groups used mathematical models where statistics or queueing theory has been used to study the effect of various parameters on network performance. The backoff counter is adjusted during retransmissions using the dynamic backoff approach described in [10], which essentially optimizes it according to user priorities (UP). The backoff counter for UP7 and UP6 is set at CW_{min}; for other priorities, it is modified according to the nodes' number of retransmission attempts. Excluding UP2 and UP4, this method has shown improvements in data packet loss of up to 10% when 20 packets per second are sent per node and about 7% when 140 packets per second are conveyed. Although even with the throughput and latency improvements, there are still major disadvantages associated with excluding UP2 and UP4. There is a greater chance of collisions because of the equal contention window (CW) sizes as defined in the standard for these priorities, especially during retransmissions when CW boundaries may be beyond IEEE 802.15.6 restrictions.

The network of Stochastic timed automata formalism has been modeled using UPPAL-SMC, where the main objective was to improve the performance of the network in situations where the network density is high [11]. Three scenarios were modeled as follows: Scenario1, where sensor nodes access the channel using a single access phase (AP) in the super-frame; Scenario 2 where the super-frame is divided into two AP with no AP (NAP) between the access phases; Scenario 3 where there are three AP in super-frame with two NAPs. It is seen that as the number of nodes increases, the number of collisions increases and this effect is more prominent for Scenario 2 and 3, where the superframe is divided into more APs. However, the performance improves by using a proposed backoff counter update mechanism where the idle listening time of sensor nodes has been increased so that the nodes wait more patiently for the channel to become free. It is seen that the using the proposed backoff counter mechanism and dividing the super-frame into three AP, the maximum number of successful packets transmitted is highest in the case of Scenario 3 as compared to other scenarios.

The Binary Exponential Backoff (BEB) Algorithm as used in IEEE 802.15.6 standard employs an exponential increase in the contention window size to reduce collision after node failure, with the contention window doubling up to a maximum value CW_{max} [12, 13]. While this approach effectively reduces collision, it can lead to delays and lower overall Quality of Service (QoS). The Prioritized Fibonacci Backoff (PFB) method allows sensor nodes to start with a random backoff count within a range constrained by a minimum contention window size, denoted as CW_{min}. This method then increases the contention window (CW) size gradually, following the Fibonacci series. The increase in CW is based on user priorities with higher-priority users being allowed smaller contention windows to reduce their waiting time. This approach balances collision avoidance with priority-based access, using the Fibonacci series to incrementally adjust the CW size after each collision or retransmission with the help of the number of collisions. Although this method reduces idle listening, it presents problems such as contention window size overlap, which causes the superframe to be underutilized and may result in a greater number of node collisions. [11–13].

Table 3. Comparison in backoff counter algorithms

Algorithms	Comparison Parameters	
	Methodology	Observations
Binary Exponential Backoff (BEB) [12, 13]	• The value of the backoff counter is chosen at random from the range $[1, CW_{min}]$ • CW size is doubled up to CW_{max} for an even number of collisions	This algorithm exponentially increases the CW size which increases the idle listening time in between the process and affects the overall performance of the standard
Prioritized Fibonacci Backoff (PFB) [11–13]	• Assign the backoff counter's value from the interval $[1, CW_{min}]$ • Based on priorities, the CW value is updated	Since the node density anticipated by the IEEE 802.15.6 standard is lower than that of other IEEE standards, overlapped contention windows in the PFB algorithm result in collisions that underutilize the superframe
Non-overlapping Backoff (NOBA) [12, 13]	• Select the backoff counter's value from the range $[CW_{min}, CW_{max}]$ • The sliding window was added to the modified CW values	Elevated lower bounds of contention windows result in extended listening times for lower user priority
PBCR [14]	• Backoff value calculation based on the network parameter index	Consider all parameters with equal weights
Unique Backoff technique [15]	• A unique backoff value from the array from one to CW_{max}	Nodes participation in the channel is considered only for one time

A Non-Overlapping Backoff Algorithm (NOBA) addresses these issues by avoiding priority conflicts and inefficiency associated with fixed slot size [13, 14]. The backoff counter value in NOBA is chosen at random from the range defined by a sliding window factor which adjusts CW_{min} and CW_{max} based on user priority and offers a more flexible and efficient approach to reduce idle listening as compared to BEB and PFB.

A Unique backoff technique has been employed, which uses a defined contention window size to assign unique backoff counter values to each sensor node according to its user priority and CW_{max} size for the node. Specifically, this approach can be used in the Random-access phase and has a specific condition that a node could only transmit once in a super frame, which results in less-than-ideal performance [15]. A hybrid backoff technique has been proposed where the contention window (CW) is reduced to half when a collision takes place for UP6 and UP7 and for the other priorities the minimal value between CW_{max} and 2 x cw is used to choose the backoff counter value for the remaining user priorities. The primary focus of this work is on UP6 and UP7, to improve the performance of these higher user-priority nodes [16]. A comparison between the different backoff counter algorithms have been presented in the Table 3.

Various algorithms have been developed to update back-off counter values in the CSMA/CA mechanism, while numerous researchers have focused on analytical models to evaluate the impact of back-off counters and additional parameters on the throughput and reliability of MBANs. Using Markov chain-based analytical models, researchers have examined how variations in network size, Bit Error Rate (BER), packet lengths, and path lengths affect the Quality of Service (QoS) of MBANs [17–19]. Additionally, non-Markovian stochastic studies have been conducted to determine the maximum throughput and minimum delay for sensor nodes operating under different frequency bands and data rates. These studies indicate that larger contention windows for the same node lead to better-normalized throughput compared to smaller contention windows, though the analysis was limited to ideal conditions with idle channels, which are not typical of real-world scenarios [20, 21]. Both Markovian and non-Markovian models contribute significantly to improving the CSMA/CA mechanism by recommending optimal contention window and back-off counter values. These adjustments lead to reduced collisions, resulting in higher throughput and minimal delay.

3 Channel Access and Sensor Priority

Sensor node prioritization is crucial for minimizing channel contention and ensuring reliable data transfer. Higher-priority nodes are more likely to access the channel immediately, as they often need to transmit emergency data without delay, potentially limiting the transmission opportunities for lower-priority nodes. According to IEEE 802.15.6 guidelines, MBAN sensor nodes are classified into eight user priority levels (UP0-UP7), with higher-priority nodes having smaller contention window (CW) values than lower-priority nodes. Assigning priority to sensor nodes is crucial to manage network efficiency and reduce potential issues. When only a few nodes are assigned high priority while many others are given low priority, retransmissions become necessary, increasing the likelihood of collisions. Under under-saturation conditions, where nodes are distributed across all priority levels, a significant gap between the minimum contention windows (CW) of high and low-priority nodes can lead to starvation for lower-priority nodes [22–24]. This disparity often results in lower-priority nodes losing their chances to access the channel. In MBANs, where wearable sensors have limited battery life, efficient priority assignment is essential to minimize retransmissions from collisions and prevent starvation, thereby prolonging the life of these critical sensors.

Priority-based Load Adaptive MAC (PLA-MAC) protocol divided patient data in four categories as shown in Fig. 3 [25]:

The super-frame is comprised for the following periods: Contention-Access Period (CAP) which is further divided into Data Transfer Slots (DTSs) and Emergency Data Transfer Slots (ETS). Emergency sensors can successfully communicate using the ETS, whereas other sensors using DTS. Since there are only three user priority which do not include the emergency sensor (CP), there is contention for the channel which

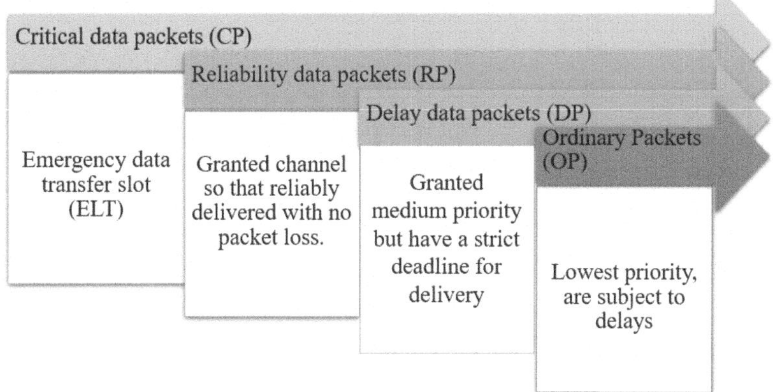

Fig. 3. Priority Levels of PLA-MAC

impairs the MAC's performance, increasing energy consumed by sensors, delaying packet transmission and decrease of data reliability.

The Preemptive and Non-Preemptive MAC (PNP-MAC) protocol classifies patient data into five categories: file transfer, emergency alert, medical continuous, medical routine, and non-medical continuous. The suggested MAC super frame consists of an advertisement, a beacon, a data transmits slot (DTS), and an emergency data transmit slot (ETS) as seen in Fig. 4 during the Contention Access Period (CAP), which is shared by the DTS and ETS, every node fights for channel access. The body coordinator first allots ETS slots to emergency sensor and remaining slots as DTS slots to other sensors. When a new emergency sensor becomes ready, the body coordinator preempts low-priority data, reallocates the remaining DTS slots to the high-priority data. When this happens, the body coordinator notifies every node by request message to de-allocate their DTS slots and change their status appropriately. If all DTS slots are taken, then ETS spaces are allotted for life-critical situations. The PNP-MAC protocol has limitations as it can lead to data loss for preempted nodes when non-essential data is removed from DTS slots to make way for essential data [26].

A non-cooperative game framework aimed at enhancing the performance of the IEEE 802.15.6 MAC protocol has been studied by another group. It proposes an improved utility function that considers both throughput and delay during CSMA/CA contention. In this framework, sensor nodes act as players, adjusting their contention window size to maximize this utility function. The contention window is minimized so that the channel access probability increases, which in turn increase the throughput and latency [27].

An analytical model focusing on mean response time and normalized throughput to evaluate the performance of the IEEE 802.15.6 CSMA/CA access method has been proposed by a group of researchers. In this work the EAP and RAP durations are adjusted based upon two probabilities, namely the probability that the medium is idle in RAP when backoff counter is decrementing and the probability of successful access and acknowledgement. It was seen that if EAP is fixed, and RAP is varied, more sensors are able to access the channel, and throughput as well as reliability improves. However, the

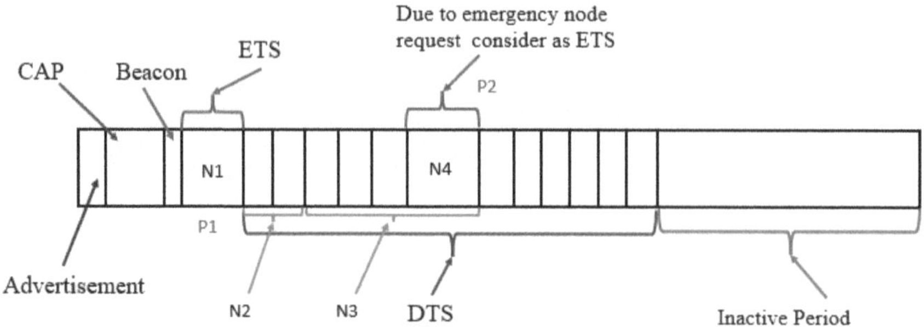

Fig. 4. Super frame in PNP-MAC

study's scope was limited to three user priorities—controlled load, medical data, and emergency—without considering additional priority nodes [28].

An analytical model has been presented by the research group, with consideration of saturated and lossy channel conditions, where they calculated probabilities of packet loss, channel busy states, and bit error rates. The study specifically examined how packet loss probability affects throughput under lossy conditions, finding that high-priority nodes effectively utilize the channel due to their smaller contention windows (CW). This, however, restricts low-priority nodes from accessing the channel, negatively impacting their throughput. While the model provides valuable insights, since it has been used for only two user priorities, its applicability is limited [29].

A hybrid node prioritizing strategy, where the Contention Window (CW) is modified after normalization has been used and throughput is observed to improve [30]. The analytical and simulation results also show that the energy consumption of hybrid nodes is reduced to 25% as compared to the standard CSMA-CA nodes.

Criteria Importance through Inter Criteria Correlation (CRITIC) has been developed for computing priority of sensor nodes based upon weights which depend on parameters like packet generation rate, data transmission rate, buffer size, packet size. The research shows that combined with dynamic slot allocation, the CRITIC yield reliability improvement by more than 50% [31]. Sixty-four sensors have been arranged in eight different priority queues, and CRITIC has been used to find local user priorities of sensors in every queue and the sensors transmit data using this local priority. This study shows that the efficiency of lower user priority nodes improves up to 50% and throughput is maintained in sustainable range, even when the channel traffic increases [32].

Several strategies have been proposed to enhance traffic allocation and user prioritization within the IEEE 802.15.6 standard, ensuring data packets reach their destinations effectively [33–37]. These include protocols like Saturation Aware for the User Priorities (SAUP), Saturation Aware for the Highest user priority (SAH), and various adaptive MAC algorithms that prioritize traffic under different conditions. For example, some protocols improve channel access for high-priority users, while others dynamically adjust priorities based on traffic or slot prediction. Although these protocols offer effective traffic prioritization, they have not been tested in scenarios involving health-related anomalies.

Along with sensor node priority and backoff counter value, slot allocation is another crucial factor that significantly impacts IEEE 802.15.6 performance. Dynamic slot allocation provides flexibility and prevents the superframe from being over or underused by altering the slot allocations to nodes.

4 Dynamic Slot Allocation for Enhanced Performance

MBAN sensor nodes have constraints on energy consumption and low transmission latency and demand high transmission probability to maintain high throughput. Considering that these sensors deal with life-critical vitals, it is crucial to support Quality of Service (QoS) and one of the important variables in determining the QoS is the superframe time utilization factor. Various dynamic slot allocation protocols are run on the central coordinator to optimize the throughput and energy efficiency [38–40].

The Traffic Aware Dynamic (TAD) MAC protocol is designed to optimize wake-up intervals (WUInt) for nodes in a wireless network by stabilizing these intervals for variable and constant traffic. The protocol operates in two stages: initially, nodes wait for a coordinator's beacon to determine which node can transmit, with others entering sleep mode to minimize idle listening. The coordinator dynamically adjusts its WUInt schedule based on observed traffic patterns, and receiving nodes align their wake-up schedules to account for hardware delays and clock drift. Each node uses a Traffic Status Register (TSR) to track recent traffic, influencing future WUInt calculations. This approach reduces unnecessary wakeups, collisions, idle listening, and wasteful broadcasts, thereby improving network performance and conserving power. However, the protocol is not ideal for WBANs as it relies too much on the preamble method, does not consider traffic categorization, and lacks prioritization for emergency data nodes. [41].

The Radio Frequency identification (RFID)-enabled MAC (RMAC) protocol dynamically modifies the wake-up and sleep modes of nodes in response to traffic, therefore mitigating the problems of overhearing and idle listening. The protocol uses two different approaches for channel access: a pre-scheduled technique for normal traffic and a RFID awakening mechanism for emergency traffic. This strategy minimizes power consumption by only waking nodes when necessary. Emergency traffic is prioritized via the RFID wakeup mechanism, which enables quick resource allocation even on a busy main channel as shown in Fig. 5. A synchronizing beacon, a customizable idle time for energy saving, and a Contention-Free time (CFP) for periodic communication are all part of the protocol's framework. Findings show that the RMAC protocol grows well with a growing number of nodes and greatly decreases power consumption when compared to IEEE 802.15.4 MAC while maintaining low latency. The impact of different traffic priorities and diverse traffic types handling is not included in this study, which might affect the protocol's performance for heterogenous network. [42].

Throughput and Channel-Aware (TCA) based dynamic scheduling methods have been simulated where the packet error rates, or signal-to-noise ratios are estimated for

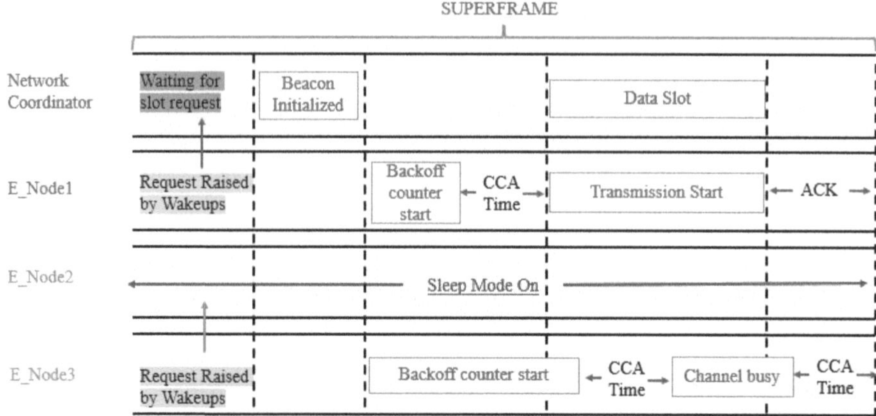

Fig. 5. Architecture of Superframe for RMAC protocol.

nodes using biomedical mobility modeling. The technique assigns the number of slots to nodes depending on the channel condition and therefore this method is known as channel aware dynamic algorithm. According to the results, some sensors that experience time-varying traffic and low data rates operate noticeably better, with a Packet Delivery Ratio (PDR) of up to 99%. Conversely, some high data rate sensors have a PDR of 95%. The main cause of this variation in performance is the fact that memory constraints cause packet drops to happen as new packets arrive [43]. The study compared static slot allocation with variable allocation, where slots are dynamically assigned when a node transmits data at a rate exceeding a threshold. The results of three medical cases—heart, neurology, and respiratory disorders—showed that variable allocation improved performance metrics, including packets received per node and packet loss rate. This improvement is attributed to the algorithm's ability to allocate more slots to sensors transmitting at higher data rates [44].

The research group introduced an improved CSMA/CA proposal featuring two new super frame segments: one for slot reallocation and another for traffic management, particularly handling increased emergency traffic. The results indicate a 2% improvement in energy efficiency compared to the standard and reduced latency. However, the technique's focus on emergency traffic limits, it is effective in scenarios with high emergency traffic volumes, making it less suitable for diverse traffic conditions [45].

Another study modifies the contention window (CW) values based on transmission success or failure. An anomaly occurs when high-priority frames use CW values meant for lower-priority traffic, causing delays and reduced transmission success. To address this, study fixes include ensuring acknowledgment requests for high-priority frames and preventing CW from exceeding maximum values. Results showed that these changes improved network performance, reducing back-off times and access delays. Additionally, modifying CW boundaries for each user priority, while reducing wait times, has led to increased energy consumption, despite the standard already defining CW boundaries based on packet priority. [46].

Another research group proposed a priority-based superframe architecture with five key segments: beacon period, Uplink Control for Emergency Traffic (UCE), Uplink Control for Normal Traffic (UCN), TimeSlots Reserved for Emergency Medical Data (TSRE), TimeSlots Reserved for Normal Data (TSRN), and TimeSlots Reserved for On-Demand Data (TSROD). This architecture incorporates three priority levels: emergency, medical, and controlled load. While intended to manage different traffic types, this approach exacerbates low-priority traffic starvation in the IEEE 802.15.6 CSMA/CA access mechanism, leading to long waiting times for low-priority traffic and creating challenges for WBAN-based eHealth applications where urgent traffic, although critical, is infrequent [47].

Several research works have emphasized the necessity of dynamic slot allocation in Wireless Body Area Networks (WBANs), tackling several issues related to conventional static allocation techniques. There are some more studies such as: A scheduling strategy based on optimum slot allocation was presented in [40]. It included a threshold-based technique to control the transmission order of nodes. To depict the WBAN channel, they used a Markov model. The only two states that are accessible for on-body linkages in this model—good and bad—which insufficiently depict the complexity of WBAN settings, is a limitation of the model.

To handle emergency packets, authors in [48] suggested a MAC protocol that adds mini-slots to a beacon-enabled superframe. For regular packets, they offered a data-rate-based planned slot allocation system. The plan has a major shortcoming despite its novel approach: high data rate nodes often consume a large amount of energy, which presents a serious challenge to its sustainability and efficiency. Authors in [49] proposed two TDMA-based scheduling systems to improve energy economy and reliability: dynamic scheduling and adaptive scheduling. Under both regular and emergency conditions, the adaptive scheduling approach dynamically allots time slots to nodes based on a study of their channel characteristics and buffer state. By contrast, time slots are only assigned according on the buffer status when using the dynamic scheduling approach. Nevertheless, both methods overlook the node priority during the slot allocation procedure, which may affect the network's overall performance. The Dynamic Slot Scheduling (DSS) technique, which makes use of a temporal autocorrelation model based on actual on-body data gathered via customized wireless transceivers, has been presented by another research group [50]. This method offers a more realistic solution for slot scheduling, but it has a drawback in that it assumes that all nodes have the same transmission power, which may not be realistic in a variety of WBAN circumstances.

Other pertinent approaches include the lost packet estimating methodology developed by authors in [51], which aims to decrease communication channel waste in the IEEE 802.15.6 MAC caused by static phase time by dynamically changing the superframe structure. The development of The MAC, a superframe structure that allows discontinuous times for various traffic types to assure Quality of Service (QoS) provisioning, including an emergency data management mechanism, in [52] further developed this idea. It is crucial to remember that these schemes in [51, 52] did not undergo real-time healthcare scenario evaluation, which leaves a gap in their efficacy and practical application in dynamic, real-world settings.

Game theory principles are also utilized to enhance MBAN QoS by improving performance metrics like packet delays, channel access probability, throughput, etc. Energy-aware cooperative game theory strategies have been explored to reduce the superframe interleaving delays when two or more hubs coexist and share the same operating channel. Shapley value-based resource allocation mechanisms have been deployed and fair bandwidth distribution amongst flow classes of multimedia services has been observed for Long Term Evolution [LTE] communication systems [53]. Nash bargaining solution in the median access control layer has been recommended for allocating time slots in WBANs with improved reliability and throughput [54].

Game theory-based time slot allocation with unique Nash equilibrium has been used for fair assignment of the transmitting slots in multi WBANs and preventing reckless resource usage with a well-organized payoff structure [55]. Stackelberg game and Bayesian game models have been used to regulate the overall interference of the coordinator and maximize the data rate of sensor transmission [56]. Inter-WBAN interference issues have been investigated using the QoS-based adaptive power regulation (QPC) system in combination with the Nash bargaining game model. The study discovered that in addition to achieving the Pareto optimum solution, it also made sure that rival participants were treated fairly [57].

A summary of the dynamic slot allocation algorithm is shown in Table 4, showing a summary of methodology used and pros and cons of the method.

Table 4. Summary of some dynamic slot algorithms

Algorithm	Comparison	
	Methodology	Observation
Traffic-Aware Dynamic (TAD) MAC [41]	Wakeup intervals optimization using flag status in a register	Energy consumption is minimized as idle listening time, overhearing, collisions and unnecessary wake up is reduced
Radio Frequency identification enabled (RFID) RMAC [42]	Dynamic modification in wakeup and sleep time, which helps to save energy and reduce average delay time for packets. Suitable for emergency sensors where number of nodes is large	The study considers the prescheduled method for allocating channels to normal traffic and considers the normal traffic at a single priority level
Throughput and Channel Aware (TCA) [43]	Slot allotment depends on the channel conditions	Leads to data loss due to memory limitations
varySchedSlots [44]	Scheduling of slots based on the nodes' data rates	The study allocates slots based on the data rate threshold value; nevertheless, it does not address the situation in which numerous nodes have the same user priority

(continued)

Table 4. *(continued)*

Algorithm	Comparison	
	Methodology	Observation
Optimum Slot allocation [47]	Slot allocation is done dynamically according to QoS which depends on data rate, delivery probability, and latency	Classify the nodes into just two categories: good and bad based on the threshold limits of QoS
Mini-Slot allocation [48]	Slots in RAP are subdivided into mini slots. and Emergency packets are sent through these mini slots while the remaining normal slot can be used for emergency or normal packets. The packet delivery ratio is improved, and energy consumption is reduced	If emergency sensor nodes are not ready for data transmission, then the mini slots which are 25% of the time are wasted
TDMA based scheduling technique [49]	Slot allotment is done in two parts: a) Emergency node slots b) Regular traffic slots	The end delay increases when the channel conditions are non-ideal as nodes are forced to sleep under fading channel conditions and packets are scheduled for the next TDMA slot
Dynamic EAP based MAC protocol [58]	The length of EAP and RAP is calculated a) EAP slot length: Based on the requirement for transmission of all Data packets b) RAP slot length: Length calculated by remaining time in the superframe and weighting them by length of EAP	Eight data priorities are categorized into three levels: a) Always Important – UP7 b) Never Important – UP0 c) Sometimes Important – UP1 to UP6 Since all priorities from UP1 to UP6 are grouped into the same category, they are treated uniformly, leading to increased collisions in the channel because these nodes are not distinguished from one another

5 MBAN Extension Using Relay Nodes

Alongside their efforts to enhance performance improvement parameters, researchers are also exploring the potential of extending the network using relay nodes. This approach aims to boost network coverage and reliability by strategically placing relay nodes to assist in data transmission. Researchers are working to overcome limitations related to signal range and interference, ultimately leading to a more robust and efficient network. The integration of relay nodes represents a promising avenue for further development and optimization in network performance.

A Group-based MAC (G-MAC) protocol, which adds a relay node to assist the central coordinator hub in handling emergency data has been suggested [59]. This relay node relieves the central hub from nonemergency data and handles all the data transmission/collision of these nodes by acting as the cluster head. The approach reduces the latency of the emergency node relieving the primary hub from overheads of the entire traffic and reserving it for the highest priority node traffic.

Cross-layered energy-aware resource allocation (CLEAR) protocol for Integrated Sensor Hubs has been introduced [60]. The findings of the study reveal that the CLEAR protocol delivers the quality of service (QoS) through interleaving the super frames and enhancing system energy efficiency. The researchers in [61] have developed an Energy-Efficient and Emergency-Aware Media Access Control (MAC) protocol (EEEA-MAC). This protocol divides the super-frame into three parts: the beacon component, the contention-free period (CFP), and the contention access period (CAP). In this case, each node has a distinct channel access strategy designed so that the source node uses the carrier sense multiple access collision avoidance (CSMA/CA) and the relay nodes adopt the hybrid CSMA/CA-TDMA. When the source node generates less data, this study helps in lowering collision, and the introduction of TDMA (time division multiple access) reduces conflicts and energy consumption at the relay node. A Joint Weight-Optimizing timeslot allocation protocol with a relay mechanism has been studied and shown to increase the throughput [62]. The weights for various sensors are determined using a hierarchical method and sensors are placed so that the most important sensor is either nearest or farthest from the sender and accordingly the transfer link is either a direct link or a relay transfer link.

6 Conclusion

This study of the state of art offers a detailed examination of the latest developments in Medical Body Area Networks (MBANs), with a special focus on various key areas including the design of dynamic slot allocation algorithms, the prioritization of sensor nodes, the optimization of backoff counter values, and the extension of network capabilities through the use of relay nodes. The research demonstrates how these advancements contribute to improvements in throughput (reaching several Mbps) and reliability. These enhancements are achieved through mechanisms that enable more efficient channel access and utilization, as well as by implementing node prioritization strategies. In MBANs, sensors are typically low-power devices with a limited wireless transmission range, generally confined to a few tens of meters. However, the introduction of relay nodes significantly extends this transmission range to several hundreds of meters. The effectiveness of this extended range is highly dependent on the strategic placement and number of relay nodes used.

MBANs are designed to operate with low power and at low data rates, primarily focusing on the transmission of critical health data such as vital signs, rather than high-bandwidth data. While MBANs might not provide the same level of throughput as other wireless technologies, they are optimized for their specific applications, emphasizing reliable and real-time transmission of medical information with minimal energy consumption. Tables 3 and 4 highlight that, although there has been considerable research aimed at improving the IEEE 802.15.6 MAC protocol, there is still a gap in studies that focus on utilizing node parameters as key decision-making factors for performance enhancement. Future research should address this gap by exploring how node parameters can be used to optimize MBAN performance. Such studies will demonstrate the practical feasibility of MBANs in real-world settings and support their ongoing development as technology and medical devices continue to evolve.

References

1. Benmansour, T., Ahmed, T., Moussaoui, S., Doukha, Z.: Performance analyses of the IEEE 802.15.6 Wireless Body Area Network with heterogeneous traffic. J. Netw. Comput. Appl. **163**, 102651 (2020). https://doi.org/10.1016/j.jnca.2020.102651
2. Yuan, X., et al.: Performance analysis of IEEE 802.15.6-based coexisting mobile WBANs with prioritized traffic and dynamic interference. IEEE Trans. Wirel. Commun. **17**(8), 5637–5652 (2018). https://doi.org/10.1109/TWC.2018.2848223
3. Benmansour, T., Ahmed, T., Moussaoui, S.: Performance analyses and improvement of the IEEE 802.15.6 CSMA/CA using the low latency queuing. In: 2017 IEEE 22nd International Workshop on Computer Aided Modeling and Design of Communication Links and Networks (CAMAD), Lund, Sweden, pp. 1–6 (2017). https://doi.org/10.1109/CAMAD.2017.8031623
4. Hernandez, M., Mucchi, L.: Survey and coexistence study of IEEE 802.15.6TM -2012 body area networks, UWB PHY. In: Body Area Networks Using IEEE 802.15.6, pp. 1–44. Elsevier (2014). https://doi.org/10.1016/B978-0-12-396520-2.00001-7
5. Cavallari, R., Martelli, F., Rosini, R., Buratti, C., Verdone, R.: A survey on wireless body area networks: technologies and design challenges. IEEE Commun. Surv. Tutor. **16**(3), 1635–1657 (2014). https://doi.org/10.1109/SURV.2014.012214.00007
6. Ullah, S., Mohaisen, M., Alnuem, M.A.: A review of IEEE 802.15.6 MAC, PHY, and security specifications. Int. J. Distrib. Sens. Netw. **9**(4), 950704 (2013). https://doi.org/10.1155/2013/950704
7. Raghavan, P., Morgan, T.: Wireless medical room control arrangement for control of a plurality of medical devices, 22 August 2017, US Patent 9,740,826. https://patentscope.wipo.int/search/en/detail.jsf?docId=WO2009151535
8. Bandyopadhyay, B., Das, D., Chatterjee, A., Ahmed, S.J., Mukherjee, A., Naskar, M.K.: Markov chain-based analysis of IEEE 802.15. 6 mac protocol in real life scenario. In: Proceedings of the 9th International Conference on Body Area Networks, pp. 331–337 (2014). https://doi.org/10.4108/icst.bodynets.2014.257202
9. Tavera, C.A., Ortiz, J.H., Khalaf, O.I., Saavedra, D.F., Aldhyani, T.H.H.: Wearable wireless body area networks for medical applications. Comput. Math. Methods Med. (2021). https://doi.org/10.1155/2021/5574376
10. Fourati, H., Idoudi, H., Saidane, L.A.: Intelligent slots allocation for dynamic differentiation in IEEE 802.15. 6 CSMA/CA. Ad Hoc Netw. **72**, 27–43 (2018). https://doi.org/10.1016/j.adhoc.2018.01.007
11. Touijer, B., Maissa, Y.B., Mouline, S.: IEEE 802.15. 6 CSMA/CA access method for WBANs: "performance evaluation and new backoff counter selection procedure". Comput. Netw. **188**, 107759 (2021). https://doi.org/10.1016/j.comnet.2020.107759
12. Khan, P., et al.: Performance analysis of different backoff algorithms for WBAN-based emerging sensor networks. Sensors **17**(3), 492 (2017). https://doi.org/10.3390/s17030492

13. Saboor, A., et al.: Dynamic slot allocation using non overlapping backoff algorithm in IEEE 802.15. 6 WBAN. IEEE Sens. J. **20**(18), 10862–10875 (2020). https://doi.org/10.1109/JSEN.2020.2993795
14. Das, K., Moulik, S.: PBCR: parameter-based backoff counter regulation in IEEE 802.15. 6 CSMA/CA. In: 2021 International Conference on COMmunication Systems & NETworkS (COMSNETS), pp. 565–571. IEEE (2021). https://doi.org/10.1109/COMSNETS51098.2021.9352747
15. Saboor, A., Ahmad, R., Ahmed, W., Alam, M.M.: A unique backoff algorithm in IEEE 802.15. 6 WBAN. In: 2018 IEEE 88th Vehicular Technology Conference (VTC-Fall), pp. 1–5. IEEE (2019). https://doi.org/10.1109/VTCFall.2018.8690812
16. Fourati, H., Idoudi, H., Saidane, L.A.: A novel IEEE 802.15. 6 CSMA/CA service differentiation. In: 2016 IEEE/ACS 13th International Conference of Computer Systems and Applications (AICCSA), pp. 1–7. IEEE (2016). https://doi.org/10.1109/AICCSA.2016.7945686
17. Preethichandra, D.M.G., Piyathilaka, L., Izhar, U., Samarasinghe, R., De Silva, L.C.: Wireless body area networks and their applications—a review. IEEE Access **11**, 9202–9220 (2023). https://doi.org/10.1109/ACCESS.2023.3239008
18. Waheed, T., Karim, F., Ghani, S.: QoS enhancement of AODV routing for MBANs. Wirel. Pers. Commun. **116**, 1379–1406 (2021). https://doi.org/10.1007/s11277-020-07558-x
19. Alkama, L., Bouallouche-Medjkoune, L., Bachiri, L.: Modeling and performance evaluation of the IEEE 802.15. 4K CSMA/CA with priority channel access mechanism under fading channel. Wirel. Pers. Commun. **115**(1), 527–556 (2020). https://doi.org/10.1007/s11277-020-07584-9
20. Ullah, S., Kwak, K.S.: Throughput and delay limits of IEEE 802.15. 6. In: 2011 IEEE Wireless Communications and Networking Conference, pp. 174–178. IEEE (2011). https://doi.org/10.1109/WCNC.2011.5779126
21. Ullah, S., Chen, M., Kwak, K.S.: Throughput and delay analysis of IEEE 802.15.6-based CSMA/CA protocol. J. Med. Syst. **36**(6), 3875–3891 (2012). https://doi.org/10.1007/s10916-012-9860-0
22. Herculano, J., et al.: MAC approaches to communication efficiency and reliability under dynamic network traffic in wireless body area networks: a review. Computing 1–25 (2024). https://doi.org/10.1007/s00607-024-01307-9
23. Dadhich, K., Kataria, D.: Wearable IoT using MBANs. In: Applied Intelligence in Human-Computer Interaction, pp. 113–127. CRC Press (2023). https://doi.org/10.1201/9781003415466-7
24. Khan, P., Ullah, N., Alam, M.N., Kwak, K.S.: Performance analysis of WBAN MAC protocol under different access periods. Int. J. Distrib. Sens. Netw. **11**(10), 102052 (2015). https://doi.org/10.1155/2015/102052
25. Anjum, I., Alam, N., Razzaque, M.A., Mehedi Hassan, M., Alamri, A.: Traffic priority and load adaptive MAC protocol for QoS provisioning in body sensor networks. Int. J. Distrib. Sens. Netw. **9**(3), 205192 (2013). https://doi.org/10.1155/2013/205192
26. Yoon, J.S., Ahn, G.S., Joo, S.S., Lee, M.J.: PNP-MAC: preemptive slot allocation and non-preemptive transmission for providing QoS in body area networks. In: 2010 7th IEEE Consumer Communications and Networking Conference, pp. 1–5. IEEE (2010). https://doi.org/10.1109/CCNC.2010.5421718
27. Shankar, A.V., Jacob, L.: A game theoretic approach for performance enhancement of IEEE 802.15. 6 based WBAN. In: 2016 International Conference on Signal Processing and Communication (ICSC), pp. 37–42. IEEE (2016). https://doi.org/10.1109/ICSPCom.2016.7980543

28. Bradai, N., Fourati, L.C., Kamoun, L.: New analytical model for IEEE 802.15. 6 under saturation condition and noisy channel. In: 2014 9th International Symposium on Communication Systems, Networks & Digital Sign (CSNDSP), pp. 243–248. IEEE (2014). https://doi.org/10.1109/CSNDSP.2014.6923833
29. Ullah, S., Tovar, E.: Performance analysis of IEEE 802.15. 6 contention-based MAC protocol. In: 2015 IEEE International Conference on Communications (ICC), pp. 6146–6151. IEEE (2015). https://doi.org/10.1109/ICC.2015.7249302
30. Shakir, M., et al.: Performance optimization of priority-assisted CSMA/CA mechanism of 802.15. 6 under saturation regime. Sensors **16**(9), 1421 (2016). https://doi.org/10.3390/s16091421
31. Das, K., Moulik, S., Chang, C.Y.: Priority-based dedicated slot allocation with dynamic superframe structure in IEEE 802.15. 6-based Wireless Body Area Networks. IEEE Internet Things J. **9**(6), 4497–4506 (2021). https://doi.org/10.1109/JIOT.2021.3104800
32. Dadhich, K., Kataria, D.: Performance evaluation of saturated medical body area network using priority reassignment. In: 3rd International Conference for Innovation in Technology (INOCON), Bangalore, India, pp. 1–6 (2024). https://doi.org/10.1109/INOCON60754.2024.10511875
33. Sadra, S., Abolhasan, M.: On improving the saturation performance of IEEE802.15.6-based MAC protocols in wireless body area networks. In: 2017 13th International Wireless Communications and Mobile Computing Conference (IWCMC), pp. 1233–1238. IEEE (2017). https://doi.org/10.1109/IWCMC.2017.7986461
34. Issaoui, L., Horrich, A., Sethom, K.: Improved MAC access under IEEE 802.15.6 WBAN standard. In: 2017 Ninth International Conference on Ubiquitous and Future Networks (ICUFN), pp. 416–420. IEEE (2017). https://doi.org/10.1109/ICUFN.2017.7993819
35. Miyazaki, T., Fukuya, T., Kohno, R.: A MAC protocol with slot prediction algorithm for wireless Body Area Network. In: 2017 11th International Symposium on Medical Information and Communication Technology (ISMICT), pp. 11–14. IEEE (2017). https://doi.org/10.1109/ISMICT.2017.7891756
36. Kim, E.J., Kim, H., Kim, D., Kim, D.: Adaptive priority-based medium access control protocol for IEEE 802.15.6 wireless body sensor networks. Sens. Mater. **30**, 1707 (2018). https://doi.org/10.18494/SAM.2018.1863
37. George, E.M., Jacob, L.: Multi-class delay sensitive medical packet scheduling in inter-WBAN communication. In: 2019 IEEE 1 3 International Conference on Advanced Networks and Telecommunications Systems (ANTS), pp. 1–5. IEEE (2019). https://doi.org/10.1109/ANTS47819.2019.9117925
38. Wang, J., Xie, Y., Yi, Q.: An all dynamic MAC protocol for wireless body area network. In: Proceedings of the 11th International Conference on Wireless Communications, Networking and Mobile Computing (WiCOM 2015), pp. 1–6 (2015). https://doi.org/10.1049/cp.2015.0703
39. Yuan, D., Zheng, G., Ma, H., Shang, J., Li, J.: An adaptive MAC protocol based on IEEE802.15.6 for wireless body area networks. Wirel. Commun. Mob. Comput. **2019**, 1–9 (2019). https://doi.org/10.1155/2019/3681631
40. Yan, Z., Liu, B., Chen, C.W.: QoS-driven scheduling approach using optimal slot allocation for wireless body area networks. In: 2012 IEEE 14th International Conference on e-Health Networking, Applications and Services (Healthcom), pp. 267–272 (2012). https://doi.org/10.1109/HealthCom.2012.6379419
41. Alam, M.M., Berder, O., Menard, D., Sentieys, O.: Tad-MAC: traffic-aware dynamic mac protocol for wireless body area sensor networks. IEEE J. Emerg. Sel. Top. Circuits Syst. **2**(1), 109–119 (2012). https://doi.org/10.1109/JETCAS.2012.2187243

42. Ullah, S.: RFID-enabled mac protocol for WBAN. In: IEEE International Conference on Communications (ICC), pp. 6030–6034. IEEE (2013). https://doi.org/10.1109/ICC.2013.6655565
43. Alam, M.M., Arbia, D.B., Hamida, E.B.: Joint throughput and channel aware (TCA) dynamic scheduling algorithm for emerging wearable applications. In: 2016 IEEE Wireless Communications and Networking Conference, pp. 1–6. IEEE (2016). https://doi.org/10.1109/WCNC.2016.7564978
44. Soni, G., Selvaradjou, K.: A dynamic allocation scheme of scheduled slots for real-time heterogenous traffic in IEEE 802.15.6 standard for scheduled access mechanism. J. Ambient. Intell. Humaniz. Comput. **14**(1), 237–256 (2023). https://doi.org/10.1007/s12652-021-03288-5
45. Jaramillo, R., Quintero, A., Chamberland, S.: Energy-efficient MAC protocol for wireless body area networks. In: Proceedings of the International Conference and Workshop on Computing and Communication (IEMCON). IEEE (2015). https://doi.org/10.1109/IEMCON.2015.7344452
46. Bukvic, M., Misic, J.: Access anomaly of emergency traffic in CSMA/CA of IEEE 802.15.6. In: Proceedings of the International Wireless Communications and Mobile Computing Conference (IWCMC). IEEE (2015). https://doi.org/10.1109/IWCMC.2015.7289133
47. Bradai, N., Ben Elhadj, H., Boudjit, S., Chaari, L., Kamoun, L.: QoS architecture over WBANs for remote vital signs monitoring applications. In: Proceedings of the IEEE Consumer Communications and Networking Conference (CCNC). IEEE (2015). https://doi.org/10.1109/CCNC.2015.7157937
48. Muthulakshmi, A., Shyamala, K.: Efficient patient care through wireless body area networks enhanced technique for handling emergency situations with better quality of service. Wirel. Pers. Commun. **95**(4), 3755–3769 (2017). https://doi.org/10.1007/s11277-017-4024-7
49. Salayma, M., Al-Dubai, A., Romdhani, I., Nasser, Y.: Reliability and energy efficiency enhancement for emergency-aware wireless body area networks (WBANs). IEEE Trans. Green Commun. Netw. **2**(3), 804–816 (2018). https://doi.org/10.1109/TGCN.2018.2813060
50. Zhang, H., Safaei, F., et al.: Channel autocorrelation-based dynamic slot scheduling for body area networks. EURASIP J. Wirel. Commun. Netw. **1**, 246 (2018). https://doi.org/10.1186/s13638-018-1261-8
51. Azhar, M.E., Rashid, I., Kanwal, S., Bashir, F., Zia, Y.: IEEE 802.15.6 superframe adjustment by using drop packet estimation technique. In: 2016 Sixth International Conference on Innovative Computing Technology (INTECH), pp. 413–417. IEEE (2016). https://doi.org/10.1109/INTECH.2016.7845063
52. Monowar, M.M., Alassaf, M.O.: On the design of thermal-aware duty-cycle MAC protocol for IoT healthcare. Sensors **20**(5), 1243 (2020). https://doi.org/10.3390/s20051243
53. Iturralde, M., Yahiya, T.A., Wei, A., Beylot, A.L.: Resource allocation using Shapley value in LTE networks. In: 2011 IEEE 22nd International Symposium on Personal, Indoor and Mobile Radio Communications, pp. 31–35. IEEE (2011). https://doi.org/10.1109/PIMRC.2011.6139974
54. Das, K., Moulik, S.: Boss: bargaining-based optimal slot sharing in IEEE 802.15. 6-based wireless body area networks. IEEE Internet Things J. **10**(4), 2945–2953 (2021). https://doi.org/10.1109/JIOT.2021.3122819
55. Zhang, B., Zhang, Y.: An individual differentiated coexisting mechanism for multiple wireless body area networks based on game theory. IEEE Access **6**, 54564–54581 (2018). https://doi.org/10.1109/ACCESS.2018.2872746
56. Wang, J., Sun, Y., Ji, Y., Luo, S.: Priority-aware price-based power control for co-located WBANs using stackelberg and Bayesian games. Sensors **19**(12), 2664 (2019). https://doi.org/10.3390/s19122664

57. Wang, J., Sun, Y., Ji, Y.: QoS-based adaptive power control scheme for co-located WBANs: a cooperative bargaining game theoretic perspective. Wirel. Netw. **24**(8), 3129–3139 (2018). https://doi.org/10.1007/s11276-017-1521-2
58. Enkoji, A., Li, M., Brisky, J.D., Melvin, R.: Dynamic EAP based MAC protocol for wireless body area networks. In: 2019 International Conference on Computing, Networking and Communications (ICNC), Honolulu, HI, USA, pp. 531–536 (2019). https://doi.org/10.1109/ICCNC.2019.8685495
59. Zia, Y., Bashir, F., Qureshi, K.N.: Dynamic superframe adaptation using group-based media access control for handling traffic heterogeneity in wireless body area networks. Int. J. Distrib. Sens. Netw. **16**(8), 1550147720949140 (2020). https://doi.org/10.1177/1550147720949140
60. Chen, D.-R., Chiu, W.-M.: Collaborative link-aware protocols for energy-efficient and QoS wireless body area networks using integrated sensors. IEEE Internet Things J. **5**(1), 132–149 (2017). https://doi.org/10.1109/JIOT.2017.2775048
61. Liang, B., Liu, X., Zhou, H., Leung, V.C.M., Liu, A., Chi, K.: Channel resource scheduling for stringent demand of emergency data transmission in WBANs. IEEE Trans. Wirel. Commun. **20**(4), 2341–2352 (2021). https://doi.org/10.1109/TWC.2020.3041471
62. He, M., Hu, F., Ling, Z., Mao, Z., Huang, Z.: A dynamic weights algorithm on information and energy transmission protocol based on WBAN. IEEE Trans. Veh. Technol. **70**(2), 1528–1537 (2021). https://doi.org/10.1109/TVT.2021.3053964

Optimizing Photon Sources and QEC in Quantum WBANs

Vikram Singh Thakur(✉) and Atul Kumar

Department of Electronics Engineering, IIT (BHU) Varanasi, Varanasi 221005, India
{vikramsinghthakur.rs.ece23,atul.ece}@iitbhu.ac.in

Abstract. Secure data transmission in healthcare-based Wireless Body Area Networks (WBANs) is increasingly vulnerable in the face of advancing quantum computing. Quantum Key Distribution (QKD) offers a solution, but its implementation in resource-constrained WBANs requires highly efficient and reliable single-photon sources. This work addresses a critical bottleneck in such sources: the inefficient population of excited states in quantum emitters like semiconductor quantum dots under conventional off-resonant excitation. We propose the Swing-UP of the quantum Emitter population (SUPER) scheme, a coherent control technique using frequency-modulated, highly-detuned pulses to achieve near-complete population inversion, resulting in single photons with high purity and indistinguishability. Crucially, we extend this physical-layer advancement to the system level by formulating a joint optimization framework for the photon source and Quantum Error Correction (QEC). This co-design methodology is essential for mitigating the high bit-error rates in lossy WBAN channels, enabling the practical realization of secure Quantum WBANs for next-generation medical applications.

Keywords: Quantum Technologies · Quantum Emitters · Single-Photon Sources · Coherent Excitation · Frequency Modulation · Quantum Dots · Excited State Population · Rabi Scheme · QEC

1 Introduction

The integration of wireless body area networks (WBANs) into healthcare promises a revolution in continuous patient monitoring and personalized medicine. However, the wireless transmission of sensitive biomedical data presents a critical security vulnerability. With the advent of quantum computing, classical encryption methods protecting this data are becoming increasingly susceptible to attacks. Quantum Key Distribution (QKD) offers a solution based on the laws of quantum mechanics, providing information-theoretic security. Implementing QKD within a WBAN-creating a Quantum WBAN (Q-WBAN)-is therefore a strategic imperative for future-proof medical data security [1,2].

The practical realization of Q-WBANs is fraught with unique physical-layer challenges. The on-body environment is inherently lossy, with signal attenuation due to body tissue absorption and dynamic channel conditions from user

K. Atul et al. (Eds.): BodyNets 2024, LNICST 666, pp. 206–223, 2026.
https://doi.org/10.1007/978-3-032-16099-7_17

movement. Furthermore, WBAN nodes are severely constrained in size, power, and computational resources. These factors contribute to high quantum bit error rates (QBER), which directly degrade the secure key rate and can compromise the entire QKD protocol [3]. Two components are paramount for overcoming these errors, a high-quality photon source and an efficient Quantum Error Correction (QEC) code. However, these components are typically optimized in isolation.

- **Photon Source Perspective:** Advanced excitation schemes, such as off-resonant, frequency-modulated pulses, are being developed to generate near-ideal single photons from quantum dots-characterized by high brightness, purity, and indistinguishability [4,5]. Operating these sources below the bandgap can help mitigate decoherence from phonon interactions, a crucial consideration for solid-state emitters [6].
- **QEC Perspective:** QEC codes are designed to correct errors, but their performance and resource overhead are typically analyzed against abstract error models, disconnected from the specific, non-ideal characteristics of a physical photon source.

This disjointed approach is fundamentally suboptimal for Q-WBANs. A high-performance QEC code is inefficient if it must correct for excessive errors from a poor source, while a near-perfect source is impractical if the QEC code's computational overhead exceeds the node's capabilities. This paper bridges the gap by introducing a co-design methodology that jointly optimizes photon sources and QEC for Quantum WBANs. We posit that for a system to be practical under stringent WBAN constraints, the physical-layer properties of the photon source must directly inform the selection and configuration of the QEC code, and vice-versa.

Our specific contributions to develop a cross-layer model that quantifies how key photon source parameters-such as indistinguishability and multi-photon probability, influenced by excitation schemes like frequency-modulated pulses-affect the logical error rate after QEC decoding. Furthermore, a joint optimization framework is formulated to determine the optimal photon source configuration and QEC code, aiming to maximize the secure key rate within given power and latency constraints. Simulation results demonstrate that the proposed co-optimized system significantly outperforms conventional, independently optimized designs, ensuring robust QKD performance in realistic, lossy WBAN channels [7]. By tightly coupling the physical and logical layers, this work provides a critical pathway towards building efficient and secure Q-WBANs, a cornerstone for the future of trustworthy digital healthcare.

The remainder of this paper is structured as Sect. 2 provides an overview of quantum emitters. Section 3 details the SUPER Scheme for Population Inversion in Two-Level Quantum Systems. Section 4 presents quantum-enabled WBAN system model and an overview of quantum gates, while Sect. 5 discusses about methodology and implementation of QEC Codes. Section 6 outlines the results and discussion. The paper concludes in Sect. 7 with a summary of findings.

2 Review of Quantum Emitters

Quantum emitters play a crucial role in the development of quantum technologies, driving advancements in quantum communication, computation, and sensing. These systems, which include atoms, molecules, and quantum dots, emit quantized energy in the form of photons. Their unique properties, governed by the principles of quantum mechanics, are essential for various applications in Q-WBANs. Quantum emitters possess discrete energy levels, allowing transitions that result in photon emission or absorption. These transitions can be described by the time-dependent Schrödinger equation [3] and are analyzed through Fermi's golden rule [1]. Consider a simple two-level quantum system where the energy levels are expressed as

$$E_0, E_1 = E_0 + \hbar\omega$$

Here, E_0 is the ground state energy, E_1 is the excited state energy, $\hbar$ is the reduced Planck constant, and ω represents the angular frequency of the emitted photon. Photon emission occurs during the transition from the excited to ground state and can be modeled using the Schrödinger equation

$$i\hbar\frac{d}{dt}\begin{pmatrix} c_1(t) \\ c_2(t) \end{pmatrix} = \begin{pmatrix} E_0 & 0 \\ 0 & E_1 \end{pmatrix}\begin{pmatrix} c_1(t) \\ c_2(t) \end{pmatrix} + \begin{pmatrix} 0 & \Omega(t) \\ \Omega^*(t) & 0 \end{pmatrix}\begin{pmatrix} c_1(t) \\ c_2(t) \end{pmatrix}$$

In this equation, $c_1(t)$ and $c_2(t)$ are the probability amplitudes for the ground and excited states, respectively, and $\Omega(t)$ is the Rabi frequency of the driving field.

As a key component in quantum communication protocols, such as QKD, single photons generated by quantum emitters establish secure communication channels [7]. The security of these protocols can be quantified using the Holevo bound, making high-quality photon sources essential for Q-WBAN security. In quantum computing, quantum emitters serve as qubits, leveraging superposition to enable parallel processing, far surpassing the capabilities of classical computing [2]. Their integration into scalable architectures is crucial for practical quantum information processing. Quantum emitters are vital in quantum sensing, offering high-precision measurements, as demonstrated by nitrogen-vacancy (NV) centers in diamond [6]. This capability is particularly relevant for biomedical sensing applications within WBANs.

Coherent excitation, which refers to the process of driving a quantum system into an excited state while maintaining the phase relationship between the field and the quantum state, is essential for quantum state manipulation. This is especially significant in semiconductor nanostructures like quantum dots, which exhibit discrete energy levels and are widely used in quantum optics and nanotechnology. The energy levels of quantum dots can be modeled using the particle-in-a-box approximation

$$E_n = \frac{h^2 n^2}{8m^* L^2}$$

where h is Planck's constant, m^* is the effective mass, and L is the quantum dot's confinement length. Single-photon sources, which emit photons one at a time with high efficiency and indistinguishability, are critical for quantum communication, quantum cryptography, and quantum computing. The indistinguishability of single photons is often evaluated using the Hong-Ou-Mandel (HOM) effect.

To enhance the interaction between the excitation field and the quantum emitter, frequency modulation (FM) can be employed, represented as:

$$E(t) = E_0 \cos(2\pi f_c t + \Delta f \sin(2\pi f_m t))$$

Here, f_c is the carrier frequency, Δf is the frequency deviation, and f_m is the modulation frequency. Detuning, which refers to the difference between the applied electromagnetic field frequency and the resonant frequency of the quantum system, is crucial for determining the excitation and emission dynamics.

This paper introduces a novel excitation method—the Swing-UP of the quantum Emitter population (SUPER) scheme-which uses highly detuned laser pulses to achieve high single-photon purity, indistinguishability, and output. The SUPER scheme overcomes the limitations of traditional excitation techniques by utilizing periodic modulation of the Rabi frequency, inducing a "swing-up" effect in the emitter's population dynamics.

The effectiveness of single-photon sources is evaluated based on metrics such as photon purity, indistinguishability, and brightness. Early analyses suggest that the 2C-SUPER scheme achieves near-unity values for these metrics, positioning it as a competitive alternative to conventional single-photon sources. Despite potential decoherence effects caused by phonon interactions, preliminary results indicate that the 2C-SUPER scheme remains a robust candidate for generating high-quality single photons. This advancement is expected to enhance QEC techniques and facilitate fault-tolerant quantum computations [4]. Moreover, it improves the fidelity of quantum communication channels by reducing the impact of noise and decoherence. One of the key challenges in quantum emitters is decoherence, where environmental interactions degrade the quality of emitted photons, impacting the performance of quantum applications. For Q-WBANs specifically, this challenge is amplified by the constrained operating environment and need for miniaturization.

As advancements in quantum dot technology and excitation protocols continue, the potential for more reliable and robust quantum systems grows, contributing to improved error correction methodologies and the broader field of quantum information processing. The integration of optimized quantum emitters with tailored QEC codes, as proposed in this work, represents a significant step toward practical Q-WBAN implementations.

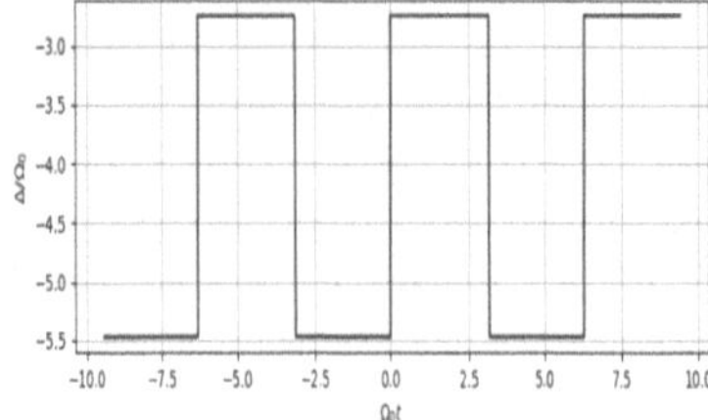

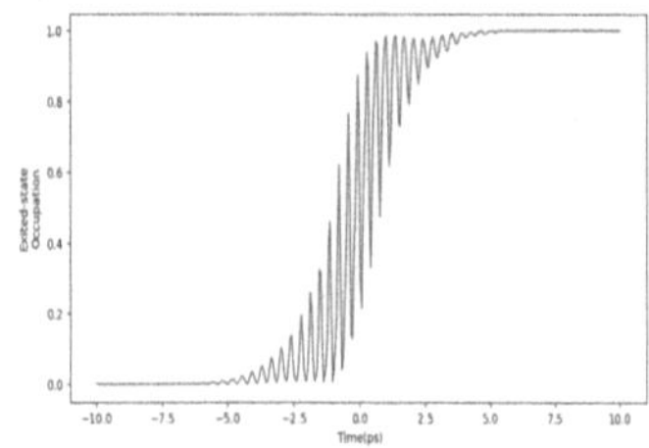

Fig. 1. (a) Detuning modulation protocol and (b) resulting population dynamics of the SUPER (Swing-UP of quantum Emitter population) scheme. The frequency-modulated pulses enable robust excitation while operating below the bandgap to minimize phonon-induced decoherence, making it particularly suitable for quantum dot-based sources in WBAN applications.

3 The SUPER Scheme for Population Inversion in Two-Level Quantum Systems

The SUPER (Swing-UP of the quantum Emitter population) scheme achieves population inversion in a two-level quantum system (quantum emitter) by modulating the detuning between two specific values, Δ_{high} and Δ_{low}. By switching between these detunings at precisely timed intervals during the Rabi oscillation cycle, the population of the excited state gradually increases, ultimately resulting in complete population inversion. This technique exploits the variation in Rabi frequencies and amplitudes associated with different detunings, ensuring efficient population transfer to the excited state through careful pulse modulation. A two-level quantum system driven by a laser field undergoes Rabi oscillations, where the population oscillates between the ground and excited states with a frequency Ω_R given by $\Omega_R = \sqrt{\Omega_0^2 + \Delta^2}$ Here, Ω_0 is proportional to the laser amplitude, and the detuning Δ is defined as the difference between the laser frequency ω_L and the transition frequency ω_0 of the quantum system $\Delta = \omega_L - \omega_0$. The system dynamics can be described using the time-dependent Schrödinger equation, which governs the coherent evolution of the quantum state under external driving fields. Figure 1a illustrates the Bloch vector representation and the temporal dynamics of the SUPER scheme utilizing rectangular pulse modulation. The mechanism for achieving population inversion involves alternating between two distinct detuning levels, denoted as Δ_{high} and Δ_{low}. An analytical expression for the dynamics under rectangular modulation has been recently established [4].

During periods when the population of the excited state rises, we employ the lower detuning Δ_{low}, which corresponds to a higher amplitude of the Rabi oscillation. Conversely, when the population in the excited state decreases, we switch to the higher detuning Δ_{high}, leading to a reduced amplitude of the Rabi oscillation. This precise timing of detuning transitions enables each oscillation cycle, as depicted in Fig. 1b, to facilitate a gradual increase in the population of the excited state, thereby promoting oscillatory behavior in the occupation levels. The SUPER scheme offers significant advantages for quantum information processing applications, *Enhanced Photon Quality,* the controlled population inversion enables generation of high-purity single photons with improved indistinguishability, crucial for quantum communication protocols [1,7], *Robustness to Decoherence,* by operating with optimized detuning parameters, the scheme minimizes sensitivity to environmental noise and phonon-induced decoherence effects [6], and *Compatibility with Quantum Dots,* the scheme is particularly well-suited for semiconductor quantum dots [2], where precise control over excitation parameters is essential for high-performance photon generation, and *Scalability,* the modular pulse structure facilitates integration with existing quantum optical setups and future quantum network architectures.

The gradual population transfer achieved through the SUPER scheme results in several key performance benefits are Near-unity population inversion efficiency through cumulative swing-up effect, Reduced multi-photon emission probability through controlled state preparation, Enhanced photon coherence properties through maintained phase relationships and Adaptability to various quantum emitter platforms through parameter optimization. The SUPER scheme represents a significant advancement in quantum state control methodologies, providing a robust and efficient approach for population inversion that is particularly valuable for quantum WBAN applications where reliable single-photon generation under practical constraints is essential.

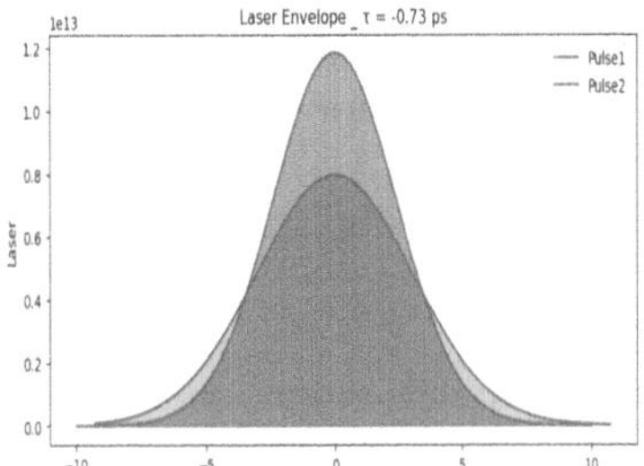

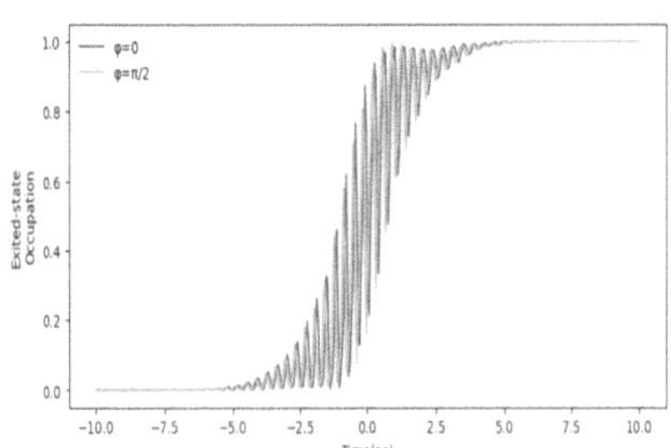

Fig. 2. (a) The normalized temporal envelope of the laser pulse sequence employed in the 2C-SUPER scheme, showing the precise timing and amplitude modulation of the excitation pulses. (b) The time-dependent evolution of the excited-state population under the 2C-SUPER scheme, demonstrating the characteristic "swing-up" behavior that leads to near-complete population inversion through controlled detuning modulation.

This Fig. effectively illustrates the key components of our 2C-SUPER scheme such as subfigure (a) shows the laser pulse envelope that drives the quantum emitter. The normalized representation clearly displays the pulse timing, duration, and relative amplitudes that are crucial for implementing the detuning modulation strategy described in your SUPER scheme section, and subfigure (b) demonstrates the resulting population dynamics, which is the core achievement of your method. The "swing-up" behavior visible in this plot shows how the excited-state population gradually increases with each pulse cycle, ultimately approaching complete population inversion. This visual evidence supports your theoretical claims about the scheme's effectiveness. explores the concept of the SUPER scheme, designed to achieve full population inversion in two-level quantum systems, such as quantum dots, using highly detuned laser pulses. The SUPER scheme modulates the laser detuning periodically, allowing the system to incrementally build excitation through controlled Rabi oscillations. The study examines two implementations, one using rectangular pulses and another employing frequency-modulated Gaussian pulses (FM-SUPER). Both approaches demonstrate effective population inversion even with laser frequencies far from resonance with the quantum transition frequency. Furthermore, the paper introduces a practical two-color SUPER scheme, using two Gaussian laser pulses with different detunings to create a beat frequency, mimicking amplitude modulation. This two-color approach achieves efficient state inversion and offers potential for experimental realization with existing laser technology. The results confirm the robustness of the SUPER scheme across various parameters, making it applicable in quantum emitters such as quantum dots, and suggesting its possible extension to other systems like superconducting circuits. Figure 2, depicts The normalized temporal envelope of the laser for the applied pulse sequence (a) and (b) The time-dependent evolution of the excited-state population under the 2C-SUPER scheme. Rabi oscillations describe the coherent transitions between the two states of the system when driven by an external field with a frequency close to resonance. The frequency of oscillations between the ground and excited states depends on the Rabi frequency (Ω_0), which is influenced by the amplitude of the applied field and detuning (Δ), the difference between the driving frequency and the system's natural frequency. The system is perturbed by Gaussian-shaped pulses. These pulses are characterized by the pulse widths s_1 and s_2, the amplitude parameters a_1 and a_2, and a central time parameter τ. Each pulse introduces a time-dependent detuning that leads to changes in the system's transition probabilities over time. The final population of the excited state as a function of varying pulse areas and pulse durations, where the pulse area remains constant for both pulses are depicted in Fig. 3.

Figure 4, depicts the coherent oscillation between two quantum states ($|0\rangle$ and $|1\rangle$) under the influence of a driving field. These oscillations describe the periodic exchange of population between the ground state $|0\rangle$ and the excited state $|1\rangle$ when subjected to a coherent external field. The frequency of these oscillations, known as the Rabi frequency, is determined by the strength of the driving field and the coupling between the two states. The system is modeled as two quantum states interacting with an external field, represented by a Hamiltonian H, which induces transitions between the states $|0\rangle$ and $|1\rangle$. The Hamiltonian H used in the code is defined as:

$$H = \frac{w_x}{2} \cdot \sigma_x$$

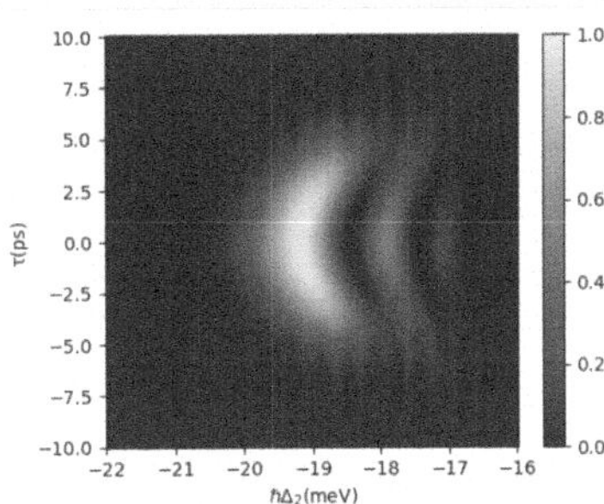

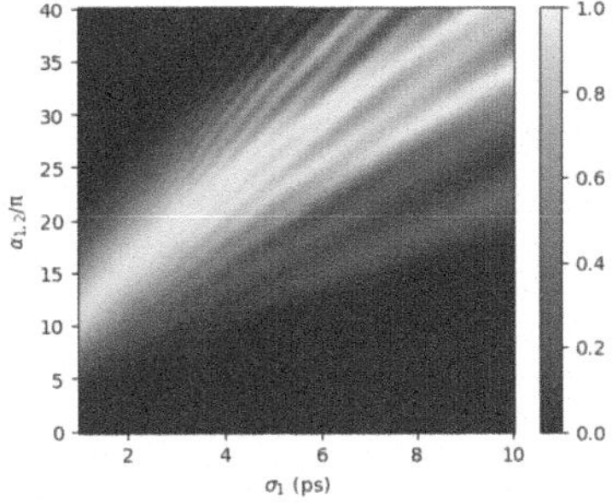

Fig. 3. (a) The final population of the excited state as a function of varying detunings and temporal delays between the two pulses. A negative time delay corresponds to the second pulse preceding the first (b) The final population of the excited state as a function of varying pulse areas and pulse durations, where the pulse area remains constant for both pulses.

where w_x is the angular frequency of the driving field, and σ_x is the Pauli-X operator, which acts as a bit-flip gate in quantum systems, flipping between the states $|0\rangle$ and $|1\rangle$. The Pauli-X operator is given by:

$$\sigma_x = \begin{pmatrix} 0 & 1 \\ 1 & 0 \end{pmatrix}$$

The Hamiltonian governs the time evolution of the quantum system under the influence of this driving field. The time evolution of the system's quantum states is determined by solving the Schrödinger equation. This solver computes the evolution of the initial states $|0\rangle$ and $|1\rangle$ over a given time interval. The behavior of the system is described by the time-dependent wavefunction $\psi(t)$, with the probability of finding the system in a particular state (either $|0\rangle$ or $|1\rangle$) given by the square of the amplitude of the corresponding state component.

The results, result0.expect[0] and result1.expect[0], provide the probabilities of the system being in the ground and excited states, respectively, as functions of time, which are plotted as Rabi oscillations. The graph illustrates the state probabilities of the ground state $|0\rangle$ and excited state $|1\rangle$ over time, with the blue curve representing the probability of being in the ground state and the orange curve representing the probability of being in the excited state. The periodic oscillations of these curves show the continuous exchange of population between the two states due to the driving field. This oscillatory behavior is characteristic of Rabi oscillations, where the system oscillates between the two states with equal time spent in each if the oscillation is fully coherent. This simulation demonstrates the behavior of a two-level quantum system under a coherent driving field, where the population oscillates between the ground and excited states at the Rabi frequency. Understanding Rabi oscillations is critical for grasping how quantum bits evolve under external control, a fundamental concept in quantum computing and related quantum technologies [8].

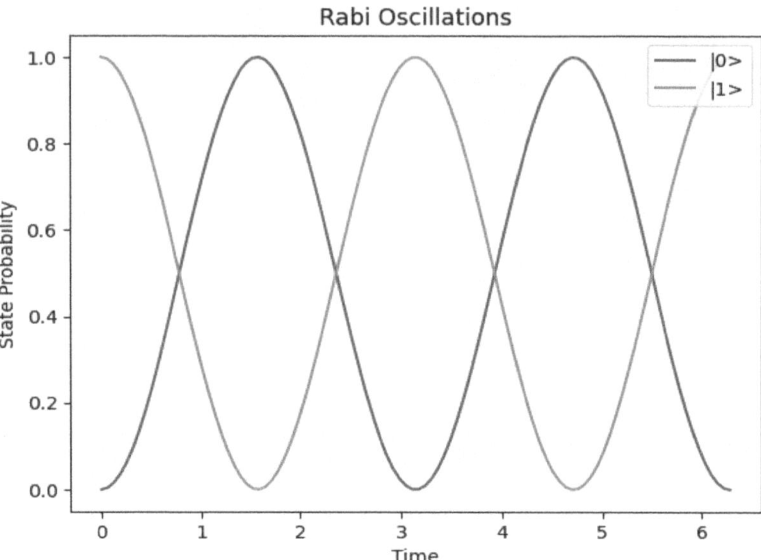

Fig. 4. The plot illustrates the coherent oscillatory behavior of the state probabilities as a function of time, indicative of the dynamics between the two quantum states under resonant excitation.

4 Quantum-Enabled WBAN System Model

The proposed system model as shown in Fig. 5, outlines an end-to-end architecture for quantum-enabled WBANs tailored for secure and high-fidelity health monitoring. The model emphasizes how optimizing photon sources and implementing QEC mechanisms can dramatically enhance data reliability and security in WBAN environments, which are subject to frequent noise and mobility-induced errors. At the sensing layer, quantum sensors collect physiological signals and encode them into quantum states. These states are generated by a photon source specifically engineered for high fidelity and controlled emission, ensuring the initial quantum information maintains integrity. The quantum encoder then prepares the sensor data as qubits for transmission over the quantum channel-this is where most external noise and error sources are encountered.

Upon transmission, the qubits pass through a quantum error detection circuit which identifies potential errors induced by environmental noise, device imperfections, or transmission faults [9]. To mitigate these errors, the quantum error correction module applies advanced QEC codes such as the Surface or Steane code, restoring the original quantum information as accurately as possible. The corrected quantum states are decoded by a dedicated module, converting them back into classical health data usable by healthcare analytics platforms. Finally, the quantum health monitoring analysis stage interprets this data for clinical decision support, integrating quantum-derived information into standard health-

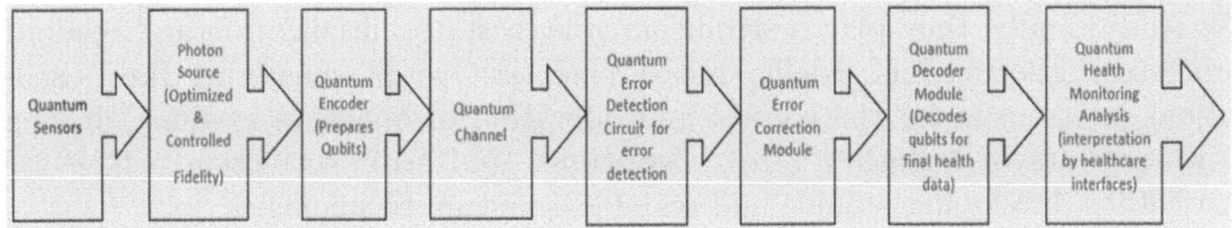

Fig. 5. Proposed end-to-end architecture for quantum-enabled WBANs designed for secure, high-fidelity health monitoring. The system integrates a high-fidelity photon source for quantum state generation, quantum sensors for physiological signal acquisition, and a quantum encoder for qubit preparation. Transmission over the quantum channel is safeguarded by error detection circuits and QEC codes to mitigate noise and mobility-induced errors. Corrected quantum states are decoded into classical health data for clinical analysis, enabling resilient, secure, and accurate health monitoring in next-generation WBAN environments.

care workflows. By strategically optimizing photon source fidelity and deploying robust QEC techniques, this system model delivers resilient, secure, and efficient health monitoring suitable for next-generation WBAN applications.

We explore advancements in photon generation and their implications for quantum technologies and QEC techniques. Reliable single-photon sources are crucial for applications in quantum communication, cryptography, and computing. As these generation techniques improve, they enhance the efficiency and reliability of quantum systems, facilitating broader adoption [10]. QEC is vital for maintaining the integrity of quantum information, which is prone to errors from environmental factors like noise and decoherence. By encoding quantum information into resilient states, QEC enables error detection and correction without disrupting computations, ensuring the accuracy of quantum systems. Moreover, these advancements extend to practical applications such as WBANs, which use wearable sensors to monitor vital health data. Integrating quantum techniques like QEC into WBANs can enhance the reliability and security of transmitted data, particularly important in medical settings where precision is critical [11]. Incorporating quantum processing into WBANs exemplifies how quantum technologies can improve classical systems. Encoding sensor data into quantum states allows for advanced error correction and efficient transmission, enhancing overall system reliability. Thus, the advancements in photon generation and QEC not only enhance quantum computing but also benefit traditional technologies like WBANs, highlighting the interdisciplinary potential of quantum innovations in healthcare and other essential fields.

Rabi oscillations are fundamental to quantum computing, enabling precise qubit manipulation and control. They describe the coherent evolution of quantum states under a driving field, allowing for the implementation of quantum gates with high precision. The Rabi frequency governs state transitions and is crucial for operations like the Pauli-X gate and complex algorithms such as Shor's and Grover's. In QEC, Rabi oscillations facilitate error detection and correction, mitigate noise impacts, and assist in gate calibration and pulse shaping

[3]. Additionally, they play a significant role in state initialization and readout processes, ensuring high-fidelity measurements. Overall, mastering Rabi oscillations is essential for the control and operation of quantum systems, driving advancements in quantum gates, algorithms, and error correction, which are critical for developing reliable and scalable quantum technologies.

4.1 Types of Quantum Gates

Quantum logic gates as shown in Table 1 form the fundamental building blocks of quantum circuits, manipulating qubits by leveraging superposition and entanglement [12,13]. Key single-qubit gates include the Pauli operators, which perform rotations on the Bloch sphere and serve as essential components for universal quantum computation.

4.2 Types of Errors in Qubits

Quantum errors arise from decoherence, hardware imperfections, or environmental disturbances such as thermal noise and electromagnetic interference, leading to undesired changes in qubit states [9]. The primary error types are bit-flip error (X error), Flips the state of a qubit, transforming $|0\rangle \leftrightarrow |1\rangle$. Phase-flip error ($Z$ error)- Changes the phase of the $|1\rangle$ state, resulting in $|1\rangle \rightarrow -|1\rangle$ while leaving $|0\rangle$ unchanged. Combined error (Y error)- A simultaneous occurrence of both bit- and phase-flip errors.

5 Methodology and Implementation of QEC Codes

A QEC code must detect and correct both bit- and phase-flip errors without directly measuring or cloning quantum states. The general process involves the following steps:

Step 1: Encoding: Logical qubits (here we write Q-bit for message qubit) are encoded using multiple physical (ancilla) qubits to protect information against errors.

Step 2: Quantum Channel: The encoded qubits are transmitted through a noisy channel (e.g., optical fiber or free-space), where errors may occur.

Step 3: Error Detection: Using syndrome measurements and quantum gates, errors are identified without collapsing the quantum state.

Step 4: Error Correction: Based on the syndrome information, corrective gates are applied to restore the qubits to their intended states.

Step 5: Decoding: The corrected logical qubits are decoded to recover the original information.

Table 1. Quantum Gate Representations and Functions

Gate	Matrix	Description
X	$\begin{bmatrix} 0 & 1 \\ 1 & 0 \end{bmatrix}$	Bit-flip: swaps $\lvert 0\rangle \leftrightarrow \lvert 1\rangle$
Y	$\begin{bmatrix} 0 & -i \\ i & 0 \end{bmatrix}$	Rotates around Y-axis by π
Z	$\begin{bmatrix} 1 & 0 \\ 0 & -1 \end{bmatrix}$	Phase-flip of $\lvert 1\rangle$
H	$\frac{1}{\sqrt{2}}\begin{bmatrix} 1 & 1 \\ 1 & -1 \end{bmatrix}$	Creates superposition
S/P	$\begin{bmatrix} 1 & 0 \\ 0 & i \end{bmatrix}$	Phase shift $\pi/2$
T	$\begin{bmatrix} 1 & 0 \\ 0 & e^{i\pi/4} \end{bmatrix}$	Phase shift $\pi/4$
SWAP	$\begin{bmatrix} 1 & 0 & 0 & 0 \\ 0 & 0 & 1 & 0 \\ 0 & 1 & 0 & 0 \\ 0 & 0 & 0 & 1 \end{bmatrix}$	Swaps two qubits
CNOT	$\begin{bmatrix} 1 & 0 & 0 & 0 \\ 0 & 1 & 0 & 0 \\ 0 & 0 & 0 & 1 \\ 0 & 0 & 1 & 0 \end{bmatrix}$	Flips target if control is $\lvert 1\rangle$
CCNOT	$\begin{bmatrix} 1 & 0 & 0 & 0 & 0 & 0 & 0 & 0 \\ 0 & 1 & 0 & 0 & 0 & 0 & 0 & 0 \\ 0 & 0 & 1 & 0 & 0 & 0 & 0 & 0 \\ 0 & 0 & 0 & 1 & 0 & 0 & 0 & 0 \\ 0 & 0 & 0 & 0 & 1 & 0 & 0 & 0 \\ 0 & 0 & 0 & 0 & 0 & 1 & 0 & 0 \\ 0 & 0 & 0 & 0 & 0 & 0 & 0 & 1 \\ 0 & 0 & 0 & 0 & 0 & 0 & 1 & 0 \end{bmatrix}$	Flips target if both controls are $\lvert 1\rangle$
CZ	$\begin{bmatrix} 1 & 0 & 0 & 0 \\ 0 & 1 & 0 & 0 \\ 0 & 0 & 1 & 0 \\ 0 & 0 & 0 & -1 \end{bmatrix}$	Phase flip if control is $\lvert 1\rangle$

5.1 Implementation of QEC Codes

During transmission, qubits are mainly affected by bit-flip and phase-flip errors. This section presents the mathematical analysis of QEC codes that individually and jointly address these error types [14].

5.2 Bit-Flip Error

A bit-flip error occurs when a qubit transitions between $\lvert 0\rangle$ and $\lvert 1\rangle$. Such errors are mitigated using the *three-qubit repetition code*, which encodes one logical qubit into three physical qubits. This method serves as the quantum analog of the classical repetition code and enhances the fidelity of quantum information transmission.

Figure 6 depicts the Quantum circuit for bit-flip error and the mathematical description of the circuit expressed in the following step. Initial quantum state, $\lvert \Psi\rangle = \alpha\lvert 0\rangle + \beta\lvert 1\rangle$ state preparation, $\lvert \Psi\rangle = \alpha\lvert 000\rangle + \beta\lvert 100\rangle$ entanglement or

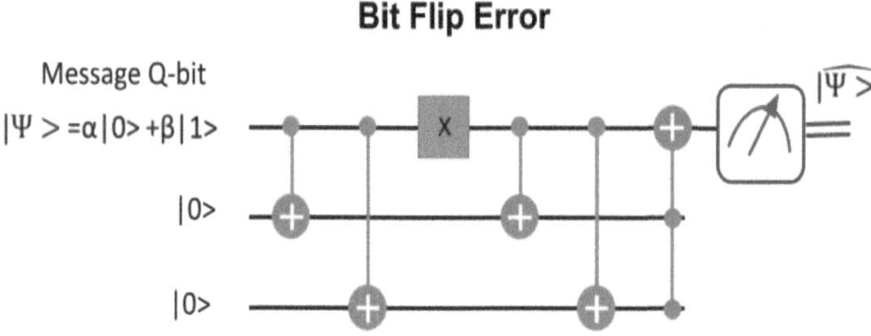

Fig. 6. Quantum circuit for bit-flip error.

encoding $|\Psi\rangle = \alpha|000\rangle + \beta|111\rangle$, introducing bit-flip error in the first qubit, $|\Psi\rangle = \alpha|100\rangle + \beta|011\rangle$,decoding, $|\Psi\rangle = \alpha|111\rangle + \beta|011\rangle$, and error correction $|\Psi\rangle = \alpha|011\rangle + \beta|111\rangle$. The estimated output states are $|\Psi\rangle = \alpha|0\rangle + \beta|1\rangle$.

5.3 Phase Flip Error

A phase-flip error occurs when the phase of the qubit changes. The quantum circuit incorporating a quantum gate designed for addressing Phase-Flip errors is presented in Fig. 7. Let us designate a Qubit for transmission in the ensuing process.

Initial quantum state,$|\Psi\rangle = \alpha|0\rangle + \beta|1\rangle$ State preparation,$|\Psi\rangle = \alpha|000\rangle + \beta|100\rangle$, Entanglement,$|\Psi\rangle = \alpha|000\rangle + \beta|111\rangle$, expressing the above state in phase form,

$$|\Psi >= \alpha| + ++\rangle + \beta| - --\rangle \tag{1}$$

Introduction of phase flip error in first qubit - $|\Psi\rangle = \alpha| - ++\rangle + \beta| + --\rangle$ Therefore, $|\Psi\rangle = \alpha|100\rangle + \beta|011\rangle$, decoding,$|\Psi\rangle = \alpha|111\rangle + \beta|011\rangle$,correction, $|\Psi\rangle = \alpha|011\rangle + \beta|111\rangle$, estimated output state - $|\Psi\rangle = \alpha|0\rangle + \beta|1\rangle$.

5.4 Both Bit-Flip and Phase Flip Error

Now, we shall elucidate the implementation of a quantum error correction code. This code is designed to concurrently address phase-flip errors (Z errors) and amplitude-flip errors (X errors) within quantum computing systems [15]. The rows symbolize the three basis states as shown in Fig. 8: $|0\rangle$, $|1\rangle$, and $|2\rangle$. Concurrently, each column is indicative of the specific qubits employed in encoding the logical qubit, denoted as $|\Psi\rangle$. The rows align with the basis states $|0\rangle$, $|1\rangle$, and $|2\rangle$, and the columns correspond to the qubits utilized in the encoding process.

$$|\Psi\rangle = \alpha|0\rangle + \beta|1\rangle \tag{2}$$

Here, X and Z are Pauli operators corresponding to bit-flip and phase-flip operations, respectively Row 1 ($|0\rangle$): The logical qubit $|\psi\rangle$ is placed in the first row. The

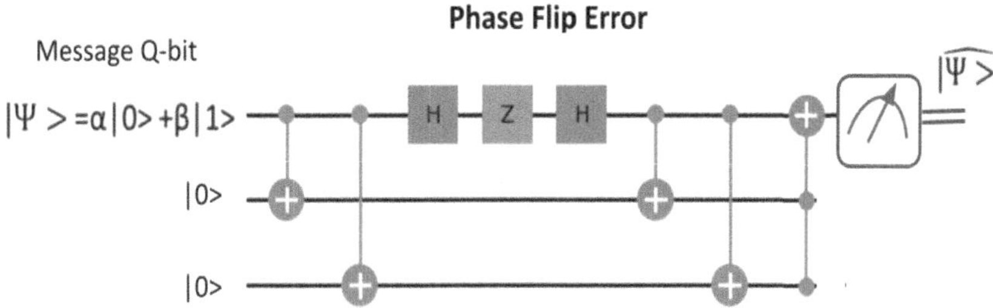

Fig. 7. Common single- and multi-qubit quantum gates used in computation and error correction.

ancillary qubits also referred to as auxiliary qubits, are strategically employed for error detection purposes. When an error manifests on a physical qubit, it induces alterations in the state of the ancillary qubits. Subsequently, measurements of the ancillary qubits provide insights into the presence of errors. furthermore, for error detection, the quantum code activates precise quantum gate operations to rectify the identified error. For instance, in the case of a detected Z error, the code applies specific operations to restore the original state of the logical qubit. A general representation of both types of errors, namely bit-flip error, and phase-flip error, in terms of quantum gates, is denoted as Bit Flip Error (X):

$$\text{Bit Flip Error}[X] = [H] - [Z] - [H]$$

Phase Flip Error (Z):

$$\text{Phase Flip Error}[Z] = [H] - [X] - [H]$$

The process of quantum communication with error correction begins with an initial qubit $|\Psi\rangle = \alpha|0\rangle + \beta|1\rangle$, which is encoded into a three-qubit state $|\Psi\rangle = \alpha|000\rangle + \beta|100\rangle$, and entangled using CNOT and Hadamard gates to form $|\Psi\rangle = \alpha|000\rangle + \beta|111\rangle$. During transmission through a quantum channel, the state may experience perturbations such as bit-flip errors, which are subsequently detected and corrected, recovering the original qubit state $|\Psi\rangle = \alpha|0\rangle + \beta|1\rangle$. In this procedure, the CNOT gate entangles the qubit with ancillary bits by designating control and target qubits: the target flips if the control is in state $|1\rangle$, otherwise no operation occurs. The Hadamard gate then induces superposition, preparing the qubits for transmission. The resulting encoded data traverses the quantum channel, where errors may occur. This demonstrates that quantum error correction ensures reliable transmission of quantum information despite channel-induced disturbances. The corresponding quantum circuit, shown in Fig. 5, is read from left to right, with gates applied earlier appearing farther to the left. The output of the Hadamard gate is written as- The initial three-qubit encoded state is

$$|\Psi\rangle = \alpha\frac{(|0\rangle + |1\rangle)^{\otimes 3}}{2\sqrt{2}} + \beta\frac{(|0\rangle - |1\rangle)^{\otimes 3}}{2\sqrt{2}}. \tag{3}$$

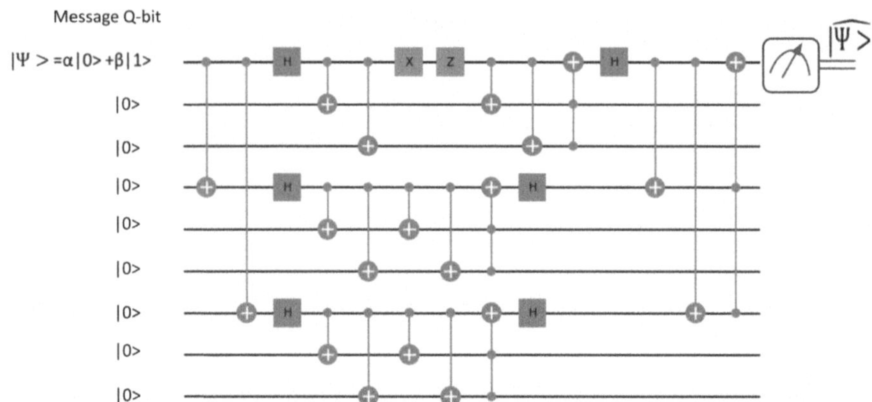

Fig. 8. The quantum circuit illustrating the a code implementation for addressing both Bit and Phase-Flip errors

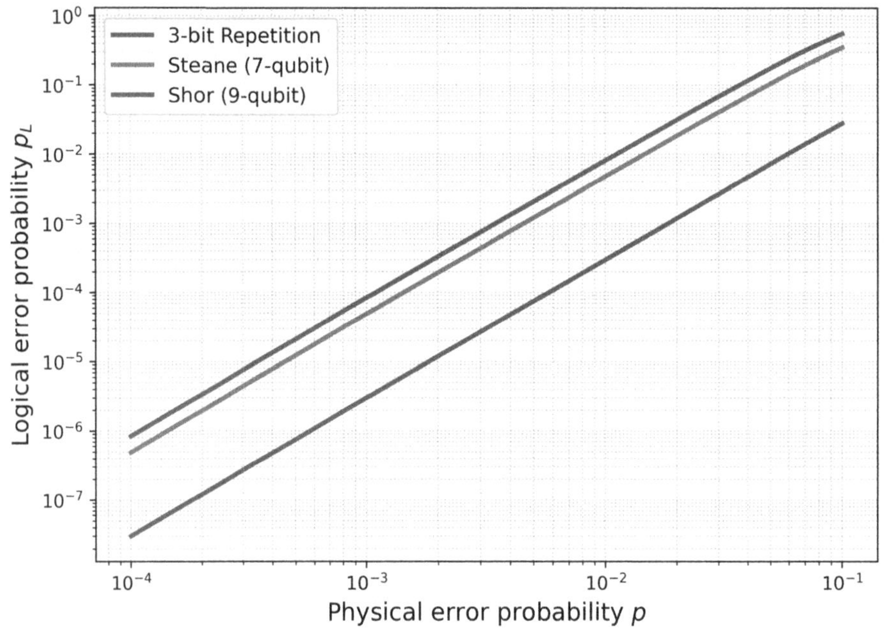

Fig. 9. Logical Error vs Physical Error of different QEC techniques.

After entanglement, it forms a GHZ-type state:

$$|\Psi\rangle = \alpha\frac{(|000\rangle + |111\rangle)^{\otimes 3}}{2\sqrt{2}} + \beta\frac{(|000\rangle - |111\rangle)^{\otimes 3}}{2\sqrt{2}}. \tag{4}$$

Introducing an error during transmission through a quantum channel, the state becomes

$$
\begin{aligned}
|\Psi\rangle = {} & \frac{\alpha}{2\sqrt{2}}(|100\rangle - |011\rangle)(|000\rangle + |111\rangle)^{\otimes 2} \\
& + \frac{\beta}{2\sqrt{2}}(|100\rangle + |011\rangle)(|000\rangle - |111\rangle)^{\otimes 2}.
\end{aligned} \tag{5}
$$

The error detection and correction process gives

$$|\Psi\rangle = \alpha|1\rangle|0\rangle|0\rangle + \beta|0\rangle|1\rangle|1\rangle, \tag{6}$$

and finally, the estimated single-qubit state is recovered as

$$|\Psi\rangle = \alpha|0\rangle + \beta|1\rangle. \tag{7}$$

6 Results and Discussion

The performance of the implemented QEC schemes was evaluated by analyzing their impact on *logical error rates* and *state fidelities* under varying physical error probabilities. Figure 9 and 10 summarize the comparative results for different QEC techniques, including the three-qubit repetition code for bit-flip errors, its Hadamard-modified version for phase-flip errors, and the Shor code for combined bit-flip and phase-flip errors and steane code.

6.1 Logical Error vs Physical Error

The curve in Fig. 9 illustrates how different QEC codes reduce the *logical error probability* as the physical error probability varies. Three-qubit repetition code- Significantly suppresses logical errors for low physical error rates, but performance degrades for higher error rates due to multiple physical errors overwhelming the correction threshold. Phase-flip QEC with Hadamard transform- Demonstrates similar improvement in phase error channels, highlighting the equivalence of phase-flip and bit-flip protection when error mapping is applied. Shor code (bit + phase-flip protection)- Exhibits the lowest logical error probability across the physical error range, especially in mixed error environments. Its multi-layer encoding delays the error rate divergence compared to simpler codes. This Fig. underscores that while simple repetition-based QEC is effective against single error types in low-noise regimes, hybrid codes like Shor and Steane offer robust performance in channels with combined error types.

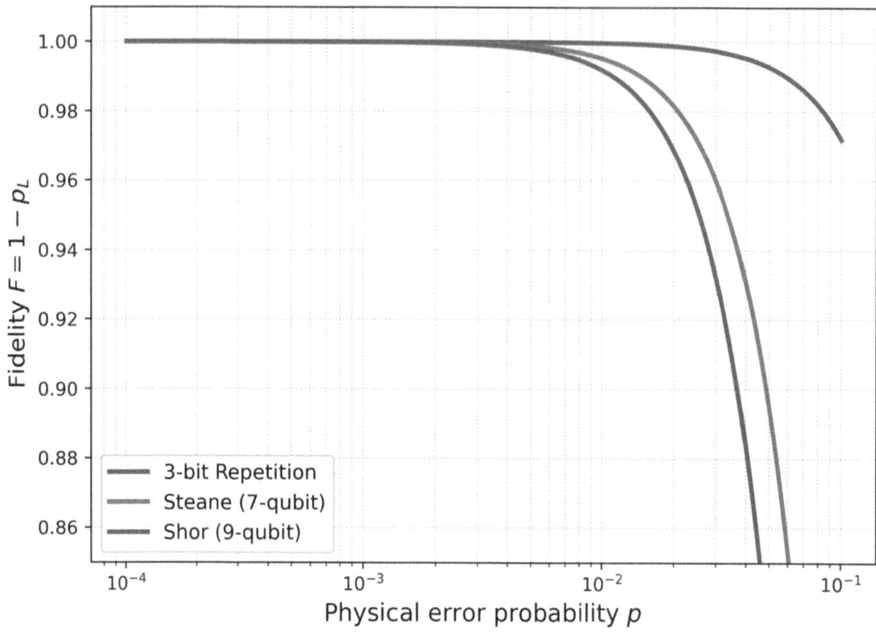

Fig. 10. Fidelity vs Physical Error for Different QEC techniques.

6.2 Fidelity vs Physical Error

Figure 10 depicts how *state fidelity*-a measure of correctness of the recovered quantum state-varies with increasing physical error rates for the different QEC methods. Fidelity is computed using

$$F(\rho, \sigma) = \left[\mathrm{Tr} \left(\sqrt{\sqrt{\rho}\, \sigma\, \sqrt{\rho}} \right) \right]^2$$

where ρ and σ are the density matrices of the ideal and corrected states, respectively. Three-qubit repetition code- Maintains fidelity above high at low error probabilities, but experiences sharp decline as error probability surpasses correction capacity. Shor and Steane code- Maintains fidelity for physical error probabilities for moderately high error rates, outperforming simpler codes due to simultaneous correction of both error types. This fidelity analysis demonstrates that optimizing photon source quality and selecting hybrid QEC strategies like the Shor ans steane code significantly improve the accuracy of recovered quantum states, even in the noisy environments typical of wireless body area networks.

7 Conclusion

The exploration and simulation of Rabi oscillations are fundamental to advancing quantum computing technology. A deep understanding of Rabi oscillation dynamics enhances the precise manipulation of qubit states, which is crucial for the design and operation of quantum logic gates. These gates form the building blocks of quantum circuits that perform complex algorithms, facilitate error correction, and generate entanglement. Insights derived from Rabi oscillations provide a robust framework for the coherent control of qubits, directly impacting the performance and reliability of quantum gates in practical quantum algorithms. By harnessing these oscillations, researchers can improve the fidelity and efficiency of quantum computations, effectively addressing critical challenges such as error correction and decoherence mitigation. Ultimately, mastery of Rabi oscillations supports the development of scalable and practical quantum computing systems, driving significant progress in quantum technology and broadening its potential applications across diverse scientific and technological fields.

References

1. Lounis, B., Orrit, M.: Single-photon sources. Rep. Prog. Phys. **68**(5), 1129 (2005)
2. Agarwal, K., Rai, H., Mondal, S.: Quantum dots: an overview of synthesis, properties, and applications. Mater. Res. Express **10**(6), 062001 (2023)
3. Dodonov, V., Man'Ko, V.: Coherent states and the resonance of a quantum damped oscillator. Phys. Rev. A **20**(2), 550 (1979)
4. Zrenner, A., Beham, E., Stufler, S., Findeis, F., Bichler, M., Abstreiter, G.: Coherent properties of a two-level system based on a quantum-dot photodiode. Nature **418**(6898), 612–614 (2002)
5. Chen, E.H., et al.: Detuning axis pulsed spectroscopy of valley-orbital states in Si/Si-Ge quantum dots. Phys. Rev. Appl. **15**(4), 044033 (2021)
6. Loss, D., DiVincenzo, D.P.: Quantum computation with quantum dots. Phys. Rev. A **57**(1), 120 (1998)
7. Gisin, N., Thew, R.: Quantum communication. Nat. Photonics **1**(3), 165–171 (2007)
8. Kukulski, R., Pawela, Ł, Puchała, Z.: On the probabilistic quantum error correction. IEEE Trans. Inf. Theory **69**(7), 4620–4640 (2023)
9. Schlosshauer, M.: Quantum decoherence. Phys. Rep. **831**, 1–57 (2019)
10. Illiano, J., Caleffi, M., Manzalini, A., Cacciapuoti, A.S.: Quantum internet protocol stack: a comprehensive survey. Comput. Netw. **213**, 109092 (2022)
11. Cornet, B., Fang, H., Ngo, H., Boyer, E.W., Wang, H.: An overview of wireless body area networks for mobile health applications. IEEE Netw. **36**(1), 76–82 (2022)
12. Yang, Z., Zolanvari, M., Jain, R.: A survey of important issues in quantum computing and communications. IEEE Commun. Surv. Tutor. **25**(2), 1059–1094 (2023)
13. Roy, P.K.: Quantum logic gates, August 2020
14. Chang, H.-H.: An introduction to error-correcting codes: from classical to quantum (2006)
15. Shor, P.W.: Scheme for reducing decoherence in quantum computer memory. Phys. Rev. A **52**(4), R2493 (1995)

Healthcare and Medical Applications

A Novel Non-invasive Wearable Hairpin Resonator-Based Electromagnetic Bio-Sensor for Early Diagnosis of Pulmonary Dense Fibrosis

Preeti Tiwari, Debarati Dutta, and Anirban Sarkar(✉)

School of Computing and Electrical Engineering, IIT Mandi, Mandi, India
{d23257,s22005}@students.iitmandi.ac.in, anirban@iitmandi.ac.in

Abstract. This work presents the design and evaluation of a novel wearable microwave sensor for real-time monitoring of lung health using a modified hairpin microwave resonator. The proposed sensor operates at a center frequency of 3.535 GHz and is capable of detecting shifts in the resonant frequency due to the changes in permittivity for different lung abnormality. The proposed sensor provides a significant shift of 46 MHz from normal lung to pulmonary dense fibrosis demonstrating its high sensitivity to detect aforementioned respiratory environment. The sensed data is then transferred to user interface incorporating a wireless module with the proposed sensor. The sensor exhibits a sensitivity of 9.79% and a figure of merit (FOM) of 288.41, along with a Q-factor of 29.46, indicating its high-performance capabilities. The simulated results of the hairpin resonator integrated with real characteristics of human tissue mimic, demonstrate its potential as a sensor for real-time monitoring of lung functions, which could aid in the early detection and management of dense fibrosis.

Keywords: Hairpin resonator · electromagnetic (EM) bio-sensor · non-invasive · pulmonary dense fibrosis · tissue dielectric properties

1 Introduction

The Escalating need for innovative healthcare solutions for an aging population is of importance for today. The global demographic shift towards an older population presents significant challenges for healthcare systems worldwide. The World Health Organization reports a dramatic increase in the population aged 60 and above, projecting a near doubling to 2.1 billion by 2050. This aging population, coupled with advancements in medical science extending lifespans, necessitates innovative and sustainable healthcare solutions, particularly in developed nations facing escalating healthcare costs [1]. To address this growing need, research efforts are increasingly focusing on leveraging technology for more effective and efficient healthcare delivery. One promising avenue lies in the development of

K. Atul et al. (Eds.): BodyNets 2024, LNICST 666, pp. 227–233, 2026.
https://doi.org/10.1007/978-3-032-16099-7_18

non-invasive, wearable sensors capable of continuous physiological monitoring. This technology holds the potential to revolutionize healthcare by enabling early detection and intervention for a range of conditions, ultimately improving patient outcomes and optimizing resource allocation within healthcare systems [2].

Pulmonary fibrosis (PF) stands as a significant challenge in respiratory medicine, characterized by the progressive and irreversible scarring of lung tissue. This insidious disease process leads to a decline in lung function, manifesting in debilitating symptoms such as shortness of breath, persistent coughing, and unrelenting fatigue [13]. While the exact etiology of PF remains multifaceted and often unclear, research points to a complex interplay of genetic predisposition, environmental exposures (e.g., toxins, dusts), and potential contributions from certain medications. A indication of PF is the excessive deposition of collagen and other extracellular matrix components within the lung parenchyma. This aberrant accumulation leads to the formation of scar tissue, disrupting the delicate architecture of the lungs and impairing their ability to expand and contract effectively during respiration [3] Consequently, individuals with PF often experience a progressive decline in respiratory function, ultimately impacting their quality of life. Diagnosis of PF requires a comprehensive and lengthy approach, integrating clinical evaluation, imaging studies (chest X-rays, high-resolution computed tomography), and pulmonary function tests. Definitive diagnosis often necessitates a lung biopsy to enable microscopic examination of the affected tissue [5]. Current management strategies for PF primarily focus on symptom control and slowing disease progression. Pharmacological interventions, including corticosteroids and immunosuppressants, aim to mitigate inflammation within the lungs. Oxygen therapy provides supplemental oxygen to alleviate breathing difficulties [4]. In advanced cases, lung transplantation may be considered as a life-prolonging measure. Despite these interventions, PF remains a serious condition with a significant impact on patient's lives. Ongoing research endeavors are crucial to unraveling the complex mechanisms underlying PF pathogenesis and developing more effective therapies to halt or reverse the fibrotic process.

In this work, a non-invasive electromagnetic resonator type bio-sensor is proposed on Rogers 4350B substrate with 1.524 mm thickness, chosen for its low-loss properties, double-sided copper cladding, dielectric constant of 3.66, and a loss tangent of 0.0037 for early diagnosis of pulmonary dense fibrosis. The sensor design features the five hairpin resonator strategically positioned on a substrate where there is also a presence of defected ground plane. This configuration, employing mixed coupling techniques, enhances electric field confinement within the central sensing region. A 50 Ω microstrip line feeds the resonator array at port 1, while port 2 is terminated with a 50 Ω load. The simulation results of the proposed hairpin resonator sensor reveal a significant shift in the resonant frequency when exposed to particularly pulmonary dense fibrosis lung condition. The sensor exhibits high sensitivity and a favorable figure of merit, enabling it to detect subtle changes in the permittivity of the lung tissue, a crucial capability for the early diagnosis and continuous monitoring of respiratory diseases.

2 Proposed Sensor Design and its Methodology

Figure 1 shows the illustration of sensing methodology using the proposed hairpin based bio-sensor and the associated wireless module based user interface. The final sensor resonator design is shown in Fig. 2, depicting all the optimized design parameters as follows W, L, g, w_1, w_2, w_s, l_1, l_2, l_3, t which are listed in Table 1.

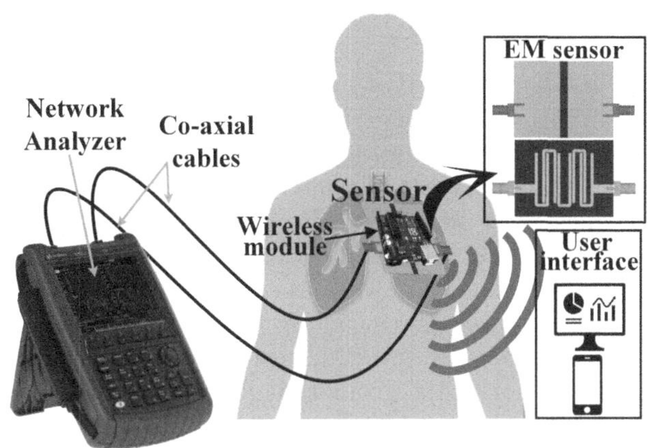

Fig. 1. Schematic of the real-time sensing of lung health monitoring system using hairpin bio-sensor.

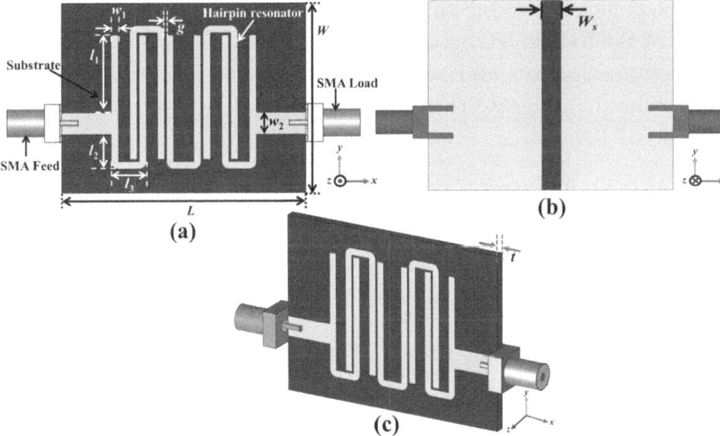

Fig. 2. Proposed hairpin resonator based bio-sensor (a) top view, (b) bottom view, (c) perspective view.

Table 1. DIMENSIONS OF THE PROPOSED SENSOR

Parameter	Dimension (mm)	Parameter	Dimension (mm)
W	35	L	40
w_1	1.20	l_1	8.25
w_2	3.50	l_2	8.25
w_s	2.00	l_3	5.70
g	0.30	t	0.035

A two-port hairpin resonator, operating at 3.535 GHz, forms the basis of the proposed non-invasive EM sensor for lung health monitoring. It is designed on a low-loss Rogers 4350B substrate (1.524 mm thickness, dielectric constant of 3.66, loss tangent of 0.0037), the sensor features five hairpin resonators loaded onto a defected ground plane. This arrangement basically employing mixed coupling, enhances electric field confinement within the central testing region. The hairpin resonator, fed by a 50 Ω microstrip line at port 1 and terminated with a 50 Ω load at port 2, incorporates two SMA connectors in its simulation model. A strategically placed slot in the ground plane mitigates unwanted resonating modes. With overall dimensions of 35 mm $\times$ 40 mm, the resonator's arm gap, set at 0.3 mm, optimizes sensitivity to dielectric property changes in the surrounding environment. Figure 3 shows the reflection-coefficient response of the proposed unloaded sensor resonator where it exhibits it's resonance at 3.535 GHz. The electric field distribution of the unloaded resonator at 3.535 GHz is shown in Fig. 4, where it is clearly visible that the field is mostly concentrated within the line segments of the hairpin structure. The design leverages a common frequency for wireless communication and sensing applications. The simulated results of the hairpin resonator integrated with real characteristics of human tissue mimic

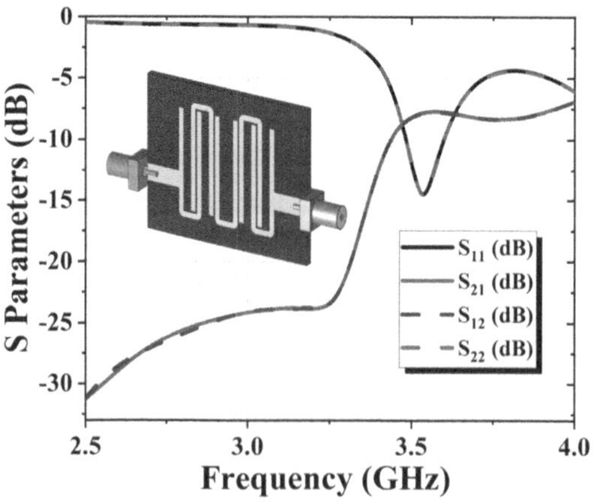

Fig. 3. S-parameters of the proposed unloaded bio-sensor resonator.

demonstrate its potential as a sensor for real-time monitoring of lung functions, which could aid in the early detection and management of dense fibrosis.

3 Results and Discussion

The performance of the sensor was evaluated by simulating its response to various lung tissue characteristics, including healthy and dense fibrosis. To do so, firstly, the healthy human tissue mimic model is loaded on top of the resonator and the shifted resonant frequency for loaded structure is obtained at 3.016 GHz as shown in Fig. 5(a). Further, the lung tissues are incorporated with the earlier used human tissue mimic model and the responses are shown in Fig. 5(b). Here, when the lung with normal permittivity ($\epsilon_r = 34.2$) is placed above the human tissue mimic (skin, fat and muscle) and in pulmonary fibrosis condition of lungs having permittivity of 49.3, the resonance shift is seen which is of 46 MHz. The change is seen from the reflection coefficients of the normal lung and pulmonary fibrosis lung which helps to detect the abnormality in the lungs.

The simulated results demonstrate the sensor's ability to effectively differentiate between normal and pulmonary lung states, making it a reliable and non-invasive tool for real-time sensing for lung health monitoring. The sensitivity [13] is defined as the shift in resonant frequency per unit change in the permittivity of the loaded tissue model in human.

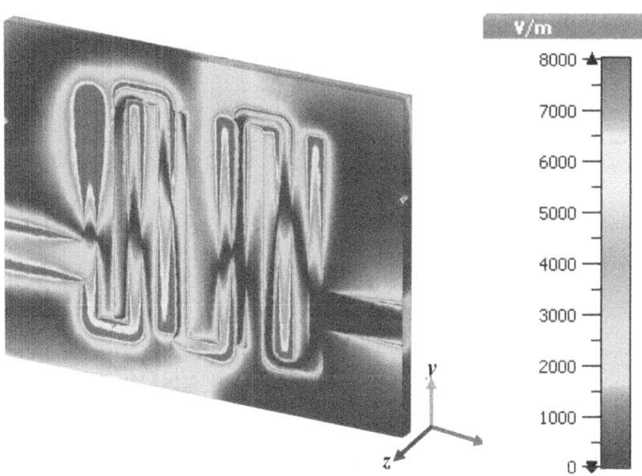

Fig. 4. Distribution of electric field within proposed bio-sensor resonator

Furthermore, the simulated results were analysed from relevant studies on wearable sensors for respiratory monitoring. The integration of the hairpin resonator [6,12] with human tissue models ensures the sensor's ability to operate in a practical, real-world setting, enhancing its potential for clinical applications [8]. Ongoing research is focused on enhancing the sensor's signal processing algorithms to improve its ability to differentiate between normal and abnormal respiratory patterns, potentially enabling the early detection of pulmonary conditions such as asthma, chronic obstructive pulmonary disease, and respiratory distress (Table 2).

Table 2. Permitivitty of Skin, Fat, Muscle, and Lungs

Permittivity	Body Part				
	Skin	Fat	Muscle	Lung(normal)	Lung(PF)
ϵ_r	41.982	5.2138	2.2216	34.2	49.3

The sensitivity for this proposed resonator can be defined using the Eq. (1).

$$Sensitivity\% = \frac{(f_2 - f_1)}{f_1(\epsilon_2 - \epsilon_1)} \times 100 \tag{1}$$

$$Q - Factor = \frac{f_r}{\Delta f} \tag{2}$$

$$FOM = Q \times S \tag{3}$$

The highest sensitivity of the proposed sensor is obtained as 9.79% using Eq. (1) and Q as 29.46 from Eq. (2). Hence, the FOM comes as 288.41.

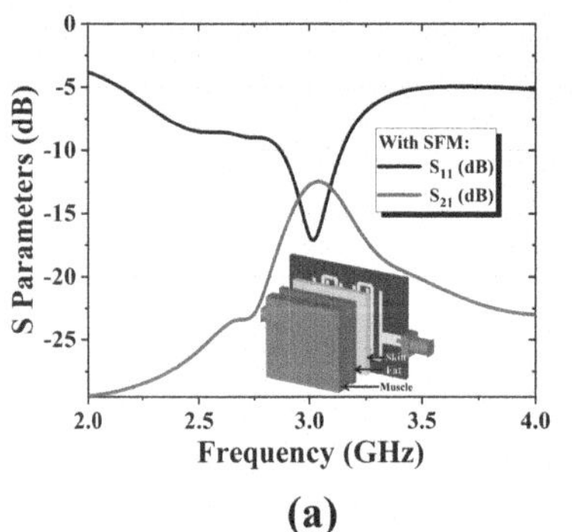

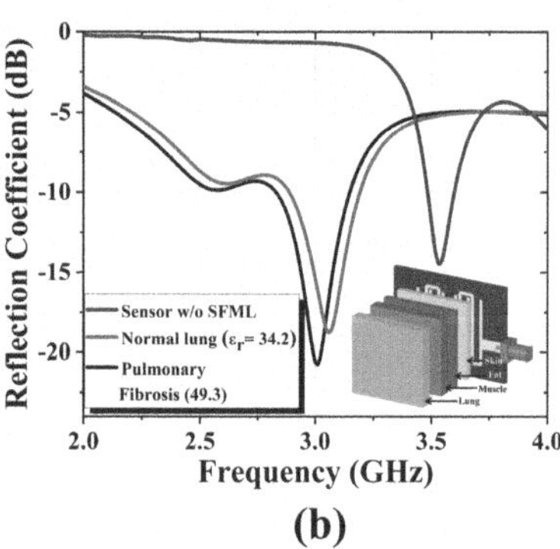

Fig. 5. S-parameters of the proposed bio-sensor resonator (a) with Skin, Fat and Muscle on top, (b) with skin, fat, muscle and both normal and pulmonary fibrosis lung segment on top.

4 Conclusion

This research proposes a novel wearable microwave sensor for real-time sensing for lung health monitoring. The sensor utilizes a modified hairpin microwave resonator with mixed coupling between its two arms, operating at a resonant frequency of 3.535 GHz. This design exhibits high sensitivity 9.79%, a Q-factor of 29.46, and a Figure of Merit of 288.41, enabling the detection of lung pulmonary fibrosis through permittivity changes while considering constant permittivity values for skin, fat, and muscle. The sensor demonstrates promising results in detecting pulmonary dense fibrosis disease and between normal healthy lung conditions. Future work aims to integrate a self-powered module, paving the way for its application in smart health systems. This is cost-effective and practical sensor design holds significant potential for continuous lung monitoring and early detection of respiratory diseases.

References

1. https://www.who.int/news-room/fact-sheets/detail/ageing-and-health
2. https://respiratory-research.biomedcentral.com/articles
3. Christodoulidis, S., Anthimopoulos, M., Ebner, L., Christe, A., Mougiakakou, S.: Multisource transfer learning with convolutional neural networks for lung pattern analysis. IEEE J. Biomed. Health Inform. **21**, 76–84 (2017)
4. Gabriel, S.M., Lau, R.W., Gabriel, C.: The dielectric properties of biological tissues: III. Parametric models for the dielectric spectrum of tissues. Phys. Med. Biol. **41**(11), 2271–2293 (1996)
5. Raabe, M.E., Davis, C.: Measuring dielectric properties of simulants for biological tissue. Merit Fair (2011)
6. Li, Y., et al.: Breathing process monitoring with a biaxially oriented polypropylene film based fiber Fabry–Perot sensor (2020)
7. Ye, J., Qu, D., Zhong, X., Zhou, Y.: Design of X-band bandpass filter using hairpin resonators and tapped feeding line. In: IEEE Symposium on Computer Applications and Communications (2014)
8. Salman, S., Psychoudakis, D., Volakis, J.L.: Determining the relative permittivity of deep embedded biological tissues. IEEE Antennas Wirel. Propag. Lett. **11**, 1694–1697 (2012)
9. Zhang, L., Wang, Z., Volakis, J.L.: Textile antennas and sensors for body-worn applications. IEEE Antennas Wirel. Propag. Lett. **11**, 1690–1693 (2012)
10. Salman, S., Wang, Z., Kiourti, A., Topsakal, E., Volakis, J.L.: A non-invasive lung monitoring sensor with integrated body-area network. In: 2013 IEEE MTT-S International Microwave Workshop Series on RF and Wireless Technologies for Biomedical and Healthcare Applications (IMWS-BIO) (2013)
11. Ye, J., Qu, D., Zhong, X., Zhou, Y.: Design of X-Band Bandpass Filter Using Hairpin Resonators and Tapped Feeding Line (2014)
12. Tayyab, M., Sharawi, M.S., Shamim, A., Al-Sarkhi, A.: A low complexity RF based sensor array for lung disease detection using inkjet printing. Int. J. RF Microwave Comput.-Aided Eng. (2019)
13. Seth, S., Banerjee, A., Tiwari, N.K., Jaleel Akhtar, M.: Frequency controlled intelligent standalone RF sensor system for dispersive material testing. J. Electromagnetic Waves Appl. **35**, 1619–1636 (2021)
14. da Costa, T.D., de Fatima Fernandes Vara, M., Cristino, C.S., Zanella, T.Z., Neto, G.N.N., Nohama, P.: Breathing monitoring and pattern recognition with wearable sensors (2019)
15. Donelli, M., Manekiya, M., Tagliapietra, G., Iannacci, J.: A Reconfigurable Pseudohairpin Filter Based on MEMS Switches (2022)

Genetic Risk Assessment for Chronic Kidney Disease: An Optimization Framework

Koshtu Hema Sravani[1], K. Swathi[1], G. Vamsi Krishna[2], N. Thirupathi Rao[1](✉), and B. Omkar Lakshmi Jagan[1]

[1] Department of Computer Science and Engineering, Vignan's Institute of Information Technology, Duvvada, Visakhapatnam, Andhra Pradesh, India
nakkathiru@gmail.com

[2] Department of Computer Science and Engineering, Dr. L. Bullayya College of Engineering, Visakhapatnam 530013, AP, India

Abstract. Non-communicable diseases can affect a considerable amount of the global population. Chronic kidney disease is one of such significant contributors to morbidity and mortality. A delay in diagnosing the disease can lead to human loss as well. Machine Learning algorithms are exhibiting remarkable interventions in the field of medicine by detecting abnormalities and performing classification tasks with proper accuracy. Employing a diverse dataset which has all the necessary features that are obtained from demographic, clinical, and laboratory data. The objective is to apply nature inspired Genetic Algorithm to obtain optimal feature subset and provide enhanced accuracy when combined with existing classifiers. Further it can be used to make clinically relevant implications that will effectively aid in the timely intervention and accurate diagnosis of the disease to potentially enhance the patient care by suitable diet and medicinal recommendations that pave the way for efficient treatment outcomes.

Keywords: Chronic kidney disease · machine learning · genetic algorithm · optimization · genetic model · risk · assessment

1 Introduction

Chronic diseases present a formidable challenge in healthcare systems worldwide, significantly affecting public health outcomes. According to medical reports, these conditions not only increase morbidity but also impose a heavy financial burden, consuming over 70% of patients' incomes for treatment. Therefore, it becomes imperative to mitigate factors that elevate patients' risk of mortality. Machine Learning (ML) [7] being a subset of Artificial Intelligence (AI) can be used to build robust algorithms [4] that will aid in solving a wide range of real-world challenges. With advancements in medical research, collecting health-related data has become easier. This data typically encompasses demographic information, medical analysis, and the patient's disease history [10]. Furthermore, considering that the prevalence and nature of diseases can vary based on geographic regions and living conditions, it is crucial to include environmental factors and

K. Atul et al. (Eds.): BodyNets 2024, LNICST 666, pp. 234–248, 2026.
https://doi.org/10.1007/978-3-032-16099-7_19

the patient's habitat within the dataset [2] for a comprehensive understanding of disease dynamics. Unstructured data, comprising doctors' records and patient-reported symptoms, complements structured data encompassing patient demographics, disease details, living conditions, and laboratory findings, enhancing diagnostic accuracy. The utilization of advanced tools such as genetic algorithms for model optimization and identification of optimal feature sets. This amalgamation of genetic algorithms with machine learning techniques aims to revolutionize CKD diagnosis by enhancing predictive accuracy and facilitating proactive healthcare interventions.

Nature inspired algorithms are those algorithms that draw patterns from nature to perform a study and analyze the evolution of certain species through generations. These algorithms can be categorized in different ways that include swarm intelligence, evolutionary algorithms, physics-based algorithms, biologically inspired algorithms [1], cultural algorithms and miscellaneous. All these categories of algorithms have their own uniqueness as each of them draw our environment which will help in solving optimization problems.

Genetic algorithms are one of the nature inspired algorithms that belong to the category of evolutionary algorithms. These evolutionary algorithms simulate the process of evolution that is inspired by the process of natural selection and genetics of human beings. Genetic algorithms can be applied on pre-processed data to obtain the optimal subset of features [5] which will thereby enhance the overall accuracy and bring in optimization. It considers the certain number of generations and population count to begin with and further it will subsequently go on working in an iterative manner that will check and heighten the fitness scores of individuals. It uses the concept of reproduction to proceed further and generates the desired set of features that will aid in the overall optimization perspective. The project aims to streamline the process of identifying relevant features associated with CKD progression [8], thereby enhancing the predictive accuracy of the model [3]. This approach not only improves the efficiency of the predictive model but also contributes to a deeper understanding [9] of the underlying factors contributing to CKD. The increasing prevalence underscores the urgency for sophisticated predictive tools to enable early detection. Late-stage CKD poses substantial health risks and escalates healthcare expenditures. Existing predictive methods often lag, resulting in delayed diagnosis and treatment initiation. Thus, the proposed system as shown in Fig. 1 aims to develop a robust machine learning model capable of early-stage prediction, thereby enhancing patient outcomes and alleviating the strain on healthcare resources.

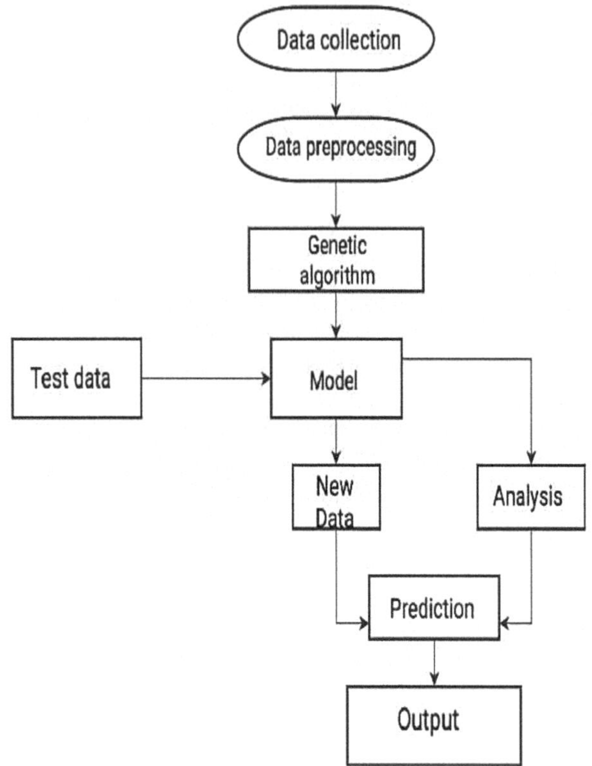

Fig. 1. Proposed model architecture

2 Literature Review

(see Table 1).

Table 1. Summary of Literature Review

References	Objective of the work	Algorithm	Accuracy (in percentage)
Nayeem Hosen et al. [11]	Prediction for Chronic Kidney Disease using Machine and Deep Learning Techniques	SVM, Random Forest and ANN	99
Khan et al. [12]	A Comparative Analysis of Machine Learning Approaches for Chronic kidney Disease Detection	Artificial Neural Network (ANN), Gaussian Naive Bayes	96.9

(*continued*)

Table 1. *(continued)*

References	Objective of the work	Algorithm	Accuracy (in percentage)
Venkatrao et al. [13]	HDLNET: A hybrid Deep Learning Network Model with Intelligent IOT for Detection and Classification of Chronic Kidney Disease	Aquila optimisation	99.18
Bn Swamy et al. [14]	An Ensemble learning Approach for detection of Chronic Kidney Disease	Random Forest, RNN	99.87
Depak K G et al. [15]	A Comprehensive Web Application for Chronic Kidney Disease Prediction with Cuisine-Centric Diet Recommendation	J48 decision tree Random Forest and ANN classification	98
Iftekhar et al. [16]	Performance Analysis of Machine Learning Algorithms in Chronic Kidney Disease Prediction	Random Forest, Ada Boost, XG Boost, Naive Bayes,	99
Drdebabrata et al. [17]	A Robust Chronic Kidney Disease Classifier Using Machine Learning	Support Vector Machine (SVM) and random forest(RF)	99.3
Ahana Bandyopadhyay et al. [18]	Alzheimer's Disease Detection Using Ensemble Learning and Artificial Neural Networks	Artificial Neural Network(ANN)	91.96
Srinivas Arukonda et al. [1]	Disease diagnosis	Grey Wolf Optimizer (GWO)-based Feature selection	98
Anurag et al. [4]	Chronic Kidney Disease Prediction Using Robust Approach in Machine Learning	Random Forest Gradient Boosting Machines (GBM) Neural Networks	98

3 Proposed System

This system aims to use genetic algorithms for feature selection and predict based on the optimal feature set. Here's a breakdown of its key components:

3.1 Data Collection and Preprocessing

A diverse dataset that includes diverse patient demographics, medical history, laboratory test results, and relevant environmental factors should be used. A variety of features are present in the dataset along with certain missing data, null values and noise. Implementation of preprocessing stepsthat include data cleaning, normalization, and feature extraction should be done to enhance the quality of input data for predictive modelling. This makes the data appropriate for predictive modelling.

3.2 Genetic Algorithm Based Feature Selection

1) Firstly, number of generations and population size should be considered in a random yet feasible manner as the algorithm is mostly dependent on these initial values for the purpose of further iteration. Then, crossover rate and mutation rate should be considered so that based on those values the evaluation fitness scores take place and values that fall within the previously mentioned constraints will be considered. Implementation of genetic operators such as mutation and selection are utilized to evolve optimal feature subsets that maximize predictive performance.
2) Evolutionary feature subset evaluation: -Fitness function evaluates feature subsets based on their contribution to predictive performance, refining the process iteratively towards optimal solutions.

3.3 Model Training and Evaluation

Incorporate the optimal feature subset selected by genetic algorithms into the machine learning model for the disease prediction. Train the machine learning model using the integrated features and evaluate its performance using metrics like f1-score, confusion matrix and accuracy.

This proposed system offers a framework for leveraging genetic algorithm combined with other machine learning techniques to obtain optimal feature set that significantly enhances the prediction accuracy.

4 Methodology

The methodology incorporates additional stages including hyperparameter optimization to fine-tune model performance, interpretability analysis for understanding the model's predictive mechanisms, and robust validation on unseen datasets to ensure reliability in diverse clinical settings. Furthermore, it emphasizes transparency and reproducibility through documentation of the entire process, promoting confidence in the developed predictive model. By integrating these components, the methodology provides a comprehensive framework which is shown in Fig. 2 for the development and deployment of an effective chronic kidney disease prediction system, poised to make a meaningful impact on healthcare delivery.

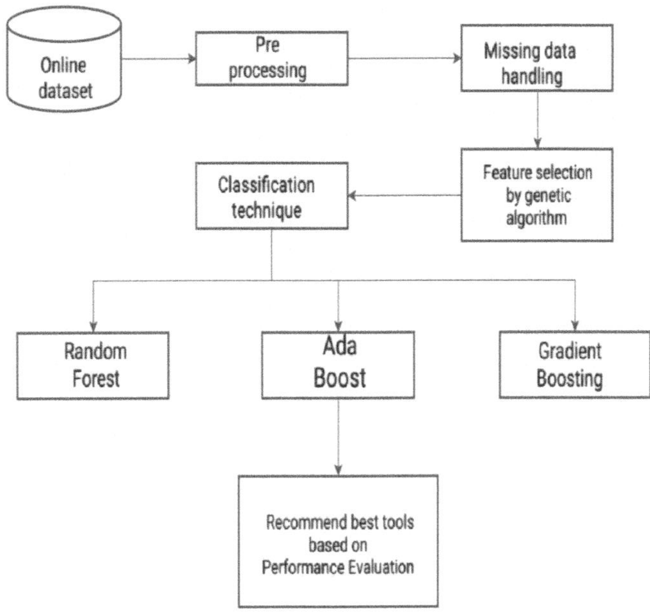

Fig. 2. Project Model

4.1 Input Patient Data

Users start by inputting patient data into the system, including demographics, medical history, laboratory test results, and environmental factors. This can be done over the system's user interface.

4.2 Data Preprocessing

The system processes the input data, conducting data cleaning, normalization, and feature extraction to prepare it for analysis. These steps ensure that the data taken is in a suitable format for subsequent modeling.

4.3 Genetic Algorithm for Feature Selection

Utilizing genetic algorithms, the system selects the most informative features from the preprocessed dataset. Through iterative optimization, the algorithm identifies key predictors of chronic kidney disease (CKD) progression, enhancing the model's predictive accuracy.

4.4 Machine Learning Model Training

Next, the system trains a machine learning model using the selected features that are obtained because of application of genetic algorithm. This process enables the trained model to learn relationships and hidden patterns which will help in making accurate predictions in the subsequent steps.

4.5 Prediction Generation

Once the model is trained, users can generate predictions for CKD progression based on the input patient data. Here we apply classifiers such as random forest classifier that is known for ensemble learning as it minimizes overfitting and increases importance of feature selection, AdaBoost classifier deals with sequential learning and lays more emphasis on misclassified data instances, Gradient Boost classifier is known for its ability to produce heightened accuracy of results, notably in classification and regression tasks. The system processes the input data through the trained model to produce predictions regarding the likelihood of CKD development or progression.

4.6 Content Display

The system displays the prediction results to the users, providing insights into the patient's CKD risk and other relevant implications identified by the model. This information laboratory technicians to produce results effectively and aids healthcare professionals in making precise decisions regarding patient care and management.

1) *System Configuration and Management*
   Data Collection Sources: Administrators have the authority to define trusted sources for acquiring CKD-related data, including healthcare databases, research repositories, and authorized medical facilities.
2) *Data Security and Privacy Controls*
   Anonymization Protocols: Implementation of protocols for anonymizing sensitive patient data during analysis.
3) *Legal and Ethical Compliance*
   Responsibility should be taken for ensuring the system's adherence to legal and ethical guidelines governing healthcare data usage, patient confidentiality, and regulatory compliance. This includes adherence to laws such as Health Insurance Portability and Accountability Act (HIPAA) to protect privacy of the patient and ensure confidentiality.

By incorporating these functionalities, administrators can effectively manage the CKD prediction system, uphold data security and privacy standards, and ensure compliance with legal and ethical regulations, thereby promoting trust and confidence in the system's operation among users.

4.7 Nature Inspired Algorithms

Nature-inspired algorithms leverage principles from biological, physical, and social systems to devise efficient problem-solving strategies. By mimicking natural processes such as evolution, swarm intelligence, and physical phenomena, these algorithms offer powerful optimization techniques for diverse applications. They operate by iteratively refining solutions through processes like genetic variation, interaction between particles, or simulated annealing. This approach allows nature-inspired algorithms to effectively explore various dimensions, obtain optimal solutions, and adapt to changing environments. With their ability to address complex optimization challenges across various domains, nature-inspired algorithms have become indispensable tools in scientific research, engineering design, and decision-making processes.

4.8 Genetic Algorithm

Genetic Algorithm is an optimization algorithm that falls under the category of evolutionary algorithms which are a classification under nature inspired algorithms. It is inspired by the process of human evolution through different generations. This algorithm is introduced by John Holland in the 1960s, it helps in obtaining optimal solutions to a problem over successive generations. The algorithm begins with a randomly generated population of individuals, each representing its own unique solution which is encoded as a string of genes. The selection of the number of generations and the population plays a crucial role in determining the overall prediction scores. Through the process of selection, crossover, mutation and reproduction individuals with identical behavior are allowed to reproduce and pass on their characteristics to the succeeding generation. Consequently, the population evolves towards better solutions by considering individuals with high fitness scores which will then participate in propagating through the next generations. Genetic algorithms as shown in Fig. 3 can be used in various fields, including health, engineering, finance, and bioinformatics, to tackle complex optimization problems where traditional methods may be time consuming, less accurate, inefficient or impractical. Their robustness to efficiently and effectively explore diverse prospects through generations and find optimal solutions by understanding hidden patterns helps them to find their application in real-world scenarios.

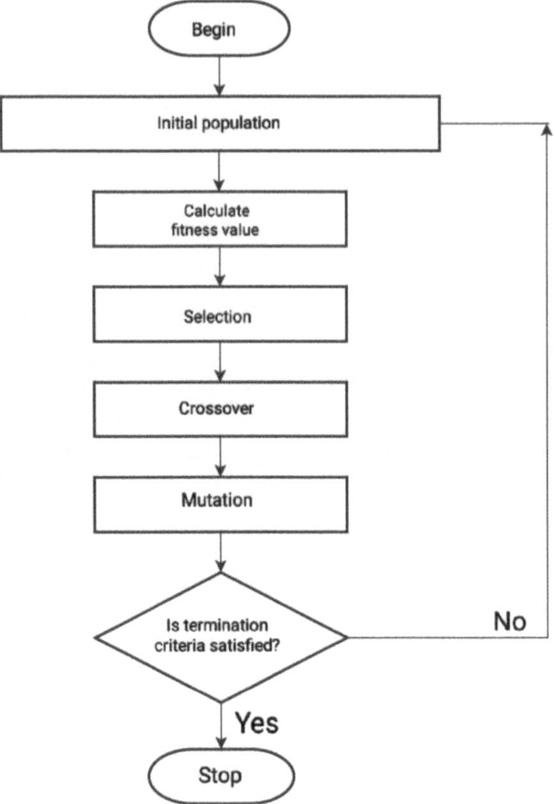

Fig. 3. Working of Genetic Algorithm

4.9 Genetic Algorithm Utilization in CKD Prediction

Genetic algorithms are crucial as it offers powerful optimization techniques to enhance feature selection and overall performance of the model. Here's an overview of key aspects of using genetic algorithms in CKD prediction:

1) *Feature Selection Optimization*
Genetic algorithms excel in optimizing feature selection processes by iteratively evolving optimal feature subsets from large datasets. By mimicking natural selection and genetic inheritance principles, GA efficiently explores the search space to identify the most informative features relevant to CKD progression prediction.
2) *Evolutionary Approach*
Genetic algorithms adopt an evolutionary approach, employing genetic operators such as crossover, mutation, and selection to iteratively evolve candidate feature subsets. This iterative process allows the algorithm to adapt and refine feature combinations over successive generations, optimizing model performance and predictive accuracy.

3) *Crossover Rate and Mutation Rate*

In genetic algorithms for CKD prediction, the crossover rate dictates the likelihood of genetic information exchange between parent chromosomes, fostering exploration and diversity. The mutation rate governs the probability of random changes, introducing diversity. Balancing these rates is critical for effective exploration of the search space while preventing premature convergence, ultimately optimizing predictive performance.

4) *Model Training Enhancement*

By integrating genetic algorithm-selected features into machine learning models for CKD prediction, developers can enhance model training and performance. The selected features serve as inputs to the model, facilitating more accurate predictions by focusing on the most relevant predictors of CKD progression.

5) *Cross-Validation and Generalization*

Genetic algorithm-based feature selection and model optimization contribute to improved cross-validation performance and generalization of CKD prediction models. By selecting robust feature subsets and optimizing model parameters, GAs helps in increasing the model's ability to study hidden patterns and features that are associated with the input data and reduces overfitting, ensuring reliable predictions in real-world applications.

5 Results and Discussions

In our project on Genetic Optimization for Chronic Kidney Disease Prognosis, we have developed a system that harnesses the power of genetic algorithms in conjunction with machine learning techniques. The system efficiently identifies key features relevant to CKD progression through genetic algorithm-based feature selection which is shown in Fig. 4. By choosing the most appropriate features as an optimal feature subset, the model achieves heightened accuracy and effectiveness in predicting CKD outcomes. Additionally, our system seamlessly integrates the selected features into the machine learning model, facilitating robust training and evaluation processes. Through this approach, we enhance the predictive capabilities of the model, providing valuable insights into CKD prognosis and facilitating proactive healthcare interventions. The prediction metrics obtained as a result of applying the genetic algorithm and the prediction metrics without applying the algorithm are given below for a comparative study from which a keen observation can be made on the optimal results delivered by the nature inspired genetic algorithm with its highest accuracy being99% in the case of AdaBoost classifier, and followed by enhanced accuracy in the case of other classifiers as mentioned in the table below. Hence, it is advisable to extend the approach of utilization of nature inspired algorithms to real-world domains as they study the hidden features and factors and work in an iterative manner to seamlessly enhance the accuracy of the models as shown in Fig. 5, 6, 7, 8 and 9.

Name	Units/Values
Specific Gravity	Nominal: 1.005, 1.010, 1.015, 1.025
Hyper Tension	Nominal: Yes/No
Hemoglobin	Numeric: in gms
Diabetes Mellitus	Nominal: Yes/No
Albumin	Nominal: 0, 1, 2, 3, 4, 5
Appetite	Nominal: good/poor
RBC Count	Numeric: millions/cmm
Pus Cell	Nominal: normal/abnormal

Fig. 4. Optimal Features obtained after applying GA

Classifiers	Accuracy before applying GA	Accuracy after applying GA
Random Forest	97.5	98.0
AdaBoost	97.0	99.8
Gradient Boost	97.5	97.5

Fig. 5. Accuracy comparison table

Gradient Boost Classifier

	Predicted: 1(Positive)	Predicted: 0(Negative)
Actual: 1(Positive)	55	3
Actual: 0(Negative)	0	62

Fig. 6. Confusion matrix of Gradient Boost Classifier

Random Forest Classifier

	Predicted: 1(Positive)	Predicted: 0(Negative)
Actual: 1(Positive)	55	3
Actual: 0(Negative)	0	62

Fig. 7. Confusion matrix of Random Forest Classifier

AdaBoost Classifier

	Predicted: 1(Positive)	Predicted: 0(Negative)
Actual: 1(Positive)	58	0
Actual: 0(Negative)	0	62

Fig. 8. Confusion matrix of AdaBoost Classifier

Classifier	Precision	Recall	f1-score
Random Forest	0.95	0.97	0.97
AdaBoost	1.00	1.00	1.00
Gradient Boost	0.95	0.97	0.97

Fig. 9. Performance Metrics

6 Conclusion and Future Scope

"Genetic Optimization for Chronic Kidney Disease Prognosis" represents a significant advancement in the field of healthcare and its related challenges. By incorporating genetic algorithms for feature selection and integrating them with machine learning techniques, we have developed a powerful predictive model capable of predicting chronic kidney disease with enhanced accuracy. This model holds immense potential and importance in aiding healthcare professionals and laboratory technicians in proper detection that helps in timely intervention to those patients who may be at risk of CKD. The successful implementation of this system can be understood by the enhanced accuracies obtained in the results. This highlights the importance of combining advanced technologies and existing knowledge to address complex medical challenges.

Moving forward, our work will pave the way for further research and innovation in predictive analytics for improved patient outcomes in chronic disease management by employing other nature inspired algorithms which include working with Ant Colony Optimization (ACO), Firefly Algorithm, Artificial Bee Colony Algorithm (ABC), Bat Algorithm and algorithms that belong to other categories of nature inspired algorithms so as to obtain optimal feature subsets and achieve overall enhanced accuracy. These algorithms can also be combined with other machine learning algorithms such as KNN, Naïve Bayes, SVM and it can also be extended to the domain of Artificial Neural Networks (ANN) and Deep Learning (DL) which can be used for an overall comparison in a broader perspective.

References

1. Arukonda, S., Cheruku, R.: A novel stacking framework with GWO-based feature selection for effective disease diagnosis. In: 2023 IEEE 20th India Council International Conference (INDICON), pp. 120–125 (2023)
2. Mamatha, B., Terdal, S.P.: Predicting chronic kidney disease using machine learning in the early stages. In: 2023 International Conference on Integrated Intelligence and Communication Systems (ICIICS), pp. 1–8 (2023)
3. Haque, Md.S., Amin, Md.S., Ahmad, S., Sayed, Md.A., Raihan, A., Hossain, M.A.: Predicting kidney failure using an ensemble machine learning model: a comparative study. In: 2023 10th International Conference on Electrical Engineering, Computer Science and Informatics (EECSI), pp. 31–37 (2023)
4. Anurag, N.V., Sharma, V., Balla, D.: Chronic kidney disease prediction using robust approach in machine learning. In: 2023 3rd International Conference on Innovative Sustainable Computational Technologies (CISCT), pp. 1–5 (2023)
5. Hassan, M.M., Ahamad, T., Das, S.: An ensemble learning approach for chronic kidney disease prediction using different machine learning algorithms with correlation-based feature selection. This paper proposes an ensemble learning approach using various machine learning algorithms with correlation-based feature selection. It develops a robust predictive model by combining multiple algorithms and selecting relevant features, to improve diagnosis accuracy (2022)
6. Hassan, Md.M., Ahamad, T., Das, S.: An ensemble learning approach for chronic kidney disease prediction using different machine learning algorithms with correlation based feature selection. In: 2022 25th International Conference on Computer and Information Technology (ICCIT), pp. 242–247 (2022)
7. Tyagi, A.K., Kumari, S.: A novelapproach to predict chronic kidney disease using machine learning algorithms. In: 2020 4th International Conference on Electronics, Communication and Aerospace Technology (ICECA), pp. 1630–1635. IEEE (2020)
8. National Institute for Health Care Excellence: Management of chronic kidney disease. This resource offers recommendations for the assessment, monitoring, and treatment of CKD in primary and secondary care settings, aiming to improve the qualityof care and outcomes for CKD patients (2021)
9. Bharath Clarke, A.L., Zaccardi, F., Gould, D.W., et al.: Association of self-reported physical function with survival in patients with chronic kidney disease. Clin. Kidney J. (2019). This study explores the association between self-reported physical function and survival in patients with chronic kidney disease
10. Arora, M., Sharma, E.A.: Chronic kidney disease detection by analyzing medical datasets in weka. Int. J. Comput. Mach. Learn. Algor. New. Adv. Mach. Learn. **3**, 19–48 (2016)
11. Hosen, N., Mozumder, Md.A.I., Sumon, R.I.: Prediction of Chronic Kidney Disease Using Machine Learning
12. Khan, R.H., Miah, J., Rahat, M.A.R., Ahmed, A.H., Shahriyar, M.A., Lipu, E.R.: A Comparative Analysis of Machine Learning Approaches for Chronic Kidney Disease Detection (2023)
13. Venkatrao, K., Kareemulla, S.: HDLNET: A Hybrid Deep Learning Network Model with Intelligent IOT for Detection and Classification of Chronic Kidney Disease (2023)
14. Swamy, B., Nakka, R., Sharma, A., Phani Praveen, S., Thatha, V.N., Gautam, K.: An ensemble learning approach for detection of chronic kidney disease (CKD)
15. Depak, K.G.A., Saikrishnan, S., Sudhakar, A.J., Kaviyarasan, K.: A Comprehensive Web Application for Chronic Kidney Disease Prediction with Cuisine-Centric Diet Recommendation (2023)

16. Ahmed, I., Ebad, T., Routh, B.B., Tasmiya, N., Sakib, S., Chowdhury, A.A.: Performance Analysis of Machine Learning Algorithms in Chronic Kidney Disease Prediction
17. Swain, D., et al.: A Robust Chronic Kidney Disease Classifier Using Machine Learning
18. Bandyopadhyay, A., Ghosh, S., Bose, M.: Alzheimer's Disease Detection Using Ensemble Learning and Artificial Neural Networks

PI-EnLLM: *P*ersonalized *I*nteractive Healthcare Assistance via *En*sembling *L*arge *L*anguage *M*odels

Aditya Dwibedi, Sreyasee Das Bhattacharjee(✉), Yu-Ping Chang, and Junsong Yuan

State University of New York (SUNY) at Buffalo, Buffalo, USA
{adwibedi,sreyasee,yc73,jsyuan}@buffalo.edu

Abstract. Personalized Assistance is critical to maintain an individual's mental health and well-being. AI-powered interactive agents demonstrate the potential to provide convenient and accessible support to individuals from diverse socio-econo-cultural backgrounds. By facilitating continual monitoring and just-in-time interventions, these agents demonstrate themselves as possible game changers in this application domain. This paper presents *PI-EnLLM*, a personalized and model-agnostic Large Language Model-based interactive healthcare assistant that can produce a context-aware response to a user query. An effective *Cooperative Optimization* process leverages the complementary strengths of multiple base LLMs to consent to a response and address a user query. In contrast to performing a tedious, resource-intensive, and task-specific LLM fine-tuning, we draft a context-aware dynamic prompt tuning technique, which can distill useful information into the prompts to generate a personalized response leveraging the user's unique past conversation context. The complementary knowledge resources of multiple LLMs are utilized to iteratively validate and enhance the response completeness and factuality in parallel. Across two large-scale publicly available datasets and our in-house *PsychEd_Care* psycho-education Question-Answer (QA) data collection, the proposed *PI-EnLLM* demonstrates consistent superior performance (e.g., $20-40\%$ improvement in F-measure of the $\mathbf{R}_L$ score reported by *PI-EnLLM*(3-Ensemble) in Psych8K dataset) compared to its individual base LLMs. This proves the effectiveness of the proposed context-aware dynamic prompt tuning toward expediting a cooperative optimization of the generated response via multiple iterations of LLM-specific validation checks. The generated response also reports impressive gain in its factuality and LLM-judge scores, exhibiting enhanced alignment with human preferences. The QA collection in the *PsychEd_Care* dataset covers essential caregiving topics including Transfer Skills, Nutrition, Dental Care, Bathing and Dressing, Toileting and Incontinence, Behavioral Issues, and Self-Care and will be available to academic researchers in the community after the work is published.

Keywords: Personalized Interactions · Large Language Models · Ensemble Model · Contextual Assistance · Dynamic Prompt Tuning

K. Atul et al. (Eds.): BodyNets 2024, LNICST 666, pp. 249–266, 2026.
https://doi.org/10.1007/978-3-032-16099-7_20

1 Introduction

Mental health well-being for an individual is of immense importance because this impacts various facets (thoughts, communications, behavior, emotional outbursts, affective states) of our lives [34]. According to the American Psychological Association, while the demand for mental health assistance continues to increase, there are hardly enough trained professionals to handle this rising demand[1]. In fact although the detection task gas received significant attention of the researchers across disciplines [3,4,21,24,54], timely intervention is critical to ensure an individual long-term mental well-being. Due to various issues including its high costs and limited resources, immediate assistance for all still seems infeasible. Artificial Intelligence (AI) has demonstrated its transformative impacts in facilitating automation in several industries and healthcare is one of them [30,32]. AI-powered health assistants have been consistently gaining popularity over the last few years, specifically among the younger generations [1]. Numerous digital platforms in this space have already shown tremendous promise to deliver an effective and just-in-time solution for the suffering population. Nonetheless, its reliability is still a concern for many, especially for the gen-X population.

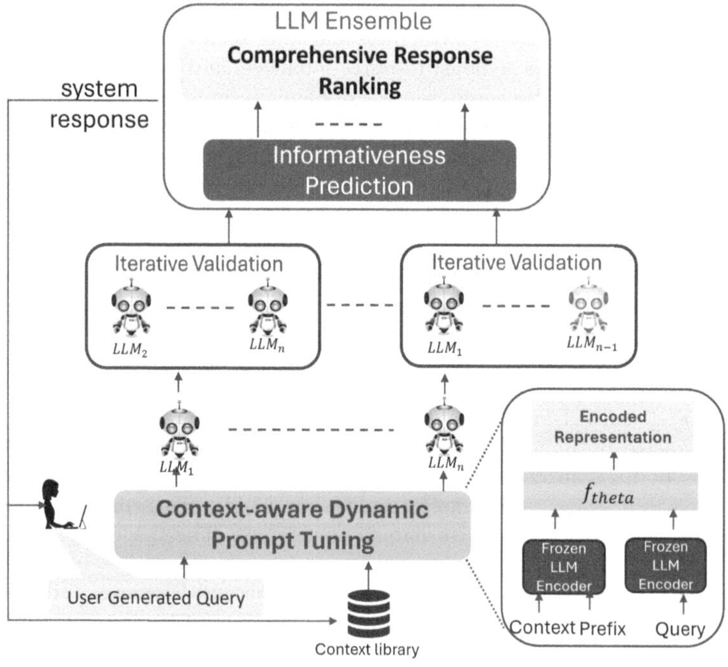

Fig. 1. Method Overview.

[1] https://www.apa.org/pubs/reports/practitioner/2022-covid-psychologist-workload.

The recent emergence of Large Language Models (LLMs) (e.g., LLaMA [42], MistralAI [17], Falcon [56]), which can generate fluent texts without any external linguistic expertise or domain-specific training, has demonstrated a significant impact in the field of AI. However, there are some fundamental limitations, which prevent them from being truly impactful in carrying out human-like meaningful conversion in a task-oriented dialogue system. *First, despite their tremendous effectiveness, the open-source LLMs exhibit distinct strengths and weaknesses, due to the variances in the underlying data collections they have been trained with, their respective architectural differences, and their unique set of hyperparameters.* Thus none of them can be tagged as the universal best over others. On the contrary, it is noted that frequently these LLMs prove themselves complementary to each other, thereby making it imperative to explore their ensembles that can better utilize their diverse skills to address a target task, e.g., answering a user query. *Second, truthfulness is often a bigger concern in the larger language models* [26]. While existing response generation systems focus primarily on securing completeness in the generated response, the aspect of truthfulness is yet to be fully explored. *Finally, to ensure task-specific context understanding within an open-source LLM, a common practice is to fine-tune it, which is significantly tedious and time-consuming* [8,43]. A set of recent works [28,38,47,55] prompt LLMs to inject the required knowledge, wherein a short and fixed text is appended with the query input to explicitly highlight the context details within the augmented query. Li and Liang [23] learn task-specific prefix to an input. Motivated by this approach, we enable the generation of an input-dependent prefix (or prompt) that can enhance the efficiency and effectiveness of the proposed *PI-EnLLM* in response generation.

More precisely, the proposed *PI-EnLLM* is a personalized and model-agnostic LLM-based interactive healthcare assistant that *given a user query, leverages the complementary strengths of multiple base LLMs to generate a more accurate and informative response.* In fact, by iterative interactions with the user, the model can present a response that fits well within the user's unique personal context. For example, by leveraging the context of a user's past conversations, *PI-EnLLM* may learn about the kind of caregiving suggestions the user may require for his grandmother, who requires help getting out of bed but does not have severe mobility issues yet. Motivated by a few recent research works, [18,27], in this work, we aim to mix the knowledge of multiple open-source base LLMs to validate and appropriately update the individual LLM responses and thereby achieve consistently superior performance. The proposed *PI-EnLLM* also aims to *improve the completeness and factuality, both in parallel*, via an effective *Cooperative Optimization* process, wherein each response generated by an initiator LLM agent is iteratively validated by a dynamic sequence of prompts to the collaborating LLM agents. *An effective context-aware prompt-tuning module is developed to incorporate the input context for carrying out a personalized conversation with the user.* The candidate responses are then ranked based on their learned reliability scores, which estimate the response factuality and completeness both within the precise problem context. To summarize, the contributions of this paper include:

- *An Effective Context-aware Dynamic Prompt Tuning* technique that can facilitate personalized response generation
- *Cooperative Optimization* that can leverage the complementary strengths of multiple LLMs to generate consensus on the response completeness and factuality, without needing to execute expensive fine-tuning.
- *Extensive Evaluation* in two large-scale publicly available psychological counseling datasets (Psych8K and OnlineTherapy4K) demonstrates the improved effectiveness of the proposed *PI-EnLLM* over the existing state-of-the-art methods.
- *Introducing PsychEd_Care, an in-house psycho-education Question-Answer (QA) Dataset* that is curated by domain experts from a series of expert-led caregiver training videos for Alzheimer's Disease and Related Dementias (ADRD) and converted into a multimodal QA collection that covers essential caregiving topics, including Transfer Skills, Nutrition, Dental Care, Bathing and Dressing, Toileting and Incontinence, Behavioral Issues, and Self-Care. Additionally, we offer *a User-friendly User Interface for seamless user study executions.*

2 Related Works

Our objective in this work is to comprehend the potential of LLM-based interactive agents in facilitating targeted machine-driven conversation. Toward this, in this section, we will briefly discuss some state-of-the-art works in two related problems: *LLM-based Response Generation System for Mental Health Assistance* and *Ensemble of LLMs.*

2.1 LLM-Based Response Generation System for Mental Health Assistance

LLM-based response generation to facilitate conversations of interactive agents has demonstrated promise in recent years. In recent work, Wang et al. [45] independently train for retrieving and reading ability. However, this impacts the model performance and results in a distribution shift between the retriever and the reader. While some works [37,46] attempt to optimize by mixing these training objectives, due to the complexity of the architectures, either learning is still inefficient and expensive or the scalability to extend on a large-scale environment remains sub-optimal. In medical science, some recent research [6,33,51] develop systems to generate consistent and knowledge-enhanced responses. Several authors [10,12,27,29,40,41,50,52] explore the potential of LLM-based interactive agents that can deliver human-like interactions with users seeking mental health support or provide some target-specific assistance (e.g., answering certain caregiving task related queries) through various platforms. However, the tendency of such LLM-based models to frequently generate factually incorrect statements is alarming [16,19,39]. In a study reported by Lin et al. [26], under human evaluation, the best-performing model GPT-3-175B was found to be correct on 58% of the questions compared to 94% correctness attained by humans. While fine-tuning and prompting have been used to elicit the domain-specific knowledge into the system [5,13,14]. *However, while fine-tuning is tedious and expensive, prompting with a fixed sequence of tokens does not demonstrate much effectiveness in designing a personalized human-like conversation. Toward this, we aim to improve the capability and reliability of the existing LLM-based models through a powerful context-aware dynamic prompt tuning technique, which can distill useful information into the prompts to generate a personalized response. The complementary knowledge resources of multiple LLMs are utilized to iteratively enhance the response completeness and factuality, both in parallel.*

2.2 Ensemble of LLMs

Like ensemble methods in machine learning [20], which are particularly impactful in improving the model biases, errors, and fundamental system uncertainties within each participant model, in a set of recent works [7,11,18,22,44,49], LLM fusion-based techniques also reported having enhanced the system's response generation ability. A few existing works [18,35,48] attempt to rerank outputs, generated for a single input, where each output is ranked based on certain target-specific criteria. However, this may not be truly effective in ensembling the complementary expertise of LLMs within the generated responses. Moreover, with the primary focus on improving the response generation capabilities in code generation and general reasoning, the existing literature do not explicitly keep track of the reliability features of a generated response. *In contrast, in this work, we extensively utilize the complementary strengths of LLMs at two phases. First, within a collaborative environment, each candidate response generated by an initiator LLM agent is further validated by a sequence of prompts to the collaborating LLM agents. This helps derive the best version of each candidate response, wherein complementary knowledge of all collaborating LLMs is incorporated via exclusive LLM-specific validation checks. Second, these validated responses are reranked based on an estimated total effectiveness score for finalizing a single comprehensive response to the user query.*

3 Proposed Method

In this section, we will describe the backbone modules of the prosed *PI-EnLLM* that can leverage the complementary strengths of multiple base LLMs to deliver a fact-checked, contextualized, and comprehensive response to a user query.

Problem Definition: A user driven conversation context with an LLM L is defined as,

$$\mathcal{U} \triangleq [q_1, a_1, q_2, a_2, ...q_{n-1}, a_{n-1}]$$

where the user's present query as q_n, we expect $L \in \mathcal{L}$ to generate a response a_n. The term $\mathcal{L}$ denotes the pool of LLMs to be ensembled for deriving a consensual, reliable, and complete response.

3.1 Cooperative Optimization

While standard models leverage the use-case-specific datasets to fine-tune each $L_i \in \mathcal{L}$ for delivering a context-relevant output, we propose a unified *context-aware dynamic prompt-tuning* module to optimize the system response within a collaborative environment parallelly.

Context-Aware Dynamic Prompt Tuning: We extend the prefix tuning approach by Li and Liang [23] for the response generation task, which appends an input $\mathbf{x}$ with a fixed set of prefix tokens $\mathbf{P}$ to obtain an augmented input $\mathbf{x}^{aug} \stackrel{\delta}{=} [\mathbf{P}, \mathbf{x}]$. In this work, we leverage the conversation context $\mathcal{U}_i$ generated by L_i to generate a learned prefixed input $\mathbf{P}_i^\theta$, defined as follows:

$$\mathbf{P}_i^\theta = f_\theta(E(\mathcal{U}_i)) \tag{1}$$

where E represents the prompt encoder function, and f_θ represents a neural network model with the learnable parameters θ. The model f_θ is trained using the traditional log-likelihood objective that can simultaneously train an encoder-decoder model to accurately decode the input from its encoded representation. For the task of response generation, the resulting context-aware user input at the nth conversation step is then defined as $\mathbf{x}_{n,i}^{aug} \stackrel{\delta}{=} [\mathbf{P}, \mathbf{P}_i^\theta, q_n]$ and the target output of the response-generating system is a_n. An overview of this module is illustrated in the Fig. 1.

In our experiments, we have employed several pre-trained seq2seq (encoder-decoder) language models (e.g., $T5$) to form the collection $\mathcal{L}$. In particular, each LLM agent in $\mathcal{L}$ acts as an initiator LLM agent and generates a candidate response that is iteratively validated by a dynamic sequence of context-aware prompts to the other collaborating LLM agents. Below, we will describe the process in more detail.

Iterative Validation: Given an initiator LLM agent $L_i \in \mathcal{L}$, the present user query q and its conversation history (if any) presented as $\mathcal{U}$, the proposed *context-aware dynamic prompt tuning* module is employed to derive $\mathbf{x}_{n,i}^{aug}$, which is fed into L_i to generate an initial response a_i^q. To mitigate the risk of the hallucination effect, we design an additional layer of response validation that employs each collaborating LLM agent $L_j \in \mathcal{L} \setminus \{L_i\}$ to fact-optimize a_i^q via a dynamically modified prompt defined as below:

$$\mathbf{P}_j^\beta = g_\theta(E(\mathcal{U}; q)) \tag{2}$$

The resulting context-aware prompt $\mathbf{P}_j^\beta$ is then used to define a context-aware input $\mathbf{y}_j^{aug} \stackrel{\delta}{=} [\mathbf{P}_j^\beta, a_i^q]$ that is fed into L_j to produce a j-validated version $(a_{i,j}^{val,q})$

of the response a_i^q. Given the query q and its candidate response collection $\{a_{i,j}^{val,q}\}_j$, we select a globally validated version $a_{i,j_{opt}}^{val,q}$ of the initial response a_i^q, where j_{opt} is defined as follows:

$$j_{opt} = \underset{j}{\text{argmax}}\{\textbf{Factool}(a_{i,j}^{val,q})\} \tag{3}$$

where the function **Factool** computes the Factuality score [26] of the generated response.

To optimize the response completeness and factuality, we iterate this process until a pre-defined stopping criteria is attained. In our experiments, this fact-optimizing process is repeated until the validated version of a_i^q generated at the end of a given iteration reports deterioration in their factuality scores, compared to that of the validated response generated in the immediately previous iteration.

3.2 LLM Ensemble

The ultimate objective of the proposed response generation system *PI-EnLLM* is to optimize the informativeness and factualities within the generated response. Toward facilitating this, we design a neural network-based *informativeness prediction* module that is trained to provide a comprehensive informativeness estimate for each candidate response $(a_i^{val,q})$.

Informativeness Prediction: Given the query q, the set of its fact-optimized candidate responses $\{a_i^{val,q}\}_i$ generated and cooperatively optimized by the LLMs in $\mathcal{L}$ and their single corresponding ground truth human-generated response a_{gt}^q, we form a regression module $\mathcal{R}()$ that estimates both Rouge-L score ($\mathbf{R_L}$) and the BLEURT (**BLEURT**) scores for each $a_i^{val,q}$. The training of $\mathcal{R}()$ involves minimizing a comprehensive loss $\mathcal{F}_{reg}$ defined as follows:

$$\mathcal{F}_{reg} = \frac{1}{||\mathcal{T}||}\sum_{q\in\mathcal{T}}\Big(Err(\boldsymbol{\alpha}_{reg}^T E(a_i^{val,q}) + \boldsymbol{\beta}_{reg}, \boldsymbol{val}_i^q)\Big), \tag{4}$$

where $\boldsymbol{val}_i^q \triangleq \Big[\mathbf{R}_L(a_i^{val,q}, a_{gt}^q)\ \mathbf{BLEURT}(a_i^{val,q}, a_{gt}^q)\Big]^T$ and $Err(,)$ is the shrinkage loss [31] that assigns more penalties for making wrong predictions on easy samples compared to the mistakes that occur in predicting the hard samples and thereby appears to be more effective compared to the standard Mean square error (MSE) loss in the presence of limited training data collection. The terms $\boldsymbol{\alpha}_{reg}^T$ and $\boldsymbol{\beta}_{reg}$ are the weight and bias terms of the network representing the regressor $\mathcal{R}$. Thus, $\mathcal{R}$ is trained to approximate the Rouge-L ($\mathcal{R}(a_i^{val,q})[0]$) and BLEURT ($\mathcal{R}(a_i^{val,q})[1]$) scores for $a_i^{val,q}$ respectively.

Comprehensive Response Ranking: During the test-time, given a query, the set of candidate responses $\{a_i^{val,q}\}_i$ generated by the LLMs in $\mathcal{L}$ are sorted based on their respective *total effectiveness scores* ($\{\mathbf{e}_i^q\}_i$) computed as:

$$\mathbf{e}_i^q = \mathbf{Factool}(a_{i,j}^{val,q}) + \mathcal{R}(a_i^{val,q})[0] + \mathcal{R}(a_i^{val,q})[1] \quad (5)$$

Then the system returns the response $a_{i_0}^{val,q}$, where $i_0 \stackrel{\delta}{=} \underset{i}{\text{argmax}}\{\mathbf{e}_i^q\}$.

4 Experiments and Observations

This section will discuss two publicly available mental-health counseling datasets and an in-house dataset that will be publicly available to academic researchers. An extensive set of experiments performed using these datasets will be described to thoroughly analyze the effectiveness of *PI-EnLLM* in different real-life problem settings.

4.1 Results and Analysis

Datasets: The performance of the proposed is evaluated using *PsychEd_Care* dataset, our inhouse psycho-education Question-Answer (QA) data collection and two large-scale publicly available psychological counseling datasets: *Psych8K* [2] and *OnlineTherapy4K*[3].

The *PsychEd_Care* dataset, a first-of-its-kind psycho-education Question-Answer dataset, consisting of 475 QA pairs, is curated from expert-led caregiver training videos focused on Alzheimer's Disease and Related Dementias (ADRD). The dataset covers essential caregiving topics including Transfer Skills, Nutrition, Dental Care, Bathing and Dressing, Toileting and Incontinence, Behavioral Issues, and Self-Care. 1000 video clips further explaining the key steps in executing the tasks related to each skill are also shared with the dataset. The conversations based on the contents covered in these training videos were led by professional nurses as well as informal caregivers, who either have prior experience of caring for a family member suffering from ADRD or have been presently taking care of someone in their personal life at present. The data was meticulously transcribed and validated by caregiving professionals with decades-long experiences, to ensure accuracy and relevance. Unlike existing datasets, which primarily focus on the mental health well-being of the *PsychEd_Care* dataset captures a conversation on a set of pre-defined topics with occasional references to the caregiver's mental health conditions also. For example, "How can I convince my grandmother to have her routine medicine? Her stubborn behavior is at times so frustrating!" To respond to such questions, the system is required to be not just considerate of the user's mental health condition and demonstrate empathy, but it is also expected to provide an accurate suggestion on the task

[2] https://huggingface.co/datasets/EmoCareAI/Psych8k.
[3] https://huggingface.co/datasets/Amod/mental_health_counseling_conversations.

she is enquiring about. Thus, the dataset reports a comprehensive coverage of critical caregiving topics, expert-led content, the inclusion of diverse dialogue lengths, and a collection of video clippings demonstrating some key caregiving tasks, which set it apart from the existing data collections, presently used by the research community. Upon publication of the paper, this dataset will be publicly available to the research community.

Psych8K is created from 260 in-depth interviews, each spanning an hour. The licensed psychological counselors directly designed and monitored the data collection process to ensure its high quality. To maintain privacy and ethical standards, the interview transcripts included in the dataset were thoroughly cleaned to eliminate any personally identifiable or sensitive information, which could have divulged the participants' identity or compromised the data integrity. Following the data processing protocol by Liu et al. [27], the segmented transcripts and their conversation summary were used to generate 8, 187 QA pairs. *OnlineTherapy4K* is another psychological counseling dataset that is obtained by scraping online forums. This dataset is a collection of 3, 510 QAs sourced from two online counseling and therapy platforms. The questions cover a wide range of mental health topics, and the answers are provided by qualified psychologists. The datasets were carefully chosen to cover various types of mental health counseling services practiced (e.g., online, in-person) these days.

Performance Metrics: To assess the effectiveness of the proposed response generation system *PI-EnLLM* in improving the performance over each of its constituent LLMs as the independent baselines, we use several metrics, which include: ROUGE-1/2/L (($R_{1/2/L}$) scores [25], Factool [9] and LLM-judge [26]. While a qualitative analysis for factuality checks using human evaluations is reported here, we also note that human evaluation is expensive. To address this, Factool and LLM-judge metrics are used as the additional metrics, popularly used as the alternative automated fact-checking. Factool is a domain-agnostic framework that detects factual errors using a given knowledge base or open-domain data source (e.g., Wikipedia) in the response generated by a Question Answering (QA) system. LLM-Judge leverages strong LLMs (e.g., Mistral) as judges to evaluate these models on more open-ended questions and predict human evaluations of the system-generated response for a test query. As shown by ZHeng et al. [53], LLM-Judge is a scalable and explainable way to approximate human preferences, which are otherwise very expensive to obtain.

For each dataset, we have chosen a random 80% of the data collection for training and the remaining 20% for testing. The experiments are repeated 3 times, each time with a random selection of train-test data distribution and the average performance is reported in Table 1.

Performance Comparison. The proposed response generation system *PI-EnLLM* leverages the pool of LLMs $\mathcal{L}$ composed of four opensource pre-trained LLM models Llama2-70B [36], Falcon-40B [2], Phi2 [15] and Mistral [17]. The performance of *PI-EnLLM* is compared with that of the individual performances

Table 1. The Comparative Performances of the Proposed response generation system *PI-EnLLM* against the baseline LLMs (Llama2-70B [36], Falcon-40B [2], Phi2 [15], and Mistral [17]) using the metrics: Precision (Pr), Recall (ReC), and F-Measure (F-meas) of the ROUGE-1/2/L (($R_{1/2/L}$) [25]; Factool [9]; and LLM-judge [26], Each entry in the table represented as a, b presents the performance details of the corresponding LLM (or a specific ensemble of constituent LLMs) with and without fine-tuning. For example, the third row and third column report the precision (Pr) of $\mathbf{R}_1$ score of the large language model Llama2 [36] as 0.59 (after fine-tuning) and 0.50 (before fine-tuning). The model *PI-EnLLM* (k-Ensemble) represents an ensemble of k baseline LLMs formed via*PI-EnLLM*. For $k = 2, 3$, in our experiments we have used different combinations of k base LLMs from the entire pool of n LLMs and the table reports an average performance of $\binom{n}{k}$ such k-Ensembled LLMs via *PI-EnLLM*.

Dataset	Model	R_1			R_2			R_1			Factool	LLM-Judge
		Pr.	ReC.	F-meas	Pr.	ReC.	F-meas	Pr.	ReC.	F-meas		
PsychEd_Care	Llama2 [36]	0.59, 0.50	0.31, 0.29	0.38, 0.36	0.29, 0.11	0.16, 0.14	0.20, 0.18	0.42, 0.40	0.24, 0.22	0.30, 0.28	0.97, 0.61	7.07, 5.67
	Falcon [2]	0.52, 0.33	0.30, 0.28	0.35, 0.27	0.28, 0.17	0.14, 0.15	0.13, 0.18	0.41, 0.31	0.22, 0.29	0.28, 0.25	0.90, 0.20	6.73, 5.65
	Phi2 [15]	0.38, 0.18	0.53, 0.38	0.43, 0.24	0.23, 0.08	0.32, 0.17	0.26, 0.11	0.15, 0.04	0.37, 0.20	0.19, 0.07	0.87, 0.15	6.93, 5.66
	Mistral [17]	0.56, 0.48	0.31, 0.25	0.39, 0.32	0.31, 0.21	0.16, 0.10	0.20, 0.13	0.44, 0.37	0.23, 0.18	0.29, 0.24	0.00, 0.00	6.95, 5.64
	PI-EnLLM (2-Ensemble)	0.59, 0.42	0.45, 0.31	0.49, 0.37	0.35, 0.28	0.29, 0.20	0.32, 0.23	0.43, 0.36	0.29, 0.23	0.35, 0.28	0.97, 0.91	7.57, 6.71
	PI-EnLLM (3-Ensemble)	0.78, 0.63	0.79, 0.41	0.74, 0.50	0.79, 0.29	0.78, 0.45	0.78, 0.50	0.78, 0.50	0.70, 0.28	0.69, 0.74	0.95, 0.48	7.95, 6.52
	PI-EnLLM (4-Ensemble)	0.74, 0.64	0.73, 0.50	0.74, 0.53	0.77, 0.49	0.69, 0.45	0.66, 0.38	0.77, 0.51	0.69, 0.44	0.66, 0.35	0.94, 0.56	7.13, 6.81
Psych8K	Llama2 [36]	0.27, 0.23	0.50, 0.47	0.33, 0.30	0.09, 0.07	0.18, 0.15	0.11, 0.09	0.17, 0.15	0.34, 0.31	0.22, 0.20	0.80, 0.58	7.58, 5.65
	Falcon [2]	0.37, 0.23	0.40, 0.39	0.37, 0.28	0.09, 0.04	0.11, 0.08	0.09, 0.05	0.21, 0.14	0.23, 0.23	0.21, 0.16	0.79, 0.48	7.13, 5.56
	Phi2 [15]	0.42, 0.19	0.56, 0.34	0.48, 0.24	0.19, 0.04	0.26, 0.08	0.21, 0.05	0.29, 0.11	0.39, 0.20	0.33, 0.14	0.81, 0.59	7.61, 5.66
	Mistral [17]	0.29, 0.27	0.45, 0.38	0.33, 0.29	0.07, 0.03	0.13, 0.05	0.09, 0.04	0.15, 0.15	0.27, 0.20	0.18, 0.16	0.73, 0.43	6.11, 5.64
	PI-EnLLM (2-Ensemble)	0.71, 0.45	0.65, 0.38	0.60, 0.34	0.61, 0.30	0.65, 0.35	0.63, 0.32	0.30, 0.22	0.42, 0.26	0.35, 0.24	0.82, 0.63	7.67, 6.30
	PI-EnLLM (3-Ensemble)	0.73, 0.45	0.76, 0.54	0.68, 0.38	0.72, 0.47	0.73, 0.46	0.68, 0.36	0.76, 0.50	0.74, 0.51	0.72, 0.44	0.95, 0.66	7.96, 6.96
	PI-EnLLM (4-Ensemble)	0.71, 0.47	0.79, 0.56	0.75, 0.51	0.74, 0.49	0.77, 0.50	0.72, 0.42	0.76, 0.54	0.71, 0.46	0.68, 0.41	0.78, 0.61	7.81, 6.42
OnlineTherapy4K	Llama2 [36]	0.52, 0.50	0.22, 0.20	0.26, 0.26	0.11, 0.10	0.40, 0.40	0.06, 0.06	0.29, 0.28	0.11, 0.11	0.14, 0.14	0.84, 0.61	7.51, 5.67
	Falcon [2]	0.07, 0.07	0.38, 0.38	0.11, 0.11	0.01, 0.01	0.08, 0.08	0.02, 0.02	0.05, 0.05	0.27, 0.27	0.08, 0.08	0.89, 0.63	7.31, 5.71
	Phi2 [15]	0.30, 0.21	0.37, 0.30	0.30, 0.23	0.06, 0.03	0.07, 0.04	0.05, 0.03	0.18, 0.13	0.21, 0.18	0.18, 0.13	0.85, 0.65	7.21, 5.69
	Mistral [17]	0.43, 0.35	0.32, 0.31	0.32, 0.30	0.07, 0.05	0.06, 0.04	0.21, 0.21	0.17, 0.14	0.17, 0.15	0.17, 0.15	0.47, 0.70	6.11, 5.37
	PI-EnLLM (2-Ensemble)	0.53, 0.37	0.39, 0.36	0.45, 0.36	0.15, 0.12	0.14, 0.10	0.15, 0.11	0.30, 0.28	0.29, 0.22	0.29, 0.25	0.89, 0.70	8.28, 6.37
	PI-EnLLM (3-Ensemble)	0.67, 0.46	0.64, 0.46	0.57, 0.42	0.70, 0.49	0.67, 0.50	0.62, 0.38	0.73, 0.54	0.69, 0.51	0.65, 0.42	0.89. 0.73	8.75, 6.44
	PI-EnLLM (4-Ensemble)	0.78, 0.53	0.73, 0.47	0.71, 0.39	0.77, 0.51	0.74, 0.49	0.71, 0.40	0.74, 0.48	0.84, 0.60	0.76, 0.45	0.92, 0.64	7.82, 6.79

of these base LLMs. Table 1 presents a detailed comparative study, where the performances of different versions of *PI-EnLLM* formed using varied combinations of base LLMs are compared against that of each LLM. The entire set of experiments is repeated with/without fine-tuning the constituent LLMs in the context of the dataset in consideration. The table reports the performances of various k-Ensemble versions of *PI-EnLLM* (described as *PI-EnLLM* (k-Ensemble)) and an average performance of $\binom{n}{k}$ such k-Ensembled LLMs designed via *PI-EnLLM*. For example, the 8th, 15th and 22nd row of the table reports an average performance of $\binom{4}{3}$ 3-Ensembled LLMs via *PI-EnLLM* in *PsychEd_Care*, *Psych8K*, and *OnlineTherapy4K* respectively. **As observed in the table, in the in-house *PsychEd_Care* dataset, *PI-EnLLM*(3-Ensemble) deliv-**

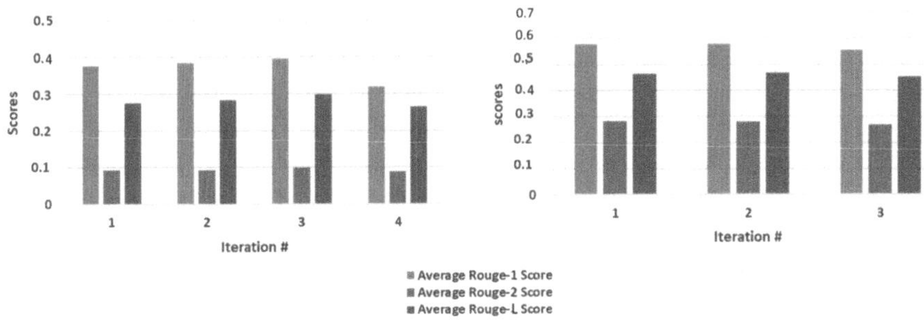

Fig. 2. An illustration of the comprehensive training of the proposed *PI-EnLLM* in a collaborative environment. At the end of 4th (and 3rd) iteration of validation by the collaborating LLM agents in $\mathcal{L}$ a response that was initially generated by Llama2-70B in left (and FalCon in the right) starts reporting deteriorated an average ROUGE F-measure (i.e. the mean of F-measures of $\mathbf{R}_1$, $\mathbf{R}_2$, and $\mathbf{R}_L$ scores) compared to that reported in its previous iteration and thereby the training iteration with this training sample stops. This figure shows the results of a 2-ensemble model, where we have 2 LLM agents in $\mathcal{L}$ (e.g., Llama2-70B, Falcon).

ers an impressive 46% **(and** 14%**) gain in the F-measure of $\mathbf{R}_1$ score when fine-tuned (or just pre-trained). It also reports** 52% **(and** 32%**) improved F-measure of $\mathbf{R}_2$ score when fine-tuned (or just pre-trained).** A similar performance trend is again reported using $\mathbf{R}_l$, another popular metric to do the quality check of a system-generated response. The trend continues as we note the average performance gains of *PI-EnLLM* in various other experimental settings (e.g. *PI-EnLLM* (2-Ensemble and *PI-EnLLM*(4-Ensemble)) in all three datasets. In fact, by pairwise comparisons of the performances of *PI-EnLLM*(3-Ensemble) and *PI-EnLLM*(4-Ensemble) reported in 8th and 9th, 15th and 16th, or 22nd, 23rd rows, we observe that while *PI-EnLLM* indeed facilitates aggregating the complementary knowledge of multiple LLMs in $\mathcal{L}$ within the generated response to enhance its completeness and contextualize features, often there is a stage of saturation, where adding more LLMs in $\mathcal{L}$ may not help further. **Also, the proposed *Cooperative Optimization* facilitated by the *Context-aware Dynamic Finetuning* proved to be significantly better than the traditional LLM fine-tuning technique, which is both computationally heavy and resource intensive.** For example, in Psych8K dataset, the best performing Phi2 reports 0.33 F-measure of $\mathbf{R}_L$ score when fine-tuned, while pre-trained *PI-EnLLM*(3-Ensemble) without fine-tuning attains an impressive 0.44 F-measure of $\mathbf{R}_L$ score in the same dataset, which proves the model's efficiency and effectiveness both simultaneously.

Ablation Study. The comprehensive training of the proposed *PI-EnLLM* in a collaborative environment is performed iteratively, where each validated system-generated response for a query in the training collection is evaluated against its ground truth human-generated response using an average ROUGE F-measure (i.e. the mean of F-measures of $\mathbf{R}_1$, $\mathbf{R}_2$, and $\mathbf{R}_L$ scores) and training iteration with the validated response is repeated if the average ROUGE F-measure at the present iteration is improved compared to that reported in its previous iteration. Figure 2 shows the results of a 2-ensemble model, where we have 2 LLM agents in $\mathcal{L}$ (e.g., Llama2-70B, Falcon). Also, the number of LLMs in $\mathcal{L}$ that are participating in the proposed *PI-EnLLM* model is a critical factor. **As observed in the table 1, while the proposed cooperative optimization process is model-agnostic and ensures an improved system-generated response compared to its constituent base LLM models, too many participant LLMs may also not be very useful to ensure continual performance gain.** In all our experiments an ensemble of 3 LLM agents appears to be performing consistently well across all datasets. **Furthermore, not only in terms of the response informativeness, the proposed *PI-EnLLM* also demonstrates its effectiveness in significantly enhancing the response factuality and reliability compared to the responses by its constituent base LLMs as pre-trained and fine-tuned.**

Qualitative Study. The examples shown in Fig. 3 demonstrate the model's ability to generate responses, that are not just factually accurate but are also designed to understand and store the user context and provide direct guidance, approval, and assurance to the user.

Human Evaluation. Users access the system via a simple user interface, the screenshot of which is shown in Fig. 4. We design an evaluation protocol that can assure its real-world applicability and reproducibility. Unlike the publicly available datasets *Psych8K* and *OnlineTherapy4K* which have larger test collections (we use a random 20% of the total data collection as the test set), for the small size and unique nature of the in-house dataset *PsychEd_Care*, human evaluation appears more important. Therefore, we perform a human evaluation using *PsychEd_Care* dataset in this work.

To evaluate the model's informativeness and truthfulness [26] we also perform the model's assessments by the real users, where the objective is to have each user provide a score against every system-generated result that represents their confidence on how true or informative this answer is. We also evaluate two additional features [27] of each system-generated response: direct guidance and approval & assurance. 10 evaluators were invited to perform this study, who were blinded of the underlying model details, which produced a specific answer to a given query. Instead of having only a True/False binary answer, we allow users to assign 10 qualitative labels. These include: True; Mostly True; Sometimes True; No true value exists; Subjective; False; Mostly False; Sometimes False; Contradiction; and Do not know. For the informativeness, we assign another 5 qualitative labels: Fully Informative; Partially Informative; Somewhat Informative; Vague; and Irrelevant. To binarize the truthfulness (and informativeness) criteria, we ensure that the response is at least subjective (and Somewhat Informative). In places, where the users were unsure of their response, a consulting expert (e.g.,

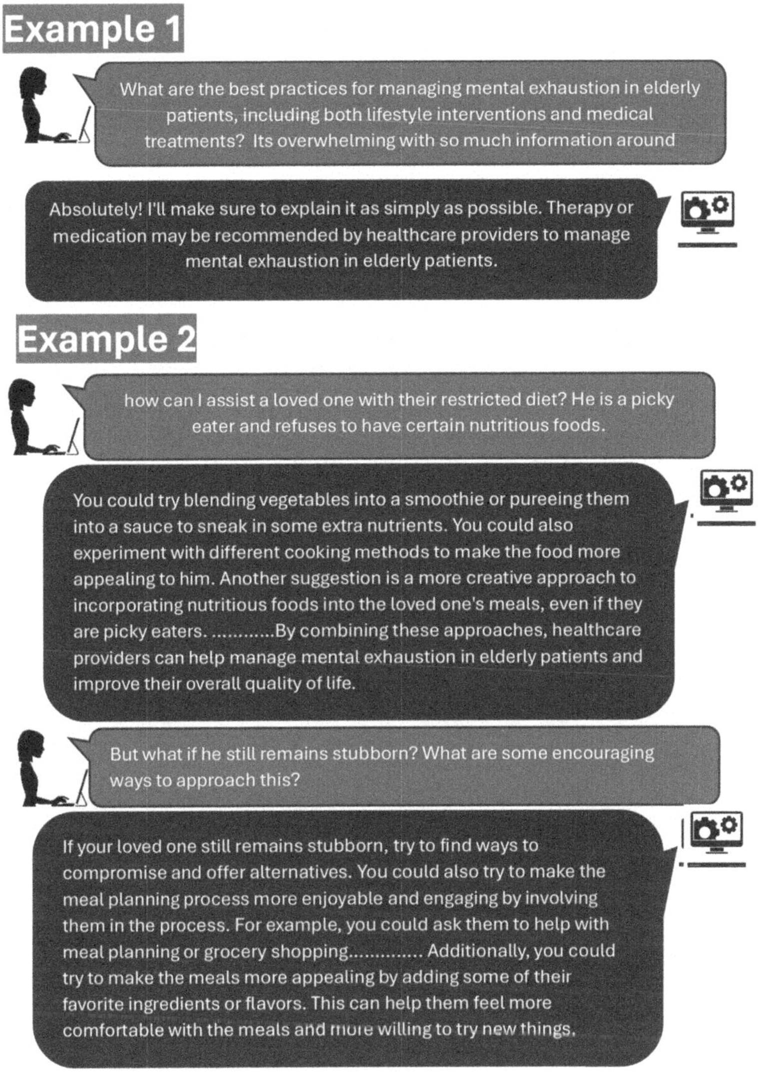

Fig. 3. The first example shown above demonstrates the proposed interactive agent *PI-EnLLM*'s ability to assure the user. The second example shown below showcases its ability to provide direct guidance while designing a context-aware response that also maintains its informativeness and truthfulness in parallel.

a senior grad student specializing in Nursing or Healthcare) was available to verify the answer. Important to note that the proposed *PI-EnLLM* retrieves the related information links to support each of its responses via pieces of evidence, which further facilitates the human evaluation. Each user is requested to interact with the system by asking 4–6 questions/caregiving skills covered in the dataset as well as a few other mental-health well-being-related questions. Each system response is then evaluated by the user on the pre-defined criteria of informativeness, truthfulness, direct guidance, approval & assurance, and answer relevance.

While *PI-EnLLM* demonstrates impressive performance in attaining an improved truthfulness (90.7%) and informativeness (95.2%) scores, and approval & assurance (98.4%), the model often lags in their ability in direct guidance (67%). Upon manual evaluation, we realize that the responses generated by the LLM models are often lengthy, and are not liked by many users. While they still find the lengthy answers informative, their lack of succinctness impacts their effectiveness in providing direct guidance.

Since human evaluation is costly, we also use LLM-Judge, which is frequently used as an alternative automated metric as a proxy in the literature [26,27,53]. As observed in the 13th column of Table 1, **the proposed *PI-EnLLM* also delivers responses that are highly aligned with human preferences. Compared to the base LLMs, *PI-EnLLM* as a fine-tuned (or just pre-trained) response generation system, demonstrates an enhanced capability of producing human-like responses in various discussion settings covered in multiple datasets using our experiments.** Impor-

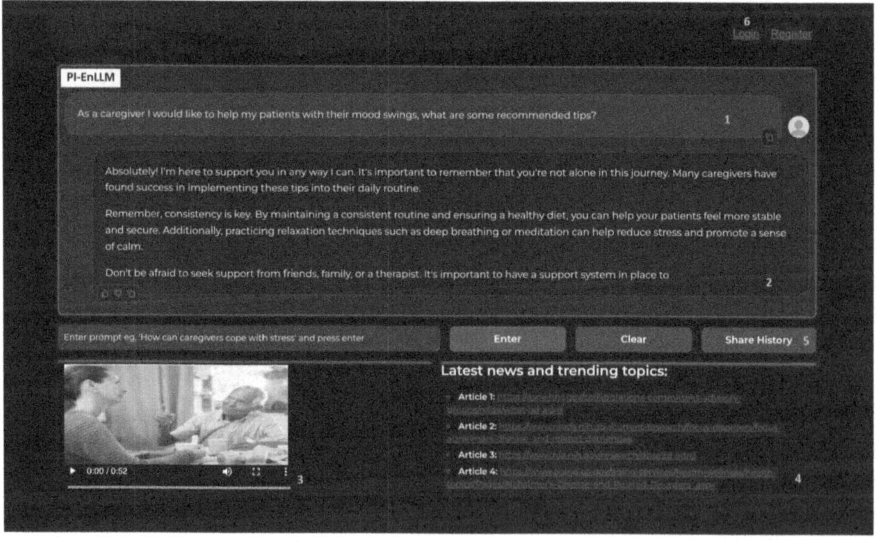

Fig. 4. A snapshot of the User Interface (UI) for *PI-EnLLM*. The annotated regions display the functionality in the UI. 1: The query inserted by the user, 2: The system-generated response, 3: the recommended video clipping elaborating some key ideas conveyed by the response, which are retrieved from the dataset repository, 4: supporting materials/articles for fact-checking, 5: allowing the user to provide permission to preserve the interaction history for future references, and 6: user can choose to register and log in or can continue as a guest.

tant to note that the effectiveness of *PI-EnLLM* prevails against various system configurations, where a varied number of LLMs are ensembled by *PI-EnLLM*. For example, in *OnlineTherapy4K* dataset, *PI-EnLLM*(3-ensemble) reports the best LLM-judge score as fine-tuned (or just pre-trained). Nevertheless, the performance reported by *PI-EnLLM*(2-ensemble) or *PI-EnLLM*(4-ensemble) also demonstrates considerable improvement compared to its base LLMs, which justifies the model stability and robustness.

5 Conclusion

In this paper, we propose *PI-EnLLM*, a personalized and mode-agnostic large language model-based interactive agent that leverages the complementary strengths of multiple LLMs to deliver a system-generated response to use-query that is both context-aware and factually rich. In a collaborative environment, the model deploys an effective context-aware dynamic prompt-tuning module that can distill useful prompting signals to deliver a personalized response. The model demonstrates significant performance gains in experiments using multiple large-scale public datasets compared to its base LLMs. The paper also introduces *PsychEd_Care*, a task-specific dataset that covers essential caregiving topics including Transfer Skills, Nutrition, Dental Care, Bathing and Dressing, Toileting and Incontinence, Behavioral Issues, and Self-Care and will be available to the academic researchers in the community after the work is published. A critical limitation of this model, which would also be our future research direction, would be to transfer it to a non-English language dataset or a dataset covering conversations in multiple languages.

References

1. Alanzi, T., et al.: Ai-powered mental health virtual assistants acceptance: an empirical study on influencing factors among generations x, y, and z. Cureus **15**(11) (2023)
2. Almazrouei, E., et al.: The falcon series of open language models. arXiv preprint arXiv:2311.16867 (2023)
3. Anand, S., Devulapally, N.K., Bhattacharjee, S.D., Yuan, J., Chang, Y.P.: Amuse: adaptive multimodal analysis for speaker emotion recognition in group conversations. In: 2023 IEEE Ninth Multimedia Big Data (BigMM), pp. 40–47. IEEE (2023)
4. Arumugam, B., Bhattacharjee, S.D., Yuan, J.: Multimodal attentive learning for real-time explainable emotion recognition in conversations. In: 2022 IEEE International Symposium on Circuits and Systems (ISCAS), pp. 1210–1214. IEEE (2022)
5. Bai, Z., Wu, N., Cai, F., Zhu, X., Xiong, Y.: Finetuning large language model for personalized ranking. arXiv preprint arXiv:2405.16127 (2024)
6. Bao, Z., et al.: Disc-medllm: bridging general large language models and real-world medical consultation. arXiv preprint arXiv:2308.14346 (2023)
7. Chang, Y.P., Dwibedi, A.K., Joshi, S., Bhattacharjee, S.D.: Development of an ai-powered emotionally intelligent, interactive agent prototype to support informal caregivers. Innov. Aging **7**(Suppl 1), 1019 (2023)

8. Chen, S., Wong, S., Chen, L., Tian, Y.: Extending context window of large language models via positional interpolation. arXiv preprint arXiv:2306.15595 (2023)
9. Chern, I., et al.: Factool: factuality detection in generative ai–a tool augmented framework for multi-task and multi-domain scenarios. arXiv preprint arXiv:2307.13528 (2023)
10. Demszky, D., et al.: Using large language models in psychology. Nat. Rev. Psychol. **2**(11), 688–701 (2023)
11. Fang, C., et al.: Llm-ensemble: optimal large language model ensemble method for e-commerce product attribute value extraction. arXiv preprint arXiv:2403.00863 (2024)
12. Gabriel, S., Puri, I., Xu, X., Malgaroli, M., Ghassemi, M.: Can ai relate: testing large language model response for mental health support. arXiv preprint arXiv:2405.12021 (2024)
13. He, Z., et al.: Large language models as zero-shot conversational recommenders. In: Proceedings of the 32nd ACM International Conference on Information and Knowledge Management, pp. 720–730 (2023)
14. Hou, Y., et al.: Large language models are zero-shot rankers for recommender systems. In: European Conference on Information Retrieval, pp. 364–381. Springer, Heidelberg (2024). https://doi.org/10.1007/978-3-031-56060-6_24
15. Javaheripi, M., et al.: Phi-2: the surprising power of small language models. Microsoft Research Blog (2023)
16. Ji, Z., et al.: Survey of hallucination in natural language generation. ACM Comput. Surv. **55**(12), 1–38 (2023)
17. Jiang, A.Q., et al.: Mistral 7b. arXiv preprint arXiv:2310.06825 (2023)
18. Jiang, D., Ren, X., Lin, B.Y.: Llm-blender: ensembling large language models with pairwise ranking and generative fusion. arXiv preprint arXiv:2306.02561 (2023)
19. Kaddour, J., Harris, J., Mozes, M., Bradley, H., Raileanu, R., McHardy, R.: Challenges and applications of large language models. arXiv preprint arXiv:2307.10169 (2023)
20. Kunapuli, G.: Ensemble methods for machine learning. Simon and Schuster (2023)
21. Li, J., Wang, X., Lv, G., Zeng, Z.: Ga2mif: graph and attention based two-stage multi-source information fusion for conversational emotion detection, pp. 1–14 (2023). https://doi.org/10.1109/TAFFC.2023.3261279
22. Li, J., Zhang, Q., Yu, Y., Fu, Q., Ye, D.: More agents is all you need. arXiv preprint arXiv:2402.05120 (2024)
23. Li, X.L., Liang, P.: Prefix-tuning: optimizing continuous prompts for generation. arXiv preprint arXiv:2101.00190 (2021)
24. Li, Z., Tang, F., Zhao, M., Zhu, Y.: Emocaps: emotion capsule based model for conversational emotion recognition. arXiv preprint arXiv:2203.13504 (2022)
25. Lin, C.Y.: Rouge: a package for automatic evaluation of summaries. In: Text Summarization Branches Out, pp. 74–81 (2004)
26. Lin, S., Hilton, J., Evans, O.: Truthfulqa: measuring how models mimic human falsehoods. arXiv preprint arXiv:2109.07958 (2021)
27. Liu, J.M., Li, D., Cao, H., Ren, T., Liao, Z., Wu, J.: Chatcounselor: a large language models for mental health support. arXiv preprint arXiv:2309.15461 (2023)
28. Liu, P., Yuan, W., Fu, J., Jiang, Z., Hayashi, H., Neubig, G.: Pre-train, prompt, and predict: a systematic survey of prompting methods in natural language processing. ACM Comput. Surv. **55**(9), 1–35 (2023)
29. Liu, S., Deng, N., Sabour, S., Jia, Y., Huang, M., Mihalcea, R.: Task-adaptive tokenization: Enhancing long-form text generation efficacy in mental health and

beyond. In: The 2023 Conference on Empirical Methods in Natural Language Processing (2023)
30. Loh, E.: Medicine and the rise of the robots: a qualitative review of recent advances of artificial intelligence in health. BMJ Leader 2018 (2018)
31. Lu, X., Ma, C., Ni, B., Yang, X., Reid, I., Yang, M.H.: Deep regression tracking with shrinkage loss. In: Proceedings of the European Conference on Computer Vision (ECCV), pp. 353–369 (2018)
32. Minerva, F., Giubilini, A.: Is ai the future of mental healthcare? Topoi **42**(3), 809–817 (2023)
33. Qian, Y., Zhang, W.N., Liu, T.: Harnessing the power of large language models for empathetic response generation: empirical investigations and improvements. arXiv preprint arXiv:2310.05140 (2023)
34. Raphael, B., Schmolke, M., Wooding, S.: Links between mental and physical health and illness. Promoting mental health (2005)
35. Ravaut, M., Joty, S., Chen, N.F.: Summareranker: a multi-task mixture-of-experts re-ranking framework for abstractive summarization. arXiv preprint arXiv:2203.06569 (2022)
36. Roumeliotis, K.I., Tselikas, N.D., Nasiopoulos, D.K.: Llama 2: early adopters' utilization of meta's new open-source pretrained model (2023)
37. Rubin, O., Berant, J.: Long-range language modeling with self-retrieval. arXiv preprint arXiv:2306.13421 (2023)
38. Shin, T., Razeghi, Y., Logan IV, R.L., Wallace, E., Singh, S.: Autoprompt: eliciting knowledge from language models with automatically generated prompts. arXiv preprint arXiv:2010.15980 (2020)
39. Shuster, K., Poff, S., Chen, M., Kiela, D., Weston, J.: Retrieval augmentation reduces hallucination in conversation. arXiv preprint arXiv:2104.07567 (2021)
40. Song, I., Pendse, S.R., Kumar, N., De Choudhury, M.: The typing cure: experiences with large language model chatbots for mental health support. arXiv preprint arXiv:2401.14362 (2024)
41. Spitale, M., Axelsson, M., Gunes, H.: Appropriateness of llm-equipped robotic well-being coach language in the workplace: a qualitative evaluation. arXiv preprint arXiv:2401.14935 (2024)
42. Touvron, H., et al.: Llama: open and efficient foundation language models. arXiv preprint arXiv:2302.13971 (2023)
43. Tworkowski, S., Staniszewski, K., Pacek, M., Wu, Y., Michalewski, H., Miłoś, P.: Focused transformer: contrastive training for context scaling. Adv. Neural Inf. Process. Syst. **36** (2024)
44. Wan, F., et al.: Knowledge fusion of large language models. arXiv preprint arXiv:2401.10491 (2024)
45. Wang, H., et al.: Large language models as source planner for personalized knowledge-grounded dialogue. arXiv preprint arXiv:2310.08840 (2023)
46. Wang, H., et al.: Unims-rag: a unified multi-source retrieval-augmented generation for personalized dialogue systems. arXiv preprint arXiv:2401.13256 (2024)
47. Wang, Y., Xia, C., Wang, G., Philip, S.Y.: Continuous prompt tuning based textual entailment model for e-commerce entity typing. In: 2022 IEEE International Conference on Big Data (Big Data), pp. 1383–1388. IEEE (2022)
48. Xie, Q., Zhou, J., Peng, Y., Wang, F.: Factreranker: fact-guided reranker for faithful radiology report summarization. arXiv preprint arXiv:2303.08335 (2023)
49. Yang, H., Li, M., Zhou, H., Xiao, Y., Fang, Q., Zhang, R.: One llm is not enough: harnessing the power of ensemble learning for medical question answering. medRxiv (2023)

50. Yao, X., Mikhelson, M., Watkins, S.C., Choi, E., Thomaz, E., de Barbaro, K.: Development and evaluation of three chatbots for postpartum mood and anxiety disorders. arXiv preprint arXiv:2308.07407 (2023)
51. Zhang, C., et al.: Cpsycoun: a report-based multi-turn dialogue reconstruction and evaluation framework for Chinese psychological counseling. arXiv preprint arXiv:2405.16433 (2024)
52. Zhang, Q., Naradowsky, J., Miyao, Y.: Ask an expert: leveraging language models to improve strategic reasoning in goal-oriented dialogue models. arXiv preprint arXiv:2305.17878 (2023)
53. Zheng, L., et al.: Judging llm-as-a-judge with mt-bench and chatbot arena. Adv. Neural Inf. Process. Syst. **36** (2024)
54. Zheng, W., Yu, J., Xia, R., Wang, S.: A facial expression-aware multimodal multi-task learning framework for emotion recognition in multi-party conversations. In: Proceedings of the 61st Annual Meeting of the Association for Computational Linguistics, vol. 1: Long Papers, pp. 15445–15459 (2023)
55. Zhu, Q., Li, B., Mi, F., Zhu, X., Huang, M.: Continual prompt tuning for dialog state tracking. arXiv preprint arXiv:2203.06654 (2022)
56. ZXhang, Y.X., Haxo, Y.M., Mat, Y.X.: Falcon llm: a new frontier in natural language processing. AC Invest. Res. J. **220**(44) (2023)

Recent Advancements in Optical Fibers Biosensors for Cancer Diagnosis

Sumeer Khajuria[1,3], Pradeep Teotia[2], and Daljeet Singh[3](✉)

[1] Department of ECE, Govt. College of Engg. and Tech., Jammu, India
[2] Telecommunication, BSNL, U.P(W), Meerut, India
[3] School of Electronics and Electrical Engineering, Lovely Professional University, Phagwara, Punjab, India
daljeetsingh.thapar@gmail.com

Abstract. Cancer is considered one of the deadliest diseases in the world mainly caused by impairments due to malfunctioning of cells in the human body. An early detection of cancer cells will lead to a reduced death rate in the long run. Conventional methods for the detection of cancer cells such as mammography, Magnetic Resonance Imaging (MRI), ultrasound, Computerized Tomography (CT), and biopsy have limitations in terms of cost, real-time fast processing, safety, and size. Both governments and companies are working hard during the last few decades in the development of biosensors for continuous checking of biological parameters which can reduce extra costs to the patients as well as to the administration. This has been made possible with the advancement made using optical fiber technology, which have lately amalgamated to the development of bio-sensors. This paper reviews the various types of OFS and their recent applications in healthcare in order to help doctors/clinical technocrats to understand OFS technology in better manner with an overview about the challenges involved in designing of OFS technology in healthcare. OFS yet needs to fulfil their great potential in healthcare and methods of increasing the adoption of medical devices based on optical fibers are discussed. These factors are important for successful translation of the developed sensors in the device development process in healthcare.

Keywords: Optical fiber sensor · surface plasma resonance · cancer diagnosis · fiber Bragg grating · detection accuracy

1 Introduction

The term cancer means the formation of a tumor in a particular region due to factors like environmental, genetic, or bacterial and viral infections. Due to the increase in tumors, there is an abnormal and unregulated growth of cells that spreads on all sides of the organ, thus decreasing its defense against cancer, which becomes incurable at later stages. According to the data provided by the American Cancer Society (ACS), there were 50% of cancer patients in 1975–1977 and then this rate increased to 66% in the years 1996–2004. Now in today's scenario, the death rate of cancer patients continuous to grow

K. Atul et al. (Eds.): BodyNets 2024, LNICST 666, pp. 267–281, 2026.
https://doi.org/10.1007/978-3-032-16099-7_21

and the number of deaths in the year 2024 is 15 million. Cancer is generally caused by three factors i.e. environmental factors: Chewing Tobacco and drinking alcohol, smoke and, radiation from industry, dangerous chemicals from factories, drinking Alcohol; genetic factors: Inherited mutations along with autoimmune dysfunction bacterial and viral infections: Stomach as well as cervical cancer [1].

With the increase in pollution and other genetic problems, prostate cancer, breast cancer, lung cancer is the most common type of cancer in both men and women. Small children are also in this group of cancer. The development of new technologies with better treatment and diagnosis thus provides better relief with enhanced quality of life to the patient even with a diagnosis of cancer in later stages [2]. Many types of cancer can be categorized and where it begins. Mainly, there are four categories of cancers are as shown in Fig. 1. In the case of biosensors, a biological entity like proteins, DNA, and RNA is converted by a biological analyte into an electrical signal for cancer detection with proper analysis techniques. Cancer biomarkers are used for the detection of cancer at the pre-stage level, its treatment, and by using chemotherapy to monitor, treat, and stopping of cancer progression. Such types of biomarkers are found in serum, blood, urine or tumor cells, etc. [3, 4].

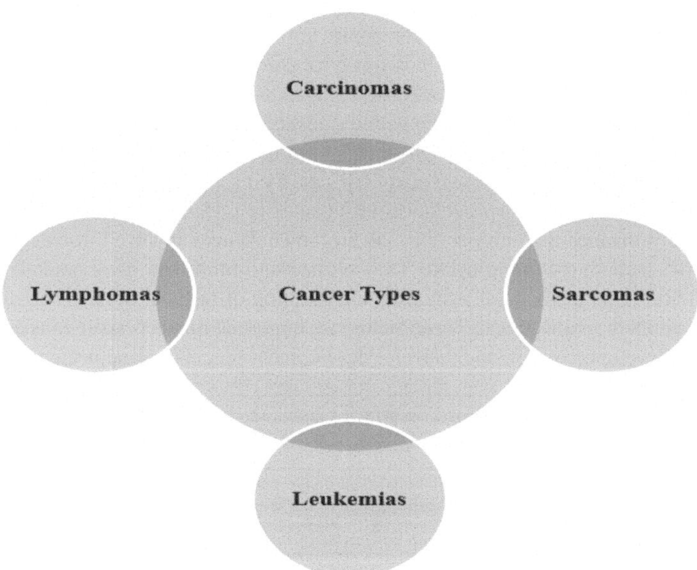

Fig. 1. Four main categories of Cancer

A biosensor may be either a reagent type or a non-reagent type. The typical biosensor shown in Fig. 2 is a non-reagent type indicates that it does not require any chemical to detect the required analyte. Such type of biosensor consists of the receptor as a first part whose purpose is to provide the selectivity of the sensor and the detector as the second part whose purpose is to convert the analyte's physical and chemical change into corresponding electrical signal thus Cancer Types Carcinomas Sarcomas Leukemias

Lymphomas play the role of the transducer. The pH electrode, piezoelectric electrode, or oxygen electrode are some examples of the detector [11]. Similarly, enzymes, antibodies, and lipid layers are some examples of receptors. By reaction, specific adsorption, or any physical or chemical process, the biological molecule of interest is sensed by the biological sensing element, and converted by the transducer (optical, electrooptical, or electrochemical) into a signal which is recognizable and usable [5–10]. For example, when a sample of blood is taken for glucose measurement which can be directly measured by a bi sensor by immersing the tip of the sensor in the sample.

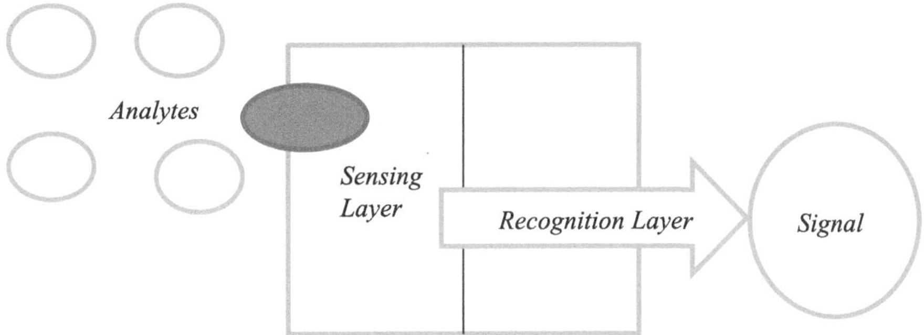

Fig. 2. Non-Reagent Biosensor

2 Optical Biosensors for Cancer Diagnosis

The term optical means light, and the biosensors that use light for detection are called optical biosensors. As such, they are immune to noise, provide good performance with high stability, have less interference and disturbance from other physical/chemical signals. These types of biosensors are widely used in various applications, which may include the drugs for patients, different food control techniques, and monitoring environmental conditions. [12]. The various optical biosensor components are shown in Fig. 3. Working of the biosensors is based on the principle of sensing the analyte with the help of an evanescent field, and they are useful for the measurement of the analyte in a medium up to ~300 nm. The amplitude of the wave with the same wavelength of light decreases with the increase in distance from the interface surface. [14]. The energy of the evanescent wave is dissipated in the form of heat, and the light is refracted because the different media have different velocities for photons [15]. Because of the change in velocity (momentum), the angle of incident light at which the resonance occurs changes as shown in Fig. 4

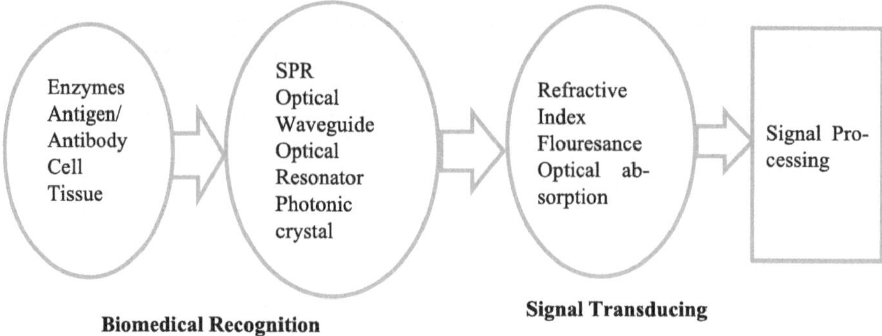

Fig. 3. Optical biosensor components [13]

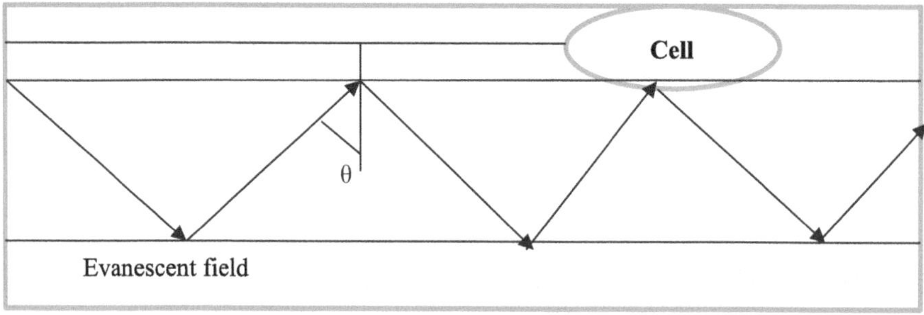

Fig. 4. Evanescent field sensing [13]

2.1 Optical-Waveguide-Based Biosensors

The material used for the construction of optical waveguides is silica/polymer materials having a small thickness and refractive index. Waveguides are of two types, namely slab and stripe [16].

Slab waveguide: Confinement of waves in the direction of thickness is called a slab waveguide.
Stripe waveguide: When the waves are confined in the direction along the waveguide is called a stripe waveguide, which is further classified as shown in Fig. 5.

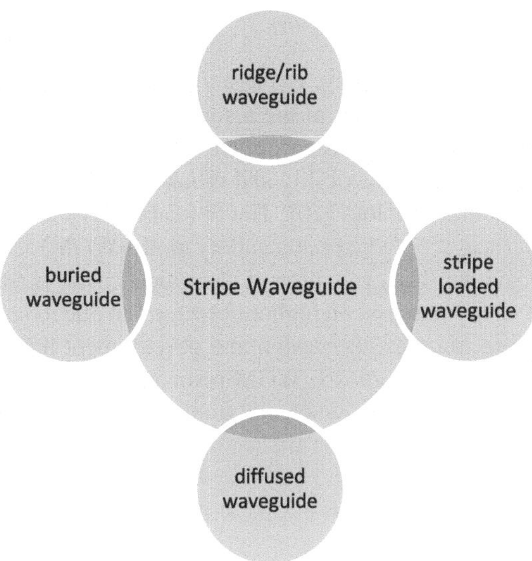

Fig. 5. Stripe Waveguide and its types [16]

The detection mechanism involves a change in the refractive index of the molecules under test with the help of an evanescent field, responsible for the detection of analyte present in bulk or by sensing molecules of interest by the passing of an optical wave into the film-forming waveguide. An evanescent field of high magnitude is produced that depends upon the dimensions of the waveguide and the material. In addition to the material used in processing technology, silicon nitride is highly used so as to bring down the propagation loss as well as to achieve the maximum field confinement in and around the near-infrared region spectrum [17]. Standard micro- and nanofabrication technologies are implemented for these waveguides (Table 1).

Table 1. Design parameters of Optical waveguide-based biosensors

Sr. No	Sensor Name	Refractive index shift	Sn (nm RIU-1)	Methodology	Applications
1	Grating coupled SPR sensors using off the shelf compact discs	1.3–1.36	319.96, 1477.74 and 2077.26	Three gratings with periods of 314 nm, 1470 nm and 6733 nm by stripping commercial optical discs or photolithography	Multiple analytes [18]
2	On-Chip Oval-Shaped Nanocavity GaAs/Si based PCW Biosensor	1.39–1.43	1.5518 (GaAs) 0.51043 (Si)	E. Coli on the surface ISFET with Sio2. E. coli length = 2.192 and diameter = 0.57 μm	Food grains Pathogens [19]

2.2 Optical-Resonator-Based Biosensors

The optical cavity, called a microcavity, acts as a transducer that provides light intensity as output by changing the parameters of the resonance due to the heating effect of the cavity. The oscillation of light due to an optical cavity has many advantages, which include a very high speed, better flexibility and minimal cost, compatibility, and detection of multianalytes with lesser loss [20]. The optical cavity classification consists of Fabry–Perot (FP) microcavities, whispering gallery mode (WGM) resonators, asymmetric cavities, and PC cavities. The evaluation of the optical cavity is done by the Q factor [21]. The Fary Perot cavity possesses a higher Q-factor, but due to some drawbacks like complex stabilization techniques, the design and development have not gained much. For biomedicine and clinical diagnosis, WGM resonators are widely used. The material used for construction is glass, polymer, and semiconductor materials. Microspheres, toroid's, and disks of Cavity geometries are available in different shapes [22] (Table 2).

Table 2. Design parameters of Optical-resonator-based biosensors

Sr. No	Sensor Name	Pressure/Thrombin Range	Sn (nm/ul)	Metals used	Methodology	Applications
1	A High Precision Fiber Optic Fabry–Perot Pressure Sensor Based on AB Epoxy Adhesive Film	0–70 kPa	257.79	Fiber Core diameter = 75 μm and a cladding diameter = 150 μm, HCF core diameter = 150 μm and a cladding diameter = 363 μm	Hollow-core single-mode fiber with a core and cladding along with AB epoxy adhesive, thick HCF	In the field of biological penetration detection and applications related to marine life engineering [23]
2	Fabry-Perot Interferomic Fibre-Optic Sensor	0.5–3.4 μL	7	SMF with core diameter = 8 and cladding diameter = 125	The FP cavity of the SMF tip is generated by placing a blood layer over the optical fiber end face. Bovine Thrombin reagent and $CaCl_2$ are used	Healthcare monitoring to chemical and biological sensing [24]

2.3 Optical-Fiber-Based Biosensors (SPR-Based Biosensors)

The use of optics in fiber helps to have an SPR sensing device that consists of a prism.

at the surface-metal interface that causes TIR (Total Internal Reflection). Therefore, to design a fiber optic biosensor the cladding of the fiber is replaced by a prism mechanism and is coated by a metallic layer as shown in Fig. 6 [25]. The light from the source is sent from one end of the fiber and the light after striking the metal-surface interface generates the evanescent field which further excites the surface plasmons at the fiber core-metal layer interface. The TIR takes place depending upon the numerical aperture of the fiber and the light wavelength, other parameters involve in the reflection are the length of the sensing region, fiber core diameter, and the performance parameters (SNR and sensitivity) [27–32]. At the other end of the fiber, the detection of the spectrum transmitted after passing through the SPR region is done by the photodiode by observing the wavelength corresponding to the dip in the spectrum. This wavelength is called the resonance wavelength [26]. The most commonly used are tapered optical fibers and fiber gratings. They provide low loss due to non-electromagnetic interference and are used for remote sensing with low attenuation.

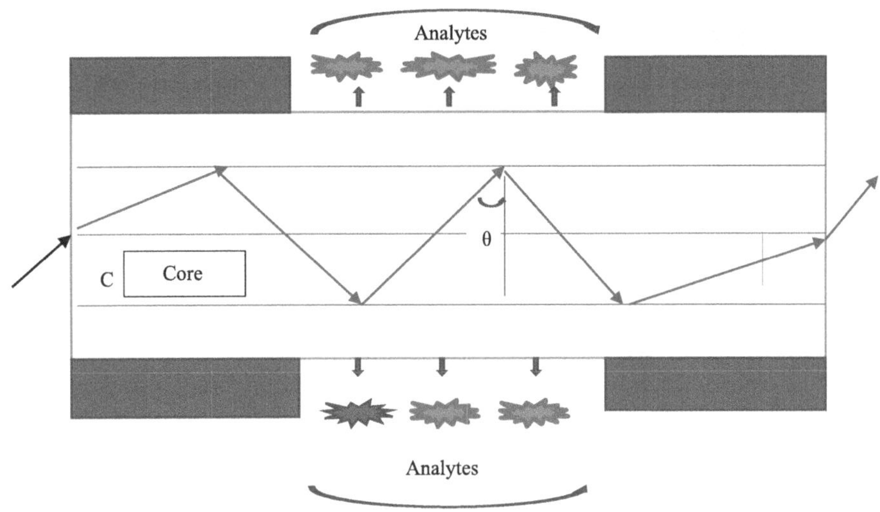

Fig. 6. Optical fiber biosensor [25]

Surface Plasmon resonance (SPR) was introduced in the early 1990s for biomolecular interaction analysis (BIA). [33]. On the other end, depending upon the modulation method used, the photo-detector detects the change in light, the wavelength used, or the angular spectrum. Phase or polarization can be detected in terms of light change. There also exists a change in the spectrum of light caused by a change in the refractive index of the dielectric Δn. [28] (Table 3).

Table 3. Design parameters of SPR-based sensors

Sr. No	Sensor Name	Refractive index shift	Sn (nm RIU-1)	Metals used	DA/LOD	Methodology	Applications
1	Highly Sensitive TiO2/Au/Graphene Layer-Based SPR	1.33–1.41	210–278.57 for various cancerous cells	Au = 50nm, TiO2 = 10nmGraphene = 0.34nm, Analyte = 1.44um	0.263	The proposed TiO2/Au/graphene-based heterostructure biosensor	Detection of cancerous cells from healthy cells [34]
2	TiO2 Coated Optical Fiber-based SPR Sensor	1.33–1.38	5000–14340	Ag = 40nm, Au = 5nm, Tio2 = 40nm	–	A bimetallic structure of silver (Ag) and gold (Au) is used, followed by (TiO2) layer	Biochemical and chemical sensing [35]

2.4 Localized Surface Plasmon (LSP)-Based Biosensors

The term LSPR means oscillation of conduction band electrons when the light gets interacted with noble metal nanoparticles. Localized surface plasmon resonance (LSPR) offers a rugged, simple, sensitive, and label-free detection technique in which the frequency of plasmons sensitivity is used to provide the change in localized refractive index at the surface of the nanoparticle. Metals having real and negative, with small positive imaginary dielectric constant are considered to be helpful in generating surface plasmons in addition to other metals like copper and aluminum. An electromagnetic field when incident upon matches at the surface of the nanoparticle oscillating electrons, a resonance condition gets satisfied. [36].

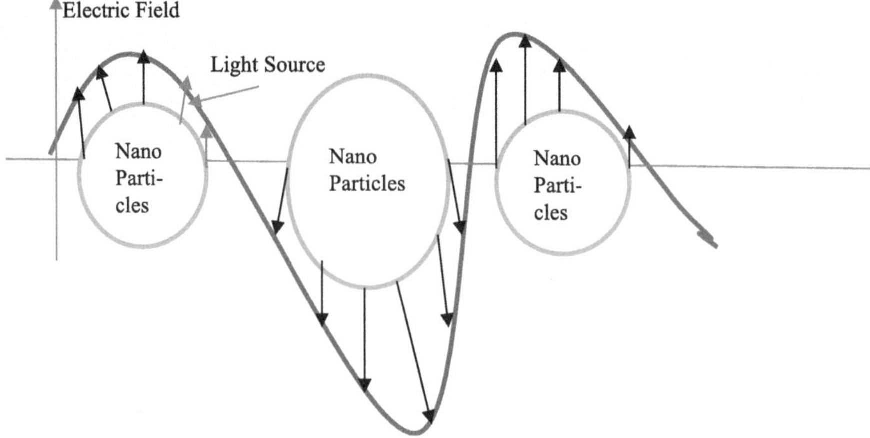

Fig. 7. Localized surface plasmon on a nanoparticle surface [36]

The Localised Surface Plasmon is a non-propagating surface Plasmon remains active in a small region near the particle surface, confined by the particle properties like size, shape, and composition. [36]. There exists a strong enhancement of electric field around the particle surface which Fastly decays with distance. At visible wavelengths, the optical extinction of particles reaches a peak value for noble metal particles at the frequency of plasmon resonance. The atmospheric medium determines the extinction peak and provides the basis of biosensors by the respective refractive index as shown in Figs. 7 and 8 [37]. To detect targets that are hard to look into, various NPs like gold or silver [38–40], magnetic [41, 42], carbon-based [43, 44], latex [45], and liposome [46] are commonly used. Out of these, metal NPs are the best ones in the market. Used. Out of these, metal NPs are the best ones in the market (Table 4).

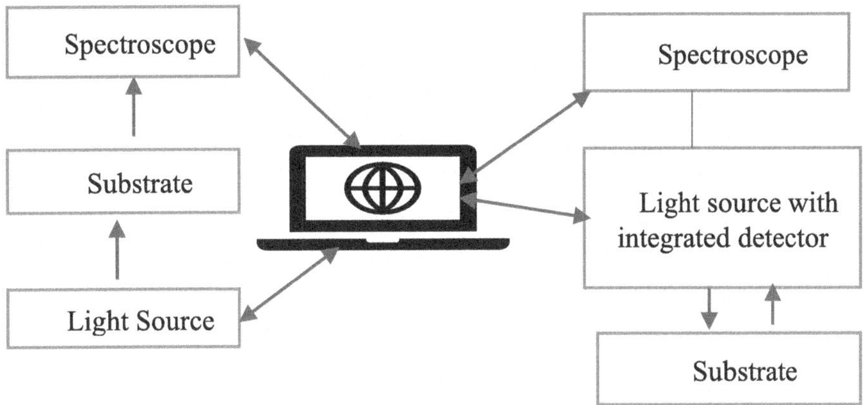

Fig. 8. LSPR transmission (left) and reflection (right) modes [49]

Table 4. Design parameters of LPSR-based biosensors

Sr. No	Sensor Name	Refractive index shift	Sn (nm RIU-1)	Metals used	DA/LOD	Methodology	Applications
1	Localized surface plasmon resonance sensors based on wavelength-tunable spectral dips	1.00, 1.33–1.37, 1.41–1.45	29.3 ± 7.8	TiO2, Ag-NO3, D20		sucrose, phosphate-buffered saline (PBS) and streptavidin type II (Mw ~ 60 000)	Immunosensors, DNA sensors, and HPLC detectors [47]
2	Localized SPR optical fibre biosensor based upon wavelength	1.33 -1.40	914 and 601	GNSs = 60 dia and GNRs aspect ratio = 4.1	1.6	Gold nanospheres and Gold nanorods	Bio-sensing applications [48]

2.5 Photonic Crystal-Based Biosensors

The term PC means Photonic crystal. It was first coined by Philip St. J. Russell in the 1990s [50] and also explained by Yablonovitch and John [51, 52]. The entire length of Photonic crystal fiber (PCF) consists of several microscopic air holes. The PCF has periodic refractive index along the axis of the fiber and is fabricated in silica glass [53]. There are two types of Photonic crystal fibers:

Holey Fiber: It consists of a solid core made up of pure silica through which light travels by the TIR mechanism which is wavelength dependent [54] It is also called Holey index fiber. [55]. It is shown in Fig. 9. Its construction consists of a hole in the center of the fiber with the diameter (D) and pitch defined as 'Λ' which represents the distance between the neighboring holes represented by 'd'.

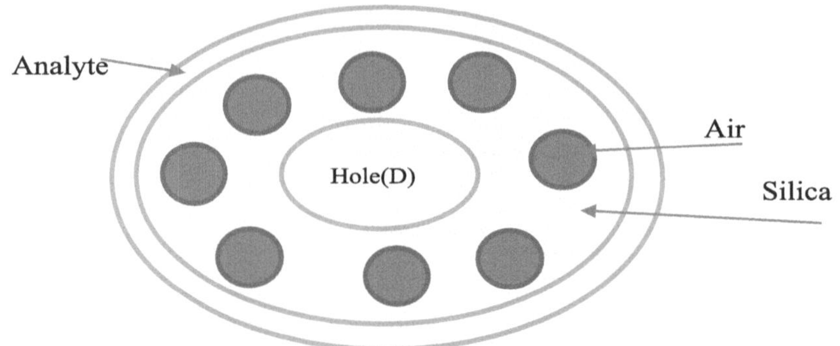

Fig. 9. Photonic crystal Holey fiber [55]

Photonic Band-Gap Fibers: Instead of light traveling in the center core, where the light is allowed to travel through the holes along the fiber core.[49]. The light follows the photonic band gap mechanism. Here the light when transmitted at a particular frequency matches the band gap frequency of the fiber, it passes through the length of the fiber after getting trapped in holes along the length of the fiber and thus the need for the greater refractive index is eliminated. It is shown in Fig. 10. It can be used for a wide range of wavelengths ranging from 300nm to 2000 nm. [55] (Table 5).

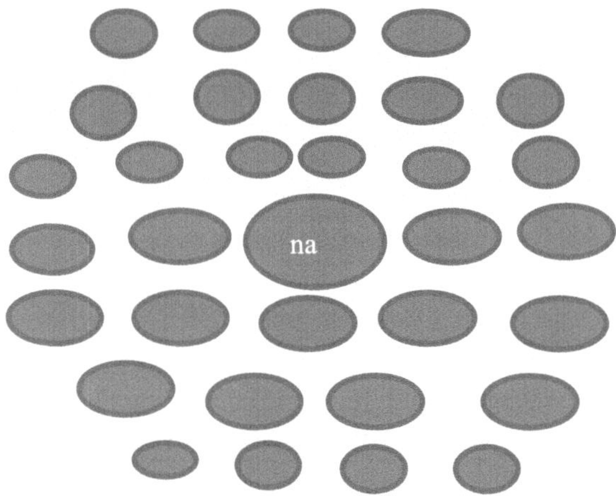

Fig. 10. Photonic Bandgap sensor [55]

Table 5. Design parameters of Photonic Crystal Fiber Sensors

Sr. No	Sensor Name	Refractive index shift	**Sn (nm RIU-1)**	Metals used	Methodology	Application
1	Graphene-Based Birefringent PCF Sensor Using SPR	1.330-1.370	860	Ag-30nm-50nm, $\Lambda = 2$um d1 = 0.4Λ, d2 = 0.2Λ	Circular PCF with air holes of different diameter as d1, d2 and pitch in different layers	Cancer detection [56]
2	High Sensitivity Photonic Crystal Fiber Refractive Index Sensor	n = 1.39 to 1.395	11000	r0 = 0.2 μm, r1 = 0.4 μm, r2 = 0.6 μm, Λ = 1.2 μm, d = 2 μm, and tg = 35 nm	Gold Coated Externally Based on SPR with	Practical biological and chemical sensing [57]

3 Challenges and Future Scope

Several parameters related to the optical structure needs to be taken in to account in regard to the classification of these main optical structures like full width at half maximum/minimum (FWHM), Q-factor, sensitivity, figure of merit (FOM) and limit of detection (LOD). In case of FOM, there exists less differences as the dependence of FOM both on the FWHM (Q-factor) and on the sensitivity. In case of different works to be compared, FOM and a low LOD relationship is difficult to establish due to different experimental conditions. However, in those cases, where the same conditions exist it is proved that by improving the FOM can achieve a better LOD. Moreover, a FOM thus can become a reasonable parameter for recognizing the performance of an optical structure as a biosensor. With more research, it will be possible to find a new exact parameter to achieve this purpose. FOM can be good indicator that can be used to compare the performance of the optical platforms in future research work. In view of the above-mentioned sensors, the main objective is to obtain the parameters like sensitivity in relation to refractive index (SRI) and the spectral bandwidth, the metals and methods used. Further, to evaluate the performance of an optical fiber biosensor, their relationship with the limit of detection (LOD) and FOM needs to be analyzed.

4 Conclusion

This work presented a review of the scientific contributions on wavelength-based optical fiber biosensors. The most prominent technologies addressing this topic are: grating-based optical fibers (tilted-FBGs and LPFGs), interferometers. This survey paper summarizes the various optical biosensors for early detection of cancer as well as the role of biosensors as a diagnostic tool, with design parameters of biosensor technology along with detection of different types of cancer cells and also for urine glucose concentration to obtain excellent sensitivity and quality factor. Different biomarkers of cancer cells present in blood can be easily detected by observing the resonance wavelength in transmission spectrum of proposed bio-sensing platform.

The mortality rate of cancers at the initial stage can be prevented by identifying the risk factors in a time-bound manner using optical biosensors. The onus lies upon keeping the standards of specific biomarkers which further suggests that there is a greater need for the exploration of biosensors in cancer detection. A biosensor is fast, accurate, and reliable in the detection of cancer cells and simultaneously keeps on checking the angiogenesis, cancer metastasis, and the effectiveness of anticancer chemotherapy agents. Yet there is a great need for further research to resolve the challenges with the application of the biosensor in cancer detection with respect to the parameters like Sensitivity, FOM and LOD. However, the difficulty in standardization of specific biomarkers demonstrates that further lines of study relating the application of biosensors in the diagnosis of cancer are still needed. No doubt, the biosensor technology has become a boon in the diagnosis, and treatment by overcoming the suffering and mortality rate of cancer patients thereby increasing the survival rate or lifespan of the cancer patient.

References

1. Tothill, I.E.: Biosensors for cancer markers diagnosis. In: Seminars in Cell & Developmental Biology, vol. 20, no. 1, pp. 55–62. Academic Press (2009)
2. Hu, Y.: BRCA1, hormone, and tissue-specific tumor suppression. Int. J. Biol. Sci. **5**(1), 20 (2008)
3. Cheng, K.Y., Chou, J.T., Tai, H.M., Huang, H.C.: The study of the fiber-optic interferometer for the calibration of PZT travel distance. In: Interferometry XII: Techniques and Analysis, vol. 5531, pp. 350–358, SPIE (2004)
4. Fabregat, I.: Dysregulation of apoptosis in hepatocellular carcinoma cells. World J. Gastroenterol.: WJG **15**(5), 513 (2009)
5. Dewa, A.S., Ko, W.H.: Biosensors, semiconductor sensors. In: Sze, S.M. (ed.) Interferometry XII: Techniques and Analysis, vol. 5531, pp. 350–358. SPIE (2004)
6. Socorro-Leránoz, A.B., Santano, D., Del Villar, I. and Matias, I.R.: Trends in the design of wavelength-based optical fiber biosensors. Biosens. Bioelectr. X, 1, p.100015, (2008–2018)
7. Diamond, D.: Principles of chemical and biological sensors., *(1998)*
8. Lowe, C.R.: An introduction to the concepts and technology of biosensors. Biosensors **1**(1), 3–16 (1985)
9. Rogers, K.R.: Biosensors for environmental applications. Biosens. Bioelectron. **10**(6–7), 533–541 (1995)
10. Turner, A.P.F.: Current trends in biosensor research and development. Sens. Actuators **17**(3–4), 433–450 (1989)
11. Guilbault, G.G., Lubrano, G.J.: An enzyme electrode for the amperometric determination of glucose. Anal. Chim. Acta **64**(3), 39–455 (1973)
12. Zanchetta, G., Lanfranco, R., Giavazzi, F., Bellini, T., Buscaglia, M..: Emerging applications of label-free optical biosensors. Nanophotonics **6**(4), 627–645 (2017)
13. Estevez, M.C., Alvarez, M., Lechuga, L.M.: Integrated optical devices for lab-on-a-chip biosensing applications. Laser Photonics Rev. **6**(4), 463–487 (2012)

14. Blaesing, F., Weigel, C., Welzeck, M., Messer, W.: Analysis of the DNA-binding domain of Escherichia coli DnaA protein. Mol. Microbiol. **36**(3), 557–569 (2012)
15. Aube, A., Breault-Turcot, J., Chaurand, P., Pelletier, J.N., Masson, J.F.: Non-specific adsorption of crude cell lysate on surface plasmon resonance sensors. Langmuir **29**(32), 10141–10148 (2013)
16. Kozma, P., Kehl, F., Ehrentreich-Förster, E., Stamm, C., Bier, F.F.: Integrated planar optical waveguide interferometer biosensors, a comparative review. Biosens. Bioelectr. **58**, 287–307 (2014)
17. Cai, Y., Chen, X., Si, J., Mou, X., Dong, X.: All-in-one nanomedicine: multifunctional single-component nanoparticles for cancer theranostics. Small **17**(52), 2103072 (2021)
18. Long, S., et al.: Grating coupled SPR sensors using off the shelf compact discs and sensitivity dependence on grating period. Sens. Actuators Rep. **2**(1), 100016 (2020)
19. Painam, B., Kaler, R.S., Kumar, M.: On-chip oval-shaped nanocavity photonic crystal waveguide biosensor for detection of foodborne pathogens. Plasmonic **13**(2), 445–449 (2018)
20. Righini, G.C., Soria, S.: Biosensing by WGM micro spherical resonators. Sensors **16**(6), 905 (2016)
21. Vahala, K.J.: Optical microcavities. Nature **424**(6950), 839–846 (2003)
22. Matthew, R., Jon, D.S., Frank, V.: Whispering gallery mode sensors. Adv. Opt. Photonics **7**(2), 168–240 (2015)
23. Zhang, Y., et al.: A high precision fiber optic Fabry–Perot pressure sensor based on AB epoxy adhesive film. In: Photonics, vol. 8, no. 12, p. 581. MDPI (2021)
24. Wu, Y., et al.: A transverse load sensor with ultra-sensitivity employing Vernier-effect improved parallel-structured fiber-optic Fabry-Perot interferometer. IEEE Access **7**, 120297–120303 (2019)
25. Lee, B.: Review of the present status of optical fiber sensors. Opt. Fib. Technol. **9**(2), 57–79 (2003)
26. Shukla, S.K., Kushwaha, C.S., Guner, T., Demir, M.M.: Chemically modified optical fibers in advanced technology, an overview. Opt. Laser Technol. **115**, 404–432 (2019)
27. Joe, H.E., Yun, H., Jo, S.H., Jun, M.B., Min, B.K.: A review on optical fiber sensors for environmental monitoring. Int. J. Precis. Eng. Manuf.-Green Technol. **5**(1), 173–191 (2018)
28. Zhao, Y., et al.: Nucleic acids analysis. Sci. China Chem. **64**(2), 171–203 (2021)
29. Maity, S., Bhattacharyya, A., Singh, P.K., Kumar, M., Sarkar, R.: Last decade in vehicle detection and classification, a comprehensive survey. Arch. Comput. Methods Eng., 1–38 (2022)
30. Hong, S., et al.: Thermo-optic characteristic of DNA thin solid film and its application as a biocompatible optical fiber temperature sensor. Opt. Lett. **42**(10), 1943–1945 (2017)
31. Huang, J., Pham, D.T., Ji, C., Wang, Z., Zhou, Z.: Multi-parameter dynamical measuring system using fiber Bragg grating sensors for industrial hydraulic piping. Measurement **134**, 226–235 (2019)
32. Teng, C., et al.: Refractive index sensor based on twisted tapered plastic optical fibers. In: Photonics, vol. 6, no. 2, p. 40. MDPI (2019)
33. Bo, L., Nylander, C., Lunström, I.: Surface plasmon resonance for gas detection and biosensing. Sens. Actuators **4**, 299–304 (1983)
34. Mostufa, S., Akib, T.B.A., Rana, M.M., Islam, M.R.: Highly sensitive TiO2/Au/graphene layer-based surface plasmon resonance biosensor for cancer detection. Biosensors **12**(8), 603 (2022)
35. Singh, Y., Raghuwanshi, S.K.: Titanium dioxide (TiO2) coated optical fiber-based SPR sensor in near-infrared region with bimetallic structure for enhanced sensitivity. Optik **226**, 165842 (2021)

36. Rhemrev-Boom, M.M., Jonker, M.A., Venema, K., Jobst, G., Tiessen, R., Korf, J.: On-line continuous monitoring of glucose or lactate by ultraslow microdialysis combined with a flow-through nanoliter biosensor based on poly (m-phenylenediamine) ultra-thin polymer membrane as enzyme electrode. Analyst **126**(7), 1073–1079 (2001)
37. Paredes, P.A., Parellada, J., Fernández, V.M., Katakis, I., Domínguez, E.: Amperometric mediated carbon paste biosensor based on D-fructose dehydrogenase for the determination of fructose in food analysis. Biosens. Bioelectr. **12**(12), 1233–1243 (1997)
38. Sacchi, S., Pollegioni, L., Pilone, M.S., Rossetti, C.: Determination of D-amino acids using a D-amino acid oxidase biosensor with spectrophotometric and potentiometric detection. Biotechnol. Tech. **12**(2), 149–153 (1998)
39. Pundir, C.S.: Determination of serum lactate with alkylamine glass bound lactate oxidase (2005)
40. Andreou, V.G., Clonis, Y.D.: Novel fiber-optic biosensor based on immobilized glutathione S-transferase and sol-gel entrapped bromcresol green for the determination of atrazine. Analytica Chimica Acta **460**(2), 151–161 (2002)
41. Sercan, D.E.D.E., Altay, F.: Biosensors from the first generation to nano-bio sensors. Int. Adv. Res. Eng. J. **2**(2), 200–207 (2018)
42. Khadilkar, P., Kelkar, V., Khan, A.: An optical biosensor employing phenylalanine ammonia lyase-immobilized films for phenylketonuria detection (2013)
43. Horibe, T., Kikuchi, M., Kawakami, K.: Interaction of human protein disulfide isomerase and human P5 with drug compounds. Anal. Using Biosens. Technol. Process Biochem. **43**(12), 1330–1337 (2008)
44. Moreira, F.T., Dutra, R.A., Noronha, J.P., Sales, M.G.F.: Novel sensory surface for creatine kinase electrochemical detection. Biosens. Bioelectr. **56**, 217–222 (2014)
45. Müllner, M., et al.: Creatine kinase-MB fraction and cardiac troponin T to diagnose acute myocardial infarction after cardiopulmonary resuscitation. J. Am. Coll. Cardiol. **28**(5), 1220–1225 (1996)
46. Liu, S., Pang, S., Na, W., Su, X.: Near-infrared fluorescence probe for the determination of alkaline phosphatase. Biosens. Bioelectr. **55**, 249–254 (2014)
47. Kazuma, E., Tatsuma, T.: Localized surface plasmon resonance sensors based on wavelength-tunable spectral dips. Nanoscale **6**(4), 2397–2405 (2014)
48. Cao, J., Tu, M.H., Sun, T., Grattan, K.T.: Wavelength based localized surface plasmon resonance optical fiber biosensor. Sens. Actuators B: Chem. **181**, 611–619 (2013)
49. Hammond, J.L., Bhalla, N., Rafiee, S.D., Estrela, P.: Localized surface plasmon resonance as a biosensing platform for developing countries. Biosensors **4**(2), 172–188 (2014)
50. Wang, Y., Meng, S., Liang, Y., Li, L., Peng, W.: Fiber-optic surface plasmon resonance sensor with multi-alternating metal layers for biological measurement. Photonic Sens. **3**(3), 202–207 (2013)
51. Gribi, S., du Bois de Dunilac, S., Ghezzi, D., Lacour, S.P.: A microfabricated nerve-on-a-chip platform for rapid assessment of neural conduction in explanted peripheral nerve fibers. Nat. Commun. **9**(1), 1–10 (2018)
52. Zhang, J.L., Wang, Y.H., Huang, K., Huang, K.J., Jiang, H., Wang, X.M.: Enzyme-based biofuel cells for biosensors and in vivo power supply. Nano Energy **84**, 105853 (2021)
53. Raut, N., O'Connor, G., Pasini, P., Daunert, S.: Engineered cells as biosensing systems in biomedical analysis. Anal. Bioanal. Chem. **402**(10), 3147–3159 (2012)
54. Bosch, M.E., Sánchez, A.J.R., Rojas, F.S., Ojeda, C.B.: Recent development in optical fiber biosensors. Sensors **7**(6), 797–859 (2007)
55. Lee, B.: Review of the present status of optical fiber sensors. Opt. Fiber Technol. **9**(2), 57–79 (2003)
56. Dash, J.N., Jha, R.: Graphene-based birefringent photonic crystal fiber sensor using surface plasmon resonance. IEEE Photonics Technol. Lett. **26**(11), 1092–1095 (2014)

57. Yasli, A., Ademgil, H., Haxha, S., Aggoun, A.: Multichannel photonic crystal fiber-based surface plasmon resonance sensor for multi-analyte sensing. IEEE Photonics J. **12**(1), 1–15 (2019)

Revolutionizing Healthcare 5.0 with Digital Twins

Sarthak Acharya[1(✉)] and Daljeet Singh[2,3]

[1] M3S Research Unit, Faculty of Information Technology and Electrical Engineering, University of Oulu, Oulu, Finland
sarthak.acharya@oulu.fi

[2] Research Unit of Health Sciences and Technology, Faculty of Medicine, University of Oulu, Oulu, Finland
daljeet.singh@oulu.fi

[3] Infotech Oulu, Univesity of Oulu, Oulu, Finland

Abstract. The proliferation of digitization, Internet of Medical Things (IoMT) technology, and consumer electronics has significantly increased the quantum of medical data, giving rise to the inclusion of Digital Twins (DTs) in the healthcare and medical fraternity. DTs enhance the operational efficiency of consumer electronics used in healthcare and aid in optimizing medical data processing, storage, and sharing. New opportunities and applications in healthcare can be unlocked by harnessing the full potential of DTs leading to ameliorated productivity, cost saving, and overall development of society. Most of the available DT architectures and frameworks are derived from other manufacturing industries which are not suitable for healthcare. Several key challenges associated with DTs are overlooked in such architectures which struggle to deal with challenges pertaining to privacy, security, standardization and interoperability. This paper presents a comprehensive overview of DT technology (DTT) for healthcare applications acknowledging key research findings from the literature. The challenges associated with implementing DTT and their possible solutions are highlighted. Several use cases of DT in healthcare are elaborated and dowelled upon. Additionally, the future aspects of DT in the healthcare sector in conjunction with consumer electronics are presented.

Keywords: Digital twin · Artificial intelligence · Healthcare · Edge computing · Internet of Medical Things · Cyber-Physical Systems

1 Introduction

Evolution of healthcare services and facilities from Healthcare 1.0 to Healthcare 5.0 represents a profound transformation. Initially characterized by manual processes, this progression has included the advent of electronic health records (EHRs), the integration of advanced imaging and telemedicine, and the emergence of interconnected health systems driven by innovative consumer electronics technologies. Today, the focus has shifted towards personalized, predictive,

K. Atul et al. (Eds.): BodyNets 2024, LNICST 666, pp. 282–292, 2026.
https://doi.org/10.1007/978-3-032-16099-7_22

and preventive care, enabled by contemporary technological paradigms. The recent incorporation of key technologies like artificial intelligence (AI), Machine Learning (ML), Internet of Things (IoT), metaverse, and Cyber-Physical Systems (CPS) has transformed every sector. Furthermore, Digital Twin technology (DTT) facilitated by enhanced data analytics and global connectivity is at the vanguard of this transformation which is not only limited to the production industry but has also sprung into consumer healthcare [9]. The use of twins is not new in the healthcare sector wherein various types of twin models are utilized such as animal trials, phantom models, computer simulation environments, etc. [20,22]. These twin models accelerate the development of medical device design, biomarker, and drug discovery models, surgical planning, methods for personalized medicine, and the development of wellness applications. However, these conventional twin models are prone to ethical issues and have circumscribed accuracy in mimicking the behavior and properties of actual biological tissue. Additionally, these twin models are generally static systems unable to replicate the complex dynamics associated with the human brain. On the other hand, the use of DTT in healthcare is demonstrated to cater to these challenges by offering seamless two-way connectivity between the consumer electronics (physical system) and its digital counterpart [19,21,24].

Motivated by the success of Digital Twin (DT) in other industries and the challenges associated with conventional twins in healthcare, this paper presents a comprehensive overview of DT technology for healthcare applications with a special focus on consumer electronics. It is observed that most of the available DT architectures and frameworks are derived from other manufacturing/production industries which are not suitable for healthcare [2]. Therefore, a standard DT architecture specially designed for healthcare is proposed in this work. Further, the challenges associated with the implementation of DT technology in current consumer electronics utilized in healthcare are highlighted. Some of these challenges include but are not limited to security and privacy of personal data in cloud computing, computing capability v/s power consumption tradeoff at edge devices, interoperability of data among different layers of DT architecture, anonymizing the healthcare data, and assurance of data availability at extremely low latency and very high speeds. Thereafter, several use cases of DT in healthcare are elaborated and dowelled upon. Finally, the future aspects related to DT in the healthcare sector in conjunction with consumer electronics are presented.

2 State-oF-tHE-Art DT-Healthcare Services

In 2002, at the University of Michigan, the concept of DT was introduced in a presentation, entitled "Conceptual Ideal for Product Lifecycle Management (PLM)" [10]. Since then, DTs have been utilized effectively in conjunction with consumer electronics in every sector. One of the core research areas in the field of DT for healthcare is the model creation which merges the human anatomy, its physiology, biological aspects, and other related fronts to the digital technology [1]. This process is usually accomplished through extensive data collection trials, image processing, and mathematical modeling along with other technologies

Table 1. Comprehensive list of some Digital Twin projects in Healthcare Facilities and Services in last 6 years.

Project Name (Country, Duration)	Organization (Funding)	Focus Area	Future Scopes	Technologies Utilized
Virtual Physiological Human (VPH) (EU)(2018–2022)	VPH Institute (EU)	Multiscale modeling of human physiology	Expansion to personalized medicine and predictive analytics	IoT, Big Data
INTEGRATE (US) (2018–2023)	INTEGRATE Consortium (NIH, Private Sector)	Integration of clinical data	Integration with AI for enhanced clinical decision-making	Cloud Computing
Virtual Liver Network (Germany) (2018–2023)	Virtual Liver Network Consortium (BMBF)	Liver disease modeling	Application to other organ systems and diseases	ML
My Digital Twin (Netherlands) (2019–24)	Philips Healthcare (Private Sector)	Personalized healthcare	Expansion to global markets, integration with consumer health apps	AI, Wearable Tech
Digital Twin for Cardiovascular Health (Global) (2019–24)	Siemens Healthineers (Public-Private)	Cardiovascular health monitoring	Real-time monitoring and predictive maintenance for personalized care	Cloud Computing
Project OSPEN (UK) (2019–24)	NHS Digital (Public Sector)	Electronic health records integration	Nationwide implementation of EHR systems	Blockchain
Living Heart Project (France) (2020–25)	Dassault Systèmes (EU, Private)	Heart disease simulation	Simulation of other organ systems and integration with patient-specific data	3D Simulation, VR
Digital Twin for Oncology (US) (2020–25)	GE Healthcare (NIH, Private)	Cancer treatment optimization	Expansion to other types of cancer and integration with genetic data	Genomics, AI
Virtual Cancer Patient (Canada) (2021–26)	Virtual Cancer Patient Consortium (CIHR)	Cancer patient modeling	Personalized treatment plans and integration with wearable tech	AI, Wearable Tech
DT4Health (Australia) (2021–26)	DT4Health Consortium (Public-Private)	General healthcare improvement	National rollout and integration with telehealth services	Telehealth, AI
SMARTsurg (EU) (2022–27)	European Commission	Surgical training and planning	Incorporation of AR/VR technologies for immersive training	AR/VR, Robotics
SIMCor (EU) (2022–27)	SIMCor Consortium (Horizon 2020)	Cardiovascular implant simulations	Simulation of other implants and devices	3D Simulation, IoT
CuraDigit (Italy) (2023–28)	CuraDigit Consortium	Digital healthcare solutions	Expansion to other EU countries and integration with AI	AI, IoT
AI4HealthSec (EU) (2023–28)	AI4HealthSec Consortium (Horizon 2020)	AI in healthcare security	Broader applications in cybersecurity across various healthcare sectors	AI, Cybersecurity
Cancer Twin for Precision Medicine (Israel) (2021–26)	Technion(ISF, Private Sector)	Cancer Treatment	Integration with National Healthcare Systems	AI, Genomics
OPTOMICS (EU)(2021–26)	Horizon 2020 (FET)	Diabetes Treatment	New Phenotyping Measurements for Type-2 Diabetes	AI, Genomics
DIGIPREDICT (EU) (2021–26)	Horizon 2020 (FET)	Prediction on Progression of Diseases	Early detection of Infectious & Cardiovascular diseases	Edge AI, ML
NeuroTwin Project (EU) (2021–26)	Horizon 2020 (FET)	Non-invasive Brain Simulations	Innovative therapy in Clinical Neuroscience	AI, Biophysics

involving mechanics, mechanical, and statistical modeling of the biological tissue/organ. These models often need regular recalibration to suit patients from different genders, ages, ethnicity, or medical conditions. This necessitates the requirement of perfect interoperability among the digital twins and their physical counterparts. One of the initial DT models for neocortical column is developed by Ecole Polytechnique Fédérale de Lausanne and International Business Machines in the Blue Brain Project [14]. In terms of diagnosis and treatment of chronic diseases, Philips has developed a DT model named HeartNavigator tool which is based on computed tomography (CT) images [18]. Another such model is the HeartFlow Analysis technology developed for diagnosis of coronary artery disease [12]. The HEARTguide module developed by FEops Institute is also an excellent example of DT technology in healthcare. DTs are also utilized in surgical procedures to create a virtual patient model for surgery planning and damage assessment. The Intelligent Maps developed by Cydar is a DT with the capability of surgical visualization [15].

In project named BreathEasy [17], a consortium of multiple entities developed patient-specific DT models of lungs of COVID-19 patients using medical images and simulations. The primary aim of this project is to forecast air circulation requirements for patients. A DT heart model was developed in the Living Heart Project by Dassault Systems [6] to simulate the physiological and structural functionalities of human heart. The designed heart model can be used for heath monitoring and therapy planning for patients. In another project, Mater Private Hospital (Dublin) and Siemens Healthineers partnered to develop Mater Private's digital twin for radiologic image processing and evaluation [11]. The development of this DT model resulted in a significant reduction in wait time for patients and improved system utilization. In [16], a DT model for Transcatheter Aortic Valve Replacement (TAVR) was developed by Obaid et al. using the HeartNavigator III software. This model was utilized to simulate virtual TAVR implementations for surgery planning.

Badano et al. [5] developed Virtual Imaging Clinical Trial for Regulatory Evaluation (VICTRE) for breast tomosynthesis. The results obtained from VICTRE were verified using clinical trials and were found consistent. Researchers from Cleveland Clinic and MetroHealth developed a DT model to reduce health disparities among citizens based on their location [7]. The project is funded by the National Institutes of Health with a grant of $3.14 million. In recent years, the deployment of DTs for healthcare sectors has gained momentum with several international projects. A non-exhaustive list of such projects is shown in Table 1. This table shows the involvement of diverse technologies related to consumer electronics with specific focuses on numerous applications. Several use cases of DT in healthcare and its practical applications are visualized in [4,13]. Coorey et al. presented a brief discussion on the use of DT technology for cardiovascular disease in [8]. Sun et al. discussed the advantages and limitations of DT technology in the medical field [23].

3 Conceptual DTT-Healthcare Framework

A conceptual framework targeting diverse healthcare services using DTs is illustrated in Fig. 1. This framework for the healthcare system comprises three integral layers. The innermost "Twinning Layer" digitally replicates four key healthcare components, i.e., infrastructure, personnel, pharmacy, and medical research facilities. Encircling this is the "Assisted Technology Layer," which harnesses advanced computational methods and technologies, including AI, ML, blockchain, federated learning, 5G/6G communication, IoT, IIoT, AR/VR, and CPS, for data processing and decision-making. All these technologies are backed by consumer electronics which plays a vital role in their implementation. The outermost layer illustrates various healthcare applications enabled by these DTTs. This framework underscores the synergy between digital twins, consumer electronics, and emerging technologies to optimize healthcare solutions.

The development of health monitoring systems and other medical applications using consumer electronics undergo a lot of experimentation before they

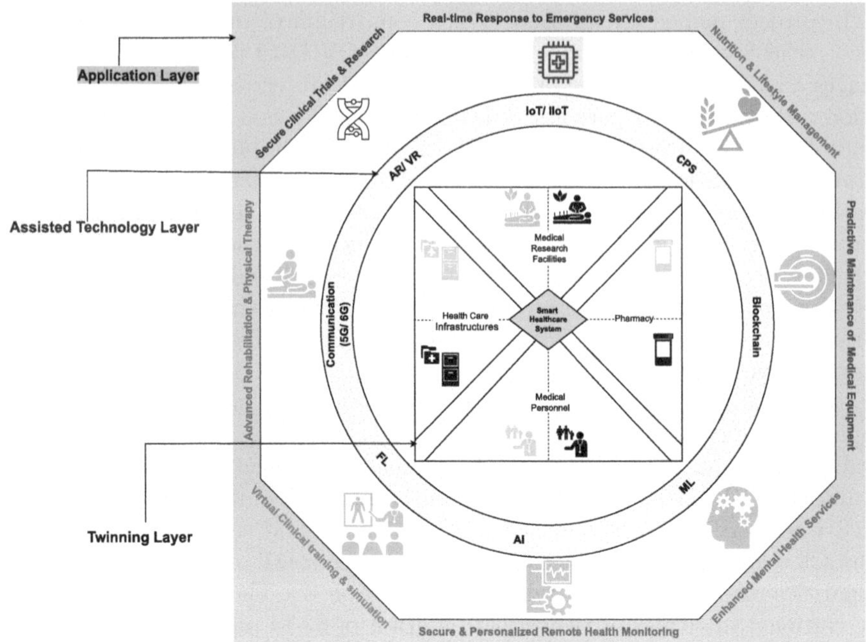

Fig. 1. The Conceptual Framework for DT-enabled Healthcare System.

can meet the requirements for clinical applications. DTs offer an excellent platform for these investigations. Potential applications of DTs in healthcare include surgery: surgery planning and damage assessment, patient recovery assessment, and digital platform for remote surgery using gesture assistance; medical education: DT-oriented hyper-realistic simulations, extended reality (XR), and Virtual Reality (VR) based training on DT patient models, digital drug discovery models, and DT-based phantom trials; medical therapeutics: virtual physiotherapy, haptic feedback in remote therapy, virtual counseling by DT models and wireless Brain Computer Interface (BCI); patient monitoring: automatic alert, feedback and actuation, early investigation and prevention using DT, virtual remote diagnosis and autonomous assessment using real-time vital monitoring. Therefore, DT along with its associates has gigantic potential in transforming the healthcare sector.

Every development comes along with its challenges. DT technology (DTT) also faces severe challenges regarding medical and personal data security, privacy, interoperability, and standardization. Health and biomedical data collected from patients during and after medical procedures is vital in foreseeing the patient's response to the procedure and recovery. Additionally, this data has enormous potential for secondary use but requires effect anonymization. The majority of this data is stored, shared, and analyzed digitally in the form of electronic health records (EHR) and genomics data on consumer electronics devices. The inclu-

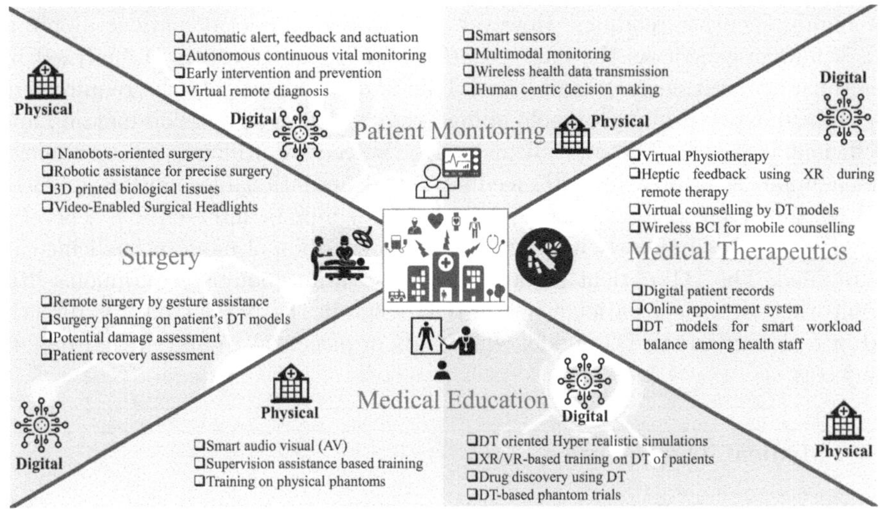

Fig. 2. Use cases of DT in healthcare: A comparison of physical and digital worlds.

sion of DT in this process increases the system complexity but allows for the safe sharing and storage of medical data for secondary use. Personalized DTs of patients offer an additional layer of privacy which ensures that the data is accessed only by its intended user. Further, another major challenge for DT is interoperability between different consumer electronic devices using separate communication protocols and working on independent standards. Therefore, a generalized framework for DTs in healthcare is the need of the hour. Finally, lack of standardization also poses a major problem in the use of DT for healthcare systems.

4 DT-Enabled Healthcare System: Use-Cases

As the DT ties information to the individual asset in the plant, it is a chief enabler of Industry 4.0's benefits. Enabling novel use cases, which are not probable with static, non-individualistic documentation together with data, is possible with context-specific information available at the right time in the right place [1]. Since the physical assetsy' digital representations are the base for decision-making, they are key components in industrial applications. This section presents several key use cases of DT in healthcare and compares the physical and digital worlds. An overview of these use cases is presented in Fig. 2.

4.1 Patient Monitoring

With the advancements in medical devices and sensor technology utilized in consumer electronics, smart sensors have evolved as an excellent solution for prolonged monitoring of patients in hospitals and generic health monitoring applications in casual settings. These smart sensors utilize multimodal measurements for highly accurate readings. However, this system model of patient monitoring is human-centric as the data generated from smart sensors is analyzed by healthcare practitioners or end users. This is accompanied by the requirement for clinical expertise, unavoidable human errors, delays in decision-making, and inefficient feedback. These problems can be solved by utilizing DT technology which imbibes automatic alert, feedback, and actuation mechanisms in medical consumer electronics devices with minimal human intervention. Thereby, the long-term goal of early intervention and prevention of modern medicine can be fulfilled. The DT patient models also assist in autonomous continuous vital monitoring of critical patients in the ICU wherein the patient data is directly fed in real-time to the DT model which aids in patient care and virtual remote diagnosis.

4.2 Medical Therapeutics

Digitization has empowered medical therapeutics using digital patient records and online appointment systems. DT technology can be utilized for smart workload balance among healthcare staff and infrastructure by predicting and channeling the resources effectively. DT patient models driven by Extended Reality (XR) can forge a virtual therapy environment wherein haptic feedback of touch, smell, and taste are incorporated into traditional voice and video communication. This results in the creation of a very realistic therapeutic environment for remote therapies and the patient feels more connected to the health staff thereby boosting the confidence of the patient in the physician. Utilization of a Wireless Brain-Computer Interface (BCI) along with DT models will further enhance the user experience for medical consumer electronics.

4.3 Medical Education

The success of the healthcare sector depends massively on the training of medical staff which currently relies on supervision assistance-based models wherein the new medical staff learns mainly by assisting experienced doctors. DT-oriented XR systems can be utilized to elevate medical education to new heights by embedding state-of-the-art consumer electronics. DT technology also aids in hyper-realistic simulations of patient models for drug discovery. Another interesting area that can benefit from DT technology is phantom creation and trials. The synergy between biological tissue-DT model-phantom trio can truly elevate the medical education experience.

4.4 Surgery

Similar to other use cases, surgical procedures can be ameliorated using DT technology, especially for remote surgery. 5G Advance and 6G have opened the gates for remote surgery by offering Ultra-Reliable and Low Latency Communications (URLLC) between medical electronics equipment and doctors at remote locations. The use of nanobots, video-enabled surgical headlights, and advanced robotic assistance in consumer electronics has empowered robotic surgery. Doctors have initiated the use of DT patient models for surgery planning and damage assessment. This also aids in the patient-specific 3D bio-printing of cells, tissues, and organs. Further, DT models also support comprehensive postoperative follow-up for patient recovery assessments.

5 Challenges and Future Directions

DT technology holds the capability to transform the healthcare sector into a truly state-of-the-art institution but it is still in its evolving phase of research and has some challenges and limitations. Unlike other applications involving consumer electronics and DTT, healthcare is hypersensitive to the concerns that arise with the inclusion of DT between doctor and patient.

5.1 Privacy and Security

The usage of personal medical data of patients must adhere to stringent regulations such as the General Data Protection Regulation (GDPR). The big question of "Who will use the data and How?" induces hesitation among patients. The involvement of multiple data processing layers: edge, fog, and cloud computing further complicates tracing data flow. This requires a very strong autonomous system to make user data anonymous. The system should be transparent to patients sharing their data which will boost their confidence in the system. The seamless and secure interoperability of data among different layers of DT healthcare architecture in a cloud computing framework of medical electronics is an open area of research.

5.2 Interoperability

Diverse technologies with heterogeneous data sources often restrict the seamless integration of the physical and digital worlds. Legacy systems, lack of standardization, ontology misalignment, inconsistent data, and compatibility issues are the main interoperability silos in the current DT-driven healthcare ecosystem [3].

5.3 Composability and Modularity

Composability refers to the dynamic composition of services which mostly faces issues such as service orchestration, reliability, and secure communication of composable services. Modularity is related to the integration of diverse modules from various sources (e.g. EHRs, imaging systems, IoT devices). Maintenance and up-gradation of consumer electronics systems hamper these factors significantly.

5.4 Scalability

Healthcare systems deal with large volumes of data. Thus, DT-enabled healthcare systems should manage and process the vast amount of data efficiently. However, such an ecosystem still faces challenges including network infrastructure (5G/6G), latency, data anonymization, legal compliance, regulatory adaptation, power requirements for electronic devices, etc.

5.5 Power Optimization

Another challenge arises in the form of a trade-off between computing capability and power consumption. The inclusion of edge computing offers versatility in terms of data processing but also imposes restrictions on power consumption due to the small size and mobility of sensor nodes utilized as medical electronics. Therefore, the multi-tier computing architecture for DT in healthcare should be optimized in terms of cross-domain data analysis and processing, especially in delay-sensitive tasks. Future AI-tailored wireless hospitals will utilize DT technology imbibed in the Intelligent Internet of Medical Things (IIoMT) for advanced data compression, information extraction, processing, and decision-making.

6 Concluding Remarks

An advanced DTT-assisted healthcare framework is proposed in this work that extends beyond traditional models by integrating comprehensive aspects like health monitoring, emergency services, nutrition, research, lab facilities, and training. Four pivotal use cases of DTT in healthcare along with their relationship with consumer electronics have been discussed. Despite its roots in intelligent manufacturing and other industrial sectors, DTT significantly enhances healthcare privacy, security, and overall quality. Nevertheless, substantial efforts are still required to realize its full potential and ensure its efficient operation with medical consumer electronics in the healthcare system. Continued research and collaboration are essential to leveraging DTT for improved healthcare outcomes.

Acknowledgment. The authors would like to thank Prof. Tero Paivarinta and Prof. Teemu Myllylä for providing research resources. The authors are thankful to Tauno Tonning Sattio for assisting with individual grants.

References

1. Abiodun, A.S., Anisi, M.H., Khan, M.K.: Cloud-based wireless body area networks: managing data for better health care. IEEE Consum. Electron. Maga. **8**(3), 55–59 (2019)

2. Acharya, S., et al.: Interoperability challenges and opportunities in vehicle-in-the-loop testings: insights from nuve lab's hybrid setup. In: 65th International Conference of Scandinavian simulation Soceity, SIMS 2024, and Second SIMS EUROSIM Conference on Modelling and Simulation, SIMS EUROSIM 2024 (2024)
3. Acharya, S., Wintercorn, O., Tripathy, A., Hanif, M., Van Deventer, J., Päivärinta, T.: Twins interoperability through service oriented architecture: a use-case of industry 4.0. In: Proceedings of the Annual Symposium of Computer Science 2023 co-located with The International Conference on Evaluation and Assessment in Software Engineering (EASE 2023). R. Piskac c/o Redaktion Sun SITE, Informatik V, RWTH Aachen (2023)
4. Attaran, M., Celik, B.G.: Digital twin: benefits, use cases, challenges, and opportunities. Decis. Anal. J. **6**, 100165 (2023)
5. Badano, A., et al.: Evaluation of digital breast tomosynthesis as replacement of full-field digital mammography using an in silico imaging trial. JAMA Netw. Open **1**(7), e185474–e185474 (2018)
6. Baillargeon, B., Rebelo, N., Fox, D.D., Taylor, R.L., Kuhl, E.: The living heart project: a robust and integrative simulator for human heart function. Eur. J. Mech.-A/Solids **48**, 38–47 (2014)
7. Clinic, C.: MetroHealth: Digital Twin Neighborhoods. https://news.metrohealth.org
8. Coorey, G., et al.: The health digital twin to tackle cardiovascular disease–a review of an emerging interdisciplinary field. NPJ Dig. Med. **5**(1), 126 (2022)
9. Garge, G.K., Balakrishna, C., Datta, S.K.: Consumer health care: current trends in consumer health monitoring. IEEE Consum. Electron. Maga. **7**(1), 38–46 (2017)
10. Grieves, M., Vickers, J.: Digital twin: mitigating unpredictable, undesirable emergent behavior in complex systems. In: Transdisciplinary Perspectives on Complex Systems: New Findings and Approaches, pp. 85–113 (2017)
11. Healthineers, S.: The value of digital twin technology. https://www.siemens-healthineers.com/perspectives/mso-digital-twin-mater.html
12. HeartFlow: Heartflow one. https://www.heartflow.com/portfolio/
13. Khan, L.U., Saad, W., Niyato, D., Han, Z., Hong, C.S.: Digital-twin-enabled 6G: vision, architectural trends, and future directions. IEEE Commun. Mag. **60**(1), 74–80 (2022)
14. Markram, H.: The blue brain project. Nat. Rev. Neurosci. **7**(2), 153–160 (2006)
15. Medical, C.: Surgical augmented intelligence. https://cydarmedical.com/
16. Obaid, D.R., Smith, D., Gilbert, M., Ashraf, S., Chase, A.: Computer simulated "virtual tavr" to guide tavr in the presence of a previous starr-edwards mitral prosthesis. J. Cardiovasc. Comput. Tomogr. **13**(1), 38–40 (2019)
17. Onscale: Project breatheasy: Digital twins of lungs to improve covid-19 patients outcomes. https://onscale.com
18. Philips: Heartnavigator: Insightful planning and guidance for structural heart disease procedures. https://www.usa.philips.com/healthcare/product/HCOPT201/heartnavigator
19. Ramu, S.P., Srivastava, G., Chengoden, R., Victor, N., Maddikunta, P.K.R., Gadekallu, T.R.: The metaverse for cognitive health: a paradigm shift. IEEE Consum. Electron. Maga. **13**(3), 73–79 (2023)
20. Särestöniemi, M., Singh, D., Dessai, R., Heredia, C., Myllymäki, S., Myllylä, T.: Realistic 3d phantoms for validation of microwave sensing in health monitoring applications. Sensors **24**(6), 1975 (2024)

21. Särestöniemi, M., Singh, D., Heredia, C., Nikkinen, J., von und zu Fraunberg, M., Myllylä, T.: Digital twins for development of microwave-based brain tumor detection. In: Nordic Conference on Digital Health and Wireless Solutions, pp. 240–254. Springer, Heidelberg (2024). https://doi.org/10.1007/978-3-031-59080-1_18
22. Singh, D., Vihriälä, E., Särestöniemi, M., Myllylä, T.: Microwave technique based noninvasive monitoring of intracranial pressure using realistic phantom models. In: Nordic Conference on Digital Health and Wireless Solutions, pp. 413–425. Springer, Heidelberg (2024). https://doi.org/10.1007/978-3-031-59091-7_27
23. Sun, T., He, X., Song, X., Shu, L., Li, Z.: The digital twin in medicine: a key to the future of healthcare? Front. Med. **9**, 907066 (2022)
24. Sundaravadivel, P., Kougianos, E., Mohanty, S.P., Ganapathiraju, M.K.: Everything you wanted to know about smart health care: evaluating the different technologies and components of the internet of things for better health. IEEE Consum. Electron. Maga. **7**(1), 18–28 (2017)

Smart Walker for Rehabilitation

V. Mythily[1], G. T. Bhuvaneshwari[2(✉)], S. Divyashree[2], and S. Madumitha[2]

[1] Department of Biomedical Engineering, Anna University, Chennai, India
mythily.bme2021@jerusalemengg.ac.in

[2] Department of Biomedical Engineering, Jerusalem College of Engineering Chennai, Chennai, India
{bhuvaneshwarigtbme2021,divyashrees234bme2021,madumithasbme2021}@jerusalemengg.ac.in

Abstract. The Intelligent Walking Aid is an innovative mobility solution designed to assist a diverse range of users, including the elderly, accident victims, specially-abled individuals, and those recovering from sports injuries. The project aims to enhance the efficiency of traditional walking aids by integrating advanced technology for real-time health monitoring and feedback. Utilizing Arduino and Node MCU microcontrollers, the system reads data from force sensors, pulse sensors, body temperature sensors, and accelerometers and uploaded to the Thing speak IoT platform for analysis and monitoring of gait pattern and posture during walking. Key features include a haptic feedback mechanism that alerts users through vibration motors when excessive force is applied, ensuring its safe use. Additionally, an accelerometer-based fall detection system activates a DC motor to mimic inflating, minimizing risk of injury during falls. To further aid in recovery, a separate posture detection device monitors walking posture and provides feedback for corrective actions. This comprehensive approach not only offers physical support but also enhances user safety and helps in faster recovery by monitoring vital health parameters, walking posture and effective feedback.

Keywords: IOT integration · fall detection · vital monitoring · force control · elderly assistance

1 Introduction

Rehabilitation plays a critical role in the treatment of patients recuperating from operations, injuries, or age-related mobility impairments. As the world's population ages quickly, mobility issues are become more common. This is especially true for the elderly, who often struggle with strength, balance, and coordination, leaving them more susceptible to falls and injuries. By 2050, there will be twice as many persons 60 years of age and older roughly 2.1 billion—according to the World Health Organization (WHO). The need for cutting-edge rehabilitation tools that not only help people move more freely but also speed up their healing and enhance their general quality of life is rising in response to these mounting worries. Conventional walkers and mobility aids are beneficial, but they

K. Atul et al. (Eds.): BodyNets 2024, LNICST 666, pp. 293–305, 2026.
https://doi.org/10.1007/978-3-032-16099-7_23

frequently lack the elements that are required to offer complete support throughout rehabilitation, like fall avoidance, posture correction, and real-time monitoring of vital signs. These restrictions create the need for a more advanced solution, and recent advances in healthcare technology are leading the way towards smart, sensor-based devices that interface with the Internet of Things (IoT) to give real-time data and individualized care. The problem statement for doing this project arises from the limitations of existing rehabilitation tools, which often fail to provide comprehensive support for individuals with mobility impairments. Traditional walkers lack features like posture correction, gait monitoring, and fall detection, leaving users vulnerable to improper movement, falls, and slower recovery times. Moreover, caregivers and healthcare professionals lack real-time data on users' health and mobility, making it difficult to track progress or intervene in case of emergencies. For elderly users and those with significant mobility challenges, these gaps can lead to increased injury risk and a prolonged recovery process.

The proposed Intelligent Walking Aid system is designed to significantly enhance traditional mobility aids by integrating advanced sensor and IoT technologies. The system reads data from various sensors to monitor vital health parameters and detect any unusual events in real time. The collected data is transmitted to an IoT platform, where it can be stored, analyzed, and monitored remotely. One of the key features of the system is its ability to detect the amount of force applied to the walking aid. If excessive force is detected, haptic feedback is provided through integrated vibration motors, alerting the user to adjust their usage and preventing potential injury. The system also continuously monitors the user's vital signs, providing timely alerts in case of abnormal readings. To address the risk of falls, the system uses sensors to detect sudden movements indicative of a fall. Additionally, the system includes a separate posture detection device to monitor and correct the user's walking posture. This feature is particularly beneficial for users undergoing rehabilitation, as it aids in quicker recovery by ensuring proper posture is maintained during movement.

One of the main obstacles is to guarantee that the walker remains accessible to users, especially elderly individuals who may lack familiarity with complex technology. It is essential for the walker to find a harmonious balance between providing advanced functionalities and ensuring a straightforward user interface. Another significant challenge is to maintain the precision and dependability of the sensors and algorithms, particularly in the context of fall detection, where inaccuracies or missed alerts could result in adverse consequences. Furthermore, the walker must be robust enough to endure daily usage while preserving the reliability of its sensors. Looking ahead, the smart walker has the potential to incorporate more advanced artificial intelligence systems to forecast rehabilitation outcomes and facilitate features such as telemedicine, allowing users to engage in virtual consultations with healthcare providers through the device.

The Smart Walker for Rehabilitation represents a significant advancement in the field of mobility aids and rehabilitation tools. By integrating modern technologies such as IoT, wearable sensors, and AI algorithms, the smart walker addresses critical gaps in traditional rehabilitation devices. Its features, such as fall detection, real-time feedback, posture correction, and vital sign monitoring, contribute to a safer, more effective rehabilitation process. The smart walker empowers users to take an active role in their recovery while ensuring that healthcare professionals can provide personalized, data-driven care.

As healthcare technology continues to evolve, the Smart Walker for Rehabilitation is poised to play a crucial role in shaping the future of assistive care and rehabilitation for individuals with mobility challenges.

2 Literature Review

Jacob Thompson et.al., (2023) suggested about the usage of soft continuum robotic airbag system in mobility aid for passive walkers reduces fall impact by deploying in various directions, demonstrating consistent performance, and enhancing safety and confidence. The proposed system will overcome the challenges of advanced algorithms and efficient components to improve sensor accuracy and battery life limitations.

Tushar Bhatia et.al., (2023) discussed about a Smart Walking Stick with features like step counting, heart rate monitoring, and fall detection. While effective, it may face issues with sensor accuracy, battery life, and connectivity. Future we overcome the limitations with accuracy, longer battery life, and reliable connectivity.

Gyung-Hwan Yuk et.al., (2019) presented a posture control system for a smart mobile walker that utilizes four linear actuators to maintain balance on uneven terrains based on orientation and ground force measurements. Despite its effectiveness, the system encounters issues with sensor noise, actuator performance, and PID control wind-up.

Nikita Prajapati et.al., (2021) proposed about the Various rehabilitation are using analysis of gait in order to check the effect of treatment on one's body. The aim of this research is to review various approaches for Gait Analysis and specifically clinical gait analysis. This paper includes the discussion on the background details of gait, related terminology and parameters, followed by the detail discussion on the approaches from subjective assessment used in the early times for analysis of gait to vision-based approaches used nowadays for analysis of gait.

Mario F. Jimenez et.al., (2024) discussed two multimodal interaction strategies for smart walkers designed to assist post-stroke patients. The first strategy uses haptic feedback and visual cues, which is more suitable for patients with higher independence but requires more effort. The second strategy combines haptic feedback with virtual torque, allowing for faster movement and providing better guidance.

A.Tereso et.al., (2022) examined how different assistive devices—crutches, standard walkers, and rollators with forearm supports—affect walking and stability in patients after knee surgery. Using accelerometers to measure gait and fall risk, the results show that while the devices produce different signals, the rollator with forearm supports offers the most stability. This suggests that the rollator can be particularly effective for improving stability and movement in patients recovering from knee surgery.

Carlos Nave Et.al., (2018) addressed the need for accessible and cost-effective rehabilitation tools, particularly for the elderly and those with motor impairments. The smart walker improves the quality of rehabilitation by providing precise metrics and real-time feedback. The experimental results show that the system can detect deviations in gait and balance, enabling physiotherapists to tailor treatment to individual needs and reduce recovery time Future enhancements could include big data analytics to predict patient outcomes and adaptation of the system to other physiotherapy tools.

Mariam Ibrahim et.al., (2023) proposed project focuses on creating an airbag-based fall detection and alerting system to protect elderly individuals from injuries caused by falls. Installed on a waist belt, the system uses a gravity sensor to detect falls, triggering airbag inflation via an air valve. Alerts are sent to the user's mobile application via Bluetooth, providing GPS location and an emergency SMS to their chosen contact. With a 90% accuracy, quick response time of 150ms, and low power consumption of 11.1w, this system ensures timely protection and notification.

Santhana Lakshmi. P et.al., (2017) discussed the development of a wearable posture correction system designed to prevent back pain by detecting and correcting poor posture. It utilizes a flex sensor placed on the lower back to monitor posture, with a buzzer providing biofeedback when deviations occur. If the user fails to adjust their posture, DC motors in a belt automatically correct the slouching position. The system is aimed at students and heavy computer users, offering a simple, low-cost solution for maintaining proper posture and preventing long-term health issues. Simulation and testing confirmed the system's effectiveness in real-time posture correction.

Kabalan Chaccour et.al., (2015) discussed the development of an electronic walker designed to assist visually impaired elderly individuals in navigating their environment safely. The system integrates various sensors, including ultrasonic and optical sensors for obstacle detection, and an accelerometer for fall and vibration detection. It provides audible notifications to guide the user around obstacles. The walker is designed to be low-cost, lightweight, and suitable for both indoor and outdoor use. Unlike many existing solutions, this walker focuses on ease of use, reliability, and the potential for future expansion with additional features.

Param Malhotra et.al., (2023) addressed the serious consequences of falls among elderly individuals, including fractures and fatalities. Existing fall protection devices, such as mobile walkers and wearable airbags, are reactive and primarily mitigate injuries after a fall occurs, lacking proactive prevention capabilities. Proposed is a solution involving two pneumatically actuated compliant continuum robots attached to the user's back. These robots proactively grasp nearby objects when a fall is detected, helping prevent impact with the ground. Fall detection relies on onboard sensors that monitor user posture and movements. Preliminary tests on mannequins in various fall scenarios show promise for enhancing fall prevention and reducing injury risk.

Toshiyo Tamura et.al., (2010) proposed wearable airbag system faces limitations, including the need for miniaturization of the inflation mechanism and the potential for false activations during daily activities. To address these challenges, further development is required to enhance the responsiveness and size of the airbag system, ensuring it activates solely during actual falls. Additionally, refining the fall-detection algorithm to differentiate between falls and similar acceleration signals from routine movements can improve accuracy and reliability.

3 Methodology

3.1 Block Diagram

The following block diagram depicts the construction of a Smart walker for rehabilitation to enhance mobility (Fig. 1).

The proposed walking assistance system is built around Arduino and Node MCU microcontrollers, which gather real-time data from several sensors such as a force sensor,

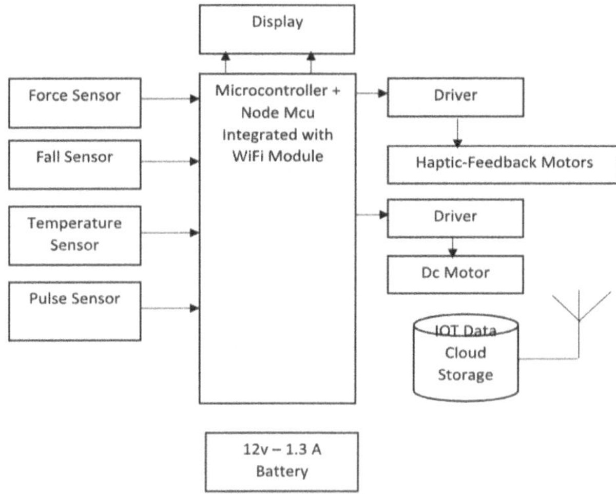

Fig. 1. Block diagram of Smart walker

fall sensor, temperature sensor, and pulse sensor. These sensors continuously monitor the user's vitals. The gathered data is then transmitted via WIFI to the Thing Speak IoT platform, where it is analyzed and stored for long-term monitoring. The force sensor detects the amount of pressure exerted on the walking aid, and when excessive force is applied, haptic-feedback motors provide vibration alerts to the user, ensuring they maintain safe usage levels.

In addition, the fall sensor continuously monitors the user's movements and issues an alert if a fall is detected, setting up a timely intervention. A temperature sensor and a pulse sensor monitor the user's vital signs such as body temperature and heart rate, while an ultrasound sensor detects obstacles in the user's path, and more safety when walking. The LCD display connected to the system provides real-time information on the user's vitals and the status of the walker, including gait stability and sensor feedback.

In the event of a drop or abnormal reading of vital signs, an alert will be sent to the cloud, and caregivers or medical personnel will be notified, so that they can respond quickly. This system not only helps in physical recovery, but also includes important safety features such as fall detection and obstacle avoidance, making walking a smart tool to improve mobility and mobility. Safety during the recovery process.

3.2 Circuit Diagram

The Arduino Uno board serves as the central processing unit (CPU) for a smart walker system, featuring various pins including analog, digital, ground, VCC, TX, and RX. Integrated with an LM35 temperature sensor, it monitors body temperature, while a pulse sensor tracks pulse rates. An ultrasonic sensor connected to the digital pins facilitates distance measurement and obstacle detection. Additionally, a force-sensitive resistor (FSR) detects applied pressure, providing haptic feedback to ensure even pressure distribution. A motor driver enables motor operations for responsive actions, complemented by a

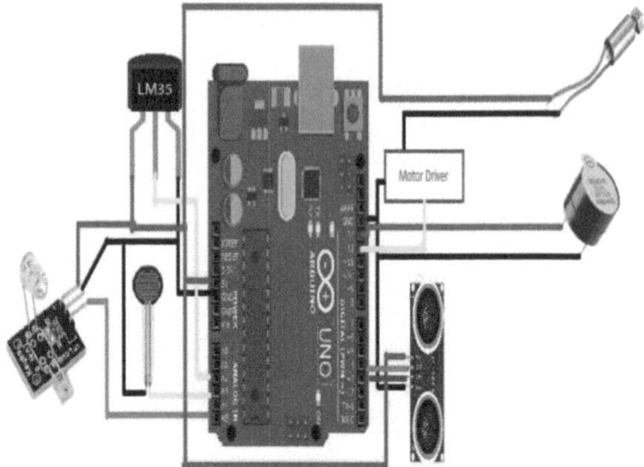

Fig. 2. Circuit diagram of developed system

buzzer that emits auditory alerts when triggered by the ultrasonic sensor. The microcontroller processes sensor data and controls output devices based on programmed logic. An accelerometer detects tilts or falls, activating appropriate responses, and an LCD displays real-time data on temperature, pulse, distance, and fall detection. Utilizing Think Speak technology, this system monitors vital signs and other parameters, storing the data in the cloud for real- time access. This setup is particularly suited for smart walkers or rehabilitation devices, where immediate data feedback and responsive control are essential for user assistance (Fig. 2).

4 Results and Discussion

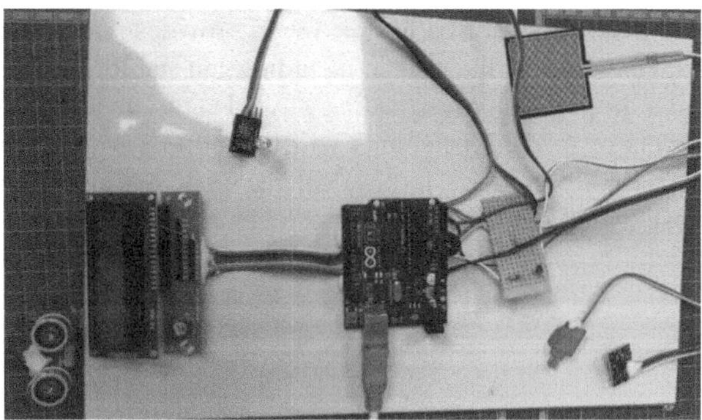

Fig. 3. Hardware setup of prototype

The Fig. 3 shown below represents the experimental setup of smart walker for rehabilitation. The force sensor (A502) integrated into the crutch is designed to measure the mechanical load applied during use. When the applied force exceeds a predefined threshold, the sensor sends an electrical signal to the microcontroller (Fig. 3).

The microcontroller, pre-programmed with the threshold limit, processes this input and activates a haptic feedback mechanism, usually a vibration motor. The intensity and duration of the haptic feedback can be modulated based on the force level detected. This real-time feedback ensures that the user is notified to redistribute their weight, preventing over-reliance on the crutch and potential harm to the body.

When users applied force to the crutch, the force sensor measured the applied load and displayed the real-time force values on the LCD screen (Fig. 4).

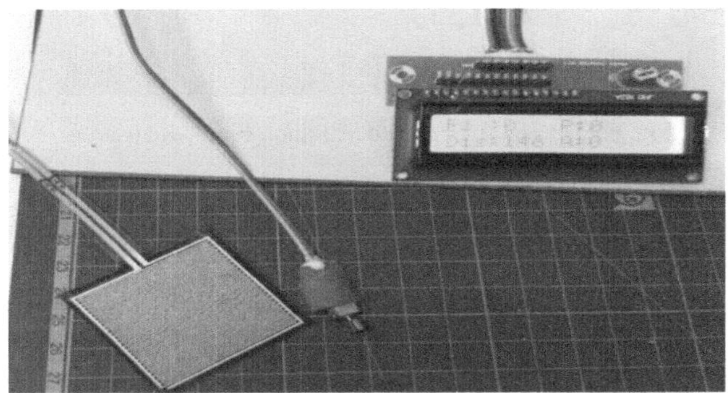

Fig. 4. Initial output of force sensor f = 0

During the initial trials, when the applied force was below the threshold, the LCD indicated that F = 459 N (Fig. 5).

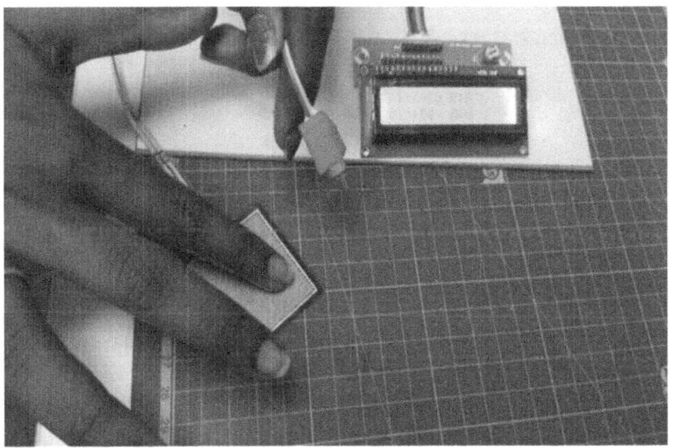

Fig. 5. Force- Responsive LCD Display Output

Once the force exceeded the set threshold, the LCD displays "force is detected" (Fig. 6).

This message, paired with the activation of the haptic feedback (vibration motor), prompted the user to redistribute their weight. This combination of tactile feedback and

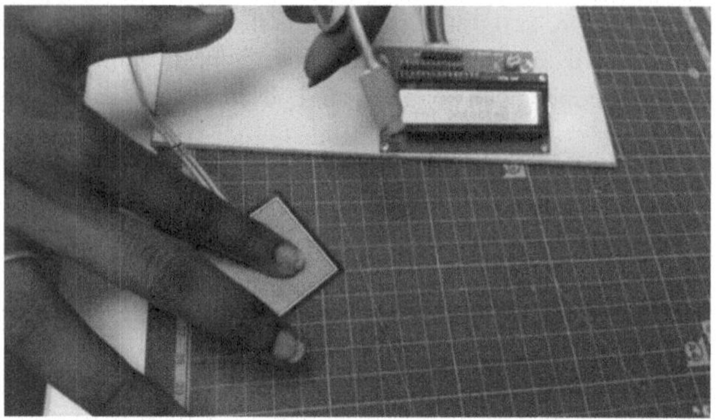

Fig. 6. Threshold-Triggered Vibration Motor Activation

clear visual cues on the LCD enhanced user safety and ensured proper uniform load balancing.

The ultrasonic sensor (HC-SR04) works on the principle of sending out ultrasonic waves and measuring the time it takes for the reflected waves (echo) to reflect back after hitting an obstacle. This time delay is used to calculate the distance between the crutch and the obstacle. When the sensor detects an object within a range of 20 cm, it triggers the buzzer via the microcontroller. The buzzer emits a sound alert to notify the user of an impending obstacle, ensuring they can navigate safely (Fig. 7).

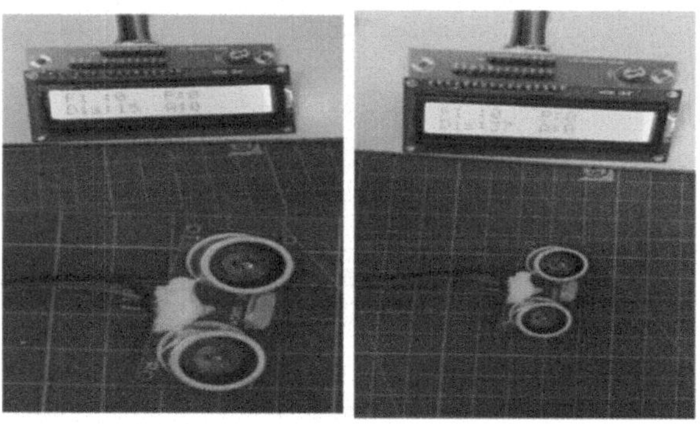

Fig. 7. The buzzer sounds when an obstacle is within 20 cm.

If there is no obstacle is within the 20 cm range, the LCD displayed the measured distance and the alert system is not activated.

After Reaching the Threshold, once an object is detected within 20 cm, visual clues is created through LCD display and simultaneously, the buzzer created an audio alert to the user. The combination of visual and auditory clues ensure that the user could get sufficient time to known the presence of obstacles in their path.

The accelerometer (MPU 9250) measures the crutch's acceleration across its x and y axis. If a sudden and significant deviation from the normal movement pattern is detected like changes in the posture during fall or slip, the accelerometer generates a signal. This signal is fed into the microcontroller, which continuously monitors for such deviations based on preset threshold values (min 9000–15000). Upon detecting a posture prone to fall at a orientation above the threshold (max 49000–57000), the microcontroller (ATmega328p) activates the buzzer, alerting the user or nearby individuals about the event, thereby potentially preventing the risk of fall and injury (Fig. 8).

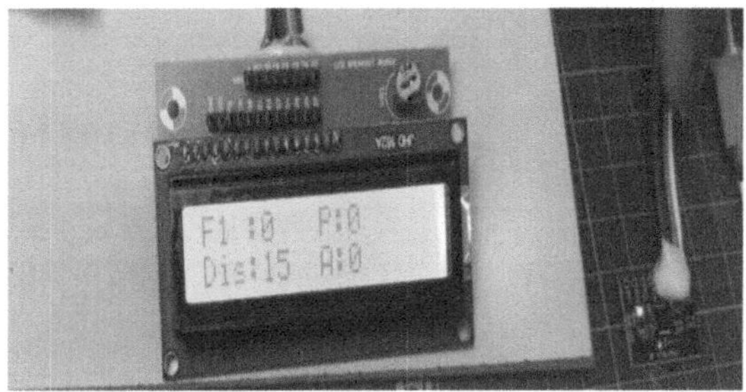

Fig. 8. The LCD displays "A = 0" when the system is at rest

During normal operation, the accelerometer monitored the crutch's movement and displays the orientation of the person. Initially, the orientation is displayed in LCD as A = 0 when the person at the static right posture (Fig. 9).

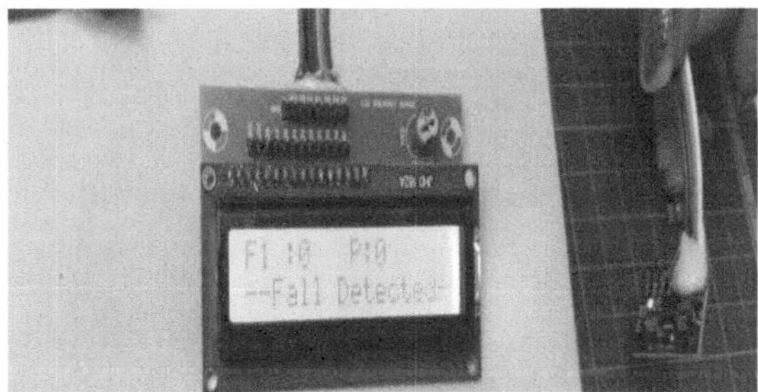

Fig. 9. The LCD shows "Fall detected" upon unusual movement

If the accelerometer detected some sudden and unusual movement patterns (i.e., deviation in orientation during potential falls above or below threshold), the LCD screen showed: "Fall Detected!" and activates the buzzer.

The LCD message paired with the buzzer alert, warned the user and those nearby about the incident, helping to initiate an immediate response. This clear visual cue on the LCD enhanced the system's reliability in providing fall alerts.

The IR pulse sensor (KY-039) uses an infrared LED and a photodetector to measure the variations in blood flow through the skin, typically at the fingertip. As blood volume changes with each heartbeat, the amount of reflected IR light fluctuates, which is detected by the sensor. These fluctuations are converted into a signal corresponding to the heartbeat rate, which is then processed by the microcontroller. The microcontroller (Atmega328p) can further calculate the heart rate per minute (BPM) and compare it against normal ranges(60-100bpm). If the heart rate exceeds or falls below a safe threshold (60), it can trigger an alert, either through visual cue and send message to care giver through IOT.

During normal operation, the pulse sensor monitored the pulse rate and displays the output. Initially, the pulse rate is displayed in LCD as p = 0 (Fig. 10).

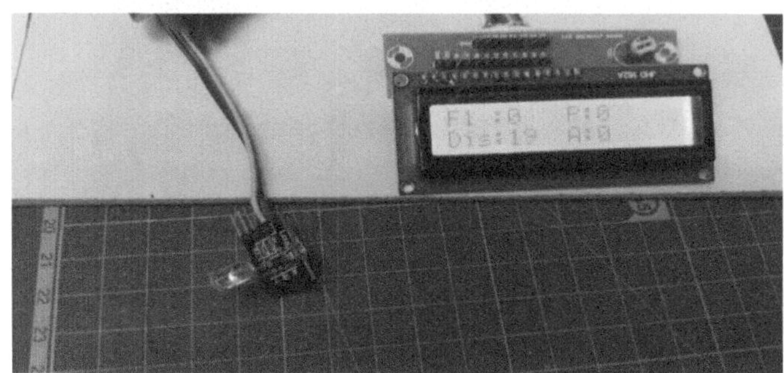

Fig. 10. The system displays the initial pulse rate as "P = 0."

During continuous monitoring, the IR pulse sensor measured heartbeats and displays "P: 104" (Fig. 11).

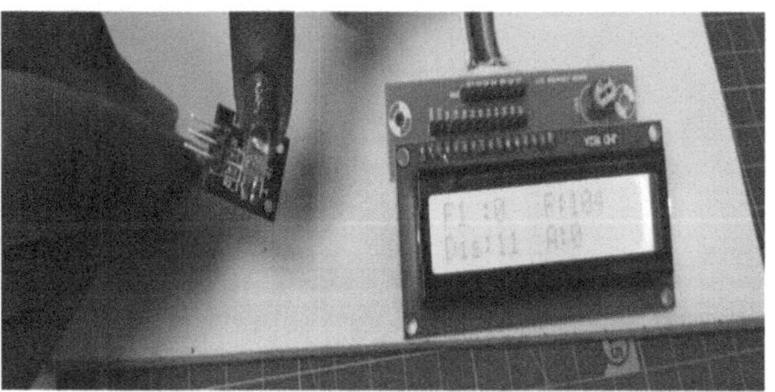

Fig. 11. The system measures the pulse rate as "P = 104."This constant feedback on the LCD reassured the user that their heart rate was within normal limits.

If the user's heart rate crossed the safe threshold (either too high or too low), the LCD will display "P: 110 - Out of Range!" (Fig. 12).

If the user's heart rate crossed the safe threshold (either too high or too low), the LCD will display "P: 110 - Out of Range!".

During continuous monitoring, temperature sensor measures the temperature and LCD displays (Fig. 13, 14 and 15).

The technology used in thinkspeak which measure the vital signs and store in the cloud. During continuous monitoring, if the vital parameters exceed the normal range, it gives an alert message to the caregiver.

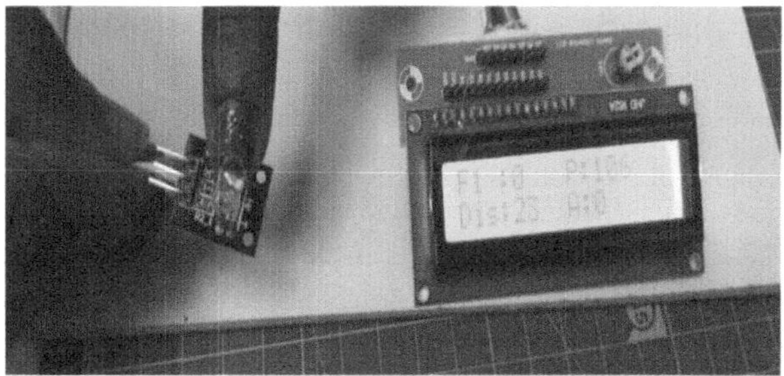

Fig. 12. LCD Displays High Pulse Rate, Activates Buzzer

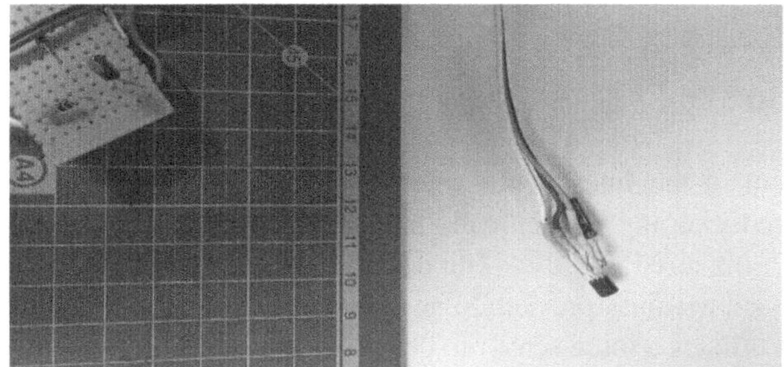

Fig. 13. System measures the temperature

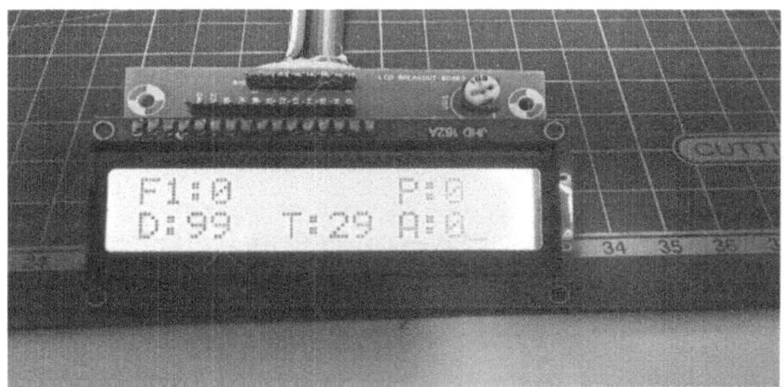

Fig. 14. Output of temperature sensor

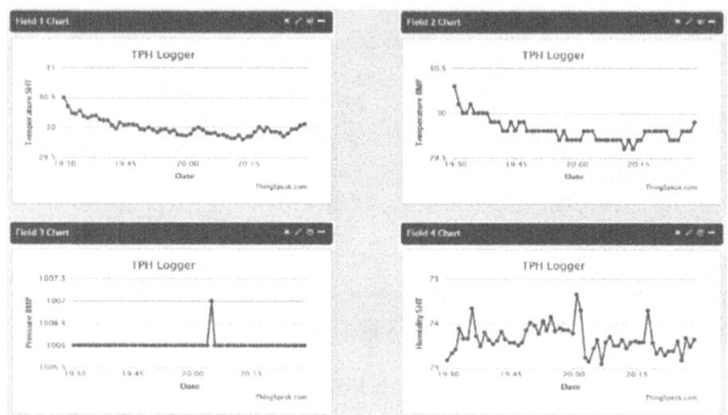

Fig. 15. IOT output

5 Discussion

The development of the Intelligent Crutch Tool demonstrates a significant advancement in assistive technology, specifically tailored to enhance the mobility and safety of individuals with impaired mobility. The design integrates multiple sensors to ensure a proactive approach to injury prevention and health monitoring for the user.

The system utilizes a force sensor to detect abnormal pressure on the crutch, which could indicate incorrect usage or excessive weight bearing of walker. If the force exceeds a predefined threshold, haptic feedback is triggered, alerting the user to adjust their weight distribution, thus reducing the risk of falls or strain.

Incorporating an accelerometer enhances the safety of the user by monitoring the crutch's movement. If the movement along the x or y axis exceeds the threshold, which may indicate instability or the user losing balance, a buzzer is activated. This real-time alert system ensures the user can correct their posture or movements immediately, preventing accidents.

The ultrasonic sensor adds another layer of security by detecting obstacles or objects within a 20 cm range. When such an object is detected, a buzzer alerts the user, allowing them to avoid collisions or missteps, particularly in environments with uneven terrain or obstacles.

Finally, the integration of an IR pulse sensor addresses the health monitoring aspect of the tool. By continuously measuring the user's heart rate, the system can detect irregularities or potential health issues, providing an alert if abnormal heart rates are detected. This feature is especially important for elderly users or those with pre-existing heart conditions, ensuring that their well-being is constantly monitored while using the crutch.

6 Conclusion

The Intelligent Crutch Tool represents a novel approach to assistive technology, combining force, motion, proximity, and health sensors into a single, multifunctional device. The inclusion of haptic feedback, buzzers, and real-time monitoring provides a robust system designed to ensure the safety, mobility, and health of the user.

This project showcases how sensor integration can significantly improve the quality of life for individuals with limited mobility. By providing immediate feedback and alerts, the tool minimizes the risk of injury, promotes better posture and balance, and ensures that users are constantly aware of their surroundings and physical well-being. Future iterations of the project could explore wireless connectivity for remote monitoring by healthcare providers and further refining the system's sensitivity for enhanced performance.

References

Vellas, B.J., Wayne, S.J., Romero, L.J., Baumgartner, R.N., Garry, P.J.: Fear of falling and restriction of mobility in elderly fallers. Age Ageing **26**(3), 189–193 (1997)

Zhong, Z.: A real-time pre-impact fall detection and protection system. In: 2018 IEEE/ASME International Conference on Advanced Intelligent Mechatronics (AIM), pp. 1039–1044. IEEE (2018)

Fukaya, K., Uchida, M.: Protection against impact with the ground using wearable airbags. Ind. Health **46**(1), 59–65 (2008)

Narayanan, S.: IoT based smart walking cane for typhlotic with voice assistance. In: 2016 Online International Conference on Green Engineering and Technologies (IC-GET). IEEE (2016)

Alwan, M., et al.: A smart and passive floor-vibration based fall detector for elderly. In: 2006 2nd International Conference on Information & Communication Technologies, vol. 1. IEEE (2006)

Reilly, D.S., Woollacott, M.H., et al.: The interaction between executive attention and postural control in dual-task conditions: children with cerebral palsy. Arch. Phys. Med. Rehabil. **89**(5), 834–842 (2008)

Alattas, R.: Postuino: bad posture detector using Arduino. Int. J. Innov. Sci. Res. **3**(2), 208–212 (2014). ISSN 2351-8014

Farella, E.: A wireless body area sensor network for posture detection. In: International Symposium on Computers and Communications (2006)

Harbouche, A.: Model driven flexible design of a wireless body sensor network for health monitoring. Comput. Netw. **129**(2), 548–571 (2017)

Yew, H.T., Ng, M.F., Ping, S.Z., Chung, S.K., Chekima, A., Dargham, J.A.: IoT Based real-time remote patient monitoring system. In: 2020 16th IEEE International Colloquium on Signal Processing & Its Applications (CSPA), pp. 176–179 (2020)

Tamilselvi, V., Sribalaji, S., Vigneshwaran, P., Vinu, P., GeethaRamani, J.: IoT based health monitoring system. In: 2020 6th International Conference on Advanced Computing and Communication Systems (ICACCS), pp. 386–389 (2020)

Manisha, M., Neeraja, K., Sindhura, V., Ramya, P.: IoT on heart attack detection and heart rate monitoring. Int. J. Innov. Eng. Technol. (IJIET) **7**(2) (2016). ISSN: 2319 – 1058

Hughes, C.T., Thompson, A.L., Collins, M.A.: Blood pressure assessment practices of dental hygienists. J. Contemp. Dental Pract. **7**, 55–62 (2007)

Saleh, M., Murdoch, G.: In defence of gait analysis: observation and measurement in gait assessment. J. Bone Joint Surg. Brit. **67**(2), 237–241 (1985)

Chambers, H.G., Sutherland, D.H.: A practical guide to gait analysis. JAAOS-J. Am. Acad. Orthopaedic Surg. **10**(3), 222–231 (2002)

Transforming Military Healthcare: Advanced Soldier Health Monitoring with Real-Time Analytics

Anirudh Chaturvedi, Sneha Pradhan, Niranjan Kumar, and Varun Gupta(✉)

Department of Electronics and Communication Engineering, National Institute of Technology Sikkim, Namchi, Sikkim, India
varungupta@nitsikkim.ac.in

Abstract. In today's world, national security depends on strong military forces and effective border control. Soldiers play a key role and their health is a priority, especially during high-risk missions. They often face real dangers, stress, and harsh conditions. To improve safety, long-range health monitoring systems using biosensors and GPS are essential. The M-Wellbeing system uses wearable tech and GSM communication to track soldiers' health and location, sending data back to base. However, identifying real threats becomes harder near enemy lines, especially with added medical and environmental challenges. This article proposes using such systems for real-time monitoring and early health assessments.

Keywords: GPS · M-Wellbeing · GSM · soldier tracking · biosensors

1 Introduction

Wellbeing telematics is an evolving field that enhances healthcare for the elderly, disabled, and chronically ill. Advances in information and communication technologies, along with mobile web capabilities, are vital to modern healthcare [1–3]. Mobile health (m-Health) enables healthcare delivery across time and location barriers, addressing chronic disease growth, high public healthcare costs, and the need for patient self-care and anytime-anywhere access [4–9].

Since the 1990s, smartphones have enabled physicians to access medical data and patients to stay informed about their health. With the rise of 3G and 4G networks, mobile computing has become central to developing effective m-Health solutions [10–12]. M-Health is transforming healthcare by improving monitoring, data collection, service delivery, information access, and medication management. Web-based m-Health architectures allow seamless interaction between doctors and patients, enabling both to access medical records anytime via smartphones, tablets, or computers. Patients can contact doctors during emergencies and manage appointments without time or location constraints [13–16].

In below some of the past literatures are reviewed to know the essence of m-health-

K. Atul et al. (Eds.): BodyNets 2024, LNICST 666, pp. 306–316, 2026.
https://doi.org/10.1007/978-3-032-16099-7_24

Mdhaffar et al. [5] implemented an IoT-based health monitoring system using the LoRaWAN protocol, known for its low-cost, low-power, and secure communication. Biosensor data, including heart rate, body temperature, and blood glucose, was transmitted to an analysis module via the LoRaWAN framework.

Walker et al. [2] designed a mobile-based health monitoring system using compact, lightweight wearable biosensors, measuring heart rate, temperature, and gas levels. These sensors were attached to soldiers to track their health in real time.

Nikam et al. [17] developed a system using IoT and GPS to monitor health and track the location of soldiers.

Gondalic et al. [4] used machine learning and IoT for monitoring soldiers' health and location, employing sensors like GPS, temperature, and heart rate. Data was wirelessly shared with nearby soldiers via ZigBee. They also proposed using LoRaWAN for communication between the warzone leader and base station in areas lacking cellular coverage or where clustering algorithms aren't feasible.

In 2019, Jasvinder Singh et al. [1] introduced a GPS and IoT-based system for soldier tracking and health monitoring. It ensures constant communication among soldiers and uses low-power, lightweight components with ARM processors to minimize energy use. The system provides vital health data and global positioning to enhance soldier safety.

Mobile technology is reshaping healthcare by changing how information is accessed and managed. Cloud computing supports this shift by enabling faster and broader healthcare delivery. Its adoption in healthcare is already underway. Advances in 4G mobile networks are driving the growth of new m-Health services and applications.

Researchers predict a shift from individual-focused to group-based services using social networks. As social platforms become integral to daily life, m-Health can use these networks to encourage healthy behaviors and raise awareness within patient communities.

Market research on m-Health highlights ongoing challenges in mobile and pervasive computing. A key issue is enabling collaboration among different m-Health applications, allowing doctors and patients to work toward shared goals. Enhancing mobile device performance, battery life, storage, and connectivity is also important.

Since collaborative m-Health systems share sensitive data over wireless networks, ensuring data privacy and security is essential. Additional research is required to evaluate how mobile technologies influence daily routines, lower healthcare expenses, and affect public and private healthcare sectors.

2 Innovation and Need

The core aim of this effort is to closely monitor soldiers operating in hostile environments to ensure national security. While effective tracking is essential, achieving high accuracy remains challenging due to terrain and technological limitations [17].

Innovation is essential, and this work aims to address key challenges in soldier monitoring. Earlier methods relied on a single soldier carrying a radio set for location updates, which failed during sudden events like avalanches, causing troop disorientation and untracked casualties. To solve this, we propose a device that tracks a soldier's location and vital signs, even without their input. The system uses NavIC a regional satellite navigation system for accurate real-time positioning across India and nearby regions. Additionally, we suggest using self-powered boots with piezoelectric crystals to generate energy to run the device.

Thus, with the assistance of this proposed system, headquarters can easily track and provide assistance to soldiers in need.

3 Proposed System

Soldiers risk their lives daily, serving in harsh terrains like mountains, forests, and fields to protect the nation [18]. Their sacrifice is unmatched, and it's our duty to support them [19]. To aid in this, we propose a system that provides real-time health updates and ensures medical support during critical battlefield situations.

Our system monitors vital signs, especially heart rate, to detect when a soldier is unconscious or critically injured [20]. If the heart rate crosses a danger threshold, a GSM modem sends an alert to the server, while a GPS tracker shares the soldier's location for immediate medical response. The system also sends SMS alerts to nearby hospitals or the base station. Figure 1 illustrates the proposed model, which includes a soldier node and a control unit.

This research aims to create a compact, low-power, cost-effective, and non-intrusive system for monitoring soldiers' health and tracking their location via longitude and latitude. The approach uses non-intrusive sensors to measure vital signs, with signal conditioning circuits to filter and amplify the signals. All components are energy-efficient and affordable. Real-time data is processed through an ADC and sent to a microcontroller [21, 22].

Soldier tracking is one of the latest GPS-based idea, and various essential blocks of the system are outlined below:

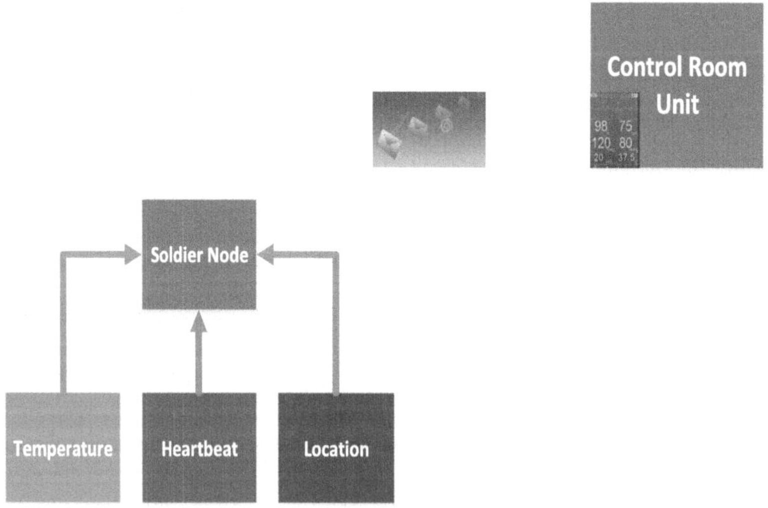

Fig. 1. Proposed model containing soldier node and control unit.

Soldier Node: This unit is affixed to the soldier's gear and comprises mainly four components [23–25]:

Biomedical Sensors: This includes a temperature sensor and a pulse oximeter, which are employed to assess the soldier's physiological condition. These sensors continuously monitor the soldier's body temperature and pulse rate, with the data being stored in the microcontroller's memory.

4x1 Keypad: Four keys are provided to the soldier, enabling them to transmit four predefined values to the base control unit for various purposes.

GPS Receiver: The GPS receiver is employed to determine the soldier's precise longitude and latitude coordinates, which are subsequently stored in the microcontroller's memory.

GSM Modem: The GSM modem facilitates communication by sending SMS messages to the army base control unit, conveying the soldier's current health status along with their exact location.

Base Control Unit: Upon receipt of the SMS, the text message on the designated phone displays the soldier's GPS coordinates. Army officials can effectively monitor the location and health status of all their soldiers through this system.

Contents of Text SMS are as Below:

- Soldier = Mr. ABC XYZ
- Temperature = 027
- Heartbeat = 065
- Longitude = 18 38.6878 N
- Latitude = 73 45.3423 E

4 Design and Implementation

A reliable and accurate positioning system with consistent indoor and outdoor coverage is crucial for military and emergency operations. GPS-based algorithms are commonly used in rescue missions to determine the positions and orientations of rescuers and those in need. By processing GPS data through GIS-based algorithms, the system calculates relative distance, elevation, and direction essential for guiding movement between two soldiers.

Integrating a GSM module allows remote data transmission, enhancing soldiers' situational awareness through reliable communication. GPS modules typically use serial communication, following NMEA standards. Figure 2 presents the proposed design model, while Fig. 3 displays the GSM and GPS configuration.

For example, during avalanches in mountainous areas, large amounts of snow can trap soldiers, including security personnel. Quick evacuation after such events is critical, and knowing the exact locations of the trapped individuals is essential. In these cases, our device will help by supplying accurate location data to the nearest rescue team. The device also notifies the command center if a soldier's vital signs reach a critical level, guiding the search team to the exact location and depth for efficient and safe rescue.

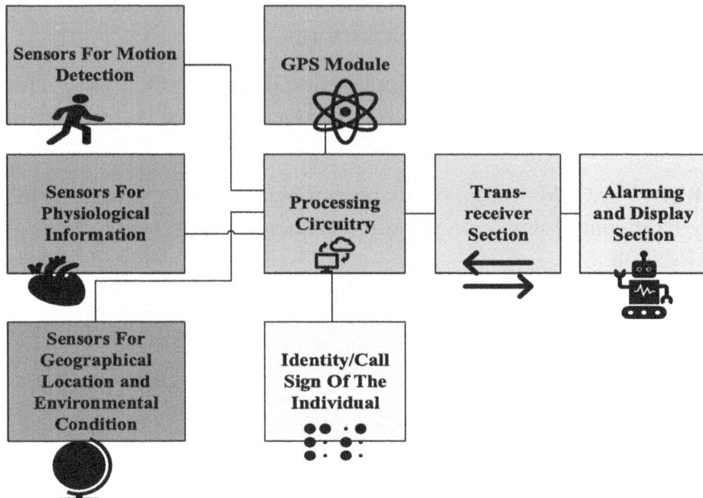

Fig. 2. Proposed design and implementation model

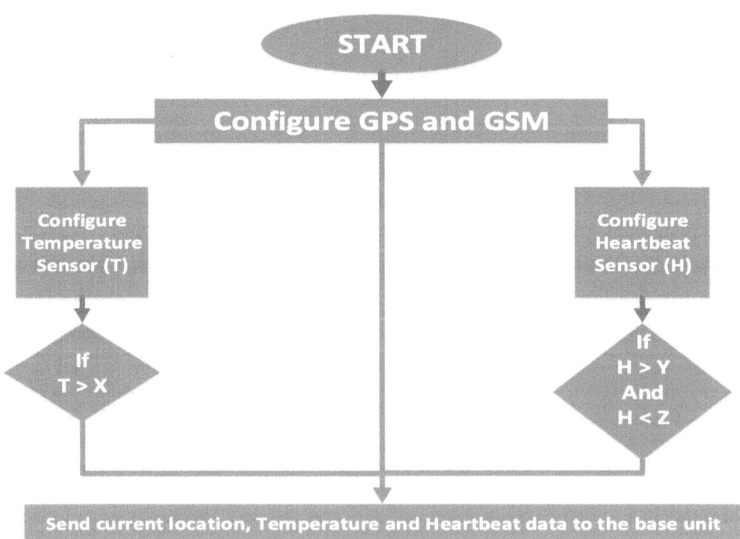

Fig. 3. Configuration of GSM and GPS

This feature is crucial not only in avalanches but also when soldiers are trapped in dense forests or captured by militant groups. Figure 4 shows the different sensors used in the system.

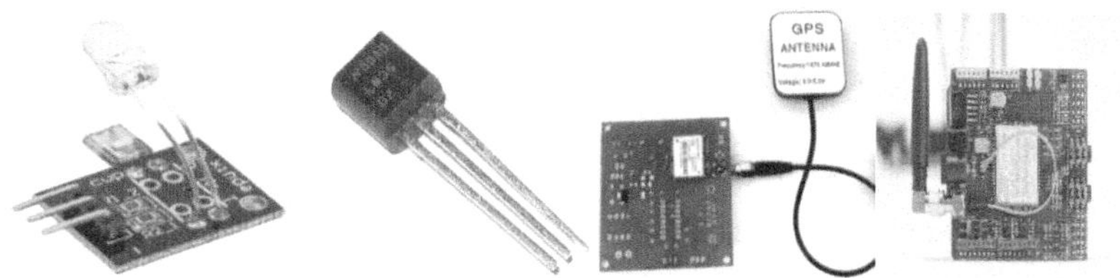

Fig. 4. a) Heartbeat sensor, b) Temperature Sensor LM35, c) GPS Module, d) GSM Module

4.1 Heartbeat Sensor

Heart rate sensors provide an easy way to evaluate cardiac activity by detecting blood flow in the finger. Blood volume in the finger changes with each heartbeat as blood is pumped through the vessels.

The sensor uses a high-brightness LED to emit light through the user's finger and measures the transmitted light with an LDR. The resulting pulse signal is then amplified, filtered, and sent to the ADC for processing.

4.2 Temperature Sensor

The LM35 is a precise temperature sensor that outputs a voltage directly proportional to the temperature in Celsius. It provides real-time readings with no delay, quickly detecting any changes from normal temperature levels.

Operating with an input voltage of 5 V, the LM35 sensor is capable of detecting temperatures ranging from −55 °C to 150 °C. Its output voltage exhibits a linear relationship with temperature, wherein a 1 °C increase in temperature corresponds to a 10 mV (0.01 V) rise in output voltage. The sensor boasts an impressive accuracy level, with deviations limited to ± 0.5 °C.

4.3 GPS Module

A GPS modem enables effective tracking of soldiers by receiving satellite signals, calculating their coordinates, and sending the data as serial input to the controller.

GPS (Global Positioning System) is a satellite-based navigation system known for its reliability in all weather conditions and global coverage. It provides accurate location and time data anywhere on Earth, typically using signals from at least four satellites.

Specifications for the GPS modem are as follows:

Supply voltage: 3.6 V.
Maximum navigation update rate: 5Hz
Operating temperature range: −40 °C to 85 °C
Operational limits: Gravity – 4 g, Altitude – 50000 m, Velocity – 500 m/s

4.4 GSM Module

The GSM modem plays a key role in sending soldiers' data to the base unit. Unlike regular mobile phones, it supports serial communication, allowing direct integration with microcontrollers to send and receive messages using AT commands.

Control of the GSM modem is facilitated through AT commands, adhering to standards such as GSM 07.07, 07.05, and SIMCOM enhanced AT Commands. Key specifications of the GSM modem include: Weight which is 3.4 g.

4.5 LCD Unit

The LCD unit is essential for displaying key output information, including the soldier's heart rate, temperature, date, time, and location [26].

5 Result

The image shows a belt containing several embedded devices as a prototype to demonstrate the model's functionality. For military use, the system will be miniaturized onto a compact PCB for convenient attachment by soldiers. Next to the belt, a shoe is shown that generates a small voltage using a dynamo and capacitors, demonstrating its ability to power the device. Figure 5 provides a real-world view of the proposed approach.

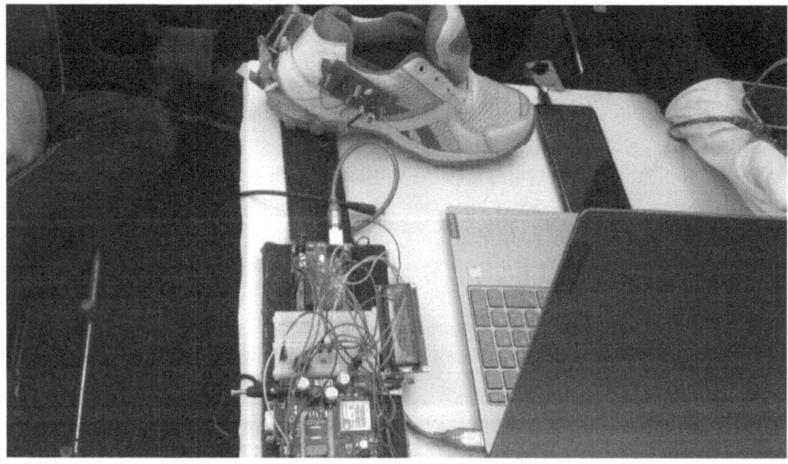

Fig. 5. Actual image of the work

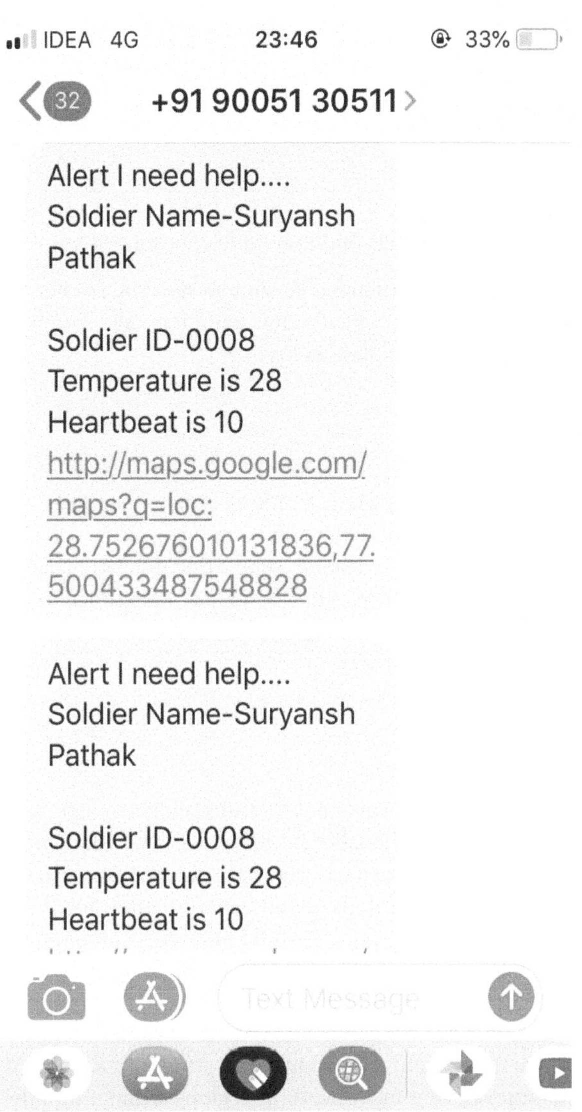

Fig. 6. Demonstration of the proposed work

The circuits in this system are powered by energy generated from walking, using motion-based charging in the soldier's shoe. As they move, power is stored in a battery, creating a self-sustaining system that removes the need for external charging or downtime. A 9V battery, fully charged by walking 15 km within 3 h, powers the circuit. Real-time monitoring of soldiers' vital signs, including heartbeat, body temperature, and location, is enabled by the circuit. This real-time information is critical for preserving the lives of our courageous soldiers. Additionally, the belt features an alarm button that, when activated, alerts the base unit of the soldier's need for assistance. The information transmitted from the device to the mobile, acting as the central unit, includes:

Soldier's name
Unique ID assigned by the base
Soldier's temperature
Soldier's heartbeat
Soldier's precise location in latitude and longitude coordinates

The device transmits data automatically without needing soldier input. However, if the soldier chooses to send data manually, the same message format is used. Figure 6 illustrates the system's proposed functionality.

6 Conclusion

Once implemented, this framework will monitor soldiers' health by tracking heart rate and body temperature, and determine their location using GPS or GSM modems. These modems transmit vital data to a base station, supporting timely decisions and emergency response. Designed for use in both wartime and rescue missions, the system integrates easily without logistical issues. By leveraging GPS and GSM, it significantly improves soldier safety and operational support.

7 Future Scope

The proposed system offers several avenues for future enhancement. Incorporating gyroscopes and accelerometers could enable AI-driven activity recognition, while adding blood pressure and electrodermal sensors may help detect distress in soldiers. Improved steering algorithms can enhance reliability and energy efficiency. Ubiquitous processing blending physical and digital systems would provide a complete view of a soldier's condition without overwhelming them with devices.

Currently, group leadership is static; dynamic head selection algorithms could improve coordination. Power management is critical, especially in harsh environments. A shoe-embedded energy system using capacitors, transistors, and a dynamo can sustainably charge batteries during movement. In regions without mobile networks, High Altitude Platforms (HAPs), unmanned aircraft at 20 km altitude, can provide secure communication, networking, and remote sensing. Interest from companies like Google and Facebook highlights HAPs' potential for secure, remote connectivity.

References

1. Singh, J., Chahajed, A., Pandit, S., Weigh, S.: GPS and IOT based soldier tracking and health indication system. Int. Res. J. Eng. Technol. 2395–0056 (2019)
2. William Walker, A.L.. Aroul, P., Bhatia, D.: Mobile health monitoring systems. In: 31st Annual International Conference of the IEEE EMBS, Minneapolis, Minnesota, USA, pp. 5199–5202 (2009)

3. Pranav Sailesh, M., Vimal Kumar, C., Cecil, B., Mangal Deep B.M., Sivraj, P.: Smart soldier assistance using WSN. In: International Conference on Embedded Systems - (ICES 2014), pp. 244–249. IEEE (2014)
4. Gondalic, A., Dixit, D., Darashar, S., Raghava, V., Sengupta, A.: IoT based healthcare monitoring system for war soldiers using machine learning. In: International Conference on Robotics and Smart Manufacturing, vol. 289, pp. 323–467 (2018)
5. Mdhaffar, A., Chaari, T., Larbi, K., Jamaiel, M., Freisleben, B.: IoT based health monitoring via LoRaWAN. In: International Conference of IEEE EUROCON, vol. 115, no. 89, pp. 2567–2953 (2018)
6. Wararkar, P., Mahajan, S., Mahajan, A., Banerjee, A., Madankar, A., Sontakke, A.: Soldier tracking and health monitoring system. Int. J. Comput. Sci. Appl. **2**(02), 81–86 (2013)
7. Govindaraj, A., Sindhuja Banu, S.: GPS based soldier tracking and health indication system with environmental analysis. Int. J. Enhan. Res. Sci. Technol. Eng. **2**(12), 46–52 (2013)
8. Pramod, P.: GPS Based advanced soldier tracking with emergency messages & communication system. Int. J. Adv. Res. Comput. Sci. Manag. Stud. **2**(6), 25–32 (2014)
9. Limbu, R., Kale, V.V.: GPS based soldier tracking and health monitoring system. Int. J. Technol. Res. Eng. **1**(12), 1485–1488 (2014)
10. Kumar, P., Rasika, G., Patil, V., Bobade, S.: Health monitoring and tracking of soldier using GPS. Int. J. Res. Advent Technol. **2**(4), 291–294 (2014)
11. Sharma, S., Kumar, S., Keshari, A., Ahmed, S., Gupta, S., Suri, A.: A real time autonomous soldier health monitoring and reporting system using COTS available entities. In: Second International Conference on Advances in Computing and Communication Engineering (ICACCE), Deharadun, India, May 2015, pp. 683–687 (2015)
12. Kumar, R., Rajasekaran, M.: An IoT based patient monitoring system using raspberry Pi. In: International Conference on Computing Technologies and Intelligent Data Engineering, Kovilpatti, India, January 2016, pp. 1–4 (2016)
13. Shaikh, R.A., Nikilla, S.: Real time health monitoring system of remote patient using arm7. Int. J. Instrument. Control Autom. **1**(3–4), 102–105 (2012)
14. Kumar, D., Repal, S.: Real time tracking and health monitoring of soldiers using ZigBee technology: a survey. Int. J. Innov. Res. Sci. Eng. Technol. **4**(7), 5561–5574 (2015)
15. Raj, G., Banu, S.: GPS Based soldier tracking and health indication system with environmental analysis. Int. J. Enhan. Res. Sci. Technol. Eng. **2**(12), 46–52 (2013)
16. Ashok, V., Priyadarshini, T., Sanjana, S.: A secure freight tracking system in rails using GPS technology. OIn: Second International Conference on Science Technology Engineering and Management (ICONSTEM), Chennai, India, March 2016, pp. 47–50 (2016)
17. Nikam, S., Patil, S., Powar, P., Bendre, V.S.: GPS based soldier tracking and health indication system. Int. J. Adv. Res. Electr. Electron. Instrument. Eng. **2**(3), 1082–1088 (2013)
18. Shelar, S., Patil, N., Jain, M., Chaudhari, S., Hande, S.: Soldier tracking and health monitoring systems. In: Proceedings of 21st IRF International Conference, Pune India, pp. 82–87 (2015). ISBN: 978-93-82702-75-7
19. Jaiswar, D., Repal, S.S.: Real time tracking and health monitoring of soldiers using ZigBee technology: a survey. Int. J. Innov. Res. Sci. Eng. Technol. **4**(7), 5560–5574 (2015)
20. Lim, H.B., Ma, D., Wang, B., Kalbarczyk, Z., Iyer, R.K., Watkin, K.L.: A soldier health monitoring system for military applications. In: International Conference on Body Sensor Networks, pp. 246–249 (2010)
21. Pangavne, S.M., Sohanlal, C., Bhavik, P.: Real time soldier tracking system. IOSR J. Electron. Commun. Eng. (IOSR-JECE) 21–24 ((2015))
22. Chakravarth, P., Natarajan, S., AntoBennete, M.: GSM based soldier tracking system and monitoring using wireless communication. Department of Electronics and Communication (2017)

23. Armarkar, A.V., Deepika, J., Punekar, M., Kapse, P., Kumari, S., Shelka, J.: Soldier health and position tracking system. Department of ETC Engineering, vol. 7, no. 3 (2017)
24. Akshay, P., Balaji, S., Raju, P., Mirajkar, P.P.: GPS based soldier tracking and health monitoring. Department of ETC Engineering, vol. 40, no. 03 (2017)
25. Kurhe, P.S., Agrawal, S.S.: Real time tracking and health monitoring system of remote soldier using ARM 7. Int. J. Eng. Trends Technol. **4**(3), 311–315 (2013)
26. Raza, Z., Liaquat, K., Ashraf, S.: Monitoring of soldier health and transmition of secret codes. NFC instutation of engineering, vol. 8 (2017)

Wearable Acoustic and Vibration Sensing for Early Detection of Cardiovascular and Respiratory Diseases Using Machine Learning

Sunny Gupta(✉)

Qualcomm India Pvt. Ltd., Noida, UP 201305, India
sunngupt@qti.qualcomm.com

Abstract. Wearables are becoming a tool to gather and analyze human health data. They can enable real-time insights, especially when acoustics and vibration sensing are combined with machine learning algorithms.

This paper describes the development and application of wearable devices equipped with microphones, accelerometers, and gyroscopes for capturing acoustic signals and vibration of physiological activities. The paper also describes the signal processing methodologies, feature extraction, and deployment of machine learning algorithms such as Support Vector Machines (SVM), Neural Networks, and Decision Trees to analyze obtained data. The paper also describes how these technologies effectively monitor vital signs of Cardiovascular Diseases (CVD) or Respiratory Diseases. The results give wearable acoustic and vibration sensing systems unrealized potential for early disease detection, individual health recommendations, and performance optimizations.

Keywords: Wearable acoustics · Early Detection · Cardiovascular Diseases · Respiratory Diseases

1 Introduction

Cardiovascular diseases (CVDs) remain the leading cause of mortality globally, with early detection significantly improving treatment outcomes. Wearable technology, equipped with acoustic and vibration sensors, can continuously monitor vital signs, offering real-time insights into heart and respiratory function. This capability, when paired with machine learning models, has the potential to detect early symptoms of CVDs, such as arrhythmias, valve disorders, and other anomalies, well before clinical symptoms manifest.

This paper investigates the use of acoustic and vibration sensors in wearable devices and explores their effectiveness in diagnosing CVDs. We begin by introducing the key sensors—microphones, accelerometers, and gyroscopes—used to capture physiological data, followed by a discussion on signal processing techniques, including noise filtering

K. Atul et al. (Eds.): BodyNets 2024, LNICST 666, pp. 317–322, 2026.
https://doi.org/10.1007/978-3-032-16099-7_25

and feature extraction. We then implement machine learning algorithms—SVM, NN, and DT—to analyze the data, compare their performance, and discuss the implications of our findings.

2 Sensors for Acoustics and Vibration Monitoring

Wearable devices equipped with microphones, accelerometers, and gyroscopes are capable of capturing complex physiological signals related to cardiovascular and respiratory functions. **Sample Heading (Third Level).** Only two levels of headings should be numbered. Lower level headings remain unnumbered; they are formatted as run-in headings.

2.1 Microphones

Microphones in wearable devices capture sounds produced by the human body, such as heartbeats and respiratory sounds. These signals, when processed correctly, can provide valuable insights into cardiovascular and respiratory health. Heart sounds, for example, include the distinct "lub-dub" sound that indicates the closing of heart valves. Abnormal heart sounds, such as murmurs, can indicate underlying heart issues like valve defects or irregular heartbeats, both common indicators of CVDs.

For respiratory monitoring, microphones can capture breath sounds, including wheezing or crackles, which can be early signs of respiratory diseases like asthma or pneumonia. Wearables equipped with microphones can record these sounds continuously, providing a stream of data that can be analyzed for irregular patterns.

2.2 Accelerometers

Accelerometers are sensors that measure the acceleration forces acting on a device. In wearables, accelerometers help monitor body movement, but they can also detect vibrations associated with physiological processes. In cardiac monitoring, for instance, accelerometers can detect minute chest vibrations produced by the heart beating. This data can help identify anomalies in heart function, such as arrhythmias or diminished cardiac output, both early signs of heart failure. Accelerometers can also assist in tracking respiratory rates by detecting the rising and falling movements of the chest. By providing continuous tracking of these vibrations, accelerometers can give detailed data on breathing patterns, which can help in diagnosing respiratory conditions.

2.3 Gyroscopes

Gyroscopes, which measure angular velocity, complement accelerometers by capturing rotational movements of the body. While gyroscopes are primarily used for motion detection, they can also detect subtle vibrations in the body, aiding in the monitoring of physiological activities. The combination of data from gyroscopes and accelerometers enhances the overall accuracy of detecting subtle vibrations linked to heartbeats and breathing patterns.

3 Signal Processing Techniques

Signal processing is critical in wearable devices, where raw data captured by sensors often includes noise and irrelevant information. Before this data can be analyzed, it needs to be cleaned and preprocessed to extract meaningful insights. The steps involved in signal processing include **filtering**, **segmentation**, and **transformation**.

3.1 Filtering

Filtering is used to remove noise from sensor data. Wearables, due to their close contact with the body, can capture environmental noise and motion artifacts. For acoustic signals, noise from external environments (e.g., conversations, wind) needs to be filtered out to focus solely on the sounds produced by the body. Similarly, for accelerometer and gyroscope data, filtering techniques like **low-pass filtering** are applied to eliminate high-frequency noise and preserve the physiological signals of interest.

3.2 Segmentation

Once noise is reduced, the data needs to be divided into smaller, manageable segments for analysis. Segmentation involves breaking continuous data streams into time windows (e.g., one-second or five-second windows). Each window is then analyzed individually, which is crucial for real-time monitoring applications. For instance, heartbeats or breaths occurring within a specific time frame can be analyzed for abnormalities without processing the entire data stream.

3.3 Transformation

To fully understand the signals captured by wearables, data often needs to be transformed from its raw form into the frequency domain. Techniques such as Fast Fourier Transform (FFT) or Wavelet Transform can decompose time-domain signals into frequency components, providing deeper insights into periodic patterns or irregularities. For example, an abnormal heart rhythm might manifest as irregular spikes in the frequency domain, which can be picked up more easily than in the time domain.

4 Feature Extraction

Once the signal processing phase is complete, the next step is feature extraction. Feature extraction involves identifying and quantifying relevant patterns from the preprocessed data. The extracted features serve as inputs to machine learning algorithms, which use these features to classify, predict, or detect anomalies. These features can be classified into:

- Time-domain features refer to measurements derived directly from the raw sensor data over time. Common time-domain features include:

  Mean - The average value of the signal over a given time window.

Peak - The highest value within the signal, indicating maximum intensity.
Root Mean Square (RMS) - The quadratic mean of the signal, often used in vibration analysis.

For instance, heart rate variability (HRV) is a common time-domain feature extracted from accelerometer data. A decrease in HRV can be an early indicator of cardiovascular issues such as heart failure or arrhythmias.

- Frequency-domain features, on the other hand, are derived from the transformed data and provide insights into the periodic components of a signal. These include:

  Spectral Energy: The energy contained within specific frequency bands, is useful for identifying irregularities in heart or respiratory sounds.
  Dominant Frequency: The frequency at which the signal's energy is concentrated, which can indicate abnormal physiological activity.

For example, the frequency of breathing can be a critical indicator of respiratory health. An unusually high or low breathing frequency may indicate the presence of asthma, COPD, or other respiratory conditions.

- Time-frequency features combine both time and frequency information, making them particularly useful for signals that change over time. Wavelet Transform is often used to extract such features, providing a detailed picture of how the signal's frequency content evolves. This is particularly helpful in detecting transient abnormalities in heart sounds or respiratory patterns that may occur only sporadically

5 Machine Learning Models and Practical Implementation

To classify the physiological data into normal and abnormal categories, we implemented three machine learning models: Support Vector Machine (SVM), Neural Network (NN), and Decision Tree (DT). Each model was trained using a dataset of labeled physiological signals, with features extracted from time and frequency domains.

5.1 Dataset

The dataset consisted of real-world physiological signals (heart and respiratory data) captured using microphones, accelerometers, and gyroscopes from wearable devices. The signals were preprocessed, segmented, and labeled as normal or abnormal based on clinical diagnosis.

5.2 Model Implementation

1. Support Vector Machine (SVM): A linear SVM was trained on the extracted features to classify the data into normal and abnormal categories.
2. Neural Network (NN): A multilayer perceptron (MLP) with one hidden layer of 100 neurons was used for the classification task.
3. Decision Tree (DT): A decision tree classifier was trained to make binary decisions based on the features extracted from the data.

6 Results and Comparison

The performance of the three models was evaluated using accuracy, precision, recall, and F1-score. The following table presents the results (Table 1):

Table 1. Table captions should be placed above the tables.

Algorithm	Accuracy	Precision	Recall	F1-Score	Training Time (s)	Inference Time (ms)
SVM	89.5	88.3	90.2	89.2	4.2	2.1
Neural Network	92.1	91.7	92.5	92.1	12.3	4.7
Decision Tree	86.7	85.4	88.1	86.7	0.8	1.9

7 Discussion of Results

- Neural Networks (NN): The neural network model outperformed SVM and DT, achieving the highest accuracy (92.1%) and F1-score (92.1%). This shows that NN is more effective at capturing the complex patterns present in the physiological data, making it ideal for early disease detection in wearable applications.
- SVM: SVM demonstrated competitive performance with an accuracy of 89.5% and an F1-score of 89.2%. Although not as effective as NN, SVM is a simpler model with faster inference time, making it suitable for real-time applications where immediate predictions are necessary
- Decision Tree (DT): While DT had the fastest training and inference times, it achieved the lowest accuracy (86.7%). The rule-based nature of DT makes it less capable of handling the noisy, complex data produced by wearable sensors, leading to lower classification performance.

8 Discussion of Results

Wearable devices equipped with acoustic and vibration sensors, when combined with machine learning algorithms, offer significant potential for the early detection of cardiovascular and respiratory diseases. Neural networks, in particular, showed superior performance in accurately classifying physiological signals. However, simpler models like SVM and decision trees may still be useful in real-time applications due to their faster inference times.

Future work should focus on improving the robustness of these models, incorporating additional sensor data (e.g., electrocardiograms), and addressing challenges such as sensor accuracy and data privacy. The continuous improvement of wearable technology, alongside advancements in machine learning, will play a critical role in the future of healthcare diagnostics.

References

1. World Health Organization. (2021). Cardiovascular diseases (CVDs). https://www.who.int/news-room/fact-sheets/detail/cardiovascular-diseases-(cvds)
2. Harnie, D., Rudd, J., Johnston, W., et al.: Wearable sensors for cardiovascular health: models and data analysis techniques. Sensors **21**(16), 5479 (2021). https://doi.org/10.3390/s21165479
3. Zhang, Y., Wang, L., Zhang, H., et al.: Heart sound classification based on feature extraction of time-frequency domain and convolutional neural networks. J. Healthcare Eng. **2020** (2020). https://doi.org/10.1155/2020/6235607
4. Rajput, D.S., Basha, S.M., Raja, G., et al.: Machine learning models for cardiovascular disease prediction. J. King Saud Univ. Comput. Inf. Sci. (2022). https://doi.org/10.1016/j.jksuci.2022.06.011
5. Arora, V., Nanda, S.: A comprehensive study of decision tree algorithms and its applications. Int. J. Comput. Appl. **975**(8887), 8–11 (2020). https://doi.org/10.5120/ijca2020919950
6. Jarchi, D., Salvi, D., Tarassenko, L., Clifton, D.A.: Accelerometry-based estimation of respiratory rate using machine learning techniques (2018)

AI and Machine Learning

A Low-Overhead CNN-Based Approach for Sleep Posture Recognition with Device-Free Monitoring Using UWB Radar

Braj Kishore Jha[1], Mohammad Faizan Siddiqui[1], Amit Anand[1], Abhishek Pathak[2], Ivan Fedosov[3], and Ankur Pandey[1](✉)

[1] Rajiv Gandhi Institute of Petroleum Technology, Jais, Amethi, India
{brajkj23ee,22ec3025,22cs2018,apandey}@rgipt.ac.in
[2] Department of Neurology, Institute of Medical Sciences, BHU, Varanasi, India
[3] Institute of Physics, Saratov State University Astrakhanskaya, Saratov, Russia

Abstract. The advancements in wireless technologies, artificial intelligence (AI), the internet of bio-nano things (IoBNT), and integrated electronic circuits have revolutionized the healthcare sector. Traditional device-based healthcare monitoring practices demand wearable or implantable sensing devices, with associated risks and drawbacks. An alternative safer approach involves leveraging device-free technologies. Acknowledging the significance of sleep monitoring in assessing a subject's health, in the proposed work, we introduce a Convolutional Neural Network (CNN)-based architecture for the classification of sleep-posture transition. Our approach integrates signal processing techniques with deep learning (DL) to enhance performance, achieving a promising sleep-posture recognition accuracy of **77.56%** without data augmentation on publicly available datasets demonstrating superior performance over existing state-of-the-art methods. This reduces the computational overhead of the proposed method. Moreover, after employing data augmentation techniques, the classification performance increases to **83.03%** outperforming other methods.

Keywords: Ultra-Wideband (UWB) radar · Deep Learning (DL) · Artificial Intelligence (AI) · Wireless Body Area Network (WBAN) · Internet of Bio-Nano Things (IoBNT)

1 Introduction

The recent pandemic has exerted tremendous strain on healthcare systems worldwide, pushing them beyond their limits, such that the challenges that have plagued the healthcare infrastructure for a long time have come into the limelight. This necessitated the paradigm shift in our healthcare ecosystem. Innovations in bio-nano materials have enabled targeted drug delivery. It has enhanced

K. Atul et al. (Eds.): BodyNets 2024, LNICST 666, pp. 325–336, 2026.
https://doi.org/10.1007/978-3-032-16099-7_26

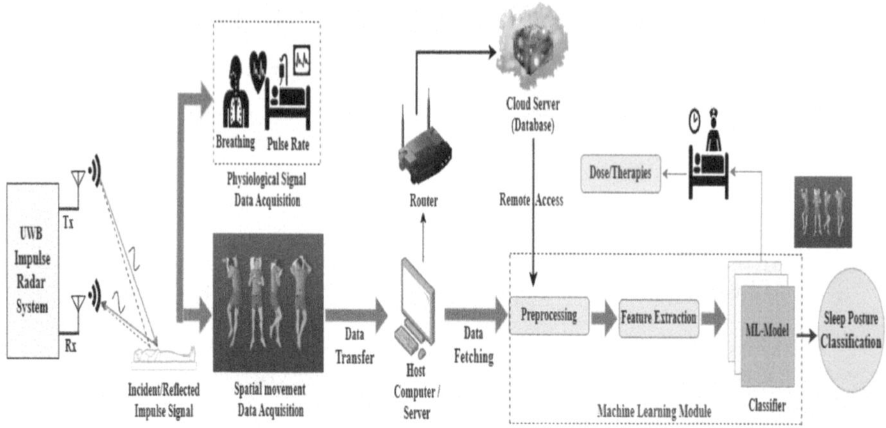

Fig. 1. Overview of the healthcare monitoring using UWB radar.

the accuracy of imaging techniques and has led to the development of biosensors that can identify disease biomarkers in minuscule concentrations. With AI-driven wireless technology, these sensors can monitor vital signs in real time, supporting proactive healthcare. Miniaturized integrated circuits further make these devices compact and efficient allowing for minimally invasive, continuous health tracking. The advancements in wireless sensor networks (WSN), micro-electromechanical systems (MEMS), metamaterials and cutting-edge deep learning technologies have further enhanced real-time and remote monitoring of patients [1]. Several device-based solutions have been proposed that record features such as heart rate, breathing rate, saturation level of oxygen and can be extended for human activity recognition, vital sign monitoring, and sleep stage estimation [2]. Despite remarkable classification accuracy, misplacement and motion artifacts reduce system performance. The costly installation of devices and their vulnerability to manual error has impeded their widespread deployment in real-world scenarios [3]. Adding to these, wearable devices reduce mobility, cause inconvenience, and can be invasive, thus setting the stage for device-free setup [4]. Thus, spotlight has shifted from device-based solutions to technology-driven, device-free approaches.

Today, considerable factions of world population are suffering from diseases somewhat correlated with one or the other type of sleep disorders. Sleep disorders affect the duration and quality of sleep, leading to a deterioration in both mental and physical health and thus serve as proven biometrics for several diseases [5]. The categories such as insomnia, breathing disorders, circadian rhythm sleep-wake disorders, and parasomnias are most common. Whereas, chronic insomnia, narcolepsy, and obstructive sleep apnea are common types of sleep disorders leading to diseases such as Type 2 diabetes, heart attack, dementia, and other cardiovascular diseases [6]. Diagnosing sleep disorders requires monitoring spatial movements of the body parts and breathing patterns, as both vary and distinguish different disorder types [7]. For instance, continuous sleep monitoring can prevent diseases like pressure ulcers in bedridden patients [8], and breath monitoring is essential to stop the spreading of infectious disease [9]. Vital signs and sleep monitoring are generally the first step of every medical examination. It ensures early diagnosis and prediction of diseases and thus facilitates the intervention of medical professionals in time.

This motivates us to introduce a contactless sleep monitoring system based on deep learning, which leverages impulse signals transmitted by UWB radar. The overview of the proposed method for sleep monitoring using UWB radar is shown in Fig. 1. The influence of bodily movement during sleep and respiratory patterns on surrounding wireless signals can be exploited for monitoring purposes. The radars measure changes in phase between the RF waves reflected by a moving object and the waves that were initially transmitted. Sleep monitoring involves the identification of posture transitions and the monitoring of vital signs. Radars detect vital signs by measuring how the phase of reflected signals is modulated by the movements of the body surface during heart and lung activities [10]. The acquired physiological signals and spatial movement data are transferred to the local host or cloud server for real-time access and remote access respectively. The data are retrieved from the server, preprocessed, and features are extracted before being fed into the deep learning model for classifying postural transitions.

1.1 Related Work

Camera-based surveillance [11] offers good monitoring but, at the cost of the subject's privacy. Additionally, the lighting, line-of-sight operation requirements, and infrastructure installation cost hinder its mass deployment [7]. The authors of [12], demonstrated a Tablet-PC-based vital sign information collection framework using wireless sensing devices and scanners. The collected data were transmitted and stored in a database server using a wireless local area network (WLAN). In [13], the author proposed a portable vital sign monitoring model using a wireless sensor network (WSN) based on a global system for mobile communication (GSM) technology. A study by [3] showcased a wireless monitoring system (Wi-Mon) using WBAN designed specifically for monitoring dengue patients. The framework achieved comparable results to that recorded by sophisticated machines. The study by [10], introduces a versatile wireless system for monitoring vital signs, utilizing microwave metamaterials and Doppler radar technology. It effectively senses respiration and heart activity through clothing, with good validation results against that recorded through an electrocardiogram device.

The Wi-Fi signal's received signal strength (RSS) and channel state information (CSI) have also been used for monitoring purposes [14]. The inability of RSS to capture fine-grained movements has shifted the focus of researchers toward utilizing CSI data of wifi [15]. Despite notable advancements in Wi-Fi-based methods, the limited availability of publicly accessible CSI datasets poses an additional challenge for researchers.

By comparing the phase of reflected radio waves to the transmitted signal, radars can identify shifts caused by the movement of an object. In the region between transmitter and receiver, alteration in amplitude, and phase shift is observed due to the presence or movement of surrounding object. These variations in signal behavior can be exploited to capture any spatial movement for monitoring purposes. Several studies proposed radar-based methods for sleep and vital sign monitoring [16–19]. In [20], the authors introduced a CW radar-based system for monitoring sleep, utilizing various handcrafted features that were fed to multiple machine learning (ML) classifiers. Due to the absence of range data and the challenges posed by multi-path interference in CW and FMCW radar, researchers have turned their attention to UWB radar. UWB radar is better suited for indoor applications because it can mitigate multi-path interference and provides high-resolution range information. The authors of [21], developed a UWB-based approach for human activity classification, in which signal spectrograms were fed to a deep convolutional neural network (DCNN) to extract features and perform classification. Specifically, the authors of [7] used UWB radar to classify various sleep postures by employing a multiview learning model along with data augmentation techniques. In [22], a time-reversal technique was deployed to estimate the breathing rate of multiple people.

The classical ML approach needsdomain expertise and manual feature extraction increases time complexities. This work presents a deep learning model aimed at improving the discriminatory capability and thus enhancing the classification accuracy. We show how the pattern learning ability of CNNs is efficiently utilized to classify various sleep postures when impulse signals from UWB radar are provided as input. Table 1 presents a brief comparison of our proposed method with the existing state-of-the-art methods.

Table 1. Comparison of the Proposed method with Existing state-of-the-art methods

Author	Methodology	Device	Accuracy
Maytus P. et al. [7]	CNN-based multiview learning	UWB radar	Medium
H. Hong et al. [20]	K-NN	CW radar	High
Chen et al. [21]	DCNN	UWB radar	High
Jesus A, Gracia et al. [14]	K-NN, SVM, QDC	Wifi-CSI	High
This work	**CNN**	**UWB radar**	**High**

QDC = Quadratic Discriminant Classifier, SVM = Support Vector Machine, K-NN = K-nearest neighbours, CNN = Convolutional Neural Network

1.2 Contributions

In this work, we propose a deep learning model that focuses on learning intricate features such as signal characteristics and behavior variations caused due to spatial movement during sleep monitoring. Our contributions include the following:

- The proposed method achieves superior performance compared to existing state-of-the-art methods in sleep and vital sign monitoring without employing any data augmentation method. Thus saving on computational cost and facilitating edge device deployment.
- Our proposed CNN-based architecture is deep and highly parameterized, it remains lightweight in terms of resource usage and time complexity.

2 Proposed Sleep Monitoring Methodology

2.1 Dataset Description

The data was collected using Xethru X4M03 commercial-grade UWB radar [7]. The dataset is divided in two sessions: Session 1 captures participants' recordings with all surrounding objects remaining still, while Session 2 involves recordings with moving objects. Each of the 12 participants performed 4 sleep postural transitions, repeating them 6 times. Participants were also asked to engage in other activities without altering their sleep position. In total, 816 samples were collected, with each sample containing a single postural transition. The dataset is publicly available at https://github.com/IoBT-VISTEC/SleepPoseNet.

2.2 Preprocessing

Once the signals are sampled, they are stored in a matrix R with dimensions $M \times N$, where M = 180 corresponds to the fast-time indices (range bins) and N = 160 to the slow-time indices. DC noise may be present in the data for each range bin index and can be removed by computing the average value across all slow-time indices. At a given instant, data includes both unrelated objects and the active target that is patients. To minimize the effect of irrelevant objects, we subtract the average value from the fast time dimension at each slow time index. Thus, both DC and background suppression are performed before feature extraction.

2.3 Feature Extraction

In this work, both time as well as frequency domain features of radar signals are extracted and utilized for model training. Assuming that all surrounding irrelevant objects are fixed and their shape is constant with time. The Time Difference (TD) involves taking differentiation along the slow time axis, capturing information specifically from moving humans. The UWB radar used has a range step size of 5.14 cm, utilizing 40 bins to cover a 2-meter range, ensuring full-body data capture. Various positions of the cropping window are selected between initial and final range bins so that the total energy of the slow-time differences in the window reaches its maximum. The cropped signal is stored in a matrix. Weighted Range-Time-Frequency Transform (WRTFT) merges spectrograms across fast-time indices by segmenting the time series and applying the Short-Time Fourier transform (STFT). These spectrograms are weighted by the energy of each fast-time index and saved in a matrix.

2.4 Data Augmentation

Firstly, we evaluate the model without data augmentation. Further, we augment the data using four augmentation techniques to make our model more robust and generalized. The time shifting (TS), range shifting (RS), time warping (TW), and magnitude warping (MW) techniques are applied to augment available data. Shifting the slow time index helps the model learn an SPT section in different positions. TS parameters are $[-10, -5, 5, 10]$, with positive and negative values indicating right and left shifts, and zero-padding for the extension section. Each sample's range bins represent body parts, and RS helps learn range position variations. RS parameters are $[2, 4]$, shifting the bins upward, with zero-padding for extensions. TW involves smoothing and randomly distorting intervals between slow time indices, and adjusting their temporal locations. Missing values are interpolated using cubic splines, with a variance parameter of 0.4 for interval distortion. Finally, MW involves generation of a random smooth curve, fluctuating around one, and each sample is scaled by this curve to introduce random amplitude changes across slow time positions. A variance parameter of 0.4 is applied, representing the degree of variation around one in the curve. Our architecture demonstrates better classification accuracy upon data augmentation.

2.5 Proposed Architecture for Sleep Monitoring

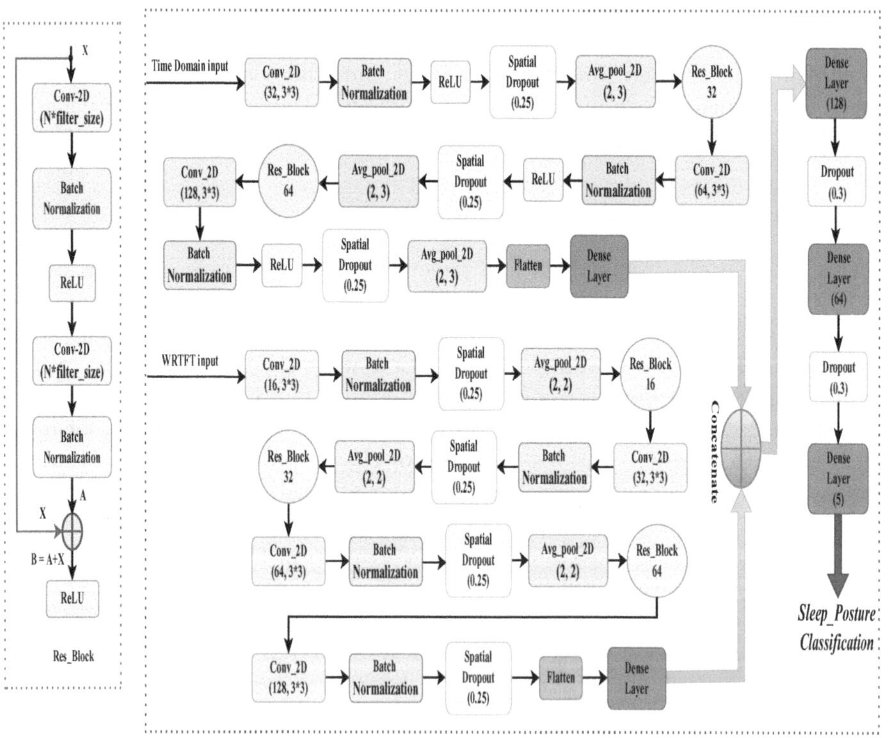

Fig. 2. The Architecture of the proposed CNN-based model for sleep monitoring.

The architecture proposed in Fig. 2 comprises two blocks: the Time Domain (TD) block and the Weighted Range-Time-Frequency Transform (WRTFT) block. The TD block comprises of three Conv2D layers, each followed by batch normalization, ReLU, spatial dropout, and average pooling layers respectively. The output of the average pooling layer is fed to the residual layer before feeding it directly to the subsequent Conv2D layer. The residual layers improve the training of deep networks by enabling better gradient flow, through skip connection, which allows for deeper and more complex models to be trained effectively. Each subsequent Conv2D layer applies twice the number of filters to learn increasingly complex patterns in the data. The batch normalization layer stabilizes and accelerates training by normalizing activations, which enhances gradient flow and speeds up convergence. The ReLU layer introduces non-linearity into the model and facilitates efficient training. The spatial dropout layer is to reduce overfitting by randomly dropping entire feature maps during training. The average pooling layer downsamples the data and extracts the most salient features. The output of the last average pooling layer is flattened to a 1D vector by flattening layer so that it can be fed to the dense layer.

The WRTFT block of our model is deeper than the work in [7], due to the addition of two more Conv2D layers, making it four in total. Each Conv2D block is followed by batch normalization, spatial dropout, and average pooling layer serving the same purpose as in the TD block. In a similar fashion, the number of filters applied doubles in subsequent Conv2D layers. The residual, flatten, and dense layer is positioned the same way as in the TD block.

The output features from the dense layer of both the blocks are fused together before they are fed to the series of three dense layers. To avoid overfitting, the output from the first two dense layers after concatenation is subjected to a dropout layer with a rate of 0.3. The rate of the spatial dropout layers in both TD and WRTFT blocks is kept at 0.25. For training the model, we have used Adam optimizer with a learning rate of 0.0001. As our model performs multi-class classification, sparse categorical cross-entropy loss is used as the loss function.

3 Results

We propose a deep CNN-based architecture for the multiclass classification task. The five sleep classes are Supine side, Supine prone, Side supine, Prone supine, and Background respectively. CNN is capable of identifying complex patterns of variations in signal behavior and characteristics on account of any bodily movement while sleeping. The extracted features in time and frequency domain were properly fed to the CNN model. The average accuracy achieved for 1000 epochs is **77.56%** for 10-fold cross-validation without data augmentation and **83.03%** for 5-fold cross-validation for 100 epochs with augmentation in our case. Our method demonstrates better performance even without augmentation, resulting in saved computational time and resources. When augmentation is applied, it further enhances generalization and robustness.

Table 2. Comparison of the validation accuracy of the Proposed method with different set of parameters

CV-Folds	No. of Epochs	Augmentation	AvgValAccuracy(%)
12	100	Yes	80.39
12	1000	No	76.41
10	100	Yes	81.93
10	1000	No	**77.56**
5	100	Yes	**83.03**
5	1000	No	76.86

Notes: CV = Cross Validation, AvgValAccuracy = Average validation accuracy

Table 3. Statistical Analysis of the proposed model with augmentation

Type	Precision	Recall	F1-score
Supine side	0.73	0.78	0.75
Supine prone	0.68	0.65	0.67
Side supine	0.86	0.85	0.85
Prone supine	0.85	0.82	0.84
Background	0.91	0.95	0.93

In this section, we have examined our CNN-based model on metrics such as Accuracy, Precision, Recall, and F1-score. We have used both sessions of the dataset. We have evaluated our model using 5, 10, and 12-fold cross-validation methods. The model achieves an **average test accuracy** of $78.86 \pm 6.9\%$ and $75.95 \pm 2.1\%$ on **Session 1 and Session 2** of the dataset respectively, using 6-fold cross-validation. The comparison of the **average validation accuracy** with different numbers of folds, and epochs, with and without data augmentation is shown in Table 2.

3.1 Statistical Analysis

In this work, the aim is to classify the various sleep postures transition categories. To examine our method, we use the standard evaluation parameters such as precision, recall, accuracy, and F1-score. The values of all four metrics are calculated using the values in the Normalized Confusion Matrix shown in Fig. 3. The calculated mean values for precision, Recall, and F1-score are 0.806, 0.81, and 0.808 respectively. Table 3 shows the comparison of precision, recall, and F1-score values for all the five classes in our classification task.

Figure 4a illustrates the convergence of Training and Validation loss with an increase in the number of epochs signifying model's ability to learn from the training data and generalize to unseen data. Figure 4b, illustrates the decreased time complexity in proposed method as compared to [7], as the latter used four augmentation techniques, each consuming $O(n^2)$ time.

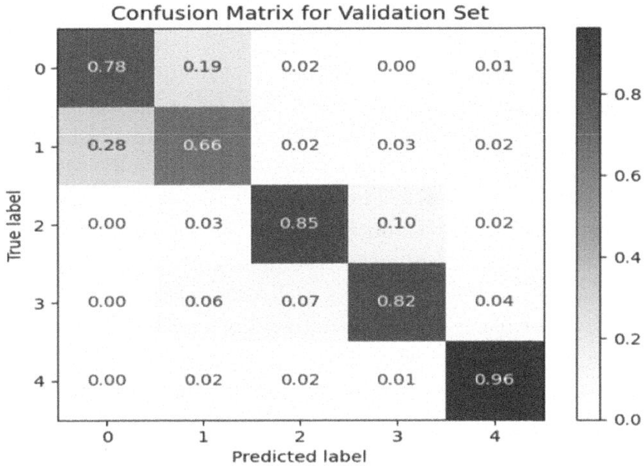

Fig. 3. Normalized Confusion Matrix for Sleep Postural Transition classification.

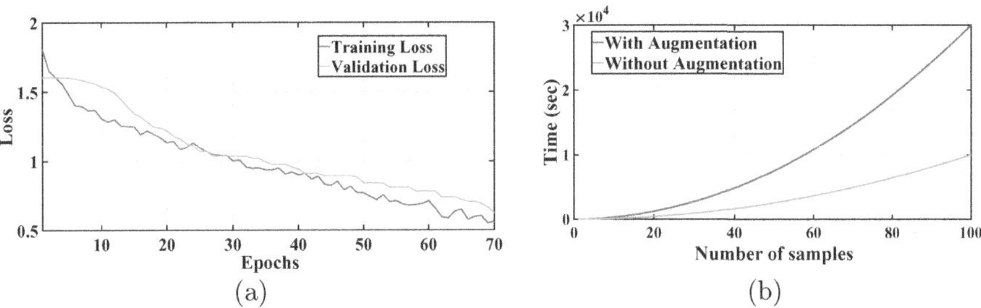

Fig. 4. Illustration of convergence of Training and Validation Loss with epochs.

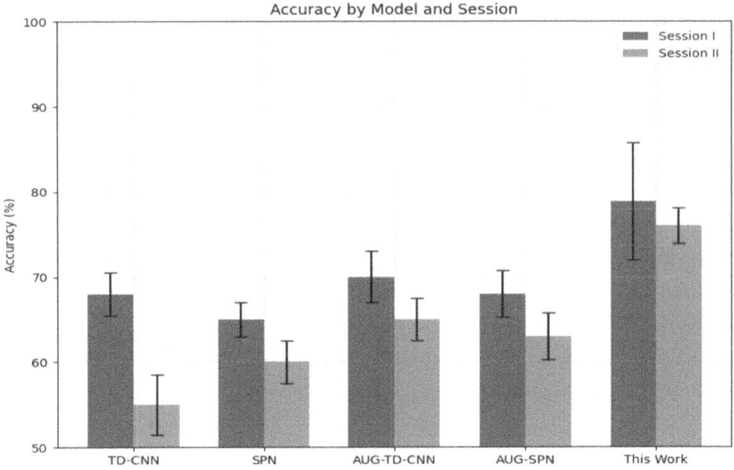

Fig. 5. Comparison of the accuracy and standard error of the proposed model with state-of-the-art models.

3.2 Comparison with the Existing State-of-the-Art Methods

Figure 5 shows the comparison of the average test accuracy of the existing state-of-the-art methods with our proposed work. The two existing approaches, under consideration are Time-Difference Convolutional Neural Network (TD-CNN) and SleepPoseNet (SPN), both without augmentation and with augmentation (AUG-TD-CNN and AUG-SPN). The average test accuracy is for 6-fold cross-validation, across both Session 1 and Session 2. Although the margin of error for Session 1 is relatively higher compared to our model's performance in Session 2, it is important to note that our model still outperforms the current state-of-the-art methods in terms of accuracy across both sessions. This demonstrates that despite the increased loss in session 1, our model achieves superior accuracy compared to existing approaches, highlighting its effectiveness and overall performance.

4 Challenges and Future Directions

Acknowledging the importance of decision-making in the medical field and the reliance of healthcare professionals on ML-based models, it is essential to develop a more generalized and accurate model before deploying it on devices. Effective sleep posture monitoring is key to diagnosing sleep disorders in which posture affects symptom severity. Device-free monitoring improves elderly and rehabilitation care by allowing caregivers to respond to posture-related risks, such as falls promptly. Despite our method shows better performance in the classification task, the aliasing effect of multiple respiratory signals can degrade its performance. Device-free sleep monitoring of multiple patients simultaneously is still a challenging task. If the breathing rates of multiple person are close to each other then the estimation may fail. Time reversal technique and analysis in doppler, angle-of-arrival (AoA), and other domains can be deployed to estimate the breathing rate of multiple person simultaneously. The transfer learning approach can be used to make the model more robust and generalized.

5 Conclusion

In this work, we propose a CNN-based method using impulse signal from low-cost commercial-grade UWB radar, for multi-class classification among five sleep postures, achieving an accuracy of **77.56%** without data augmentation. With augmentation, the accuracy increases to **83.03%**. This work also illustrates the superior performance of the proposed method as compared with existing state-of-the-art models. The higher accuracy without any augmentation technique enhances the on-device deployability of the proposed method. Future work includes the implementation of a transfer learning and exploration of other data augmentation approaches for building a more robust and generalized model to handle real-time cases for remote health monitoring systems.

References

1. Catherwood, P.A., Steele, D., Little, M., Mccomb, S., Mclaughlin, J.: A community-based IoT personalized wireless healthcare solution trial. IEEE J. Transl. Eng. Health Med. **6**, 1–13 (2018)
2. Sun, X., Qiu, L., Wu, Y., Tang, Y., Cao, G.: Sleepmonitor: monitoring respiratory rate and body position during sleep using smartwatch. In: Proceedings of the ACM on Interactive, Mobile, Wearable and Ubiquitous Technologies, vol. 1, no. 3, pp. 1–22 (2017)
3. Nubenthan, S., Shalomy, C.: A wireless continuous patient monitoring system for dengue: Wi-Mon. In: 2017 6th National Conference on Technology and Management (NCTM), pp. 23–27. IEEE (2017)
4. Choksatchawathi, T., et al.: Improving heart rate estimation on consumer grade wrist-worn device using post-calibration approach. IEEE Sens. J. **20**(13), 7433–7446 (2020)
5. Yousefi, R., et al.: Bed posture classification for pressure ulcer prevention. In: Annual International Conference of the IEEE Engineering in Medicine and Biology Society, vol. 2011, pp. 7175–7178 (2011)
6. Drager, L.F., McEvoy, R.D., Barbe, F., Lorenzi-Filho, G., Redline, S.: Sleep apnea and cardiovascular disease: lessons from recent trials and need for team science. Circulation **136**(19), 1840–1850 (2017)
7. Piriyajitakonkij, M., et al.: SleepPoseNet: multi-view learning for sleep postural transition recognition using UWB. IEEE J. Biomed. Health Inform. **25**(4), 1305–1314 (2020)
8. Lyder, C.H.: Pressure ulcer prevention and management. JAMA **289**(2), 223–226 (2003)
9. Atif, M., Muralidharan, S., Ko, H., Yoo, B.: COVID-beat: a low-cost breath monitoring approach for people in quarantine during the pandemic. J. Comput. Des. Eng. **9**(3), 992–1006 (2022)
10. Nguyen, D.T., Zeng, Q., Tian, X., Ho, J.S.: Non-contact vital sign monitoring with a metamaterial surface. In: IEEE MTT-S International Microwave Biomedical Conference (IMBioC), vol. 2022, pp. 37–39. IEEE (2022)
11. Deng, F.: Design and implementation of a noncontact sleep monitoring system using infrared cameras and motion sensor. IEEE Trans. Instrum. Meas. **67**(7), 1555–1563 (2018)
12. Chan, Y.-S., Liang, H.-J., Lin, Y.-H.: Using wireless measuring devices and Tablet PC to improve the efficiency of vital signs data collection in hospital. In: IEEE International Symposium on Bioelectronics and Bioinformatics (IEEE ISBB 2014), vol. 2014, pp. 1–4. IEEE (2014)
13. Deshmukh, V., Wagh, S.: A proposed architectural model for vital sign monitoring system. In: 2015 International Conference on Communications and Signal Processing (ICCSP), pp. 1758–1762. IEEE (2015)
14. Armenta-Garcia, J.A., Gonzalez-Navarro, F.F., Caro-Gutierrez, J., Galaviz-Yanez, G., Ibarra-Esquer, J.E., Flores-Fuentes, W.: Mining Wi-Fi channel state information for breathing and heart rate classification. Pervasive Mob. Comput. **91**, 101768 (2023)
15. Liu, J., Liu, H., Chen, Y., Wang, Y., Wang, C.: Wireless sensing for human activity: a survey. IEEE Commun. Surv. Tutorials **22**(3), 1629–1645 (2019)
16. Shyu, K.-K., Chiu, L.-J., Lee, P.-L., Tung, T.-H., Yang, S.-H.: Detection of breathing and heart rates in UWB radar sensor data using FVPIEF-based two-layer EEMD. IEEE Sens. J. **19**(2), 774–784 (2018)

17. Ding, C., Hong, H., Zou, Y., Chu, H., Zhu, X., Fioranelli, F., Le Kernec, J., Li, C.: Continuous human motion recognition with a dynamic range-doppler trajectory method based on FMCW radar. IEEE Trans. Geosci. Remote Sens. **57**(9), 6821–6831 (2019)
18. Fontana, R.J.: Recent system applications of short-pulse ultra-wideband (UWB) technology. IEEE Trans. Microw. Theory Tech. **52**(9), 2087–2104 (2004)
19. Zhang, C., Kuhn, M., Merkl, B., Fathy, A.E., Mahfouz, M.: Accurate UWB indoor localization system utilizing time difference of arrival approach. In: IEEE Radio and Wireless Symposium, vol. 2006, pp. 515–518. IEEE (2006)
20. Hong, H., Zhang, L., Gu, C., Li, Y., Zhou, G., Zhu, X.: Noncontact sleep stage estimation using a CW doppler radar. IEEE J. Emerg. Sel. Top. Circ. Syst. **8**(2), 260–270 (2018)
21. Chen, W., et al.: Non-contact human activity classification using DCNN based on UWB radar. In: 2019 IEEE MTT-S International Microwave Biomedical Conference (IMBioC), vol. 1, pp. 1–4 (2019)
22. Chen, C., Han, Y., Chen, Y., Liu, K.R.: Multi-person breathing rate estimation using time-reversal on WiFi platforms. In: 2016 IEEE Global Conference on Signal and Information Processing (GlobalSIP), pp. 1059–1063. IEEE (2016)

A Real-Time Driver Safety Assistance Proactive Accident Care Using Deep Learning and Attention Mechanisms

Shatakshi Saxena(✉), Angel(✉), Aaryaveer Gill(✉), and Shailendra Tiwari(✉)

Department of Computer Science and Engineering, Thapar Institute of Engineering and Technology, Patiala 147001, Punjab, India
{ssaxena1_be21,aangel_be21,agill_be21,shailendra}@thapar.edu

Abstract. Transport-related incidents cause $\tilde{1}$.25 million deaths annually worldwide, with driver drowsiness a major factor. In India, about 328,000 accidents yearly are attributed to drowsy driving. This paper presents a real-time driver drowsiness detection system using deep learning and attention mechanisms in Wireless Body Area Networks. The system compresses a heavy baseline model into a lightweight version using facial landmark key point detection. It employs ResNet50 for feature extraction, XAI techniques like GradCam, and a modified MobileNet with spatial attention. It uses transfer learning and considers multiple drowsiness indicators (head tilting, blinking, yawning) for robust detection across various conditions. Temporal factors are included to enhance prediction reliability. Experimental results show up to 98.4% accuracy, even with drivers wearing masks or glasses. This research demonstrates the potential of advanced driver assistance systems to reduce drowsy driving risks and improve road safety, hereby assisting in proactive accident care.

Keywords: Drowsiness · Spatial Attention · MobileNetV2 · Face detection · Deep Learning · Wireless Body Area Networks

1 Introduction

Drowsy driving is a significant and often underestimated contributor to road accidents, posing a substantial risk to public safety. Each year, approximately 328,000 crashes, 109,000 injuries, and 6,400 fatalities in India are attributed to drowsy driving, according to the latest study from the AAA Foundation for Traffic Safety [1]. While behaviors such as speeding, drinking, and distracted driving are widely recognized as dangerous, drowsy driving has only recently gained the attention it deserves. Most drowsy-driving incidents occur between midnight and 6 a.m. or during late afternoon hours when drivers are most prone to fatigue. Alarmingly, 1 in 25 drivers admits to fell asleep at the wheel, and

These authors contributed equally to this work.

K. Atul et al. (Eds.): BodyNets 2024, LNICST 666, pp. 337–354, 2026.
https://doi.org/10.1007/978-3-032-16099-7_27

driving after more than 20 h without sleep can impair performance as severely as having a blood alcohol concentration (BAC) of 0.08%, the legal limit for intoxication. Fatigue triples the likelihood of involvement in a car accident, and fatigue-related crashes resulting in injuries or fatalities cost over $109 billion annually, excluding property damage. Despite 96% of drivers acknowledging the dangers of drowsy driving, fewer than 30% believe they are at risk of being stopped for this behavior. These statistics underscore the urgent need for real-time, highly efficient, and accurate system of drowsiness detection models to enhance road safety and prevent fatigue-related accidents.

Recent advancements in driver drowsiness detection have leveraged various technological approaches. Notably, the integration of Wireless Body Area Networks (WBANs) offers a promising framework for continuous, real-time monitoring of driver alertness by utilizing a network of wearable sensors that communicate vital health and behavioral data to onboard vehicle systems or remote medical databases. Our research introduces advanced techniques for driver drowsiness detection, leveraging WBANs to create a seamless integration of wearable technology with deep learning algorithms. By employing a lightweight, modified MobileNet model, our solution enables efficient processing on devices with limited computational power, ensuring real-time performance within a WBAN framework. Trained on over 41,790 RGB images of size 227 $\times$ 227, our approach achieves superior accuracy and efficiency, addressing the critical need for reliable and non-intrusive detection systems. Our model effectively extracts relevant features such as the state of the eyes, mouth, and head tilt, incorporating time-varying signs of drowsiness. Additionally, our system is designed to maintain high accuracy even when drivers wear glasses or masks, a feature particularly relevant in the context of the COVID-19 pandemic. Henceforth, by integrating IoT and WBAN technologies, our method provides early warnings to drivers, helping to prevent unintended accidents. This study presents, compares, and evaluates various deep learning algorithms to identify the most promising approaches for detecting driver fatigue and drowsiness, establishing a robust framework for real-time applications within WBAN environments.

Once the drowsiness is detected, our proposed solution can be used for proactive accidental care. Depending on the severity of drowsiness, the system can trigger varying levels of alerts. Three distinct scenarios are identified based on the detected levels of drowsiness. In the case of low drowsiness, a mild alarm is triggered to prompt driver awareness. When the system detects medium drowsiness, a high-volume alert is initiated, indicating a need for increased caution. In instances of extreme drowsiness, the mobile app is activated for immediate intervention, ensuring prompt and necessary measures are taken to address the heightened risk. These tiered responses contribute to a proactive approach to mitigating the impact of driver drowsiness on road safety. If extreme drowsiness persists, the system activates the Mobile App. The app is automated to provide a last-call notification to the driver, allowing 5 to 10 s for the driver to respond and prevent potential accidents. If the alarm persists without intervention, the app promptly notifies local emergency services, including police, hospitals, and fire brigades, ensuring swift post-crash care and recovery. Thus, we can ensure real-time driver safety assistance care i.e., our Vahan Chakshu model using deep learning and attention mechanisms.

The remainder of the paper is structured as follows: Sect. 2 reviews related works in driver drowsiness detection, highlighting existing approaches and their limitations. Section 3 describes the methodology employed in our study, with a detailed account of the training and testing phases. In Sect. 4, we present the experimental setup and results, showcasing the performance of the proposed models. Section 5 offers a comprehensive analysis of the results, comparing our methods with recent advancements in the field. Finally, Sect. 6 concludes the paper and outlines future research directions, summarizing the essential findings and potential areas for further development.

2 Related Works

Numerous studies have been conducted to identify and mitigate driver drowsiness using various behavioral and physiological indicators. Facial signals like rapid and continuous blinking, head movements, and repeated yawning are critical indicators of drowsiness [2]. Computerized quasi-behavioral procedures are frequently employed to assess the amount of drowsiness in drivers by observing these unusual behaviors. Most research focusing on behavioral techniques emphasizes blinking [3–6] and PERCLOS [7–11], which measures the percentage of eyelid closure over the pupil over time. These studies aim to establish a drowsiness identification model that considers the varying impact of drowsiness on driving performance.

Several studies have used multiple facial expressions and ocular scans to identify signs of drowsiness [12–15]. In addition to blinking and PERCLOS, researchers have examined other behavioral indicators such as yawning [9], and head or eye position orientation to gauge the degree of drowsiness [19,22]. Magán et al. [20] proposed an Advanced Driver Assistance System (ADAS) that leverages sequences of images to detect drowsiness using recurrent and convolutional neural networks. Despite their innovative approach, the system achieved a modest 60% accuracy on test data, indicating room for improvement in detection precision. Similarly, Bekhouche et al. [21] explored the hybrid selection of deep features from video sequences to enhance detection accuracy, although integrating multiple features remains a complex challenge. Schwarz et al. [30] examined multi-sensor driver monitoring systems, combining data from various sensors to improve prediction reliability. Yet, these systems often face data synchronization and real-time processing issues. Jacobé de Naurois et al. [17] developed a model using artificial neural networks to detect and predict driver drowsiness. While this approach showed promise, it faced challenges in real-time applications due to computational demands and the necessity for extensive training data.

Stancin et al. [9] investigated using EEG signal features for drowsiness detection, demonstrating the potential for high accuracy but with significant practical limitations in non-intrusive implementation. This highlights the balance needed between accuracy and practicality in real-world applications. Quddus et al. [22] proposed using long short-term memory (LSTM) and convolutional neural networks (CNNs) for drowsiness detection, showing potential in analyzing temporal sequences of driver behavior. However, their models required substantial computational resources, which could limit real-time application. Jabbar and Shinoy [6] introduced a CNN-based model for Android applications, focusing on real-time monitoring but struggling with hardware constraints on mobile platforms, which affected processing speed and overall performance. Wijnands et al. [16] further explored real-time monitoring using 3D neural networks, achieving high accuracy but encountering challenges in processing speed and system integration, which are crucial for deployment in real-world settings.

Recent research has explored the integration of Wireless Body Area Networks (WBANs) in driver drowsiness detection systems, leveraging the capabilities of wearable sensors to provide continuous monitoring and real-time alerts. Movassaghi et al. [24] outlined the potential of WBANs in healthcare applications, highlighting their suitability for real-time physiological monitoring due to their low-power, lightweight, and non-intrusive nature. Building on this, Singh et al. [25] employed WBANs with electroencephalogram (EEG) sensors to monitor brain activity for drowsiness detection, achieving high sensitivity and specificity in detecting early signs of fatigue. Similarly, Choi et al. [26] utilized a hybrid approach that combines WBAN-based heart rate monitoring and facial feature extraction, enhancing the accuracy of drowsiness detection in real-time environments. Additionally, research by Oikonomou et al. [27] demonstrated the effectiveness of WBANs in continuously monitoring driver behaviors and physiological parameters, such as eye closure rate and heart rate variability, to detect drowsiness and provide timely interventions. These studies underscore the promise of WBANs in creating robust, scalable, and accurate drowsiness detection systems, particularly when integrated with advanced deep learning models to enhance data analysis and predictive capabilities.

In recent years, several studies have focused on enhancing driver safety and accident prevention through advanced technologies in intelligent transportation systems. Mishra et al. [32] explored accident-prone features in urban environments, offering a proactive approach to accident prevention by utilizing real-time sensing of urban places. Their work emphasizes the importance of identifying risky features in urban infrastructure for proactive driving. Similarly, Han et al. [33] proposed a novel approach using LSTM and Transformer models to evaluate real-time crash risk based on traffic flow and driver behavior data, demonstrating the effectiveness of deep learning techniques for predictive safety measures in dynamic driving environments. Koesdwiady et al. [34] provided a comprehensive review of recent trends in driver safety monitoring systems, identifying the key challenges and state-of-the-art technologies in vehicular safety, particularly in the use of sensors and machine learning for real-time monitoring. Additionally,

Qu et al. [35] conducted an in-depth analysis of driver behavior monitoring systems, leveraging computer vision and machine learning techniques, which have become central to understanding and mitigating risky driving behaviors.

3 Methodology

Our methodology begins by utilizing a compressed deep learning model built upon a lightweight network architecture that incorporates facial landmark key point detection. By leveraging a conglomeration of advanced deep learning techniques, such as a MobileNetV2 with a spatial attention mechanism and transfer learning, the model effectively captures multiple drowsiness indicators, including head tilting, blinking, and yawning.

3.1 Data Preprocessing

The data preprocessing commences by verifying labels and class names, ensuring each class (Drowsy and Non-Drowsy) is accurately represented, and counting occurrences to maintain a balanced dataset. Then pixel values are normalized to a standard range to enhance training efficiency and model performance, addressing variations in lighting conditions. Next, it is checked that all images had the correct RGB channels and conformed to the expected shapes (227×227 pixels for DDD and 640×480 pixels for NTHU), resizing or converting as necessary. These steps are crucial for preparing the data and ensuring its quality and consistency for efficient and accurate model training.

3.2 Deep Feature Extraction

To extract deep facial features from the datasets, a ResNet-50 model retrained on the Driver Drowsiness Dataset (DDD) [29] and the NTHU Drowsiness Dataset [28] is employed. ResNet-50, built on a residual learning framework, reformulates some layers to learn residual mappings rather than direct mappings between inputs and outputs. This model consists of 48 convolutional layers, one Max-Pooling layer, and one Global Average Pooling layer. The latter is crucial as it captures higher-level features from deeper layers, producing a 2048-dimensional output layer considered the feature vector of the input face image. The Grad-Cam method, used for generating spatial attention maps, visualizes the last activation ReLU layer before the average pooling layer. Applying Grad-Cam as in Fig. 2 to face images using ResNet-50 trained on the DDD and NTHU datasets confirms that this model provides more detailed facial information, which is crucial for accurate drowsiness detection (Fig. 1).

To obtain the spatiotemporal feature vector for each video sequence, an observation matrix is created, where each row represents the deep features (2048 dimensions) extracted from the corresponding frame. These features are then aggregated using two operations: mean and root mean square (RMS), which were experimentally determined to yield excellent performance. Two normalized

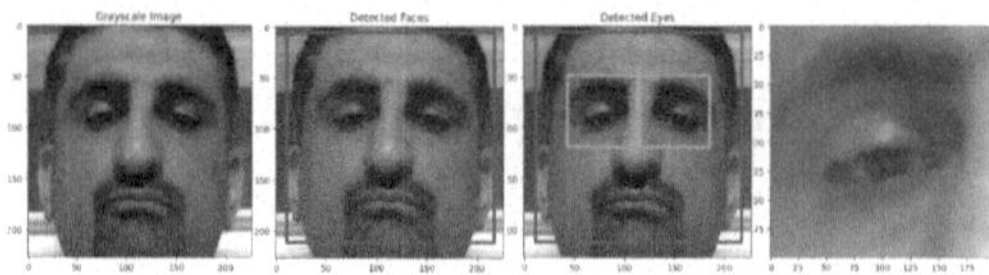

Fig. 1. Facial Features Extraction using ResNet-50 model.

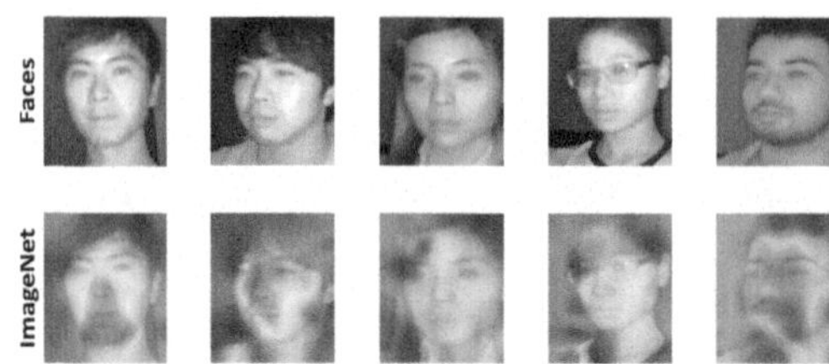

Fig. 2. Grad-CAM explanation maps for five face images are presented, with the predicted class for each face determined by the deep learning model [21].

vectors thus represent the temporal sequence of deep features concatenated into a single feature vector for the sequence. This process involves sampling frames and skipping specific frames within a sliding time window, typically set to process segments equivalent to 833 milliseconds of video. This approach ensures that decisions are frame-based and predictions can be made continuously by shifting the time window across frames, enabling real-time drowsiness detection.

3.3 Our Fine-Tuned Model

This section details the architecture and fine-tuning approach employed in our proposed model for driver drowsiness detection, focusing on enhancing feature extraction capabilities and integrating an efficient attention mechanism to improve classification accuracy. The architecture builds upon the MobileNet-V2 framework, a lightweight convolutional neural network (CNN) optimized for efficient image classification tasks, particularly on mobile and resource-constrained devices. The fine-tuning process incorporates additional layers to refine feature extraction and introduce a custom spatial attention module that emphasizes salient features while suppressing irrelevant information, thereby optimizing the model's overall performance.

MobileNet-V2, a variant of the MobileNet family, is selected due to its speed, computational efficiency, and ability to achieve high accuracy with minimal resources. The model is pre-trained on the ImageNet dataset [31], which provides a rich set of generic features learned from over a million images across 1,000 categories. This transfer learning approach allows the model to leverage these pre-learned features, thus accelerating convergence and enhancing the generalization capacity when adapted to a specific task.

For this, the pre-trained MobileNet-V2 model is fine-tuned on two dedicated datasets, the DDD and NTHU, which are tailored for driver drowsiness detection.

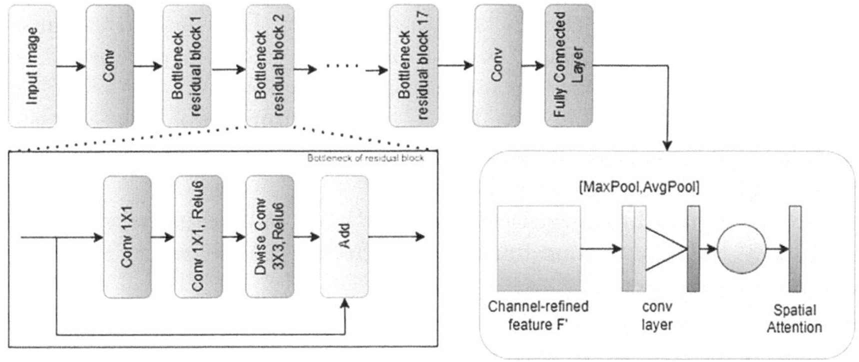

Fig. 3. Architecture of our proposed Modified MobileNetv2 in conglomeration with Spatial Attention Mechanism.

The initial layers of the MobileNet-V2, with an input shape of 224 × 224 × 3 and an alpha value of 0.75, are frozen to retain the generic features that are beneficial for the downstream task. The trainable parameters are confined to the newly added layers, which are specifically designed to adapt the model for driver drowsiness classification.

To enhance the model's feature extraction capabilities, a series of custom fine-tuned layers are appended to the base MobileNet-V2 architecture. The proposed architecture incorporates the following components:

1. **Global Average Pooling Layer (GAP):** The output of the MobileNet-V2 base model is initially passed through a Global Average Pooling (GAP) layer, which reduces the dimensionality of the feature maps by computing the average output of each feature map across its spatial dimensions. Formally, the output of the GAP layer can be expressed as:

$$x_{gap} = \frac{1}{H \times W} \sum_{i=1}^{H} \sum_{j=1}^{W} x_{ij} \tag{1}$$

where x_{ij} represents the activation at position (i, j), and H and W denote the height and width of the input feature map, respectively. This transformation condenses each feature map into a single value, preserving the most salient spatial information.

2. **Batch Normalization Layer:** Following the GAP layer, a Batch Normalization (BN) layer is applied to stabilize the learning process by normalizing the output activations to have zero mean and unit variance. This normalization can be represented mathematically as:

$$\hat{x} = \frac{x - \mu}{\sqrt{\sigma^2 + \epsilon}} \tag{2}$$

$$y = \gamma \hat{x} + \beta \tag{3}$$

where x is the input to the BN layer, μ and σ^2 are the mean and variance of the input activations, γ and β are learnable scale and shift parameters, and ϵ is a small constant added for numerical stability.

3. **Dense Layers with Leaky ReLU Activation:** Two fully connected (Dense) layers with non-linear activation functions are added to increase the model's capacity to learn complex patterns:
   - **First Dense Layer:** A Dense layer with 512 units is initialized, using a Leaky ReLU activation function to introduce non-linearity. The output can be expressed as:

$$f(x) = \begin{cases} x & if x \geq 0 \\ \alpha x & if x < 0 \end{cases} \tag{4}$$

   where α is a small constant (typically 0.01) to ensure that small negative values are allowed to pass through, mitigating the vanishing gradient problem.
   - **Dropout Layer:** To prevent overfitting, a Dropout layer with a dropout rate of 0.5 is applied, randomly setting 50% of the input units to zero during each update cycle while training. This process can be denoted as:

$$y_i = x_i \cdot Bernoulli(p) \tag{5}$$

   where $p = 0.5$ is the dropout rate, and $Bernoulli(p)$ represents a Bernoulli random variable that outputs 1 with probability p.
   - **Second Dense Layer:** Another Dense layer with 256 units and a Leaky ReLU activation function is incorporated, followed by another Dropout layer with the same configuration.
4. **Output Layer:** The final layer of the model is a Dense layer with 2 units and a softmax activation function to predict the probability distribution over the two target classes ("Drowsy" and "Non-Drowsy"). The output is given by:

$$softmax(z_i) = \frac{e^{z_i}}{\sum_j e^{z_j}} \tag{6}$$

   where z_i denotes the i-th logit corresponding to class i.

Integration of the Attention Module: To further refine the classification performance, a spatial attention module is integrated into the model architecture. This module enhances the feature extraction process by dynamically weighting salient spatial features and suppressing irrelevant ones, thereby improving the receptive field of the convolutional layers.

1. **Design of the Spatial Attention Module:** The spatial attention module is constructed with two dilated convolution layers and two 1×1 convolution layers. The dilated convolution layers are designed with dilation rates of 2 and 3, respectively, to maximize the receptive field while maintaining spatial

continuity of the feature semantics. The dilated convolution operation can be formally defined as:

$$F_i(x) = \sum_{m=1}^{K} \sum_{n=1}^{K} w_{m,n} \cdot x_{(i+d \cdot m, j+d \cdot n)} \tag{7}$$

where $F_i(x)$ represents the dilated convolution output at position i, $w_{m,n}$ is the filter weight at position (m, n), x is the input feature map, and d denotes the dilation rate. The dilated rates of 2 and 3 are chosen to strike a balance between increasing the receptive field and preserving spatial continuity.

2. **Calculation of the Receptive Field Size:** The actual receptive field size of the two dilated convolution layers is calculated iteratively. For the i-th layer, the receptive field size F_{i+1} is given by:

$$F_{i+1} = F_i + (K - 1) \cdot \prod_{j=1}^{i} S_j \tag{8}$$

where F_{i+1} is the receptive field of the current layer, F_i is the receptive field of the previous layer, S_j denotes the product of the step sizes of all preceding layers, and K is the convolution kernel size. For the proposed module, the effective receptive field size is calculated to be 12×12, denoted as $f_{12\times12}$.
3. **Attention Map Generation:** The output of the spatial attention module is represented by an attention map $\tilde{V}$, which is derived through a sigmoid activation function applied to the output of a 1×1 convolution operation on the dilated convolution output:

$$\tilde{V} = \sigma(A_{avg}) \tag{9}$$

where A_{avg} is defined as:

$$A_{avg} = Conv_{1\times1}(dilated\_conv) \tag{10}$$

and $\sigma(\cdot)$ denotes the sigmoid function, which ensures the attention weights are bounded between 0 and 1.

The inclusion of the spatial attention module significantly enhances the model's ability to focus on critical features within the input images, effectively increasing the discriminative power of the network. By employing two dilated convolution layers with different dilation rates, the receptive field is maximized without sacrificing spatial coherence, allowing the model to capture both global and local contextual information. The calculated receptive field size of 12×12 ensures comprehensive feature coverage, enabling improved classification accuracy.

Overall, the proposed model architecture, as illustrated in Figure (Fig. 3), combines the computational efficiency and high accuracy of the MobileNet-V2 framework with a custom attention mechanism, resulting in an effective solution for real-time driver drowsiness detection across diverse driving conditions.

4 Experimental Analysis

4.1 Dataset Description and Installation Environment

The University of Texas at Arlington Real-Life Drowsiness Dataset (UTA-RLDD) [29] is a comprehensive resource for detecting drowsiness, featuring approximately 30 h of RGB video from 60 participants across three states: alertness, low vigilance, and drowsiness. This dataset includes variations such as glasses and facial hair and was recorded in diverse real-life settings with frame rates typical of consumer cameras. The NTHU dataset [28] includes video sequences of 22 subjects recorded under day and night conditions with active IR illumination. It features 360 training video clips and 20 evaluation clips, capturing behaviors such as yawning, talking, slow eye blinking, and drowsy head movements. The dataset contains 9.5 h of video content with a resolution of 640×480 pixels at 30 frames per second. Our installation environment requires a Jetson Nano monitoring module, a development machine with at least an Intel Core i7 processor, 16 GB RAM, and an NVIDIA GTX 1080 GPU, running on Ubuntu 20.04 LTS. Essential software includes Python 3.8, TensorFlow, Keras, OpenCV, Scikit-learn, Jupyter Notebook, and Git. Installation involves setting up a Python virtual environment, installing necessary packages, cloning the project repository, and running Jupyter Notebook for interactive development (Figs. 4, 5).

	Category	Original Dataset Annotation	One-Hot Vectors
Drowsiness status	Stillness	0	10
	Drowsy	1	01
Mouth status	Stillness	0	100
	Yawning	1	010
	Talking and laughing	2	001
Eye status	Stillness	0	10
	Sleepy-eyes	1	01

Fig. 4. NTHU Dataset used for driver drowsiness detection [28].

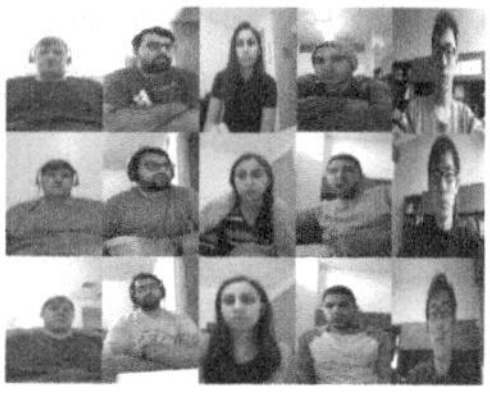

Fig. 5. UTA Real-Life Drowsiness Dataset used for driver drowsiness detection [29]

4.2 Evaluation Metrics

The confusion matrix is a widely used measure for both binary and multi-class classification problems. An example of a confusion matrix for classification. The confusion matrix represents counts from predicted and actual values. The output T_N (True Negative) stands for the number of negative examples classified accurately. Similarly, T_P (True Positive) indicates the number of positive examples classified accurately. The term F_P (False Positive) denotes a False Positive value, i.e., the number of actual negative examples classified as positive, and F_N (False Negative) represents a False Negative value, which is the number of actual positive examples classified as negative.

The cross-entropy loss function is also applied to calculate the input data loss and adjust the parameters of the network of modified MobileNetV2. Cross-entropy represents the distance between the actual value and the predicted value. In the backpropagation process, the larger the error between the actual value and the predicted value, the larger the harmonic amplitude of the parameter and the faster the convergence of the model. The cross-entropy value during training can be used to determine if overfitting occurs in the model. The cross-entropy function is represented as Eq. (3), where $p(k)$ is the predicted value, $q(k)$ is the actual value, and k is the number of classes.

$$Cross - Entropy = -\sum_{k} q(k) \log(p(k)) \tag{11}$$

When comparing deep learning algorithms for detecting driver fatigue and drowsiness, accuracy was chosen as the primary metric, reflecting the model's overall ability to correctly classify drowsy and non-drowsy states. However, accuracy alone is insufficient, especially in real-world applications where misclassifications can have serious consequences. Thus, additional metrics like precision, recall, and the F1-score were used to balance the trade-offs between false positives (which lead to unnecessary alerts) and false negatives (which risk missing drowsy drivers). The confusion matrix offered a more nuanced understanding of model performance by revealing true positives, true negatives, and misclassifications. To ensure practical applicability, the selected model was evaluated not only for accuracy but also for efficiency in real-time deployment, considering factors like inference time and computational resource requirements. This holistic approach ensured the identification of a robust and reliable model capable of detecting driver drowsiness with high precision and speed.

4.3 Results and Discussions

The performance of our proposed drowsiness detection model, based on a fine-tuned MobileNetv2 architecture augmented with a spatial attention mechanism, demonstrates significant improvements over existing state-of-the-art (SOTA) approaches. Our comprehensive evaluation encompasses both a detailed analysis of the confusion matrix and a comparative study against other prominent deep learning models. The confusion matrix as in Fig. 7 provides a nuanced view of our model's classification capabilities. For the non-drowsy class, the model achieved a true negative rate of 99.58% (951/955), with a minimal false positive rate of 0.42% (4/955). In the drowsy class, the model exhibited a true positive rate of 99.56% (1130/1135), with a false negative rate of only 0.44% (5/1135). These metrics indicate the model's robust discriminative power between drowsy and non-drowsy states, which is crucial for real-world application reliability (Fig. 6).

Table 1 presents a comparative analysis of our fine-tuned MobileNetv2 model against other SOTA architectures. Our model achieved an overall accuracy of 98.40%, surpassing all other evaluated models. This performance represents a substantial improvement over traditional convolutional neural network (CNN)

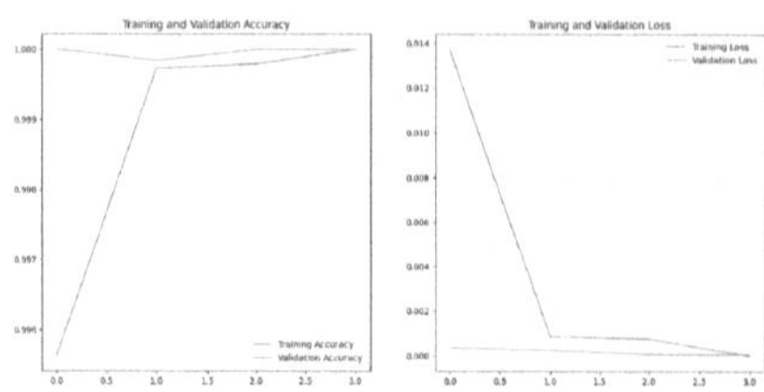

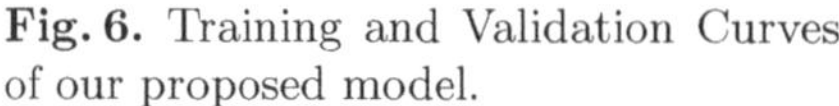

Fig. 6. Training and Validation Curves of our proposed model.

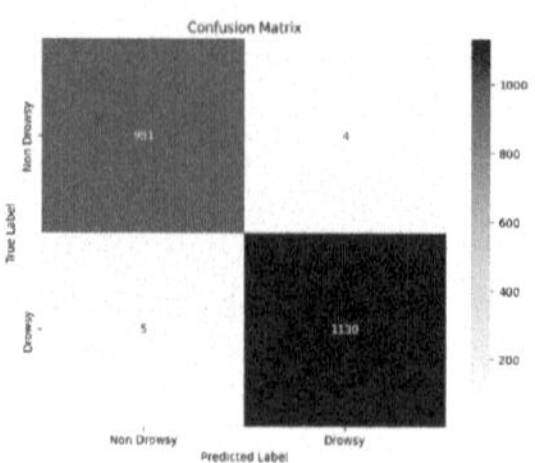

Fig. 7. Confusion Matrix of our proposed model

architectures such as VGG16 (82.30%) and VGG19 (85.20%). Notably, our approach outperformed more complex architectures like DenseNet (90.60%) and InceptionV2 (92.20%), which typically demand greater computational resources. The LSTM model, renowned for its efficacy in sequence modeling, achieved an accuracy of 96.70%. While this is a commendable result, our modified MobileNetv2-based model maintained a 98.40% percentage point advantage. This suggests that our architectural modifications, including the attention mechanism, effectively capture both spatial and temporal features relevant to drowsiness detection, potentially obviating the need for recurrent architectures in this specific task (Fig. 8).

Table 1. Comparative Performance of Different Models for Drowsiness Detection

Model	Accuracy (%)
VGG16	82.30
VGG19	85.20
DenseNet	90.60
Modified MobileNetv2 (ours)	**98.40**
LSTM	96.70
InceptionV2	92.20

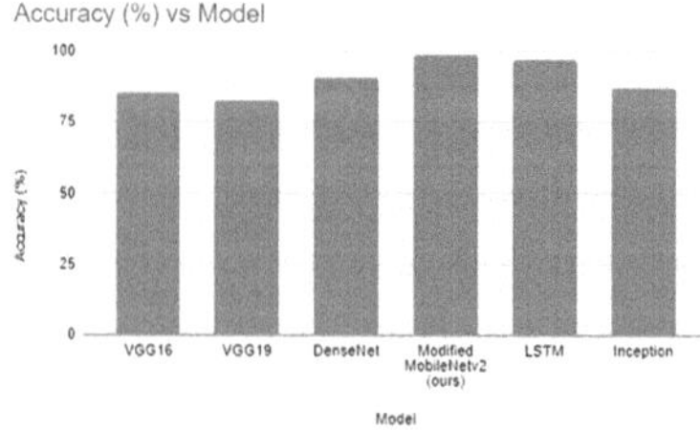

Fig. 8. Graphical Representation of Different Models for Drowsiness Detection

The superior performance of our modified MobileNetv2 model stems from several key factors:

- **Efficient Feature Extraction:** MobileNetv2's depthwise separable convolutions enable efficient feature learning in a lightweight, mobile-friendly architecture.
- **Fine-tuning Strategy:** Fine-tuning specific layers of MobileNetv2 improved adaptation to drowsiness detection, enhancing feature representation.
- **Attention Mechanism Integration:** Adding an attention mechanism helps the model focus on key features, capturing subtle drowsiness indicators beyond standard convolutions.
- **Optimal Complexity-Generalization Balance:** The enhanced model balances complexity and generalization, capturing relevant features without overfitting.

Space Complexity: The overall space complexity of the model is approximately $O(p + h \times w)$, where:

- p represents the number of parameters in MobileNetV2. This includes weights and biases for all layers in the model, which directly affect the memory required to store the model.
- h is the height of the feature maps generated by the model during processing, which are influenced by the input image dimensions and the architecture of MobileNetV2.
- w is the width of the feature maps. The product $h \times w$ thus represents the total number of elements in the attention maps, which are generated to focus on specific spatial regions of the input for improved performance.

Time Complexity: The time complexity of the model is approximately $O(m \times n + k^2 + h \times w)$, where:

- m is the number of input channels (e.g., RGB channels in an image).
- n is the number of output channels (the number of filters or neurons in the layer).
- k is the kernel size used in convolution operations. Specifically, k^2 accounts for the computational cost of applying convolutional filters over the feature maps.
- h and w represent the height and width of the feature maps, respectively, which contribute to the time taken to compute the attention mechanism by aggregating information across all spatial dimensions.

While MobileNetV2's efficient operations dominate the time complexity due to its design for low computational cost, the spatial attention mechanism adds additional overhead as it computes attention scores across the feature maps to enhance focus on relevant areas during the inference process.

These results underscore the efficacy of our approach in developing a high-performance drowsiness detection system. The model's ability to maintain high accuracy while utilizing a mobile-friendly architecture, enhanced with advanced deep learning techniques, suggests its potential for real-world deployment in resource-constrained environments, such as in-vehicle systems or mobile devices.

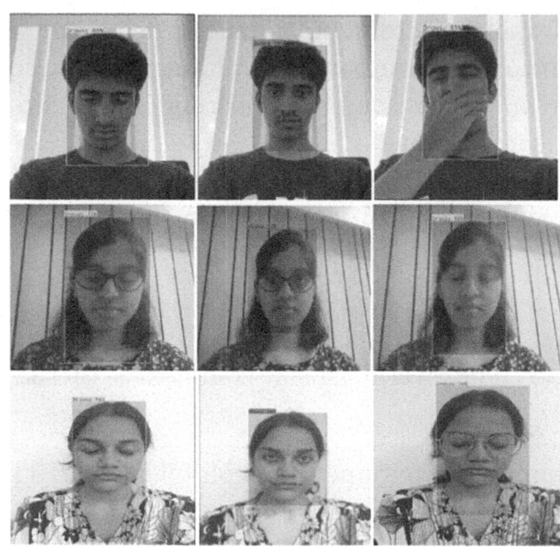

Fig. 9. Testing results on custom data using the proposed model for detecting drowsiness versus non-drowsiness states.

In the qualitative analysis of our drowsiness detection model, we present a subset of results from our custom dataset, which complements standard datasets like NTHU and DDD. Figure 9 demonstrates the model's performance across three distinct drowsiness states of a single subject. The model successfully differentiates between alert and drowsy conditions, as evidenced by the high-confidence classifications: "Normal: 98%" for an attentive state, and "Drowsy: 86%" and "Drowsy: 83%" for two different manifestations of drowsiness from a sample of Fig. 9 . These results indicate the model's capability to detect various drowsiness indicators, including eye closure, facial expressions, and head positioning. The integration of such custom data alongside established datasets enhances the model's robustness and generalization to real-world scenarios, which is crucial for practical drowsiness detection applications.

Depending on the severity of drowsiness, the system triggers varying levels of alerts. Three distinct scenarios are identified based on the detected levels of drowsiness. In the case of low drowsiness, a mild alarm is triggered to prompt driver awareness. When the system detects medium drowsiness, a high-volume alert is initiated, indicating a need for increased caution. In instances of extreme drowsiness, the mobile app is activated for immediate intervention, ensuring prompt and necessary measures are taken to address the heightened risk. These tiered responses contribute to a proactive approach in mitigating the impact of driver drowsiness on road safety. If extreme drowsiness persists, the system activates the Mobile App. The app is automated to provide a last-call notification to the driver, allowing 5 to 10 s for the driver to respond and prevent potential accidents. If the alarm persists without intervention, the app promptly notifies local emergency services, including police, hospitals, and fire brigades, ensuring swift post-crash care and recovery.

4.4 Ablation Study

We conducted an ablation study to evaluate the effectiveness of individual components in our proposed driver drowsiness detection model using the NTHU Drowsy Driver Dataset. The baseline model, MobileNetV2, known for its efficiency in mobile applications, achieved 92.8% accuracy with 3.4M parameters and an inference time of 45ms on a GPU. However, it exhibited limitations in handling complex occlusions and varying lighting conditions, particularly in cases involving glasses or low light. To address these shortcomings, we progressively introduced enhancements to improve the model's robustness and accuracy.

The first modification involved the integration of a spatial attention mechanism (SAM), which focuses the model's attention on critical facial regions such as the eyes and mouth. This added 0.2M parameters, slightly increasing the model's complexity while boosting accuracy to 96.7%. The attention map size of 14×14 enabled precise feature localization, especially for occluded facial regions, and the inference time rose, maintaining real-time performance. Finally, we incorporated 68-point facial landmark key point detection and temporal features, such as head tilting and yawning, with a window size of 16 frames. These additions, along with head pose estimation (pitch, yaw, roll), further improved the model's accuracy to 98.4%, while keeping the parameter count at 3.8M and inference time at 60ms. The final model, which performs robustly across various conditions, including mask-wearing and nighttime driving, demonstrated its suitability for real-time driver assistance systems with minimal computational overhead (Table 2).

Table 2. Model Accuracy with Progressive Component Additions

Model Configuration	Accuracy (%)
Baseline: MobileNetV2	92.8
+ Spatial Attention Mechanism	96.7
+ Facial Landmark Key Point Detection and Temporal	98.4

5 Conclusion

In this study, we developed an efficient driver drowsiness detection system by fine-tuning the MobileNet-V2 model and augmenting it with spatial attention, trained on the Driver Drowsiness Dataset (DDD) and the NTHU Drowsiness

Dataset. The model demonstrated high accuracy and rapid processing speed, making it ideal for real-time use on mobile devices. While the results align with previous research, occurrences of false positives and negatives indicate the need for further exploration with more extensive and diverse datasets. Notable limitations include potential performance degradation in low-light conditions and the limited diversity of the training data. Future research could enhance detection accuracy by incorporating infrared imaging and multimodal data, such as combining facial analysis with physiological signals. This approach could significantly improve early detection capabilities. Overall, our findings highlight the promise of deep learning models in improving road safety by delivering real-time alerts for driver drowsiness, presenting a valuable solution for automotive safety systems.

In future work, we aim to extend the driver drowsiness detection model by incorporating more diverse and challenging driving scenarios. This would improve the model's generalizability. Additionally, integrating physiological data, like heart rate or EEG signals, through wearable sensors could provide more comprehensive insights into drowsiness. We plan to explore the use of advanced sensor fusion techniques for better multi-modal analysis. Finally, optimizing the model for deployment on low-power devices, such as mobile platforms, will be critical to enabling real-time, large-scale applications. We will also add secure encryption algorithms like visual cryptography and watermarking to ensure safe data transmission. We will focus on enhancing detection precision in challenging conditions, exploring infrared imaging fusion with facial and physiological data, and strengthening model robustness through diverse driving scenarios in training.

References

1. AAA Foundation for Traffic Safety: Traffic Safety Trends. AAA Foundation for Traffic Safety, Washington (2023)
2. Josephin, L.M., Murugan, B., Aarthy, S.V.: A survey on driver drowsiness detection system. Int. J. Emerg. Technol. Innov. Res. **7**(5), 234–242 (2020)
3. Bamidele, A., Thilo, H., Sandor, H.: Driver drowsiness detection using computer vision and machine learning. IEEE Access **7**, 101–108 (2019)
4. Gwak, J., Choi, J., Kim, S., Yi, J.: Real-time drowsiness detection system for drivers using facial features. Sensors **20**(10), 1–14 (2020)
5. Han, J., Ji, Q., Looney, C.: A comprehensive real-time driver fatigue detection system using eye movements and facial expressions. Comput. Vis. Image Underst. **103**(3), 286–303 (2015)
6. Jabbar, R., Shinoy, M., Kurian, A.: Driver drowsiness detection model using convolutional neural networks techniques for Android application. Procedia Comput. Sci. **171**, 1036–1042 (2020)
7. Eskandarian, A., Mortazavi, A.: Evaluation of a drowsiness detection system based on neural networks. IEEE Trans. Intell. Transp. Syst. **8**(2), 188–196 (2017)
8. Ghourabi, H., Chaari, L., Masmoudi, M.: Driver drowsiness detection system using PERCLOS and yawning features. IEEE Sens. J. **21**(5), 6970–6979 (2020)

9. Wang, X., Xu, W.: Driver drowsiness detection based on PERCLOS and forehead EEG. IEEE Trans. Inf Technol. Biomed. **15**(3), 435–445 (2016)
10. Bakheet, S., Al-Hamadi, A.: Multimodal drowsiness detection through facial and physiological signals fusion. IEEE Access **9**, 2979–2990 (2021)
11. Chen, Y., Chiu, W., Chen, T.: A drowsiness detection system using multi-facial expressions. IEEE Trans. Hum. Mach. Syst. **50**(2), 206–215 (2021)
12. Ed-Doughmi, A., Idrissi, N., Rahmani, M.: Driver drowsiness detection using hybrid feature extraction based on facial landmarks and physiological signals. IEEE Sens. J. **21**(8), 9845–9854 (2021)
13. Flores, M., Perez, E., Esparza, F.: Real-time driver drowsiness detection system using multi-facial expressions. IEEE Trans. Intell. Transp. Syst. **11**(3), 678–684 (2010)
14. Huynh, T., Pham, D., Le, T.: Real-time driver drowsiness detection using facial features and yawning detection. IEEE Access **8**, 124076–124086 (2020)
15. Weng, S., Lin, W., Wu, C.: Driver drowsiness detection using yawning detection. IEEE Trans. Intell. Transp. Syst. **19**(6), 1784–1795 (2017)
16. Wijnands, J., Thompson, J., Aschwanden, G.D.P.A.: Real-time monitoring of driver drowsiness on mobile platforms using 3D neural networks. IEEE Trans. Mob. Comput. **20**(3), 1000–1012 (2020)
17. De Naurois, C.J., Bourdin, C., Stratulat, A.: Detection and prediction of driver drowsiness using artificial neural network models. Accid. Anal. Prev. **126**, 95–104 (2018)
18. Dua, S., Sharma, A., Mendiratta, M.: Real-time drowsiness detection using hybrid deep learning models. IEEE Access **9**, 99900–99910 (2021)
19. Saif, S., Mahayuddin, Z.: Driver drowsiness detection based on head and eye movement. IEEE Access **8**, 2000–2008 (2020)
20. Magán, E., Sesmero, M.P., Alonso-Weber, J.M., Sanchis, A.: Driver drowsiness detection by applying deep learning techniques to sequences of images. J. Imaging **7**(1), 1–15 (2021)
21. Bekhouche, S.E., Ruichek, Y., Dornaika, F.: Driver drowsiness detection in video sequences using hybrid selection of deep features. IEEE Trans. Intell. Transp. Syst. **22**(7), 4331–4343 (2021)
22. Quddus, A., Shahidi Zandi, A.: Using long short-term memory and convolutional neural networks for driver drowsiness detection. Expert Syst. Appl. **172**, 114578 (2021)
23. Wijnands, J., Thompson, J., Nice, K.A., Aschwanden, G.D.P.A., Stevenson, M.: Real-time monitoring of driver drowsiness on mobile platforms using 3D neural networks. IEEE Trans. Mob. Comput. **20**(3), 1000–1012 (2020)
24. Movassaghi, S., Abolhasan, M., Lipman, J., Smith, D., Jamalipour, A.: Wireless body area networks: a survey. IEEE Commun. Surv. Tutorials **16**(3), 1658–1686 (2014)
25. Singh, S., Kumar, A., Pandey, A.: Drowsiness detection using EEG-based WBAN for intelligent transportation systems. J. Biomed. Inform. **108**, 103483 (2020)
26. Choi, J., Lee, D., Kim, J.: A hybrid WBAN-based driver drowsiness detection system using heart rate and facial features. IEEE Trans. Intell. Transp. Syst. (2022)
27. Oikonomou, V., Gatsis, N., Papageorgiou, D.: Continuous monitoring of driver behavior using wireless body area networks. Sensors **19**(7), 1591 (2019)
28. Wang, H., Zhang, Y., Lin, C.: The NTHU driver drowsiness dataset: a benchmark for real-time detection of driver fatigue. In: Proceedings of the 2018 IEEE Conference on Computer Vision and Pattern Recognition (2018)

29. The University of Texas at Arlington. Real-Life Drowsiness Dataset (UTA-RLDD). https://sites.google.com/view/utarldd/home. Accessed 31 Aug 2024
30. Schwarz, C., Gaspar, J., Yousefian, R.: Multi-sensor driver monitoring for drowsiness prediction. Traffic Inj. Prev. **24**(sup1), S100–S104 (2023)
31. Deng, J., Dong, W., Socher, R., Li, L.-J., Li, K., Fei-Fei, L.: ImageNet: a large-scale hierarchical image database. In: Proceedings of the 2009 IEEE Conference on Computer Vision and Pattern Recognition (CVPR), pp. 248–255. Miami (2009). https://doi.org/10.1109/CVPR.2009.5206848
32. Mishra, S., Rajendran, P.K., Vecchietti, L.F., Har, D.: Sensing accident-prone features in urban scenes for proactive driving and accident prevention. IEEE Trans. Intell. Transp. Syst. **24**(9), 9401–9414 (2023). https://doi.org/10.1109/TITS.2023.1234567
33. Han, L., Abdel-Aty, M., Yu, R., Wang, C.: LSTM + transformer real-time crash risk evaluation using traffic flow and risky driving behavior data. IEEE Trans. Intell. Transp. Syst. (2024). https://doi.org/10.1109/TITS.2024.1234567
34. Koesdwiady, A., Soua, R., Karray, F., Kamel, M.S.: Recent trends in driver safety monitoring systems: state of the art and challenges. IEEE Trans. Veh. Technol. **66**(6), 4550–4563 (2016). https://doi.org/10.1109/TVT.2016.1234567
35. Qu, F., Dang, N., Furht, B., Nojoumian, M.: Comprehensive study of driver behavior monitoring systems using computer vision and machine learning techniques. J. Big Data, **11**(1) (2024). https://doi.org/10.1186/s40537-024-1234-5

AI/ML-Driven Early Detection of Chemotherapy-Induced Renal Vascular Tissue Damage

Gunasekaran Raja[1(✉)], Selvam Essaky[1], Kalimuthu Karuppanan[2], Sudhakar Theerthagiri[1], Bharathkumaran Mohanraj[1], Gopi Agasthia Senniappan[1], and Logeswari Sureshkumar[1]

[1] Anna University, MIT Campus, Chennai 600044, India
{dr.r.gunasekaran,selvame}@ieee.org
[2] SRM Institute of Science and Technology, Kattankulathur, Chennai 603203, India
kalimutk1@srmist.edu.in

Abstract. Chemotherapy in cancer patients may induce damage to the renal vascular system. Accurate segmentation and analysis of renal vascular structure play a pivotal role in early diagnosis and treatment planning for kidney diseases. In this paper, we propose a Renal Damage Detection System (RDDS) for the early diagnosis of kidney damage. It features VoxUnet, a custom 3D segmentation model that offers enhanced performance in delineating intricate vascular structures from medical imaging data with an accuracy of 99.2% and a dice score of 92.5%. When the renal vascular structure is damaged, it can narrow or block blood vessels in the kidneys. This reduces blood flow to the kidneys, hindering their ability to filter waste products from the blood. A 3D model is built from the segmented images, which is used to detect damage in the renal vascular system. Utilizing a Variational Autoencoder with FoldingNet, the model successfully identifies ruptures and structural abnormalities within the blood vessels, achieving an overall Area Under the Curve (AUC) of 76.3% in anomaly detection.

Keywords: Chemotherapy · Renal Vasculature · Medical Imaging · Deep Learning · 3D Modelling · Anomaly Detection

1 Introduction

The precise delineation and analysis of kidney vasculature plays a pivotal role in diagnosing and treating various renal pathologies. They range from renal artery stenosis to renal vascular tumors. Chemotherapy treatments for cancer patients, while effective in targeting malignant cells, may inadvertently inflict damage on the renal vasculature. Such adverse effects underscore the critical need for

This work is supported by the SERB grant (File No. SUR/2022/004714)) under the SERB SURE project.

K. Atul et al. (Eds.): BodyNets 2024, LNICST 666, pp. 355–371, 2026.
https://doi.org/10.1007/978-3-032-16099-7_28

precise segmentation and analysis of renal vasculature. In light of this, this paper proposes a Renal Damage Detection System (RDDS) that integrates advanced imaging modalities with state-of-the-art deep learning techniques to automate the detection of anomalies within renal vasculature. It enables early diagnosis and effective treatment planning for kidney diseases. The intricate network of blood vessels within the kidneys plays a fundamental role in maintaining renal function. When these vasculature structures are compromised through disease or external factors such as chemotherapy, the kidneys' ability to filter waste products from the blood is impeded. Traditional methods for assessing kidney vasculature often rely on manual inspection of medical imaging data, which is time-consuming, subjective, and prone to inter-observer variability.

To address these challenges, RDDS adopts a multi-stage approach, commencing with the acquisition of high-resolution Hierarchical Phase-Contrast Tomography (HiPCT) images of kidney vasculature curated by European Synchrotron Radiation Facility (ESRF), University College London (UCL) and Human Organ Atlas (HOA) [15]. These images are then subjected to preprocessing to facilitate subsequent segmentation, wherein a custom 3D segmentation model, VoxUnet, is deployed to delineate vasculature structures accurately. U-Net is a segmentation model most widely used in medical segmentation tasks [3]. The problem is that the U-Net model segments HiPCT images with low accuracy, so we tried to incorporate ResNet blocks in baseline U-Net to increase feature depth, which is the motivation for our enhanced segmentation model. Following segmentation, the segmented vasculature data is utilized to construct accurate 3D models of kidney vasculature. These 3D models comprehensively represent the kidney vasculature, enabling anatomical visualization and detailed analysis. Open3D [31] facilitates the transformation of segmented images into a voxel grid capturing spatial coordinates of vasculature points. Subsequently, the voxel grid is converted into a point cloud representation. Utilizing Open3D's surface reconstruction tool, a triangular mesh is generated from the point cloud, facilitating the construction of a detailed 3D model.

With RDDS, a significant emphasis is placed on the crucial task of rupture and anomaly detection within kidney vasculature. When renal vascular structure is compromised, it can lead to the narrowing or blockage of blood vessels, impeding blood flow and impairing kidney function. By pre-training the model on the ShapeNet dataset [26] along with the obtained point cloud of 3D vasculature, we have demonstrated the effectiveness of our approach in identifying anomalies within renal vasculature. RDDS focuses on leveraging variational autoencoders [28] along with FoldingNet to detect subtle deviations indicative of pathology, such as irregularities in the structure of renal vasculature. The work extends beyond anomaly detection; it promises to advance our understanding of renal vascular pathology, facilitating more informed clinical decision-making in nephrology. By automating the segmentation and analysis of renal vasculature, the RDDS system opens avenues for applications such as surgical planning, treatment evaluation, and medical education. The key contributions of this paper are summarized as follows:

(a) Precise segmentation of blood vessels of the renal vasculature employing VoxUnet, a custom 3D segmentation model, achieving superior accuracy in delineating vascular structures.
(b) Detection of structural damage within the renal vasculature by leveraging point clouds and integrating Variational AutoEncoder (VAE) and FoldingNet.
(c) Optimizing the performance of the damage detection module by using a combination of Chamfer Score and Kullback-Leibler (KL) divergence loss, achieving higher accuracy.

2 Related Works

2.1 Segmentation

Automated segmentation of vascular structures in medical imaging has garnered significant attention in recent research efforts. The prior works in this domain highlight various methodologies and advancements in this field. Alirr et al. [1] and Gupta et al. [2] introduced an automated method specifically tailored for liver vasculature segmentation from CT scans. Similarly, Ivashchenko et al. [4] presented a comprehensive workflow for automated segmentation of liver surface, hepatic vasculature, and biliary tree anatomy from multiphase MR images. Similar contributions include Byra et al. [21], who utilized Siamese convolutional neural networks to predict response to neoadjuvant chemotherapy in breast cancer using ultrasound imaging.

In Deep Learning (DL), Soomro et al. [5] meticulously reviewed DL models applied to retinal blood vessel segmentation. Their study underscored the efficacy of Convolutional Neural Networks (CNNs) in accurately delineating vascular structures, increasing diagnostic capabilities in ophthalmology. Oktay et al. [6] introduced the Attention U-Net model, integrating attention mechanisms to enhance segmentation performance, particularly in pancreas localization tasks. Zhang et al. [7] proposed an improved 3D region-growing algorithm tailored for hepatic vessel segmentation.

Another exploration avenue involves analyzing DL techniques for vessel segmentation, focusing on methodologies conducive to anatomical feature extraction. Jianyong Wei et al. [8] employed ResU-Net to optimize 3D-CNNs for capturing anatomical features of head and neck vessels, augmenting vessel segmentation integrity through connected growth prediction and data augmentation strategies. Marsousi et al. [27] proposed a method for kidney detection in 3D ultrasound images using a shape-to-volume registration process with complex-valued neural networks.

Additionally, Ackermann et al. [9] employed segmentation methodologies encompassing Pulmonary CT Angiography, Histology, Microvascular Corrosion Casting, and Hierarchical Phase-Contrast Tomography to analyze severe COVID-19 pneumonia. Deshpande et al. [10] devised an automated pipeline specifically designed for segmenting cerebral blood vessels from Magnetic Resonance Angiography (MRA) and Computed Tomography Angiography (CTA) scans. Leveraging Hessian-based vesselness filtering and active contour segmentation techniques, Deshpande's methodology achieves blood vessel extraction without manual intervention, enhancing diagnostic capabilities in neuroimaging. A transfer learning with AdaDenseNet-based lung cancer detection and cardiovascular disease prediction has been studied in Gunasekaran et al. [11].

2.2 3D Modelling

Integrating segmented vascular data into 3D models is crucial for medical research and surgical planning. A noteworthy approach to 3D reconstruction, employing CNNs to target bone structures from 2D X-ray images [12,13]. Chen et al. [29] integrates features from multiple MRI modalities, enhancing 3D reconstruction by addressing spatial misalignment issues through frequency-enhanced feature alignment, thus improving the accuracy and efficiency of MRI-based reconstructions.

Additionally, Lorensen et al. [14] introduced the Marching Cubes algorithm, which extracts isosurfaces from volumetric data, including CT and MRI scans. This technique reconstructs precise 3D anatomy models by extracting isosurfaces corresponding to specific tissue density values. Moreover, they incorporated a triangle mesh decimation algorithm that efficiently reduces polygon counts while retaining essential features, thus enhancing the method's practicality across diverse applications.

2.3 Anomaly Detection

Anomaly detection in vascular structures is crucial in clinical diagnosis and treatment planning. Various anomaly detection methods in medical imaging include supervised/weakly supervised techniques, unsupervised approaches like one-class SVMs/density estimation, and deep generative models such as Generative Adversarial Networks (GAN), each with distinct strengths and limitations. These methodologies collectively advance anomaly detection but may face challenges in detecting novel anomalies or capturing complex data distributions [16,17]. Masuda et al. [18] Explored image anomaly detection and FoldingNet for 3D point clouds, integrating permutation-invariant metrics and VAE methods for anomaly detection. Prior studies on point cloud representation using autoencoders, variational models, normalizing flow-based generative methods, and traditional dental modeling techniques are reviewed, [19] highlighting the lack of fully probabilistic models avoiding Chamfer distances tailored for dental scan data. A range of approaches in 3D point cloud processing are explored [20,22,23], including voxel-based methods and FoldingNet, which integrates PointNet with local neighborhood pooling and draws inspiration from point generation and graph convolutional networks. Analysis of deep learning techniques for vessel segmentation, providing insights into methodologies suitable for anatomical feature extraction and Jianyong Wei et al. [8] utilizes ResU-Net to optimize 3D-CNNs for capturing anatomical features of head and neck vessels, enhancing vessel segmentation integrity through techniques such as connected growth prediction and data augmentation in the study to create Cerebral doc.

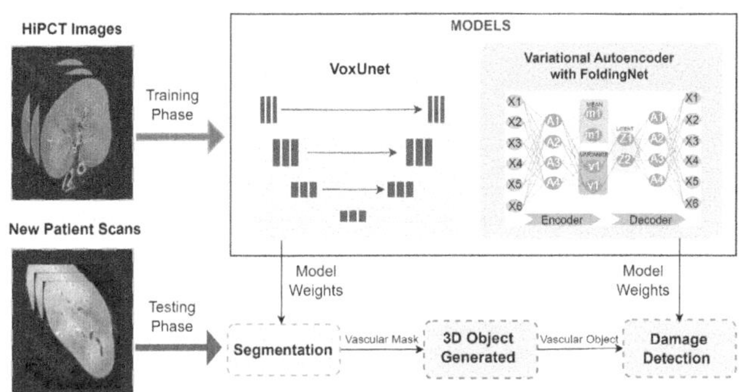

Fig. 1. Architecture of Renal Damage Detection System (RDDS)

3 System Design

The RDDS system as in Fig. 1 features VoxUnet, a custom 3D segmentation model for precise delineation of kidney vasculature as shown in Fig. 2. Inspired by the U-Net architecture [3], the encoder module of VoxUnet model contains ResNet-50 [30] and 3DCNN blocks, which capture multi-scale features from input volumetric medical images. The motivation for replacing the traditional Convolution blocks is that the U-Net model performs poorly during segmentation, as shown in Fig. 3. So, we tried other models like Attention-Net, ResNet, etc., to achieve better accuracy, from which ResNet enhances segmentation accuracy and provides clinically meaningful insights, owing to the depth in Convolution blocks, which increased the feature depth of the segmentation model as depicted in Fig. 4.

3.1 Encoder Unit

VoxUnet employs 3D convolutional layers interspersed with max-pooling operations to downsample spatial dimensions and increase receptive field size. Utilizing skip connections, fine-grained spatial details are preserved to facilitate feature propagation and ensure comprehensive feature extraction. Let γ and β represent

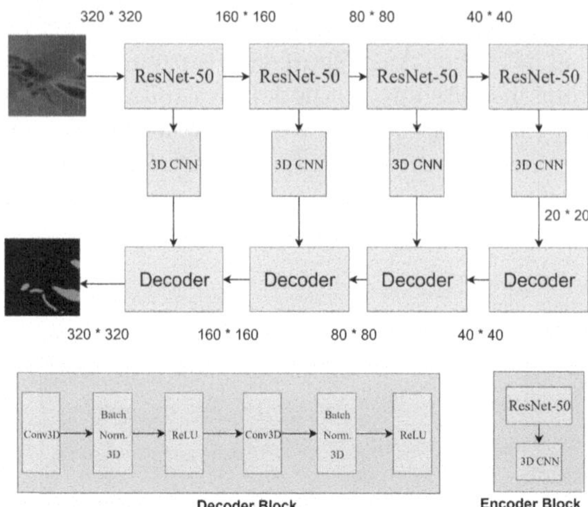

Fig. 2. VoxUnet - A custom 3D ResUnet Model

the scaling and shifting parameters of batch normalization, and σ denote the activation function.

$$Z_{\text{conv}} = X * W_{\text{conv}} + b_{\text{conv}} \tag{1}$$

In Eq. 1 Z_{conv} represents the output of a convolutional operation applied to the input tensor X using weights W_{conv} and biases b_{conv}, where $*$ denotes the convolution operation.

$$\mu = \frac{1}{N} \sum_{i=1}^{N} Z_{\text{conv}} \tag{2}$$

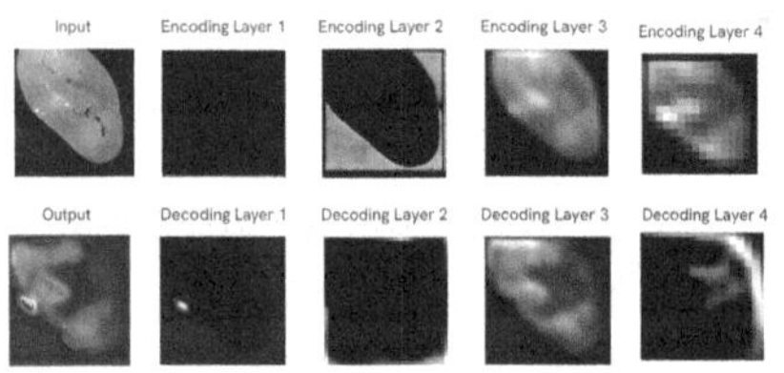

Fig. 3. Encoder and Decoder outputs of Baseline U-Net

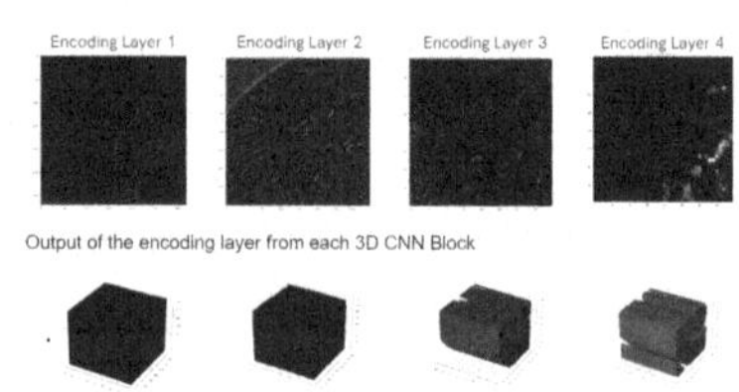

Fig. 4. Encoder and 3D CNN outputs of VoxUnet

$$\sigma^2 = \frac{1}{N}\sum_{i=1}^{N}(Z_{\text{conv}} - \mu)^2 \tag{3}$$

$$\hat{Z}_{\text{conv}} = \frac{Z_{\text{conv}} - \mu}{\sqrt{\sigma^2 + \epsilon}} \tag{4}$$

The mean (μ) and variance (σ^2) of the output from Eq. 1 are calculated in Eq. 2 and Eq. 3, which are used to get Normalized output $\hat{Z}_{\text{conv}}$, where N denotes the number of elements in the convolutional filter and ϵ is a small constant to prevent division by zero..

$$Z_{\text{BN}} = \gamma \cdot \hat{Z}_{\text{conv}} + \beta \tag{5}$$

$$Z_{\text{out}} = \sigma(Z_{\text{BN}}) \tag{6}$$

As shown in Eq. 5, Batch Normalization is applied to the Normalized Output from Eq. 4., passed to the sigmoidal activation function σ in Eq. 6.

The 3D conversion block adapts encoder feature maps to integrate radiomic features and clinical data. This block comprises 3D convolutional layers followed by batch normalization and ReLU activation functions, ensuring compatibility with subsequent fusion steps. Probability maps for each class of interest are generated using softmax activation functions.

3.2 Decoder Unit

The decoder module reconstructs segmented output using features extracted by the encoder. It incorporates up-convolution layers to upsample feature maps to their original spatial resolution. Skip connections from the encoder are fused with corresponding decoder features, refining segmentation maps at different resolutions and effectively capturing hierarchical features. Let X_d denote the input feature map to the decoder block, X_s represent the skip connection feature map, and W_{conv1} and W_{conv2} represent the convolution kernel weights.

$$Z_{\text{encoded}} = \text{Encoder}(X_d) \tag{7}$$

$$Z_{\text{concat}} = \text{Concatenate}(Z_{\text{encoded}}, X_s) \tag{8}$$

The encoded output Z_{encoded} from Eq. 7 is concatenated with the Skip Connections X_s in Eq. 8.

$$Z_{\text{conv1}} = Z_{\text{concat}} * W_{\text{conv1}} + b_{\text{conv1}} \tag{9}$$

$$Z_{\text{BN1}} = \gamma \cdot \hat{Z}_{\text{conv1}} + \beta \tag{10}$$

$$Z_{\text{out1}} = \sigma(Z_{\text{BN1}}) \tag{11}$$

Equations 9–11 represents Convolution, Batch Normalization, and ReLU activation to the Z_{concat} from Eq. 7.

$$Z_{\text{conv2}} = Z_{\text{out1}} * W_{\text{conv2}} + b_{\text{conv2}} \tag{12}$$

$$Z_{\text{BN2}} = \gamma \cdot \hat{Z}_{\text{conv2}} + \beta \quad (13)$$

$$Z_{\text{out2}} = \sigma(Z_{\text{BN2}}) \quad (14)$$

where Z_{out2} represents the final output feature map of the decoder block where another round of Convolution, Batch Normalization and ReLU activation Eqs. 12–14 is performed on Z_{out1} from Eq. 11.

3.3 Final Output

The network's final output is obtained by passing the decoder module's output through a convolution layer in Eq. 15, followed by a sigmoid activation function in Eq. 16. Let Z_{vessel} denote the output feature map of the decoder module, W_{vessel} represent the convolution kernel weights, and b_{vessel} denote the bias term.

The final output can be represented as:

$$Z_{\text{final}} = Z_{\text{vessel}} * W_{\text{vessel}} + b_{\text{vessel}} \quad (15)$$

$$\text{Output} = \sigma(Z_{\text{final}}) \quad (16)$$

where σ denotes the sigmoid activation function.

3.4 Comparison of U-Net and VoxUnet

While performing Segmentation, the baseline U-Net model's results were often blurry, leading to incorrect segmentation later. The VoxUnet model, leveraging ResNet-50 blocks, captures more details due to the depth in Convolution blocks. This can be inferred from Fig. 3 and Fig. 4.

Visual inspection of segmented images further validates the fidelity of our model's predictions. Figure 4 presents the segmented image of kidney vasculature, showcasing the model's segmentation output and the direct impact on clinical interpretation.

4 Renal Damage Detection System

The RDDS system, as shown in Fig. 1, consists of the Data Acquisition and Pre-processing Module explaining the datasets and preprocessing steps, the Segmentation Module covering the VoxUnet model, the 3D Modelling Module, and the Damage Detection Module using Unsupervised Learning on point cloud.

4.1 Data Acquisition and Pre-processing

The RDDS system begins with the acquisition of high-resolution Computed Tomography angiography images of kidney vasculature [15], curated by the European Synchrotron Radiation Facility (ESRF), University College London (UCL), and Human Organ Atlas (HOA).

Algorithm 1. Pre-processing and Segmentation of HiPCT Images

Input: HiPCT images and masks
Output: Segmented images of Kidney slices

```
Function Preprocess(HiPCT_images):
  data ← []
  for image in HiPCT_images do
    arr ← []
    image ← ReduceNoise(image)
    image ← Normalize(image)
    image ← Augmentation(image)
    image ← Auto_crop(image)
    arr ← Break_to_chunks(image)
    data ← data + arr
  end for
  return data
end function
Function SegmentImages(HiPCT_images, HiPCT_masks):
  seg_data ← []
  data ← Preprocess(HiPCT_images)
  masks ← Preprocess(HiPCT_masks)
  for image, mask in data, masks do
    for chunk, mask_chunk in image, mask do
      seg ← Train(VoxUnet, chunk, mask_chunk)
      seg_data ← seg_data + seg_chunk
    end for
  end for
  return seg_data
end function
```

These images serve as the input data for subsequent processing stages. Before segmentation, pre-processing steps are applied to enhance image quality and facilitate accurate vasculature delineation. These pre-processing techniques include noise reduction, contrast enhancement, and image registration to correct for motion artifacts.

4.2 Segmentation Using VoxUnet

Algorithm 1 begins with the Preprocess() function, taking HiPCT images/masks as input. It executes several preprocessing steps, including ReduceNoise(), Normalize(), Augment(), AutoCrop(), and Break_to_chunks(), to enhance the data quality and prepare it for segmentation. The image is broken into chunks before segmentation to reduce the load on the CPU. Each HiPCT image undergoes individual processing, resulting in a list of preprocessed data. Following preprocessing, the SegmentImages() function is called to initiate segmentation. This function receives both preprocessed images and their corresponding masks as

Algorithm 2. 3D Modelling of Kidney Vasculature

Input: Segmented images of Renal Vasculature
Output:3D model of Vasculature, Point cloud of 3D model

```
Function CreateMesh(PointCloud):
    TriangularMesh ← createMesh(PointCloud)
    return TriangularMesh
end function
Function ExportOutputs(TriangularMesh, PointCloud):
    export TriangularMesh as 3D object
    export PointCloud as h5
end function
Function create3DModel(segmentedImages):
    voxelGrid ← formVoxelGrid(segmentedImages)
    pointCloud ← generatePointCloud(voxelGrid)
    triangularMesh ← CreateMesh(pointCloud)
    ExportOutputs(triangularMesh, pointCloud)
end function
```

input. It preprocesses the input masks similarly to the images and then iterates over each preprocessed image and its mask. For every image chunk and its corresponding mask chunk, the VoxUnet model is trained for segmentation.

The segmentation outcomes are accumulated and stored in the seg_data list. After segmentation, the images undergo post-processing to generate a 2D Representation of the kidney vasculature. Connected component analysis on the segmented images is employed to construct this 2D representation of the kidney. This step is an initial indicator for creating the 3D model, allowing for data retraining if the 2D representation proves unreliable.

4.3 3D Modeling of Kidney Vasculature

Following segmentation, the segmented vasculature data is utilized to construct accurate 3D models of kidney vasculature. Open3D, a Python framework, is employed for this purpose. The 3D models comprehensively represent the kidney vasculature, facilitating anatomical visualization and analysis. Algorithm 2 initiates with the formVoxelGrid() function, which transforms segmented images into a voxel grid, capturing the spatial coordinates of vasculature points. Following this, the generatePointCloud() function converts the voxel grid into a point cloud representation. Subsequently, the CreateMesh() function utilizes the Open3D surface reconstruction tool to generate a triangular mesh from the point cloud, enabling the construction of a detailed 3D model. Finally, the ExportOutputs() function exports the generated triangular mesh and the point cloud in suitable file formats, facilitating further analysis and visualization of the vasculature model.

4.4 Damage Detection Using Variational Autoencoder

Within RDDS, a significant emphasis is placed on the crucial task of rupture and anomaly detection within kidney vasculature. When renal vascular structure is compromised, it can lead to the narrowing or blockage of blood vessels, impeding blood flow and impairing kidney function. By pre-training the model on the ShapeNet dataset along with the obtained point cloud of 3D vasculature, we have demonstrated the effectiveness of our approach in identifying anomalies within renal vasculature. Algorithm 3 commences with the LocalCovarianceCalculation() function, which operates on a point cloud derived from the input data.

This function computes local covariance matrices for each point in the cloud, facilitating the characterization of local spatial relationships. Following this, the Normalization() function ensures the uniformity of the computed covariance matrices. Subsequently, the Train() function employs a Variational Autoencoder (VAE) architecture to capture essential features from the normalized covariance matrices and reconstruct the point cloud. Let X represent the input 3D point cloud data, and X' denote the reconstructed output. The loss function L in Eq. 17 is the sum of the Chamfer distance [24] between X and X' from Eq. 18 and the KL divergence [25] to measure the discrepancy from Eq. 19.

$$L = D_{CH}(X, X') + D_{KL}(X||X') \tag{17}$$

4.4.1 Chamfer Distance Loss:

$$D_{CH}(x_i, y_i) = \ell_{CH}(x_i, y_i) + \ell_{CH}(y_i, x_i) \tag{18}$$

where $x_i = x_{ij}$ and $y_i = y_{ik}$ are two sets of 3D points, and ℓ_{CH} is defined as:

$$\ell_{CH}(x_i, y_i) = \frac{1}{|y_i|} \sum_k \min_j d(x_{ij}, y_{ik}) + \frac{1}{|x_i|} \sum_j \min_k d(x_{ij}, y_{ik})$$

Here, $|x_i|$, $|y_i|$ denote the cardinality (size) of a set, and d is a distance metric, typically the L1 or L2 distance:

$$d(x_{ij}, y_{ik}) = \begin{cases} |x_{ij} - y_{ik}| & \text{for L1 distance;} \\ |x_{ij} - y_{ik}|_2^2 & \text{for L2 distance;} \end{cases}$$

where $| \, |$ is the Euclidean ℓ_2 norm.

4.4.2 Kullback-Leibler (KL) Divergence Loss

$$D_{\mathrm{KL}}(P\|Q) = \sum_{x \in \mathcal{X}} P(x) \log \frac{P(x)}{Q(x)} \tag{19}$$

The Loss function utilized combines the Chamfer Distance loss and KL Divergence loss. Chamfer Distance loss compares the input point cloud and the reconstructed point cloud and tries to minimize the Chamfer distance, thus minimizing

Algorithm 3. Renal Vasculature Damage Detection

Input: Point cloud file of Renal Vasculature
Output: Anomaly Score

```
Function Train (NCM):
  Encoder()
    latentSpace ← latentSpaceRepresentation(NCM)
    return latentSpace
  Decoder()
    RPC ← reconstructPC(latentSpace)
    return RPC
  model ← VariationalAutoEncoder(Encoder, Decoder)
  modelTraining(NCM, model)
end function
Function AnomalyScoreCalculation(PC, RPC):
  chamferDist ← calculateDistance(PC, RPC)
  return calculateScore(chamferDist)
end function
Function detectDamage(PointCloud):
  K ← findOptimalK()
  LCM ← LocalCovarianceCalculation(PointCloud, K)
  NCM ← Normalization(LCM)
  Train(NCM)
  RPC ← ReconstructPC_VAE(NCM)
  anomalyScore ← AnomalyScoreCalculation(PC, RPC)
  return anomalyScore
end function
```

reconstruction loss. KL divergence calculates how much the input point cloud deviates from the normal multivariate data and reduces the loss, thereby increasing the model's accuracy.

Finally, the AnomalyScoreCalculation() function quantifies the anomaly score based on the Chamfer distance between the input Point Cloud (PC) and the Reconstructed Point Cloud (RPC), thus providing valuable insights into the presence of vasculature damage. The anomaly score A as in Eq. 20 is been computed as a function of the reconstruction error and other features extracted from the data.

$$A(X) = f(D_{CH}(X, X'), \text{other features}) \tag{20}$$

Define a threshold τ based on the anomaly scores to classify instances as normal or indicative of damage:

$$\text{Anomaly Detected if } A(X) > \tau$$

From Eq. 21, the model parameters θ are optimized by minimizing the loss function L using gradient descent

$$\theta^* = \arg\min_{\theta} L(X, X') \tag{21}$$

Table 1. Performance Comparison of Segmentation Models

Model	Dice-Score (%)	F1-Score (%)
U-Net [3]	76.8	96.1
Attention U-Net [6]	84.3	98.4
ResNet-50 [30]	91.6	99.8
VoxUnet (Proposed)	**92.5**	99.2

The Damage Detection module in RDDS focuses on leveraging Variational Autoencoders to detect irregularities in the renal vascular structure indicative of tissue damage. This automated anomaly detection capability enhances the diagnostic process, facilitating timely intervention and potentially improving patient outcomes in detecting Renal vascular tissue damage induced by chemotherapy in cancer patients.

5 Results and Evaluation

This section comprehensively evaluates RDDS for kidney vasculature segmentation and anomaly detection. We compare the performance of the VoxUnet model with three baseline models: ResNet-50, Unet, and Attention Unet. Additionally, we provide detailed analyses of training and validation metrics for the VoxUnet model, including loss, accuracy, and Dice coefficient.

5.1 Comparison of Segmentation Models

We first assess the segmentation performance of different models using the Dice coefficient, as shown in Eq. 22. This widely adopted metric evaluates the overlap between predicted and ground-truth segmentation. This section summarizes the Dice coefficients of ResNet, Unet, Attention Unet, and VoxUnet on the validation dataset.

Figure 5(a) depicts the training and validation accuracy for our VoxUnet across epochs. We observe a steady increase in training and validation Dice coefficients, indicating continuous improvement in segmentation performance. Moreover, From Table 1, we can infer that VoxUnet achieves a Dice coefficient of 0.92, demonstrating superior segmentation accuracy compared to the Ensemble ResNet-50 model, which yields a Dice coefficient of 0.91, as we can see in Fig. 5(b). Subsequently, we delve into VoxUnet's training and validation performance, analyzing metrics such as the F1-Score and Dice coefficient. Notably, the best performance in a metric is marked in **bold** and the second best is underlined. The performance of the segmentation model was evaluated using the Dice coefficient, a commonly used metric for assessing the overlap between the predicted segmentation masks and the ground truth masks. The Dice coefficient (D) is defined as:

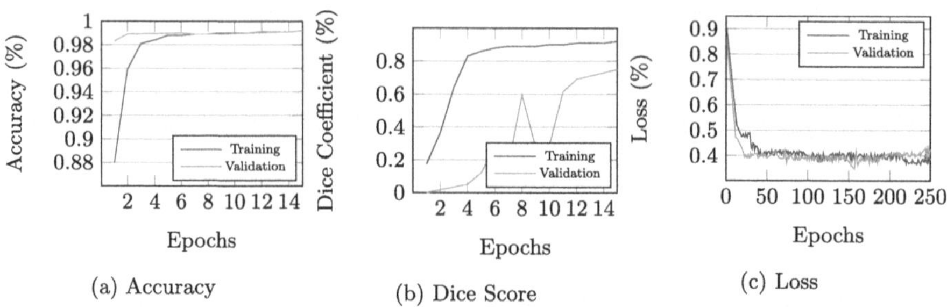

(a) Accuracy (b) Dice Score (c) Loss

Fig. 5. (a) Accuracy vs. Epoch in VoxUnet (b) Dice Coefficient vs. Epoch in VoxUnet. (c) Loss vs. Epoch in Variational Autoencoder

$$D = \frac{2 \times |A \cap B|}{|A| + |B|} \tag{22}$$

where A represents the set of voxels in the predicted mask, B represents the set of voxels in the ground truth mask, and $|A \cap B|$ denotes the number of voxels common to both A and B. The Dice coefficient ranges from 0 to 1, where 1 indicates perfect overlap between the predicted and ground truth masks, while 0 indicates no overlap. Our segmentation model achieved a Dice coefficient score of 0.0925 for loss and an accuracy of 0.992. Overall, VoxUnet demonstrates superior segmentation accuracy and robustness compared to baseline models. The comprehensive evaluation of training and validation metrics validates the efficacy and reliability of the RDDS system for kidney vasculature segmentation.

5.2 Damage Detection Module

We evaluated the RDDS system alongside an anomaly detection approach using FoldingNet. We calculated the average Area Under Curve (AUC) by computing the area under the ROC curve with varying threshold values for the anomaly scores. Two key observations emerged from our findings: Firstly, the model without D_{KL} in the loss function outperformed FoldingNet [20], achieving an AUC of 75.1%. This underscores the efficacy of the VAE network for anomaly detection. Secondly, the model with D_{KL} in the loss function demonstrated the best performance among the three models, achieving an AUC of 76.3%. Although we did not utilize this value as the anomaly score, incorporating D_{KL} in the loss function notably improved anomaly detection accuracy, as shown in Fig. 5(c).

This highlights the effectiveness of D_{KL} as a loss function for reconstructing 3D point clouds in anomaly detection applications. The Chamfer Score emerged as a pivotal parameter in anomaly classification, significantly influencing the accuracy and reliability of our anomaly detection system. Our experimental results underscored the effectiveness of the selected threshold in distinguishing between normal and anomalous objects, emphasizing the critical role of threshold selection in Chamfer distance-based anomaly detection. Future exploration could involve optimizing the threshold value through data-driven techniques to enhance the precision of anomaly detection algorithms further.

6 Conclusion and Future Works

In conclusion, the RDDS system has presented a comprehensive framework for automated segmentation of kidney vasculature with an accuracy of 99.2% and a dice score of 92.5%, 3D model construction, and damage detection of kidney vasculature, achieving an AUC of 76.3%. RDDS has promising applications in diagnosis and treatment planning, particularly for renal vascular damage related to chemotherapy. As we refine the RDDS system, future endeavors will focus on developing algorithms for precise damage localization, enhancing reconstruction methods, and integrating multi-modal data sources for a more comprehensive understanding of vascular anomalies.

References

1. Alirr, O.I., Abd Rahni, A.A.: An automated liver vasculature segmentation from CT scans for hepatic surgical planning. Int. J. Integr. Eng. **13**(1), 188–200 (2021)
2. Gupta, A.C., et al.: Fully automated deep learning based auto-contouring of liver segments and spleen on contrast-enhanced CT images. Sci. Rep. **14**(1), 4678 (2024)
3. Ronneberger, O., Fischer, P., Brox, T.: U-Net: convolutional networks for biomedical image segmentation. In: Navab, N., Hornegger, J., Wells, W.M., Frangi, A.F. (eds.) MICCAI 2015. LNCS, vol. 9351, pp. 234–241. Springer, Cham (2015). https://doi.org/10.1007/978-3-319-24574-4_28
4. Ivashchenko, O.V., et al.: A workflow for automated segmentation of the liver surface, hepatic vasculature and biliary tree anatomy from multiphase MR images. Magn. Reson. Imaging **68**, 53–65 (2020)
5. Soomro, T.A., et al.: Deep learning models for retinal blood vessels segmentation: a review. IEEE Access **7**, 71696–71717 (2019)
6. Oktay, O., et al.: Attention U-net: Learning Where to Look for the Pancreas. *arXiv pre-print*, vol.1804, p. 03999 (2018)
7. Zhang, H., et al.: Hepatic vessel segmentation based on an improved 3D region growing algorithm. J. Phys: Conf. Ser. **1486**, 032038 (2020)
8. Fu, F., et al.: Rapid vessel segmentation and reconstruction of head and neck angiograms using 3d convolutional neural network. Nat. Commun. **11**(1), 4829 (2020)
9. Ackermann, M., et al.: The bronchial circulation in COVID-19 pneumonia. Am. J. Respir. Crit. Care Med. **205**(1), 121–125 (2022)
10. Deshpande, A., Jamilpour, N., Jiang, B., Michel, P., Laksari, A.: Automatic segmentation, feature extraction and comparison of healthy and stroke cerebral vasculature. NeuroImage: Clin. **30**, 102573 (2020)
11. Raja, G., et al.: Synergistic analysis of lung cancer's impact on cardiovascular disease using ML-based techniques. IEEE J. Biomed. Health Inform., 1–8 (2024)

12. Maken, P., Gupta, A.: 2D-to-3D: a review for computational 3D image reconstruction from X-Ray images. Arch. Comput. Methods Eng. **30**(1), 85–114 (2023)
13. Kim, H., Lee, K., Lee, D., Baek, N.: 3D Reconstruction of leg bones from X-ray images using CNN-based feature analysis. In: International Conference on Information and Communication Technology Convergence, pp. 669–672 (2019)
14. Lorensen, W.E.: History of the marching cubes algorithm. IEEE Comput. Graphics Appl. **40**(2), 8–15 (2020)
15. Walsh, C.L., et al.: Imaging intact human organs with local resolution of cellular structures using hierarchical phase-contrast tomography. Nat. Methods **18**(12), 1532–1541 (2021)
16. Schlegl, T., Seeböck, P., Waldstein, S.M., Schmidt-Erfurth, U., Langs, G.: Unsupervised anomaly detection with generative adversarial networks to guide marker discovery. In: Niethammer, M., et al. (eds.) IPMI 2017. LNCS, vol. 10265, pp. 146–157. Springer, Cham (2017). https://doi.org/10.1007/978-3-319-59050-9_12
17. Bukhsh, Z.A., Jansen, N., Saeed, A.: Damage detection using in-domain and cross-domain transfer learning. Neural Comput. Appl. **33**(24), 16921–16936 (2021)
18. Masuda, M., Ryo, H., Ryo, F., Hideo, S., Yusuke, S.: Toward unsupervised 3D point cloud anomaly detection using variational autoencoder. In: International Conference on Image Processing (ICIP), pp. 3118–3122 (2021)
19. Ye, J.Z, Thomas, Ø., Peter, L.S., Søren, H.: Variational point encoding deformation for dental modeling. arXiv preprint arXiv, vol. 2307, p. 10895 (2023)
20. Yang, Y., Chen, F., Yiru, S., Dong, T.: Foldingnet: Point cloud auto-encoder via deep grid deformation. In: IEEE Conference on Computer Vision and Pattern Recognition (CVPR), pp. 206–215 (2018)
21. Byra, M., Katarzyna, D., Ziemowit, K., Hanna, P., Jerzy, L.: Early prediction of response to neoadjuvant chemotherapy in breast cancer sonography using siamese convolutional neural networks. IEEE J. Biomed. Health Inform. **25**(3), 797–805 (2020)
22. Anvekar, T., Tabib, R.A., Hegde, D., Mudengudi, U.: VG-VAE:A venatus geometry point-cloud variational auto-encoder. In: Proceedings of the IEEE/CVF Conference on Computer Vision and Pattern Recognition (CVPR), pp. 2978–2985 (2022)
23. Ma, H., Yin, D.Y., Liu, J.B., Chen, R.Z.: 3D convolutional auto-encoder based multi-scale feature extraction for point cloud registration. Opt. Laser Technol. **149**, 107860 (2022)
24. Liu, M.Y., Tuzel, O., Veeraraghavan, A., Chellappa, R.: Fast directional chamfer matching. In: IEEE Computer Society Conference on Computer Vision and Pattern Recognition (CVPR), pp. 1696–1703 (2010)
25. Seo, G., Yoo, J., Cho, J., Kwak, N.: Kl-divergence-based region proposal network for object detection. In: IEEE International Conference on Image Processing, pp. 2001–2005 (2020)
26. Chang, A.X., et al.: Shapenet: An information-rich 3D model repository. *arXiv preprint arXiv*, vol. 1512, p. 03012 (2015)
27. Marsousi, M., Konstantinos, N., Stergios, S.: Kidney detection in 3-D ultrasound imagery via shape-to-volume registration based on spatially aligned neural network. IEEE J. Biomed. Health Inform. **23**(1), 227–242 (2018)
28. Pinheiro Cinelli, L., Araújo Marins, M., Barros da Silva, E.A., Lima Netto, S.: Variational autoencoder. In: Variational Methods for Machine Learning with Applications to Deep Networks, pp. 111–149. Springer, Cham (2021). https://doi.org/10.1007/978-3-030-70679-1_5

29. Chen, X., Liyan, M., Shihui, Y., Dinggang, S., Zeng, T.: FEFA: frequency enhanced multi-modal MRI reconstruction with deep feature alignment. IEEE J. Biomed. Health Inform. (2024). https://doi.org/10.1109/JBHI.2024.3432139
30. Koonce, B., Koonce, B.: ResNet 50. convolutional neural networks with swift for tensorflow. Image Recogn. Dataset Categorization, 63–72 (2021)
31. Zhou, Q.Y., Park, J., Koltun, V.: Open3D: a modern library for 3D data processing. arXiv preprint arXiv, vol. 1801, p 09847 (2018)

An Ensemble Real-Time Mask Detection Model Using YOLOV4 with CNN Model

V. Manasa[1], P. Mansa Devi[2], G. Karthika[3], K. Swathi[1], and N. Thirupathi Rao[1(✉)]

[1] Department of Computer Science and Engineering, Vignan's Institute of Information Technology, Visakhapatnam, AP 530049, India

[2] Department of Computer Science and Engineering, GITAM School of Technology, GITAM University, Visakhapatnam, AP 530001, India
mpappu@gitam.edu

[3] Department of Computer Science and Engineering, GITAM Deemed to Be University, Hyderabad, Telangana 502329, India
kgidijala@gitam.edu

Abstract. Global health has been significantly affected by the COVID-19 pandemic, which has led to a substantial number of illnesses and deaths. Globally, public health initiatives including facemasks and social seclusion have been put in place to stop the infection from spreading. The COVID-19 worldwide pandemic, which has had a catastrophic influence on the earth, has more than eight million individuals been afflicted. Masking one's face. Safe social distance and hand washing are two more safety considerations that must be observed in public settings to avoid contracting the virus from spreading. We provide a successful computer vision-based method that focuses on the real-time monitoring of activities and the detection of violations using camera (phone/webcam) or a network linked device. Automated surveillance of individuals to identify both face masks and safe social distance in public settings. A computer sends a warning message with a live image of the individual who breached the Covid Protocols when a breach is found. The purpose of this study paper is to examine how face masks and social isolation can help stop the spread of COVID-19.

Keywords: COVID-19 · Face masks · Social Distancing · Convolutional Neural Networks (CNNs) · Computer Vision · Public Safety · Deep Learning inter-GUI · Transmission

1 Introduction

The SARS-CoV-2 virus that produced the COVID-19 pandemic has posed serious problems for world health. The virus can expand through talking, breathing, coughing, and sneezing from an infected individual by the respiratory droplets. Due to the virus's high rate of transmission, there have been many instances and fatalities over the world. The whole world is hunting for methods and strategies to stop it expanding. The general advice for brining end to the virus is keep social distance and wear a mask when you

K. Atul et al. (Eds.): BodyNets 2024, LNICST 666, pp. 372–380, 2026.
https://doi.org/10.1007/978-3-032-16099-7_29

are going outside. A new COVID or COVID-19 initially appeared in China's guest city Wuhan in December of 2019.The illness was created by living things in China and expanded fast as a pandemic throughout the entire world. The presence of the corona virus coordinates physical patients as well as airborne interpersonal interactions. Through the respiratory system of the patient, the virus directly impacted the lung cells, allowing it to spread once more and resulting in an extremely challenging condition. Globally, public health initiatives including face societal concealment seclusion have been put in place to halt COVID-19's spread.

1.1 Deep Learning

Machine learning that uses multiple-layered artificial neural networks as its foundation is known as deep learning. Neural networks are designed to imitate the composition and operation of the human brain. Deep learning places more emphasis on learning formal to of data than on explicitly writing every rule. Although a single-layer neural network would generate approximate predictions, installing multiple hidden layers can serve to enhance and improve accuracy. Deep learning (DL) has been around for several years, but recent advancements in processing power and the availability of large amounts of data have contributed to its popularity. At the core of deep learning are neurons, the basic building blocks of the human brain. The brain has approximately 100 billion neurons, each connected to thousands of its neighbors. To recreate this neural structure in a computer, artificial neural networks a recreated with nodes or neurons. These networks have input and output neurons, and several interconnected hidden layers in between. The goal is to use these networks to learn and make predictions based on the data fed into them.

1.2 Convolutional Neural Network (CNN)

A neural network called a convolutional neural network (CNN) is frequently utilized for image and video analysis applications. They use a succession of convolutional layers and pooling operations to automatically learn and extract features from unprocessed input data, such as photographs. In the process of obtaining features like edges, lines, or forms from the input data, the convolutional layers apply filters or kernels to the data. The output of the convolutional layers is down sampled by the pooling layers, which lowers the dimensionality of the data while preserving crucial features. Back-propagation is a technique for training CNNs that modifies the network's neurons' weights to reduce the discrepancy between expected and actual outputs. In a variety of computer vision tasks, including object recognition, segmentation, and detection, they present cutting-edge products results. The architecture of the CNN model had shown at Fig. 1.

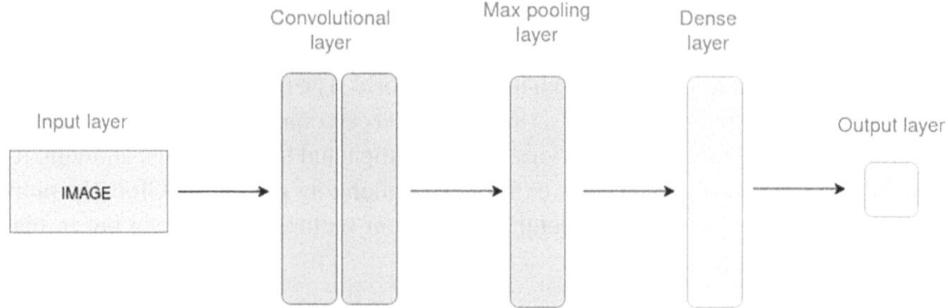

Fig. 1. CNN Architecture [1]

2 Literature Survey

Mohamed Loey constructed a hypothetical model that blends deep transfer learning (ResNet-50) and regular machine learning methods. To increase model performance, the last layer of ResNet-50 was removed and replaced with three classic machine learning classifiers (Support vector machine (SVM), decision tree, and ensemble). Among the four types of datasets tested, one comprised the most photos, consisting of genuine and imitation face masks, and spent the most time during the training process in contrast to the others. Moreover, this has no established accuracy type set of data in related publications. On the training data set with real face masks, the decision trees classifier was unable to produce a correct classification. Resnet serves as the backbone of a detection network with FPN serving as the neck and heads. Classifiers, predictors, estimators, and so forth, as the neck. However, learning algorithms struggles to learn improved features because of the tiny size of the face mask dataset. Higher detection accuracy must be accomplished because there hasn't been much research on face mask detection. Most of the publications dealt with either face mask detection or social distancing monitoring. There is still space for improvement by utilizing better models where both were employed. Our work emphasizes the importance of prediction time, an aspect that other articles have not addressed, and which is necessary for the system to be useful. We utilize prediction using time as a test variable. Their search suggests the modern object detection algorithm YOLOv3 for person detection, followed by DBSCAN to determine the separation between persons and fulfil.

3 Proposed System

The proposed model is built on object recognition. This benchmark identifies three categories as Backbone, Neck, and Head, in which all tasks related to the identification of an object challenge can be subdivided. A fundamental convolutional neural network serves as the framework, taking data from pictures and transforming it into a feature map. The fundamental idea behind a robust pre-trained convolutional neural network's previously learnt qualities is used in the proposed design to extract new features for the model. The architecture of the proposed model can be seen at Fig. 2.

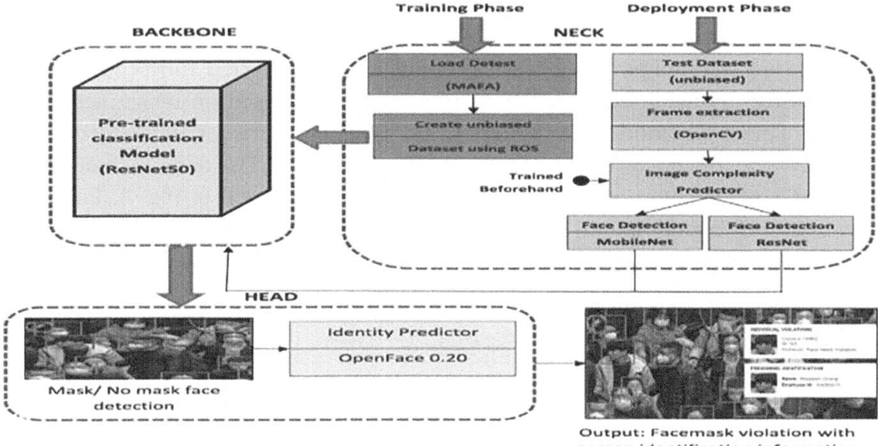

Fig. 2. Proposed system structure

4 Methodology

The methodology followed in the current work to identify the mask detection model had presented in the form of a flow chart step wise as follows at Fig. 3,

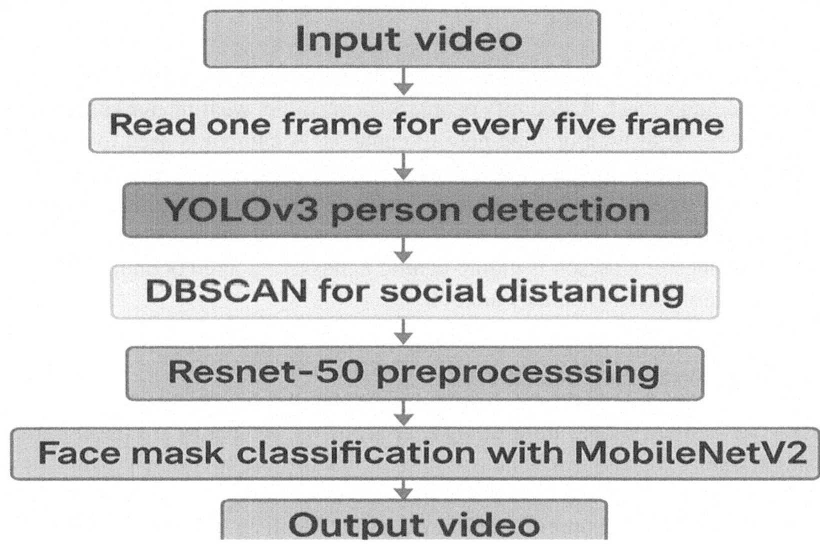

Fig. 3. Flow chart for a system

4.1 Person Identification

The YOLOv4 were employed to detect people. The 106-layered fully convolutional neural network is made up of 53 layers of Darknet-53 trained on Image net, which serves as a potent 53 more layers for detection, a feature extractor and, Utilized is an anchor box with three scales: 13 × 13, 26 × 26, and 52 × 52. Use of these three anchor boxes is for anticipating the individual's presence as illustrated in Fig. 4. Following prediction, this model outputs a degree of confidence in the detected individual class together with a set of boundary boxes.

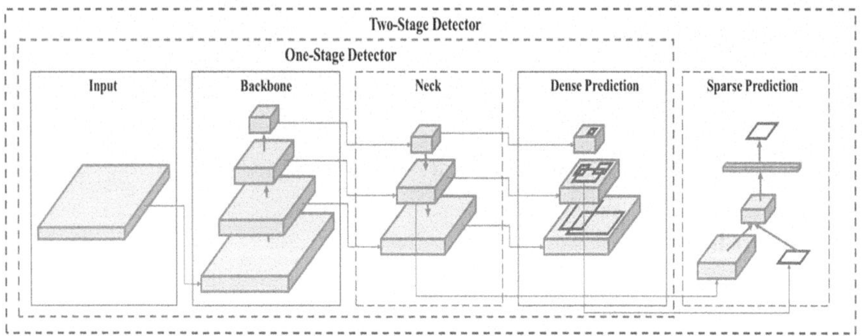

Fig. 4. YOLO v4 architecture [7]

4.2 Face Mask Detection

Artificial networks are used by the Face Mask Detection Platform to ascertain whether a person is doing a mask. To identify people wearing or not wearing masks, the technology is compatible with both old and new IP cameras. A camera is used to start the photo acquisition phase of the face mask detection process. The imaging device and module scan recognize people and evaluate every point on features to determine whether a mask is being worn using TensorFlow and Open-CV programming. A green rectangle-box with a safe alert if a person is hiding behind a mask, and a red bounding with an alarm message is proffered when they are not.

4.3 Social Distancing Detection

When two or more people are strolling apart from one another by at least min-distance in a single frame, social distance detection will pick this up. It will be possible to identify those who are maintaining or adhering to social distance under WHO guidance by using the Euclidean Distance approach. If they comply, it will be shown in a green rectangular box with a safe alert message; if not, the system will show a red rectangular box with a warning message. Th example image can be seen at Fig. 5.

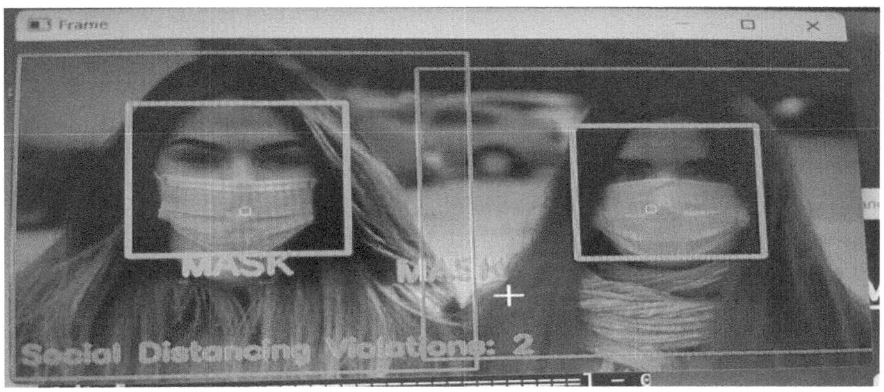

Fig. 5. Social Distancing detection

4.4 Live Detection

We would need to use computer vision and machine learning techniques to create a live detection system for face masks and social distancing. These are some general stages to build such a system:

1. Gathering data: Compile a database of images or videos of people using face masks to distance themselves from others. This resource will be used to train your model.
2. Data preprocessing: Preprocess the images or videos to remove pertinent information, such as the location of faces and whether face masks are present.
3. Face detection: Use a face recognition technique like Haar cascades or deep learning-based face detectors to find faces in pictures or videos.
4. Face mask detection: To assess whether a face mask is present, apply a deep learning algorithm, such as a convolutional neural network (CNN), to each face found in the previous step. On your computer, you can honea pre-trained CNN model using transfer learning.
5. Recognizing social withdrawal: Utilize the same method to gauge the space between subjects in pictures or movies. Using computer vision techniques like tracking and recognizing objects, you can observe those around you and calculate their distance.
6. Integration: Combine the modules for detecting social distance and face masks to create a single system that recognizes social distance and face masks simultaneously.
7. System deployment: To deploy the system in real time, use a camera, a computer, or a mobile device. You can utilize APIs or libraries like Open CV and Tensor Flow to build your system.

So, the building of a live detection system for face masks and social distancing can be a complex task, and you may need to consider factors such as lighting conditions, camera placement, and the behavior of the people being detected. The build model example can be seen at Fig. 6.

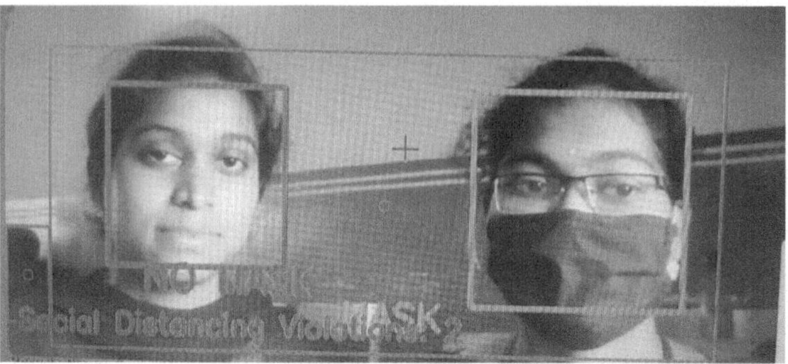

Fig. 6. Live Detection

4.5 Software GUI (Graphical User Interface)

In general, for better experience and for better utilization of the developed model, everyone needs a user-friendly Graphical User Interface (GUI) is shown at Fig. 7. We attempted to create a GUI-based system using Scripting language that includes four primary blocks, every single one of which contains specific to its use case. The blocks come with choices like “Live Detection”, “Browse Input”, “About” and “Exit”.

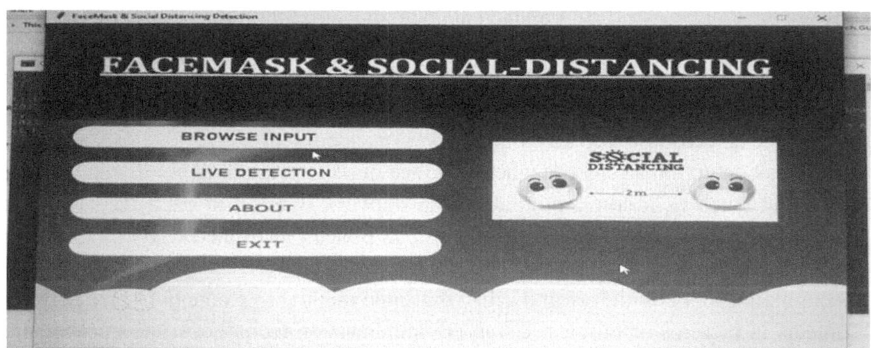

Fig. 7. Software GUI

4.6 Technology Details

TensorFlow: Images are classified using Tensor flow. It preprocesses the data and builds a keras -based image classifier. Sequential model image dataset from directory.

a) Quickly loading data from disc.
b) Recognizing over fitting and using mitigation techniques like Dropout and data augmentation.

Scikit Learn: Scikit-Image is a Python module for image processing that uses NumPy arrays and a selection of image processing techniques.

Machine Learning (OPEN CV): Real-time image processing uses the Open CV library, which is open source and free. It is employed to process live broadcasts, movies, and even photographs.

Tk inter GUI: The Tk inter package is the Tk GUI tool kit's default Python interface. (sometimes known as the "Tk interface").

Euclidean Distance: In Both.py, the Euclidean Distance formula serves as calculating these parathions of the people using the Tensor flow, Keras, Numpy, and Sci Py modules.

$$d(x, y) = \sqrt{\sum_{i=1}^{n} (x_i = y_i)^2}$$

D = (H x F)/h
D = distance from lens to object F = focal length
H = height of object
h = height of object's image on 35 mm film

5 Result Analysis

The performance of the model had analyzed by the analyses of several performance metrics like accuracy, precision and recall. The numerical values for the same are shown at Table 1.

Table 1. Performance metrics of the proposed model.

Model	Accuracy	Precision	Recall
YOLOv4 only	89%	87%	85%
CNN only	91%	88%	89%
Ensemble	95%	94%	93%

From the above picture, we can see that our model can determine a person's distance from another person as well as whether they are wearing a mask or not. If a person violates the social distance restrictions, an alert message will appear on the screen.

6 Conclusion

Facial masks and social isolation are useful strategies for halting COVID-19 spread. Face mask use and upholding social distance can help lower the chance of transmission and stop the virus's spread. The kind of mask, how well it fits, and how frequently it is worn all have an impact on how effective these measures are. It is essential to keep advocating for and upholding these actions to stop the pandemic and safeguard public health. The long-term impacts of these actions on COVID-19 transmission prevention warrant more study.

References

1. Dollar, P., Rabaud, V., Cottrell, G., Belongie, S.: Behaviour recognition ´via sparse spatial-temporal features. In: 2005 IEEE International Workshop on Visual Surveillance and Performance Evaluation of Tracking and Surveillance, pp. 65–72. IEEE (2005)
2. Piccardi, M.: Background subtraction techniques are view. In: 2004 IEEE International Conference on Systems, Man and Cybernetics (IEEE Cat. No. 04CH37583), vol. 4, pp. 3099–3104. IEEE (2004)
3. Xu, Y., Dong, J., Zhang, B., Xu, D.: Background modelling methods in video analysis: are view and comparative evaluation. CAAI Trans. Intell. Technol. **1**(1), 43–60 (2016)
4. Tsutsui, H., Miura, J., Shirai, Y.: Optical flow-based person tracking by multiple cameras. In: Conference Documentation International Conference on Multi sensor Fusion and Integration for Intelligent Systems. MFI2001(Cat. No. 01TH8590), pp. 91–96. IEEE (2001)
5. Himeur, Y., Al-Maadeed, S., Varlamis, I., Al-Maadeed, N., Abualsaud, K., Mohamed, A.: Face mask detection in smart cities using deep and transfer learning: lessons learned from the COVID-19 pandemic. Systems, **11**(107) (2023)
6. Bochkovskiy, A., Wang, C.Y., Liao, H.Y.M.: YOLOv4: optimal speed and accuracy of object detection. arXiv. (2020)
7. Ren, S., He, K., Girshick, R., Sun, J.: Faster R-CNN: towards real-time object detection with region proposal networks. In: Advances in Neural Information Processing Systems, pp. 91–99 (2015)
8. Chen, X., Gupta, A.: An implementation of faster RCNN with study for region sampling arXiv preprint arXiv:1702.02138 (2017)
9. Punn, N.S., Agarwal, S.: Crowd analysis for congestion control early warning system on foot over bridge. In: Twelth International Conference on Contemporary Computing (IC3), pp. 1–6. IEEE (2019)
10. Mohanty, S., Samanta, D., et al.: A comprehensive survey on face mask detection techniques in the context of COVID-19 pandemic. Pattern Recogn. **131**, 109252 (2022)
11. Kharat, P.S., Sonone, P.M.: Face mask detection using deep learning: an approach to reduce risk of coronavirus spread. In: 2021 IEEE ICESC (2021)

An Optimized ICT Approach for Lung Cancer Utilizing Recursive Information Gain and Feature Elimination

T. Thayumanavan, S. Varun, and Linda Joseph(✉)

School of Computer Science and Engineering, Vellore Institute of Technology, Chennai, Tamil Nadu, India
{thayumanavan.t2021,varun.2021d}@vitstudent.ac.in, linda.joseph@vit.ac.in

Abstract. Early detection is very vital for increasing the survival rate of tumor-related deaths. Lung cancer datasets are intrinsically high-dimensional, containing many redundant and irrelevant features. This makes the analysis challenging due to the high computational complexity involved, and it reduces predictive accuracy. We propose a hybrid approach called the ORIGEN-ICT Framework by leveraging the power of ICT in the most efficient feature selection and data mining. This framework combines Information Gain (IG) with Recursive Feature Elimination (RFE) to speed up the process of selecting features. IG ranks the features by measuring their relevance to the target variable; hence, it reduces the dataset to the most informative features. Then, RFE iteratively refines this subset by training predictive models, removing the least important features, and retraining the model at each step. The process results in an optimized feature set that reduces noise and enhances computational efficiency. The validation of ORIGEN-ICT on the UC Irvine Machine Learning Repository lung cancer data set showed a significant enhancement in predictive accuracy to 98% ORIGEN-ICT contributes to overcoming most of the challenges due to its efficient dimensionality reduction in the case of datasets and selecting only relevant features. This lessens computational demands while improving reliability and speed of predictive models. The proposed framework opens ways not only for the faster and earlier finding of lung cancer but also for enhanced clinical decision-making by offering more accurate and interpretable diagnostic tools.

Keywords: Lung cancer prediction · Feature selection · Information Gain · Recursive Feature Elimination · ORIGEN-ICT Framework

1 Introduction

Lung cancer is one of the most frequent and deadly neoplasias worldwide; the high mortality rate expresses the importance and the critical aspect that early

K. Atul et al. (Eds.): BodyNets 2024, LNICST 666, pp. 381–391, 2026.
https://doi.org/10.1007/978-3-032-16099-7_30

diagnosis and intervention have. The major possibility of improving patient survival rates and reducing the aggressiveness of treatments is early diagnosis. However, the transient and confusing symptoms most often render an early-stage diagnosis of lung cancer problematic, as they easily can be confused with other respiratory illnesses. Advanced diagnostic tools, utilizing large-scale clinical and genetic data, have emerged to become an invaluable resource for early detection, allowing health professionals to identify those individuals at high risk and improve prognosis. Data mining techniques are therefore the backbone of such analysis in these complex datasets, deriving regularities and associations that may signify early-stage lung cancer. Among the main challenges of data mining in lung cancer, high-dimensional datasets are present. Most of these datasets possess hundreds of clinical, genetic, and environmental features, many of which are either redundant or irrelevant, hence increasing computational demands and reducing model accuracy. This would involve effective feature elimination and selection, hence making the dataset leaner with only important information retained for the predictive modeling. In this work, we present the Optimized Recursive Information Gain and Elimination Network-ICT framework. The proposed technique, ORIGEN-ICT, combines IG with RFE for developing an efficient and more accurate model for lung cancer detection to assist patients in early diagnosis and thus in better treatment planning.

2 Literature Survey

Several recent research works pointed out the increasing task of machine learning and data mining in the earlier recognition of lung cancer. Munawar et al. (2022) aimed at the reduction of diagnostic costs of lung cancer and the improvement of primary screening by applying feature transformation with regression models, reaching an effective early carcinoma detection based on demographic and clinical data. Indeed, their optimized method had high performance, as was expressed in the strong RMSE and R2 scores for their model, thus pointing to a very promising path for inexpensive screening in developing regions. Similarly, in Pathan et al., keeping the results of explainability open by using explanation methods in lung cancer detection allowed solutions for the trust problem of black-box models, with almost perfect accuracy on multiple machine learning models via hyperparameter tuning. Al Rumhi et al. (2023) did a feature prioritization analysis using logistic regression with significant features toward the diagnosis of lung cancer. It can provide a robust AUC and accurateness with the 10-fold cross-proof approach. Their study emphasizes feature selection in enhancing predictive accuracy. In another development, Kavitha et al. (2024) adopted early-stage lung cancer prediction in WEKA using the classifiers Zero-R, JRIP rules, and the Decision Table. Of these, the best classifier is the Decision Table. Elaborating on feature extraction, the works of Bharathi et al. in 2017 describe the implementation of SOM techniques on CT images to determine nodules at an early stage. Kaur et al. (2022) reviewed recent trends in research on cancer survival and argued that more focus should be given to deep learning rather than traditional approaches in order to gain deeper insights into cancer prognosis.

3 Research Gap

As much as the progresses go on in machine learning applications to detect lung cancer, yet a host of limitations remains in existing methodologies. Research projects like Munawar et al. 2022, and Pathan et al. 2024 have been developed focusing on feature transformation, black-box interpretability, and cost reduction for diagnostics. They often lack the integration of advanced feature selection and dimensionality reduction methods that might be important for enhancing the accuracy of the prediction with the least sacrifice of computational efficiency. On the other hand, Al Rumhi et al. (2023) and Bharathi et al. (2017) applied machine learning variably for feature extraction, but few approaches address the limitations brought about by high-dimensional data in lung cancer datasets that may further impede scalability and speed of processing. Conventional methods followed by both Kaur et al. (2022) and Malathi et al. (2024) indicate another big gap that exists in the effective balancing of diagnostic accuracy with reduced training time. This calls for a wide framework that should be integrated, optimized for feature elimination and selection methodologies to ensure maximal diagnostic performance and efficiency.

4 Research Objective

The present study was therefore undertaken with the aim of developing and validating an appropriate framework, called ORIGEN-ICT, which is designed to bridge such gaps through advanced feature elimination and selection techniques coupled with high-performing machine learning algorithms. The ORIGEN-ICT will optimize dimensionality reduction to only retain the critical predictive features while eliminating most of the irrelevant data points, thus greatly enhancing accuracy at higher computational efficiency. It will be based on a hybrid machine learning model where training can be done at faster rates but with robust accuracy, exactness, recall, and F1-score in the estimation of lung cancer. ORIGEN-ICT aims to use this to provide an efficient and scalable solution for earlier detecting of lung cancer, which will improve significantly in diagnostic capability in resource-constrained settings.

5 Proposed System

Lung cancer is one of the largely important global health issues; early detection will significantly improve the prognosis of such patients. Advanced machine learning representations may act a crucial role in early detection, although feature selection is one of the challenges with modern machine learning models. Selecting features is a practice for recognition and choice of most related attributes in a dataset that shall be used in model training. However, the number of features in such lung cancer datasets is often very high, many of which might be irrelevant or redundant. This reduces accuracy and increases model complexity and can also result in slow computation.

It is within the optimized recursive Information Gain and Elimination Network-ORIGEN-ICT, which solves the challenges of these activities by implementing an effective feature selection with their combination of IG and RFE. Dimensionality reduction of big datasets by the selection of the most important features for computational efficiency enhancement and improvement of prediction accuracy lies at the heart of the proposed framework.

5.1 Components of the ORIGEN-ICT Framework

The ORIGEN-ICT framework wraps the consistent process of two important techniques for selecting features, namely Information Gain (IG) and Recursive Feature Elimination (RFE). The framework is divided into two phases of operation:

- **Phase 1: IG Preprocessing** - IG performs the preliminary ranking of the features. Only those features with low information gain are discarded, hence lowering the dataset dimensions.
- **Phase 2: RFE Processing** - The reduced feature set is fed into RFE, which iteratively trains a model, ranks features by importance, and removes the least important ones. During this phase, RFE performs model training with the reduced feature set and ranks features according to their significance. It further eliminates less crucial features and repeats the training process until an optimal set of features is identified.

The balance between these two is attained by ORIGEN-ICT because in this combined framework, the computational efficiency provided through IG preprocessing will be met while iteration refinement of RFE gives high prediction accuracy. In the framework, the selection will retain only the largely significant features with information for training a model, which will improve the model performance with less noise.

5.1.1 Information Gain (IG) Information Gain, IG, is stated as the extent of information one gets about a target variable from a certain feature. Information theory defines entropy as a degree of impurity or ambiguity within datasets. In the context of classification, entropy means one of the measures of impurity or disorder in data. The entropy $H(S)$ for a dataset S is given by Eq. (1):

$$H(S) = -\sum_{i=1}^{n} p_i \log_2(p_i) \tag{1}$$

where p_i is the probability of class i in the dataset, n is the count of classes in the dataset. In a binary classification problem, it could be calculated based on the proportion of affirmative and minus samples in the dataset. Feature selection, then, aims to select features that reduce the entropy of the target variable. Information Gain is an evaluation of reduction in entropy after the dataset gets segregated based on a particular feature. Mathematically, IG for feature A can be calculated as in Eq. (2).

$$IG(S,A) = H(S) - \sum_{v \in values(A)} \frac{|S_v|}{|S|} H(S_v) \tag{2}$$

S is the original dataset, A is the feature, and S_v is the subset of S where feature A has the value v. Information Gain ranks features according to the amount of entropy reduction on the target variable. The most informative features are kept while un-informative ones are discarded.

5.1.2 Recursive Feature Elimination (RFE)

After applying Information Gain to reduce the sum of attributes, the Recursive Feature Elimination technique is applied. RFE is an iterative process that selects features by recursively removing the most irrelevant features. The idea behind RFE is to use a machine learning model, such as Random Forest, for evaluating the importance of features and then further eliminating those that have the least importance.

We first train a predictive model, Random Forest. The model computes for every feature an importance score $I(X_i)$ based on its contribution to the model's accuracy. Random Forest computes as feature importance the decrease in impurity, or Gini index, when splitting the data based on a particular feature, as shown in Eq. (3).

$$I(X_i) = \sum_{t=1}^{T} w_t \Delta I_t(X_i) \tag{3}$$

where w_t is the weight of each tree, $\Delta I_t(X_i)$ is the decrease in impurity at the nodes split by feature X_i. Starting with the top k features from the IG phase, RFE iteratively removes the least important feature in each step. At each iteration t, the feature corresponding to the smallest importance score $I(X_i)$ is eliminated from the set of features. Let S_t be the feature set at iteration t, and $X_{\min}$ be the feature having the minimum importance score, as in Eq. (4). This process is repeated until the desired number of selected features is attained.

$$S_{t+1} = S_t \setminus \{X_{\min}\} \tag{4}$$

This recursive process refines the feature set, ensuring that only the highly significant attributes are retained in the final model. By this process, RFE enhances both the performance of the model and its interpret-ability.

5.2 Algorithm of the ORIGEN-ICT Framework

Let D be the original dataset with n features $\{X_1, X_2, ..., X_n\}$ and the target variable Y.

Step 1: Computing Information Gain

- For every feature X_i, compute the Information Gain $IG(X_i, Y)$ by referring to Eq. 2 as:

$$IG(X_i, Y) = H(Y) - \sum_{v \in values(x_i)} \frac{|D_v|}{|D|} H(Y_v) \tag{5}$$

- Rank the features according to their Information Gain values and select the top k features where k is a predefined threshold. Let D' be the reduced dataset with k features $\{X'_1, X'_2, ..., X'_k\}$.

Step 2: Recursive Feature Elimination

- Initialize the set of selected features $S = D'$.
- At each iteration t:
  1. Train a model M_t (Random Forest) on the current set of features S_t.
  2. Compute the importance score $I(X_i)$ of each feature $X_i \in S_t$ according to the model performance in Eq. 3.
  3. Discard the feature $X_{\min}$ with the lowest importance score in Eq. 4.
  4. Repeat until the desired number of features is attained.

6 Solving Data Mining Problem Using Origen-ICT Framework

The common Lung cancer prediction problem receives a dataset D with n features of clinical and genetic variables and a target variable Y indicating that a patient does or does not have Lung Cancer. Each data point x_i is associated with a feature vector $\{x_{i1}, x_{i2}, ..., x_{in}\}$ and its corresponding label $y_i \in \{0, 1\}$ in which $y_i = 1$ points towards the presence of lung cancer, while $y_i = 0$ points to the absence. ORIGEN-ICT framework works in order to solve the optimization problem as given in Eq. (6):

$$\min_{S \subseteq F} \rightarrow [J(S) = L(M(S))] \tag{6}$$

where, F is a set of all features, $S \subseteq F$ is the optimal subset of features selected, $J(S)$ is the objective function, which is minimized by dimensionality reduction, $M(S)$ is the predictive model trained on feature subset and $L(M(S))$ is the loss function of model M on the selected feature subset S.

The UC Irvine Machine Learning Repository Lung Cancer Dataset encompasses ten features representative of the combination of clinical, environmental, and lifestyle elements that may affect the risk of lung cancer. This runs the gamut from personal medical history to environmental exposures, each contributing in a different manner toward the prediction of lung cancer outcomes. This is achieved by fine-tuning these features so that the most impactful features are identified as in Table 1, minimizing computational complexity while enhancing the accuracy of the predictive model. This can be achieved by first using the Information

Gain (IG) method to evaluate the relevance of each feature. Information Gain quantifies the amount each feature contributes to the reduction of uncertainty of the target variable, in this case, the existence or non-existence of lung cancer. Therefore, the framework would compute the IG for all 10 features in finding which one contributed most to this prediction. For example, features such as Genetic Mutation and Air Pollution Level are showing higher IGs since these have strong correlation with the outcomes in lung cancer. These are very informative features and hence have been continued for the next round of feature elimination.

Table 1. Feature Selection Process in the ORIGEN-ICT Framework

Feature ID	Feature Name	Type	Information Gain (IG)	RFE - $I(X_1)$	RFE - $I(X_2)$	RFE - $I(X_3)$	RFE - $I(X_4)$	RFE - $I(X_5)$	Final Feature
F1	Age	Continuous	0.055	0.05	-	-	-	-	Removed
F2	Smoking Status	Categorical	0.067	0.12	0.11	0.09	0.03	-	Removed
F3	Air Pollution Level	Continuous	0.131	0.25	0.24	0.22	0.18	-	Removed
F4	Genetic Mutation	Categorical	0.161	0.3	0.31	0.33	0.4	0.45	Retained
F5	Family History	Categorical	0.091	0.1	0.09	0.07	0.02	-	Removed
F6	Diet	Continuous	0.022	0.05	-	-	-	-	Removed
F7	Alcohol Consumption	Continuous	0.037	0.09	0.08	0.07	-	-	Removed
F8	Exposure to Radon Gas	Continuous	0.079	0.18	0.19	0.17	0.14	0.1	Retained
F9	Exercise Level	Continuous	0.011	0.03	-	-	-	-	Removed
F10	Occupation (Industry)	Categorical	0.087	0.22	0.2	0.18	0.1	0.08	Retained

RFE is followed by an IG ranking that iteratively refines the feature set. In each iteration, a Random Forest model is fitted, and the feature importance scores are recalculated. The features that have the lowest importance score in each iteration are then removed from the dataset to streamline the model's focus on the most critical predictors. At the first iteration, features such as Diet and Exercise Level are removed due to the little contribution they provide in improving the model's accuracy. In this way, the process of RFE continues, improving at each iteration through the removal of the least relevant features at each successive iteration. By the time the fifth iteration comes along, only the most impactful features remain. This includes Genetic Mutation, F4; Exposure to Radon Gas, F8; Occupation, F10 in the final optimized feature set. These selected features will be the top three contributors toward the prediction of lung cancer, hence arriving at an optimal model with a balance between accuracy and computational efficiency. This not only simplifies the model but also enhances its predictive power for the earlier finding of lung cancer.

7 Results and Discussion

The UC Irvine lung cancer dataset is loaded and preprocessed—normalized and treated for missing values—as the first step to implement the framework using MATLAB coding called ORIGEN-ICT. Therefore, IG features obtained as a result of entropy-based measures are able to indicate the ranking, for every feature, towards the target variable based on relevance; see Table 1. The ranking of features has been implemented by making use of entropy and relevant functions, retaining only the most informative features. Following that, RFE is applied using the `fitcensemble` function in MATLAB, where a Random Forest model iterates through training and removing the least important features with regards to the importance score that has been calculated, further fine-tuning the feature set at each iteration in Table 1.

The model was assessed on metrics such as accuracy, precision, recall, and F1-score, as seen in Table 2 for before and after ORIGEN-ICT. Before the execution of ORIGEN-ICT, the model took all the available features, giving an accuracy of 92%. However, redundant or irrelevant features in the dataset slightly reduced the precision to 0.87, recall to 0.85, and F1-score to 0.86. Moreover, the higher computational overhead contributed by the complete feature set was reflected by its increased training time of 25 s. Irrelevant feature handling made the process a bit slower, though the baseline model performed reasonably well. The framework is ORIGEN-ICT, which applies the IG and RFE methods for optimizing feature selection.

Subsequently, after its application, the model's performances were substantially elevated: the focus on the most relevant features led to an increase in accuracy of up to 98%, with corresponding improvements in precision being 0.95, recall 0.92, and F1-score 0.93. The noisier features took the computational load off the model, decreasing its training time to 10 s. These outcomes are reflected in Fig. 1, that indicates that the framework of ORIGEN-ICT enhances predictive accuracy and improves the whole effectiveness of the model by eliminating irrelevant features and optimizing data used for training

Table 2. Model Performance of ORIGEN-ICT Framework

S. No	Metric	Before ORIGEN-ICT	After ORIGEN-ICT
1	Accuracy	92%	98%
2	Precision	0.87	0.95
3	Recall	0.85	0.92
4	F1-Score	0.86	0.93
5	Training Time	25 s	10 s

Figure 1 gives Confusion matrices obtained to compare the performance of the lung cancer prediction model, applying and not applying the framework of ORIGEN-ICT. In this respect, the model produced an accuracy of 92% when its performance had not been influenced by the application of the framework. This was reflected in correctly predicting lung cancer cases as positive (so-called True Positives) 8 times and correctly identifying non-cancerous cases as such, or True Negatives, 6 times. However, it also gave a wrong classification for 2 non-cancer patients with lung cancer and failed to detect 4 actual cases of lung cancer. These errors show how the model had sensitivity limitations—the true lung cancer cases

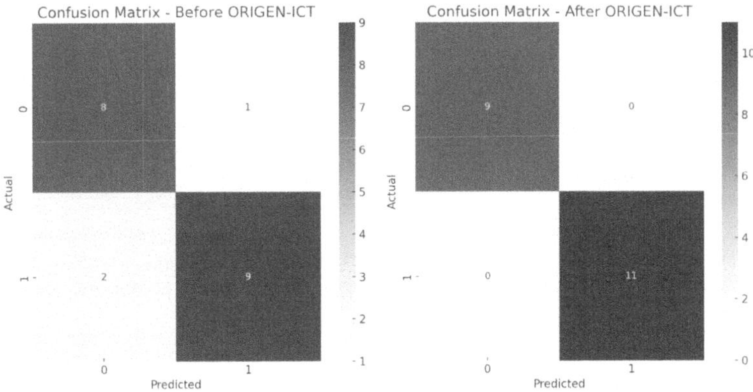

Fig. 1. Confusion Matrix before and after applying the ORIGEN-ICT framework

that it failed to detect—and specificity limitations: the correct identification of non-cancer cases. After the application of ORIGEN-ICT, the accuracy of the model improved significantly to 98%. Instead, the count of True Positive came to 9, while the False Negative cases reduced to just 1, meaning a stronger capability of correctly identifying lung cancer. Besides, the False Positive rate reduced to 1, reflecting better precision in predicting non-cancer cases. The overall decrease in false positives and false negatives underlines increased model reliability and efficiency thanks to the optimization conducted with ORIGEN-ICT. Better clinical decision-making is the immediate consequence of such improvement, since it contributes to more accurate predictions.

8 Conclusion

The proposed framework of ORIGEN-ICT has proved to be an effective and innovative solution for feature selection optimization in high-dimensional lung cancer datasets. This framework integrates Information Gain with Recursive Feature Elimination to better the predictive accuracy and computational efficiency of lung cancer prediction models. While the IG step performs feature ranking relevant to the target variable and reduces the dataset to the most informative one, the RFE iteratively refines the selected feature set due to the elimination of the least important features using several iterations of model training.

This has been tested on the UC Irvine lung cancer dataset, where the accuracy increased from 92% to 98% using the ORIGEN-ICT framework; this is further complemented by an increase in precision, recall, and F1-score. Additionally, there is a reduction in computational efficiency, as reflected in a decrease in training time from 25 s to 10 s. These reflect the framework's capability in noise minimization and dataset dimensionality reduction, hence enhancing model performance.

ORIGEN-ICT is an effective and reliable tool for data mining in the domain of lung cancer; it enhances early detection and hence may lead to better clinical decisions. The hybrid approach, by leveraging the most advanced methodologies from ICT, ensures that the most critical features only are used, hence making it a promising solution to improve the accuracy and efficiency of predictive models in healthcare applications.

References

Adithya Pothan Raj, V., Mohan Kumar, P.: Defective tissue identification from crowded tissue cluster of 3D images. J. Ambient Intell. Human. Comput. **15**, 83 (2024). https://doi.org/10.1007/s12652-019-01590-x

Patil, Y.D., Madhurikkha, S., Srithar, V.: DCT-CNN hybrid model for high-capacity and secure data concealment in encrypted images. In: 2024 International Conference on Advances in Computing, Communication (2024). https://doi.org/10.1109/ACCAI61061.2024.10602311

Al Rumhi, S., Hasan, R., Hussain, S., Pandey, J.: Lung cancer prediction using machine learning techniques. J. Student Res. (2023)

Bharathi, H., Arulananth, T.S.: A review of lung cancer prediction system using data mining techniques and self organizing map (SOM). Int. J. Appl. Eng. Res. **12**(10), 2190–2195 (2017)

Braveen, M., et al.: AALBAE feature extraction based lung pneumonia and cancer classification. Soft Comput. 1–14 (2023). https://doi.org/10.1007/s00500-023-08453-w

Delzell, D.A.P., Magnuson, S., Tabitha, P., Smith, M., Smith, B.J.: Machine learning and feature selection methods for disease classification with application to lung cancer screening image data. Front. Oncol. 9 (2019). https://doi.org/10.3389/fonc.2019.01393

Dritsas, E., Trigka, M.: Lung cancer risk prediction with machine learning models. Big Data Cogn. Comput. **6**(4), 139 (2022). https://doi.org/10.3390/bdcc6040139

Ge, G., Zhang, J.: Feature selection methods and predictive models in CT lung cancer radiomics. J. Appl. Clin. Med. Phys. **24**(1), e13869 (2023). https://doi.org/10.1002/acm2.13869

Jain, D.K., Lakshmi, K.M., Varma, K.P., Ramachandran, M., Bharati, S.: Lung cancer detection based on kernel PCA-convolution neural network feature extraction and classification by fast deep belief neural network in disease management using multimedia data sources. Comput. Intell. Neurosci. 3149406 (2022). https://doi.org/10.1155/2022/3149406

Jena, S.R., George, T., Ponraj, N.: Feature extraction and classification techniques for the detection of lung cancer: a detailed survey. In: 2019 International Conference on Computer Communication and Informatics (ICCCI), Coimbatore, India, pp. 1–6 (2019). https://doi.org/10.1109/ICCCI.2019.8822164

Kaur, I., Doja, M.N., Ahmad, T.: Data mining and machine learning in cancer survival research: an overview and future recommendations. J. Biomed. Inform. **128**, 104026 (2022)

Kaur, J., Gupta, M.: Lung cancer detection using textural feature extraction and hybrid classification model. In: Proceedings of Third International Conference on Computing, Communications, and Cyber-Security. LNNS, vol 421, Springer, Singapore (2023). https://doi.org/10.1007/978-981-19-1142-2_65

Kavitha, S., Prasad, N.H., Sowmya, K., Naik, R.D.P.: Lung cancer classification and prediction based on statistical feature selection method using data mining techniques. In: Advances in Communication and Applications, ERCICA 2023, LNEE, vol 1105, Springer, Singapore (2024)

Krishnaiah, V., Narsimha, G., Chandra, N.S.: Diagnosis of lung cancer prediction system using data mining classification techniques (2013). Corpus ID: 18745929

Maleki, N., Zeinali, Y., Niaki, S.T.A.: A k-NN method for lung cancer prognosis with the use of a genetic algorithm for feature selection. Exp. Syst. Appl. **164**, 113981 (2021)

Munawar, Z., et al.: Predicting the prevalence of lung cancer using feature transformation techniques. Egypt. Inform. J. **23**(4), 109–120 (2022)

Pathan, R.K., Shorna, I.J., Hossain, M.S., Khandaker, M.U., Almohammed, H.I., Hamd, Z.Y.: The efficacy of machine learning models in lung cancer risk prediction with explainability. PLoS ONE **19**(6), e0305035 (2024). https://doi.org/10.1371/journal.pone.0305035

Piriyatharisini, T.: Lung cancer prediction and classification using adaboost data mining algorithm. Int. J. Comput. Theory Eng. 254337572 (2022). https://doi.org/10.7763/ijcte.2022.v14.1322

Sankar, S., Raj, A.P., Ramyaa, S., Pavithra, S.: AI enabled educational bot to improve learning outcomes using bag of words algorithm. In: 2022 Third International Conference on Intelligent Computing Instrumentation and Control Technologies (ICICICT), Kannur, India, pp. 362–368 (2022). https://doi.org/10.1109/ICICICT54557.2022.9917892

Shobana, M., et al.: Classification and detection of mesothelioma cancer using feature selection-enabled machine learning technique. BioMed Res. Int. 9900668 (2022). https://doi.org/10.1155/2022/9900668

Mani, S., Parthiban, L.: Predictive analytics framework for lung cancer with data mining methods. In: Chen, J.I.-Z., Tavares, J.M.R.S., Iliyasu, A.M., Du, K.-L. (eds.) ICIPCN 2021. LNNS, vol. 300, pp. 783–800. Springer, Cham (2022). https://doi.org/10.1007/978-3-030-84760-9_67

Vinmalar, F.L., Kombaiya, A.K.: Prediction of lung cancer using data mining techniques. Int. J. Eng. Res. Technol. **7**(1) (2019)

Vinodini, S.: Analyzing sentiments in paulo coelho's literary works using VADER sentiment analysis. In: International Conference on Innovative Computing, Intelligent Communication and Smart Electrical Systems (ICSES), pp. 1–6. IEEE (2023). https://doi.org/10.1109/ICSES60034.2023.10465319

Vinodini, S.: Enhancing literary analysis through artificial intelligence and machine learning: insights from 'the alchemist'. In: International Conference on Recent Advances in Information Technology for Sustainable Development (ICRAIS), IEEE (2024)

Vinodini, S.: The analysis of language, sentiment, and themes in Paulo Coelho's 'Brida' using TextBlob. In: Ninth International Conference on Science Technology Engineering and Mathematics, pp. 1–8. IEEE (2024). https://doi.org/10.1109/ICONSTEM60960.2024.10568869

Zubi, Z., Saad, R.: Improves treatment programs of lung cancer using data mining techniques. J. Softw. Eng. Appl. **7**, 69–77 (2014). https://doi.org/10.4236/jsea.2014.72008

Comparative Analysis of ResNet50 vs. ResNet101 Architectures in Brain Tumor Classification

Jatinder Kaur(✉), Ashutosh Kumar Singh, and Neeru Jindal

Department of Electronics and Communication Engineering, Thapar Institute of Engineering and Technology, Patiala, India
{jkaur60_phd20,aksingh,neeru.jindal}@thapar.edu

Abstract. In recent years, a brain tumour has become a fatal illness. Magnetic resonance imaging (MRI) is the primary method for diagnosing brain tumors and their extent. The advancements in Deep Learning techniques for computer vision have mainly been attributed to the abundance of training data and advancements in model designs, leading to improved accuracy in supervised environments. This study aims to enhance the capability and effectiveness of Magnetic resonance images for categorizing brain tumors. This paper utilizes pre-trained models ResNet50 and ResNet101 to train our dataset of brain tumors. Regarding their accuracy, this research compares the ResNet50 and ResNet101 models, as both address the same image classification task. The accuracy scores were 90% for ResNet50, and 93% for ResNet101, respectively. These accuracies enhance the early detection of tumors, potentially preventing physical consequences like paralysis and other impairments.

Keywords: Brain tumor · Magnetic resonance imaging · ResNet50 · ResNet101

1 Introduction

Brain tumors, characterized by the unusual proliferation of cells in the brain, have emerged as the most prevalent type of cancer globally, posing significant challenges to the healthcare community. In 2020, cancer resulted in the deaths of 10 million individuals, as reported by the World Health Organization (WHO). Many cancers can be prevented by avoiding known risk factors and adopting preventive measures [1]. A brain tumor consists of abnormal cells originating from the brain's parenchyma or nearby areas. Brain cancer can result in substantial impairments that greatly disrupt a patient's everyday functioning [2]. Tumors, abnormal growths of cells within the body, can be classified into two distinct categories: Benign and Malignant. Benign tumors originate from tissues associated with the brain and are non-cancerous. But in the case of Malignant tumors, they are cancerous and proliferate, frequently resulting in fatality. Therefore, early detection of brain tumors is crucial to improving patient survival rates [3].

K. Atul et al. (Eds.): BodyNets 2024, LNICST 666, pp. 392–402, 2026.
https://doi.org/10.1007/978-3-032-16099-7_31

An imaging method that does not require invasive procedures is provided by MRI, with detailed pictures of the body's internal anatomy being created using powerful magnetic fields and radio waves, without the use of ionizing radiation. It is considered more effective for diagnosing and treating brain tumors than Ultrasound imaging or Computer Tomography (CT) [4, 5]. Identifying patterns or textures for classification in extremely diverse images requires a labour-intensive and time-consuming task, particularly with large datasets. Numerous approaches have been developed to assist radiologists in improving their diagnostic accuracy.

Convolutional Neural Networks (CNNs), which autonomously learn a progressively complex set of features from data, have recently demonstrated notable success in enhancing the accuracy of medical diagnoses and categorization of diseases [6]. Deep CNN networks face challenges like performance degradation, the vanishing gradient issue, and difficulties in optimizing the network. The residual network (ResNet) design addresses these issues and offers a very efficient method for improving recognition accuracy [7]. ResNet50 and ResNet101 are utilized to evaluate the accuracy of brain tumor detection and treatment techniques.

2 Related Work

Classifying brain tumors from magnetic resonance images is essential to medical imaging to ensure precise diagnosis and treatment strategies. Numerous research projects have concentrated on creating and assessing machine learning and deep learning algorithms for this. Mircea et al. [8] extract wavelet coefficients from images using a feature-based technique. They argue that wavelet transforms offer superior temporal resolution, enabling more precise identification of spatial and frequency characteristics within the image.

Paul et al.[9] used different classifiers, a random forest, a fully connected neural network, and a convolutional neural network, to classify MRI brain tumors. Convolutional neural networks achieved the best accuracy rate, reaching 90.26% with several layers, including convolutional, MaxPool, and completely connected. Khawaldeh et al. [10] suggested a technique for classifying glioma brain tumors without invasive procedures based on an improved AlexNet convolutional neural network. The categorization was accomplished using magnetic resonance images of the complete brain, using labels at the image level rather than the pixel level.

A CNN technique incorporating data augmentation for classifying brain tumors was proposed by Sajjad et al. [11] The approach adopted for the brain tumor classification uses segmented brain tumors based on segmented Magnetic Resonance Imaging images. They utilized VGG-19 architecture that was pre-trained for classification and obtained accuracy rates of 87.39% and 90.66% for original and augmented datasets, respectively. Afshar et al. [12] recommended a method for classifying brain tumors that integrates tumor coarse borders as supplementary inputs, which boosts CapsNet's tumor type accuracy to 90.89% on the dataset. Deep learning models that have been pre-trained are leveraged for extracting image features, providing better accuracy than traditional models.

3 Proposed Work

Pre-trained models are leveraged for extracting image features, providing better accuracy than traditional models. They also facilitate greater interpretability, understanding, and management of the data. The suggested transfer learning approach categorizes brain magnetic resonance images into tumor and non-tumor categories. Various preprocessing techniques are employed to augment and enhance the MRI images. A publicly available database on the Kaggle platform was utilized for this study [13]. The original dataset comprises 253 magnetic resonance images, including 155 images with tumors and 98 images without tumors, as shown in Fig. 1. With the help of augmentation, the dataset for MRI training has been increased by expanding the collection. After that, two pre-trained architectures, ResNet50 and ResNet101, are utilized to test and assess the suggested model. In this study, significant preprocessing steps are presented along with an elaboration on the classification model built on transfer learning techniques. Figure 2 depicts the flowchart outlining the proposed method for classifying brain tumors.

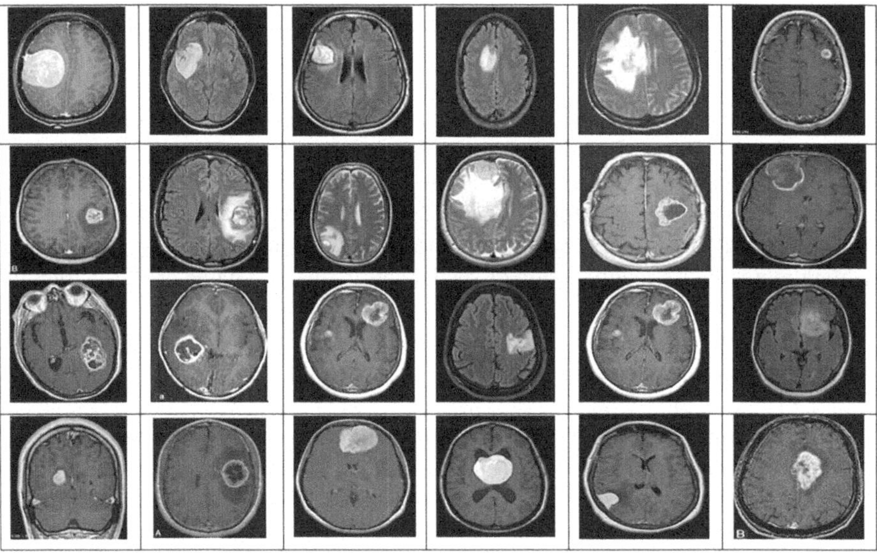

Fig. 1. Sample of Dataset Containing Brain MRI Images

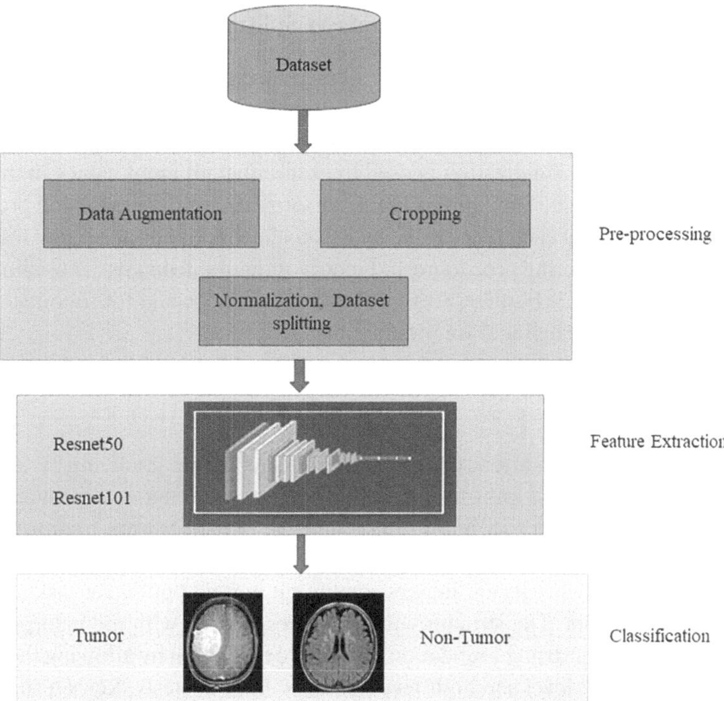

Fig. 2. Flowchart of the suggested framework for classification of brain tumor

3.1 Data Augmentation

Data augmentation is a form of regularization that helps to mitigate overfitting by expanding the training dataset with variations of the existing data. The transformations included Flip, Rotate, height, and width with varying degrees of transformation. This process improves the model's generalization and prevents overfitting. The initial dataset of images has been expanded from 253 to 2823 images through augmentation. The information shown in Table 1 displays the quantity of images in both the tumor and non-tumor classes after data augmentation.

Table 1. Data obtained after applying data augmentation

Tumor Label	No. of images
Tumor	1549
Non-Tumor	1274

3.2 Crop, Normalization, Resize, and Dataset Splitting

The first task involves using the OpenCV library to crop and identify the outermost points in the bounding boxes. It is important to note that the magnetic resonance images utilized in this research are gathered from various locations, leading to variations in image sizes. Then the normalization is used to ensure that all input values in the model fall within the same range. This impacted the performance of the model and prediction. It is achieved by dividing each pixel value by its standard deviation. Resizing the images helps to expedite the training procedure and reduce memory demands. These images are resized to $224 \times 224 \times 3$. Further, 80% of the dataset is allocated for training, whereas the remaining 20% is designated for validation.

3.3 Transfer Learning

ResNet was developed to address the problem of disappearing gradients by integrating residual connections. These links enable the training of more intricate networks to better capture complex features in brain tumor images, outperforming traditional CNNs that struggle with depth-related performance issues. The architecture has demonstrated strong performance in classifying images, making it a great option for tasks involving classifying brain tumors. The structure of ResNet, especially with the incorporation of residual blocks, offers a strong foundation for feature extraction by allowing the network to effectively learn low-level and high-level features. In initial tests, ResNet showed better accuracy and feature extraction than other models. The depth and adaptability of ResNet, coupled with its lower chance of overfitting, render it an outstanding choice.

In this study, two models, ResNet50 and ResNet101, were employed, both trained on 1.28 million images from ImageNet for classifying 1,000 categories. He et al. [14] developed ResNet, utilizing residual blocks to enhance gradient flow across the network, enabling the training of extremely deep networks. The primary concept is to implement skip connections that circumvent one or more layers, facilitating improved gradient flow and reducing training durations. The design of ResNet tackles issues of vanishing gradients and degradation in deep networks, which makes it well-suited for complex brain tumor classification tasks. In this study, both ResNet50 and ResNet101 models were employed; specifically, ResNet50 is illustrated in Fig. 3 and ResNet101 can be seen in Fig. 4 for classifying brain tumors. ResNet-101 is a modified version of the ResNet. The ResNet50 model is composed of 48 convolutional layers utilizing convolutional neural networks. There are two other layers, one being a Max Pooling layer and the other an Average Pooling layer. This network structure allows for the integration of shortcut connections and the use of residual functions, facilitating deep neural networks to minimize training errors through layer stacking.

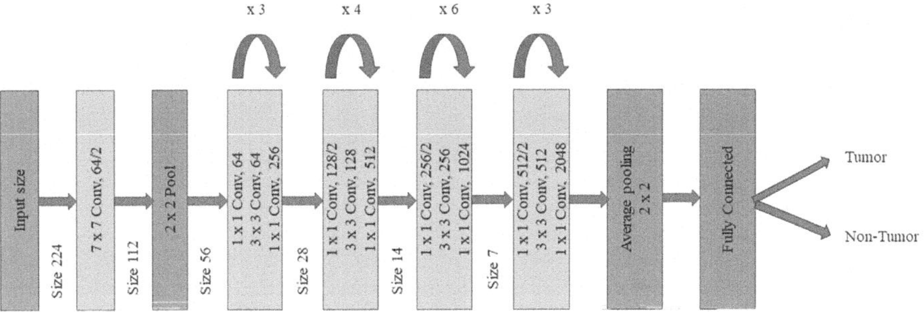

Fig. 3. Architecture of ResNet50

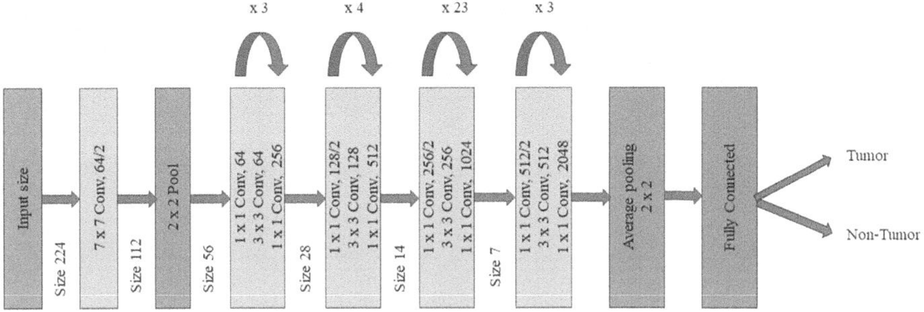

Fig. 4. Architecture of ResNet101

3.4 Performance Evaluation

Assessing a classifier's performance is crucial in machine learning since it allows us to gauge how effectively the model categorizes data accurately. To assess the performance of a classifier, the typical metrics such as accuracy, precision, F1-score, and recall are used as shown in Eqs. (1 to 4).

$$\text{Accuracy} = \frac{\text{TP} + \text{TN}}{\text{TP} + \text{TN} + \text{FP} + \text{FN}} \tag{1}$$

$$\text{Recall} = \frac{\text{TP}}{\text{TP} + \text{FN}} \tag{2}$$

$$\text{Precision} = \frac{\text{TP}}{\text{TP} + \text{FP}} \tag{3}$$

$$\text{F1 score} = \frac{2 \times \text{Precision} \times \text{Recall}}{\text{Precision} + \text{Recall}} \tag{4}$$

where, True Positive (TP), True Negative (TN), False Positive (FP), and False Negative (FN) values are achieved.

3.5 Results and Discussion

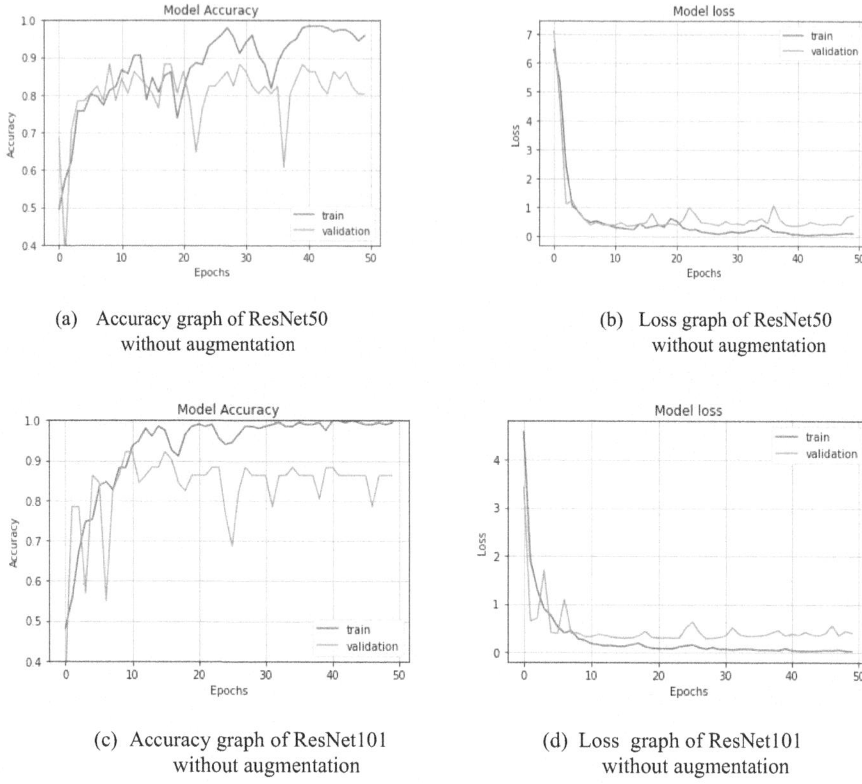

(a) Accuracy graph of ResNet50 without augmentation

(b) Loss graph of ResNet50 without augmentation

(c) Accuracy graph of ResNet101 without augmentation

(d) Loss graph of ResNet101 without augmentation

Fig. 5. Training and Validation accuracy and loss outcomes achieved using ResNet50 and ResNet101 without augmentation

The research involved conducting experiments on a brain-MRI dataset to identify tumors. All the brain tumor image classifications utilized have been executed with the libraries of Keras and TensorFlow. Each network undergoes training for 50 epochs using a batch size of 32. This experiment utilizes the Adam optimization method [15] to adjust neural weights using training data. The Adam optimizer is implemented with a learning rate set to 0.0001. ResNets are particularly effective in this domain due to their use of residual connections, which allow for very deep networks to be trained by overcoming the vanishing gradient problem. This structure enables the model to capture both low-level and high-level features essential in medical imaging, where fine details can signify tumor presence. Additionally, the depth of ResNets helps them learn complex patterns unique to tumors, such as texture variations or shape irregularities, which are challenging to detect in shallower networks. In the results, this work observed that these properties contributed to the strong performance in classifying tumor vs. non-tumor images. Figure 5(a), 5(b), 5(c), and 5(d) demonstrate the absence of augmentation in the ResNet50 and ResNet101 models through their loss and accuracy. Figure 6(a), 6(b),

6(c), and 6(d) show the performance in terms of loss and accuracy of the ResNet50 and ResNe101 models with augmentation. As demonstrated in Fig. 5 and 6, ResNet-50 was the least efficient in this system, whereas ResNet101 performed best using augmentation and no augmentation. Figure 7 and Fig. 8 illustrate the confusion matrix for ResNet50 and ResNet101 with and without augmentation.

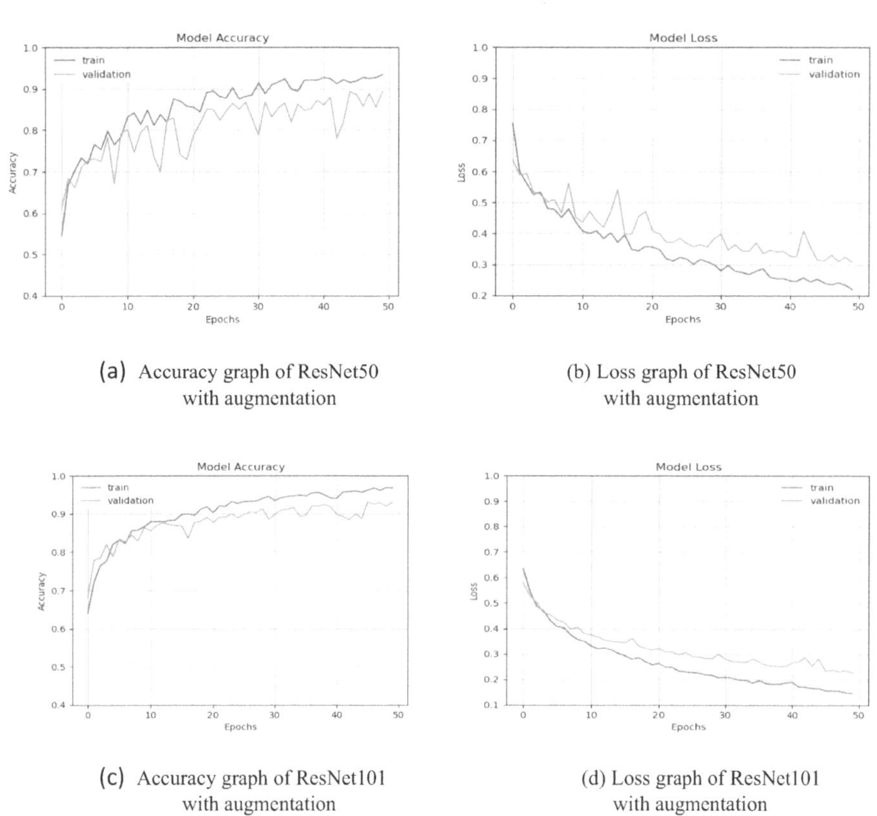

(a) Accuracy graph of ResNet50 with augmentation

(b) Loss graph of ResNet50 with augmentation

(c) Accuracy graph of ResNet101 with augmentation

(d) Loss graph of ResNet101 with augmentation

Fig. 6. Training and Validation accuracy and loss outcomes achieved using ResNet50 and ResNet101 with augmentation

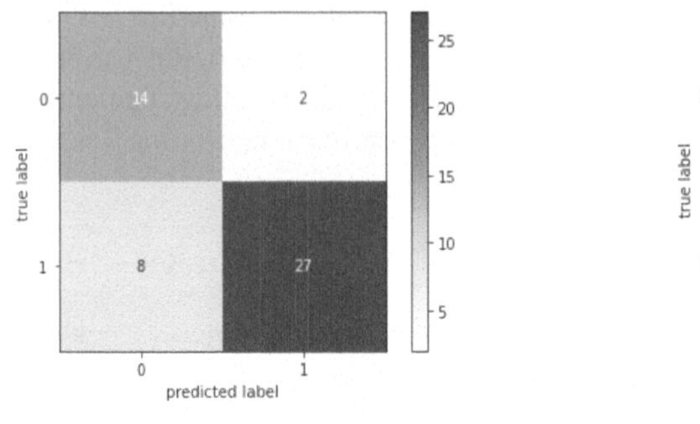

(a) Confusion matrix of ResNet50

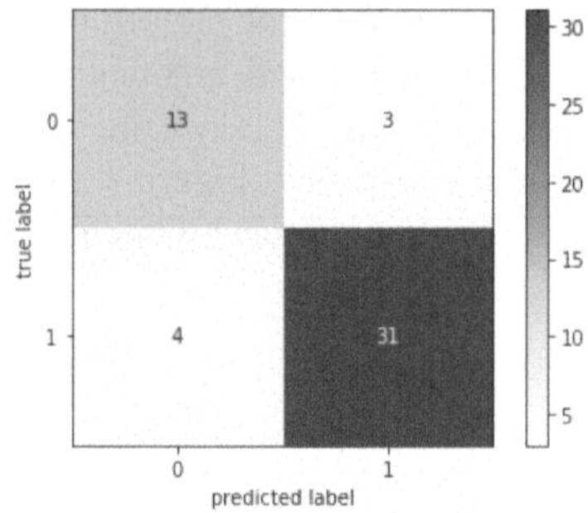

(b) Confusion Matrix of ResNet101

Fig. 7. Confusion matrix achieved using ResNet50 and ResNet101 without augmentation

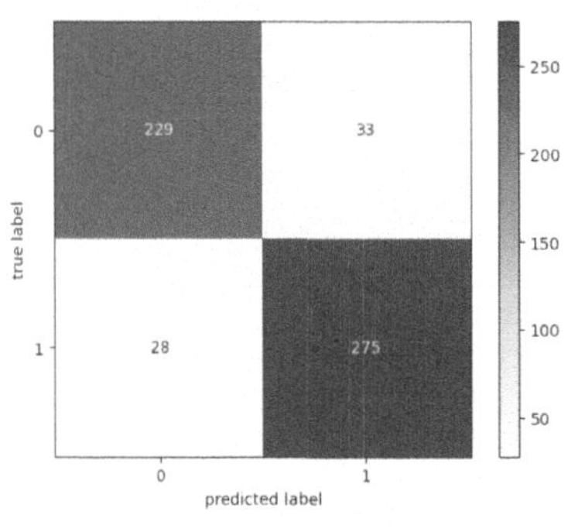

(a)Confusion Matrix of ResNet50

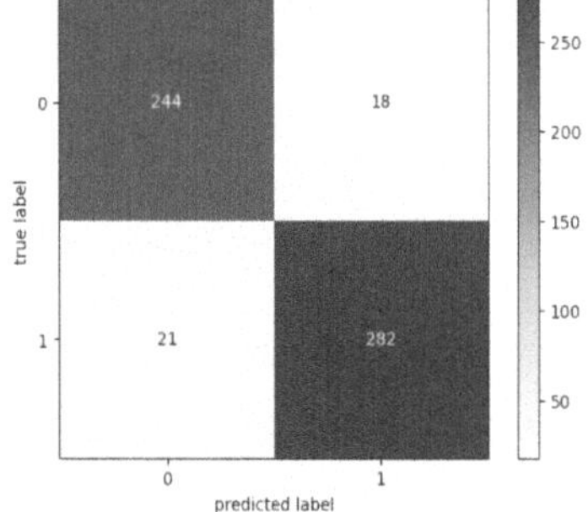

(b) Confusion Matrix of ResNet101

Fig. 8. Confusion matrix achieved using ResNet50 and ResNet101 with augmentation

Table 2 shows the precision, recall, precision, accuracy, and F1-score findings for the two examined architectures. The performance of the proposed framework, assessed without data augmentation, demonstrates encouraging outcomes for both ResNet50 and ResNet101 structures. ResNet50 achieves 80% accuracy, with a recall of 82.5%, precision of 78.5%, and an F1 score of 79%. Although the results are decent, ResNet101 outperforms them significantly, achieving an accuracy rate of 86%, a recall rate of 85%, a precision rate of 84%, and an F1 score of 85%. ResNet101's superior accuracy and balanced metrics indicate it provides improved generalization and classification performance in comparison to ResNet50. These results show that the increased complexity of ResNet101 gives a noticeable benefit in terms of accuracy and F1 score, resulting in an enhanced F1 score overall. Table 3 clearly illustrates that the ResNet101 classifier surpasses ResNet50, exceeding them by 93.5% and 93% in F1-score and accuracy correspondingly. When data augmentation was applied during evaluation, the suggested framework demonstrated a significant improvement in performance for both the ResNet50 and ResNet101 models. ResNet50 achieves a remarkable accuracy of 90%, while its recall, precision, and F1 scores are each at 89%. This suggests a reliable and consistent performance, highlighting the positive impact of augmentation on improving the model's capacity to generalize. ResNet101 outperforms ResNet50, reaching a superior accuracy of 93%. Its precision, recall, and F1 score are all at 93%, with a minor enhancement to 93.5% in the F1 score. These results confirm that the deeper ResNet101 model benefits more from data augmentation, leading to improved accuracy and more consistent performance across different metrics. Overall, the framework that includes augmentation exhibits superior outcomes, particularly with ResNet101, emphasizing its capacity to enhance model dependability and precision in classification.

Table 2. Performance metrics of the suggested framework (excluding augmentation)

Algorithm	Accuracy	Recall	Precision	F1 score
ResNet50	80%	82.5%	78.5%	79%
ResNet101	86%	85%	84%	85%

Table 3. Performance metrics of the suggested framework (including augmentation)

Algorithm	Accuracy	Recall	Precision	F1 score
ResNet50	90%	89%	89%	89%
ResNet101	93%	93%	93%	93.5%

4 Conclusion

This study demonstrates that the ResNet101 model outperforms ResNet50 in accuracy, achieving 93% compared to 90% with data augmentation. The higher performance of ResNet101 may be attributed to its deeper architecture, optimized hyperparameters, and the nature of the augmented data. Both models benefit from augmentation, but the ResNet101 model shows greater effectiveness, offering improved accuracy and consistent performance across various metrics. These findings suggest that the deeper ResNet101 model is the more effective choice for brain tumor classification in MRI scans, providing a more reliable and accurate solution. This remarkable accuracy could assist in the early identification of brain tumors, thus helping to avert serious physical consequences, such as paralysis, disability, and even mortality. These results confirm that the deeper ResNet101 model benefits more from data augmentation, improving accuracy, and consistent performance across different metrics.

Acknowledgment. The authors thank the 5G Use Case Lab of DECE, TIET Patiala, funded by the Department of Telecommunication (DoT) Government of India for providing valuable support and discussions.

References

1. Ferlay, B.F., et al.: Global Cancer Observatory: Cancer Today," Lyon, France: International Agency for Research on Cancer (2020). https://gco.iarc.fr/today. Accessed 25 Aug 2021
2. De Robles, P., et al.: The worldwide incidence and prevalence of primary brain tumors: a systematic review and meta-analysis. Neuro Oncol. **17**(6), 776–783 (2015)
3. El-Dahshan, E.A., Mohsen, H.M., Revett, K., Salem, A.M.: Computer-aided diagnosis of human brain tumor through mri: a survey and a new algorithm. Expert Syst. Appl. **41**(11), 5526–5545 (2014)
4. Khambhata, K.G., Panchal, S.K.: Multiclass classification of brain tumor in MR images. Int. J. Innov. Res. Comput. Commun. Eng. **4**(5), 8982–8992 (2016)
5. Zacharaki, E.I., et al.: Classification of brain tumor type and grade using MRI texture and shape in a machine learning scheme. Magn. Reson. Med. **62**, 1609–161 (2009)
6. J. Seetha, and S. Selvakumar Raja "Brain tumor classification using convolutional neural networks," in Biomed. Pharmacol. J. 2018, vol. 11(3), 2018
7. Feng, V.: An Overview of ResNet and its Variants. published on Towards Data Science (2017)
8. Gurbină, M., Lascu, M., Lascu, D.: Tumor detection and classification of MRI brain image using different wavelet transforms and support vector machines. In: 2019 42nd International Conference on Telecommunications and Signal Processing (TSP), Budapest, Hungary, pp. 505–508 (2019). https://doi.org/10.1109/TSP.2019.8769040
9. Paul, J.S., et al.: Deep learning for brain tumor classification. In: Medical Imaging 2017: Biomedical Applications in Molecular, Structural, and Functional Imaging, vol. 10137, p. 1013710 (2017)
10. Khawaldeh, S., et al.: Non-invasives grading of glioma tumor using magnetic resonance imaging with convolutional neural networks. Appl. Sci. **8**(1), 48–60 (2017)
11. Sajjad, M., Khan, S., Muhammad, K., Wu, W., Ullah, A., Baik, S.W.: Multi-grade brain tumor classification using deep CNN with extensive data augmentation. J. Comput. Sci. **30**(1), 174–182 (2019)
12. Afshar, P., Plataniotis, K.N., Mohammadi, A.: Capsule networks for brain tumor classification based on MRI images and coarse tumor boundaries. In: ICASSP 2019 - 2019 IEEE International Conference on Acoustics, Speech and Signal Processing (ICASSP), Brighton, UK, pp. 1368–1372 (2019). https://doi.org/10.1109/ICASSP.2019.8683759
13. https://www.kaggle.com/datasets/navoneel/brain-mri-images-for-brain-tumor-detection
14. He, K., Zhang, X., Ren, S., Sun, J.: Deep Residual Learning for Image Recognition (2015)
15. Kingma, D.P., Ba, J.: Adam: a method for stochastic optimization," arXiv preprint arXiv: 1412.6980 (2014)

Comparison of Vector Network Analyzers for On-body and In-body Measurements in Time and Frequency Domains

Daljeet Singh[1,2(✉)], Mariella Särestöniemi[1,2,3], and Teemu Myllylä[1,2,4,5]

[1] Research Unit of Health Sciences and Technology, Faculty of Medicine, University of Oulu, Oulu, Finland
{mariella.sarestoniemi,teemu.myllyla}@oulu.fi

[2] Infotech Oulu, Oulu, Finland
daljeet.singh@oulu.fi

[3] Centre for Wireless Communications, Faculty of Information Technology and Electrical Engineering, University of Oulu, Oulu, Finland

[4] Medical Research Center, Oulu, Finland

[5] Optoelectronics and Measurements, Faculty of Information Technology and Electrical Engineering, University of Oulu, Oulu, Finland

Abstract. Microwaves have immense potential in biomedical and clinical applications for monitoring and diagnosis of biological tissue and their properties. Vector Network Analyzer (VNA) is a key component for these microwave measurements. The accuracy of a microwave monitoring system depends heavily on the capability of VNAs. Apart from measurement accuracy, the size, cost, radiation power, power consumption, and robustness are other factors that need to be considered for choosing a particular VNA for biomedical applications. This paper presents a thorough comparative analysis of two commercially available VNAs, Agilent Technologies 8720ES S-parameter Network Analyzer and PicoVNA 108 by PICO Technologies. The 8720ES VNA operates at 50 MHz to 20 GHz whereas PICO VNA has an operating bandwidth of 300 kHz to 8.5 GHz. Firstly, parametric analysis is presented which compares both VNAs in terms of their statistical features. Thereafter, extensive on-body measurements are conducted using two standard antennas. Additionally, In-body measurements are also conducted for further investigation of the matter. Numerous multifold measurements on both VNAs provide a strategic comparative analysis of both VNAs.

Keywords: Brain phantom · in-body measurements · on-body measurements · microwave · S parameters · vector network analyzer

1 Introduction

The last few decades have witnessed enormous growth in the usage of microwave techniques for medical diagnosis and therapy driven by rapid research advancements in millimeter-wave and terahertz bands. As a result of non-ionizing radiations and the ability of non-invasive measurements, numerous medical and

K. Atul et al. (Eds.): BodyNets 2024, LNICST 666, pp. 403–414, 2026.
https://doi.org/10.1007/978-3-032-16099-7_32

healthcare applications of microwaves have emerged such as the diagnosis of tumors and cancer cells [9], characterization of fluid hydrodynamics in tissue [13], modeling of in-body and on-body communication in body area networks [2], health monitoring of organs [8], bio-imaging, temperature monitoring and control in thermal ablation, brain activity tracking, and measurement of vital signs [12], etc. All these applications involve accurately calculating antenna gain and phase response to characterize the object/phenomena under test. These measurements are utilized in healthcare for either diagnosis or imaging or both.

Vector network analyzers (VNAs) are a key component in any measurement setup operating in the microwave band. These measurements are based on accurate modeling of the electromagnetic properties of the dielectric materials under test by measuring the input reflection coefficients (Sxx) and reverse transmission coefficient (Sxy) as a function of frequency. Precise calculation of the antenna coefficients helps in effective system modeling, thereby reducing the risk of miscalculations. Therefore, very high-end, bulky, and costly VNAs are generally utilized for accurate measurements with minimal possible errors. However, practical healthcare applications involve measurements with patients in critical conditions which require something more than just the accuracy of measurements. The comfort level of patients and doctors is also an important aspect of this process. Therefore, the clinical use of the microwave technique requires careful selection of VNA and its accompanying system. Furthermore, this key aspect is also important to promote the use of health monitoring devices in daily life outside hospital settings.

2 Literature Survey

A lot of studies in the literature investigate the performance of VNAs. Wang et al. [18] proposed a two-tier Bayesian analysis method for analyzing the performance of a VNA. The three-step proposed method is generalized and utilizes an uncertainty propagation mechanism for n-port VNAs. The initial step involves calculating the posterior distribution of VNA uncertainties using the Bayesian approach. In the next step, Monte-Carlo simulations are applied to the data obtained in step one. Finally, statistical analysis is applied to the data from step two. The partial derivative method is proposed in [14] wherein short-open-load-through (SOLT) calibration was applied. The authors in [14] suggested that the proposed method can be utilized for modeling non-ideal calibration.

Maoliu and Yichi proposed a covariance-based method for measuring the non-linearity of VNAs, especially in polyharmonic measurements [6]. Similarly, another covariance-based method for uncertainty analysis of VNAs is presented in [5] wherein it is shown that the covariance matrix has the potential to characterize all issues related to scattering. In [1], the well-known root-squaring method is described for characterizing VNA measurement accuracy. A multiport model for error analysis of the calibration process of n-port VNA is presented in [3]. Further, analytical calculations are shown for modeling bidirectional conversion between 16 and 12-term calibration.

In another study, Marks et al. proposed a method to compare calibration accuracy of VNAs from 45 MHz–18 GHz. The study compares open short load through calibration with a sliding load calibration wherein isolation and switching errors were neglected. Recently, Shang et al. [11] presented a comparative analysis between VNA and optical methods for calculating dielectric characteristics. Time and frequency domain spectroscopy methods were used for optical measurements whereas open resonators, free-space quasioptical, and guided approaches were utilized for VNA-based measurements. The experiments were conducted on seven samples in five major laboratories throughout the globe at 2 GHz–1 THz.

2.1 Motivation and Contribution

Although numerous studies have been published on the comparison of calibration techniques for VNAs and to characterize their performance in measuring antenna parameters, this aspect of study in biomedical and clinical applications is still new. Apart from measurement accuracy, the size, cost, radiation power, power consumption and robustness are other factors that need to be considered for choosing a particular VNA for biomedical applications. The performance of VNA to characterize small dielectric changes in biological samples is still an open area of research. Therefore, this paper presents a comparative analysis of two commercially available VNAs i.e. 8720ES S-parameter network analyzer by Agilent Technologies [15] and PICO VNA 108 by PICO Technology [16]. The 8720ES VNA operates at 50 MHz to 20 GHz whereas PICO VNA has a operating bandwidth of 300 kHz to 8.5 GHz. Both of these VNAs are compared on two grounds: i) parametric analysis based on data sheet available with the device, and, ii) measurement accuracy for on-body and in-body trials for biomedical applications. Multifold measurements are conducted for an extensive analysis of time and frequency domain analysis of both VNAs to track their amplitude and phase variations for different standard samples.

The rest of the paper is organized as follows: the material and methods are presented in Sect. 3. The results and discussion are presented in Sect. 4. Section 5 holds the concluding remarks of the paper.

3 Materials and Methods

This section demonstrates the key technical parameters of two VNAs undertaken for comparative analysis in this study. Furthermore, the biological models utilized for in-body and on-body measurements are also explained. The measurement setup for measuring antenna characteristics and comparison of results consists of two commercially available VNAs Keysigght 8720ES [15] and PICO VNA 108 [16] connected with 3.5 mm high-precision cables. Three different antennas are used for the measurements. The first antenna is a Rogers5880 monopole which operates at 2–10 GHz [7]. A more detailed description of this flexible antenna design is available in [7]. This antenna is very suitable for on-body

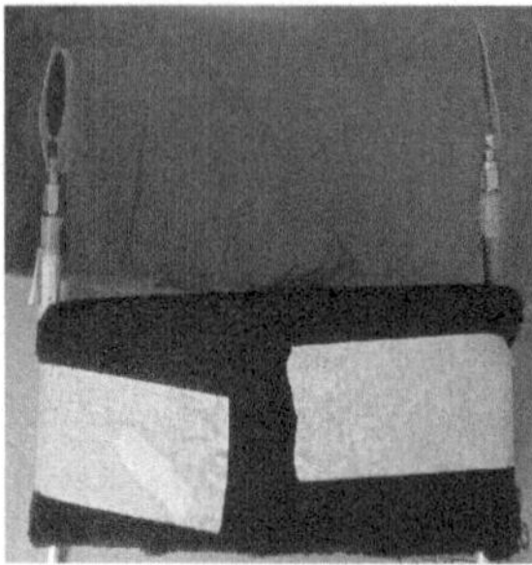

(a) Free space measurement setup.

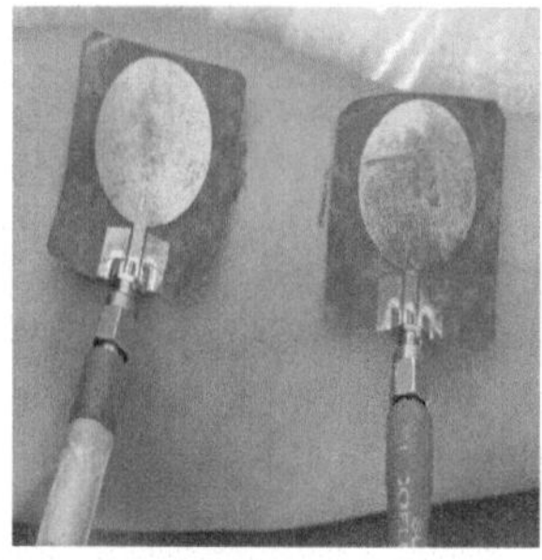

(b) On-body measurement with antenna 1

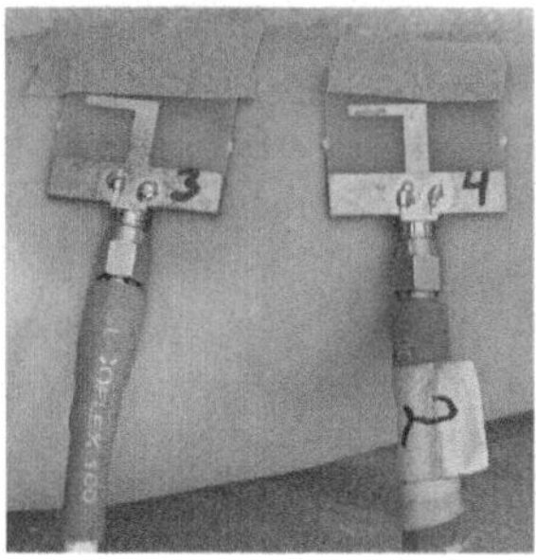

(c) On-body measurement with antenna 2

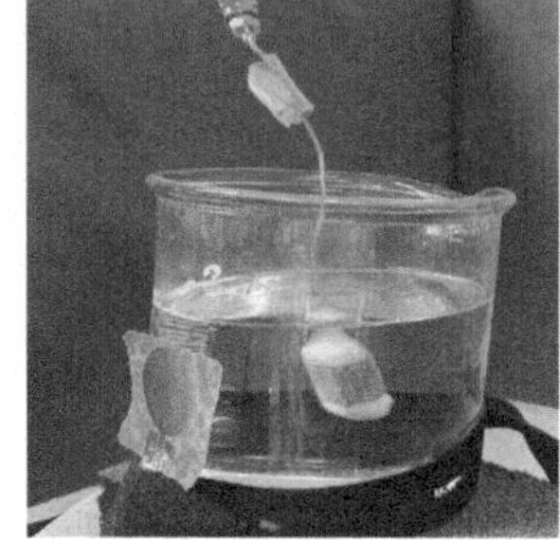

(d) In-body measurement with antenna 1

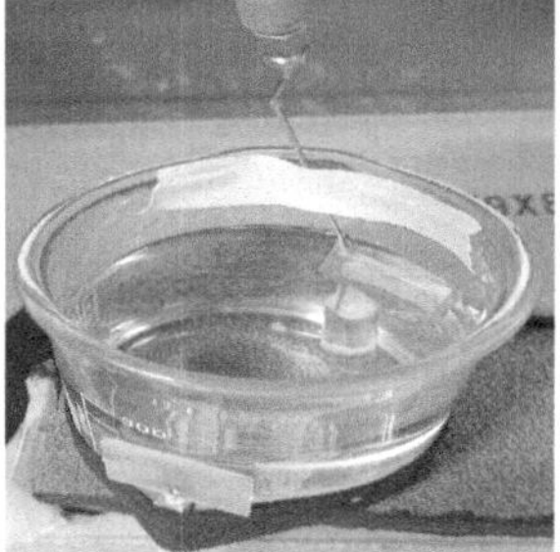

(e) In-body measurement with antenna 2

Fig. 1. Measurement setup for comparison of VNAs.

measurements because of its flexibility. The second antenna is a dipole antenna printed on FR-4 substrate with an overall dimensions of 30.3 × 25 × 1.6 mm [4]. The antenna has a free space operational bandwidth of 3.74–4.25 GHz with resonant frequency = 3.906 GHz. The performance of this antenna can be further enhanced by employing a cavity based approach which is not undertaken in this study for simplicity. The third antenna is a capsule antenna originally proposed in [10] for biomedical applications. The antenna has a diameter of 10 mm and length 15 mm which makes it suitable for in-body measurements.

The measurement schedule for this study consists of S parameter calculation in a) free space, b) on-body, and c) in-body conditions. All measurements are conducted in an anechoic chamber for removal of environmental noise and interference. For free space measurements, the antennas are placed 20 cm apart in the anechoic chamber. The setup for free space measurement is shown in Fig. 1(a). The on-body measurements are taken from the skin of the subject. The antennas are placed 2 cm apart on the arm of the subject as shown in Fig. 1(b) and (c) for antenna 1 and antenna 2 respectively. For in-body measurements, a bio-mimicking phantom is developed whose dielectric properties match with that of human brain. The phantom is prepared by mixing distilled water with sugar in a ratio (10 ml: 8.5 g). The liquid brain phantom is poured into a glass beaker for measurements and a flexible antenna is inserted 5 cm into the phantom. The other port of VNA is connected to antenna 1 or 2 for in-body measurements. The setup utilized for in-body measurements is shown in Fig. 1(d) for antenna 1 - antenna 3 and Fig. 1(e) for antenna 2 - antenna 3.

The antennas are placed in the exact spot for each measurement by carefully marking the area. For PICO VNA 108, the data is collected using proprietary software PICO VNA5 supplied with the VNA [17]. Matlab is used for data extraction from the 8720ES S-parameter network analyzer. Both the VNAs are calibrated using a standard mechanical calibration kit by Keysight Technology (85052B) with 3.5 mm connectors and a sliding load. For a fair comparison, both VNAs are calibrated for full two-port calibration from 1–8 GHz at 5 dBm with 801 sweep points. The real and imaginary values of all four S parameters (S11, S12, S21, and S22) are calculated and saved for each case. Two important parameters are calculated from these values, i.e.: magnitude of $S(dB) = 20\log(\sqrt{\Re[S]^2 + \Im[S]^2})$ and phase $\phi(degrees) = \arctan\left(\frac{\Im[S]}{\Re[S]}\right)$. The time domain results are further calculated from these measurements by taking Inverse Fourier Transform (IFFT) of the intended frequency band. The IFFT is implemented in MATLAB using standard Fast Fourier Transform (FFT) function.

4 Results and Discussion

In this section, the time and frequency domain results obtained from on-body and in-body measurements are presented. To reduce the systematic measurement error, each trial was repeated five times. The results obtained from these 5 measurements are averaged to calculate the final values for that particular trial. To improve the visualization of results, in some cases, the mean measured value is shown with a solid line, and the standard deviation between different samples and locations is shown using shading of the same color.

Table 1. Comparison of 8720ES S-parameter Network Analyzer with PicoVNA 108 Vector network analyzer.

Parameter	8720ES	PICO VNA 108
Dynamic Range	100 dB	124 dB
Frequency Range	50 MHz to 20 GHz	300 kHz to 8.5 GHz
Measurement Accuracy	10 ppm (at 23 °C ± 3 °C)	10 ppm (at 23 °C ± 3 °C)
Noise Floor	−120 dBm	−124 dBm
Trace Noise	0.04 dB	0.005 dB
Temperature Drift	± 7.5 ppm (0–55 °C)	± 0.5 ppm/°C
Resolution	1 Hz, 0.01 dB	10 Hz, 0.1 dB
Phase noise (10 kHz offset)	2 GHz: −55 dBc 20 GHz: −35 dBc	0.3 MHz–1 GHz: −90 dBc/Hz 1 GHz–4 GHz: −80 dBc/Hz > 4 GHz: −76 dBc/Hz
Sweep time*	1106 ms	72 ms
Error correction	Frequency response and isolation error correction Interpolated Error Correction	Frequency response and isolation error correction, Impedance conversion, source match correction, Averaging, smoothing, filtering, Electrical length, dielectric constant correction compensation
Software Visualization	Magnitude, phase, group delay, smith chart, polar, SWR, time domain	Log/linear magnitude, phase, Re, Im, group delay, VSWR, time domain, polar, smith
Weight	25 kg	1.9 kg
Dimensions	222 × 425 × 457 mm	286 × 174 × 61 mm
Power consumption	280 W	25 W
Maximum output power	+5 dBm	+3 dBm
Maximum input level	+10 dBm	+10 dBm

*Calculated with 201-point, 6 kHz IF bandwidth, Two-port calibration

4.1 Parametric Analysis

The parametric analysis presented in this section is based on the standard data available in the datasheet of 8720ES and PICO VNA 108. This analysis is based on key parameters that affect the measurement accuracy of a VNA and also covers other characteristics related to ease of access. A detailed summary of the parametric analysis is presented in Table 1. It can be visualized from Table 1 that PICO VNA 108 has a higher dynamic range of 123 dB as compared to 100 dB for 8720ES with the same measurement accuracy of 10 ppm (at 23 °C ± 3 °C) and noise floor of −120 dB. The frequency range of operation for 8720ES is from 50 MHz to 20 GHz which is very large as compared to PICO VNA 108 which has an operational frequency range of 300 kHz to 8.5 GHz. The trace noise is reported to be 0.04 dB and 0.005 dB for 8720ES PICO VNA 108 respectively which showcases the superior stability of PICO VNA. In terms of resolution, 8720ES (1 Hz, 0.01 dB) is almost ten times better than PICO VNA (10 Hz, 0.1 dB) and also outperforms PICO VNA in terms of lower phase noise. Due to its advanced electronics, PICO VNA 108 has a very fast sweep time of 72 ms as compared to 1106 ms for 8720ES. The sweep time in this case is calculated with 201-point, 6 kHz bandwidth, and full two port calibration settings.

PICO VNA 108 also offers more advanced error correction modules including dielectric constant compensation, source match correction, averaging, smoothing, and filtering operations. In terms of usability and ease of access, PICO VNA 108 stands tall with only 1.9 kg weight and small dimensions of 286 × 174 × 61 mm whereas 8720ES has a body weight of 25 kg with overall dimensions of 222 × 425 × 457 mm. There is also a significant difference in the power consumption of both these VNAs with PICO VNA consuming 25 W power as compared to 280 W for 8720ES.

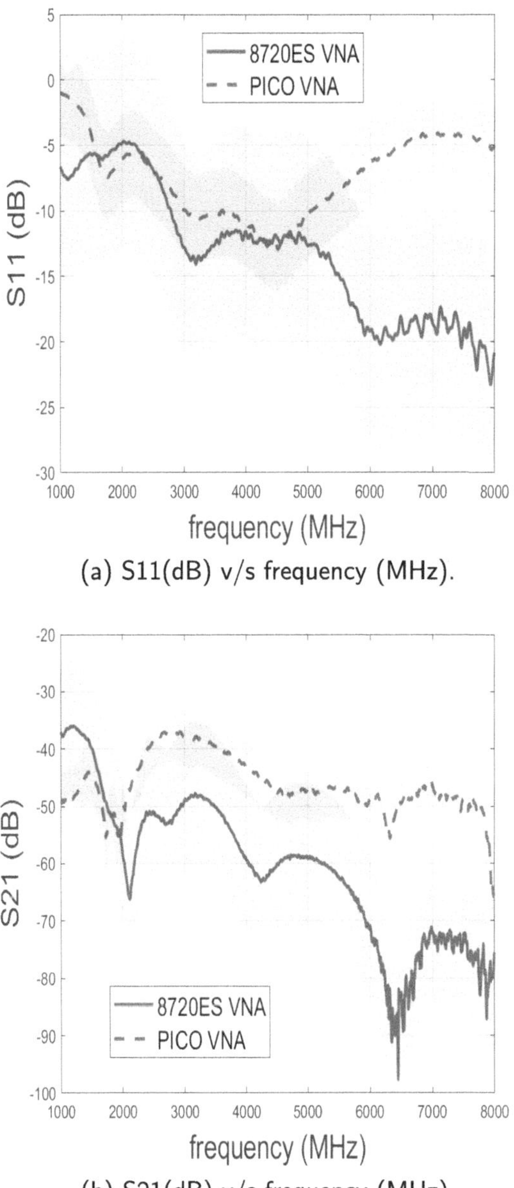

Fig. 2. S11(dB) and S21(dB) v/s frequency (MHz) for on-body measurements.

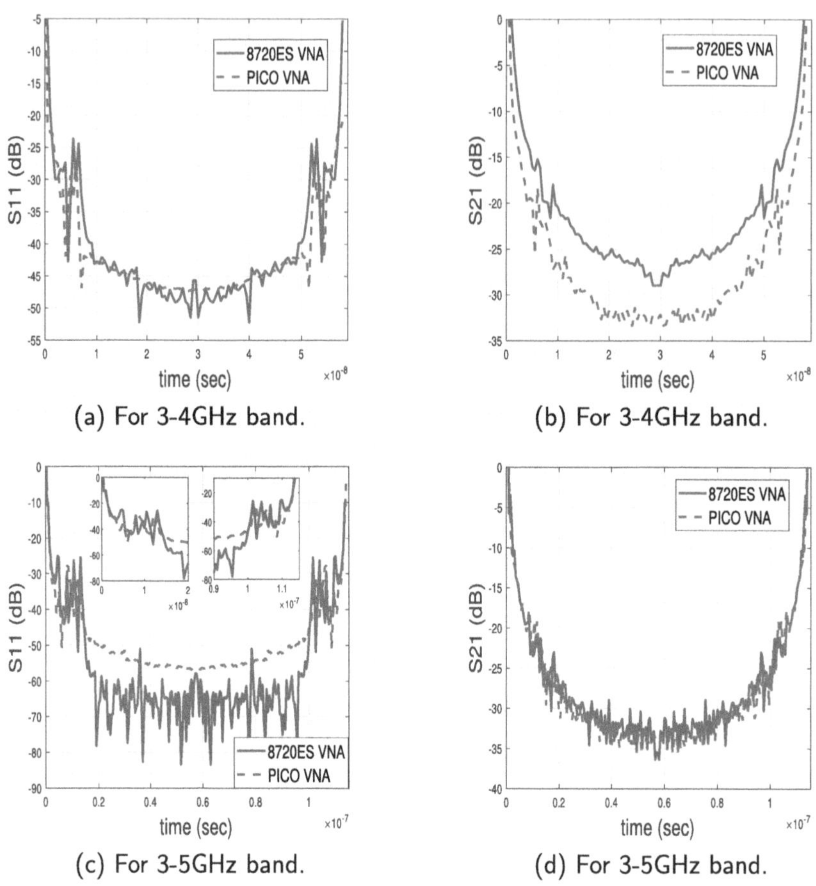

(a) For 3-4GHz band.
(b) For 3-4GHz band.
(c) For 3-5GHz band.
(d) For 3-5GHz band.

Fig. 3. S11(dB) and S21(dB) v/s time(sec) for on-body measurements.

4.2 On-body Measurements

The on-body measurements are taken by placing a pair of antenna 1 and then antenna 2 on the skin of the subject as descried in Sect. 3. The S(dB) v/s frequency plot for on-body measurements is shown in Fig. 2. It can be visualized from Fig. 2(a) that the S11 response for both VNAs has a similar trend in the lower frequency band from 1–5 GHz, whereas, the response changes from 5–8 GHz. The standard deviation (σ) for 8720ES VNA is much higher as compared to PICO VNA 108 as can be visualized from the shaded region of Fig. 2(a). Similarly, the S21(dB) v/s frequency (MHz) plot for two VNAs is shown in Fig. 2(b) wherein the curves show a similar trend. Similar to Fig. 2(a), the results from 8720ES VNA showcase a higher variance in-between trials. For a deeper insight into the comparison, time-domain results for both VNAs are shown in Fig. 3. For example, the net standard deviation of S11 for on-body measurements is $\sigma_{S11} =$ 5.1057 for 8720ES and 3.0142 for PICO VNA 108 respectively. Further the value of σ_{S21} are 12.82 and 5.1747 for 8720ES and PICO VNA 108 respectively. The results are plotted for two separate cases of 3–4 GHz (Fig. 3(a), (b)) and 3–5 GHz (Fig. 3(c), (d)). It can be visualized from Fig. 3 that both VNAs showcase correlated results.

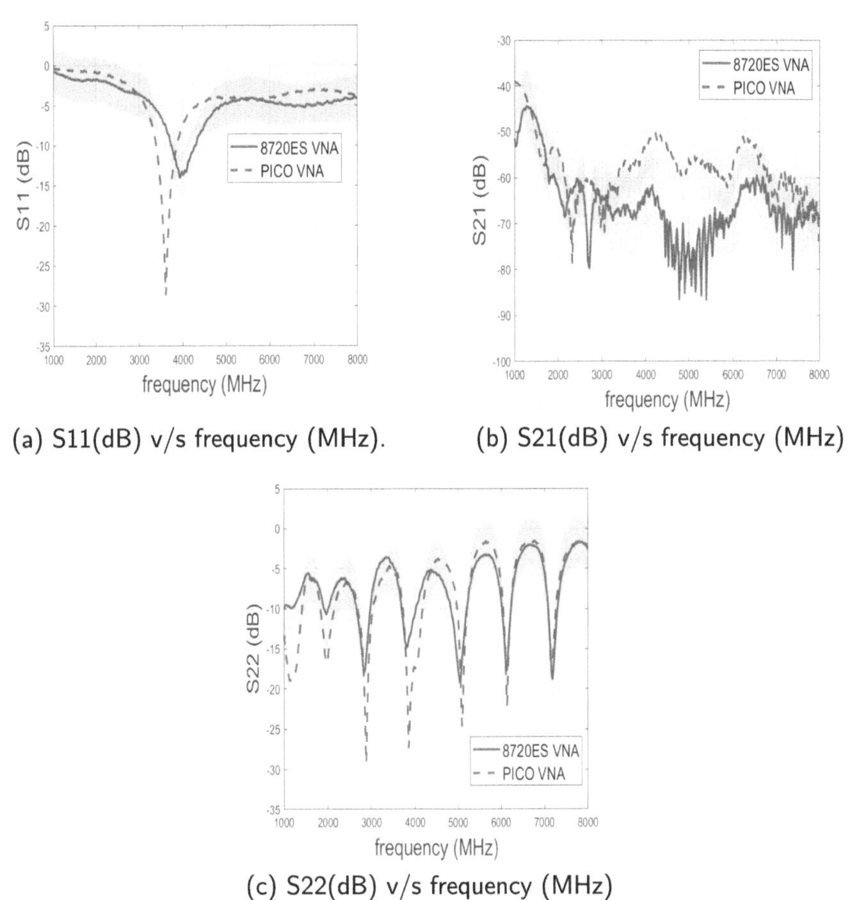

(a) S11(dB) v/s frequency (MHz).

(b) S21(dB) v/s frequency (MHz)

(c) S22(dB) v/s frequency (MHz)

Fig. 4. Comparison of antenna response v/s frequency for in-body measurements.

4.3 In-body Measurements

The in-body measurement results for antenna 2 using 8720ES VNA and PICO VNA 108 are shown in Fig. 4. It can be visualized from S11 (dB) v/s frequency (MHz) plot of Fig. 4(a) that the antenna response with PICO VNA 108 is sharper and is able to characterize the channel with more resolution as compared to 8720ES VNA. For instance, the resonating frequency (min S11) for 8720ES VNA is at 3948.75 MHz with S11 = −13.73 whereas for PICO VNA, the minimal of

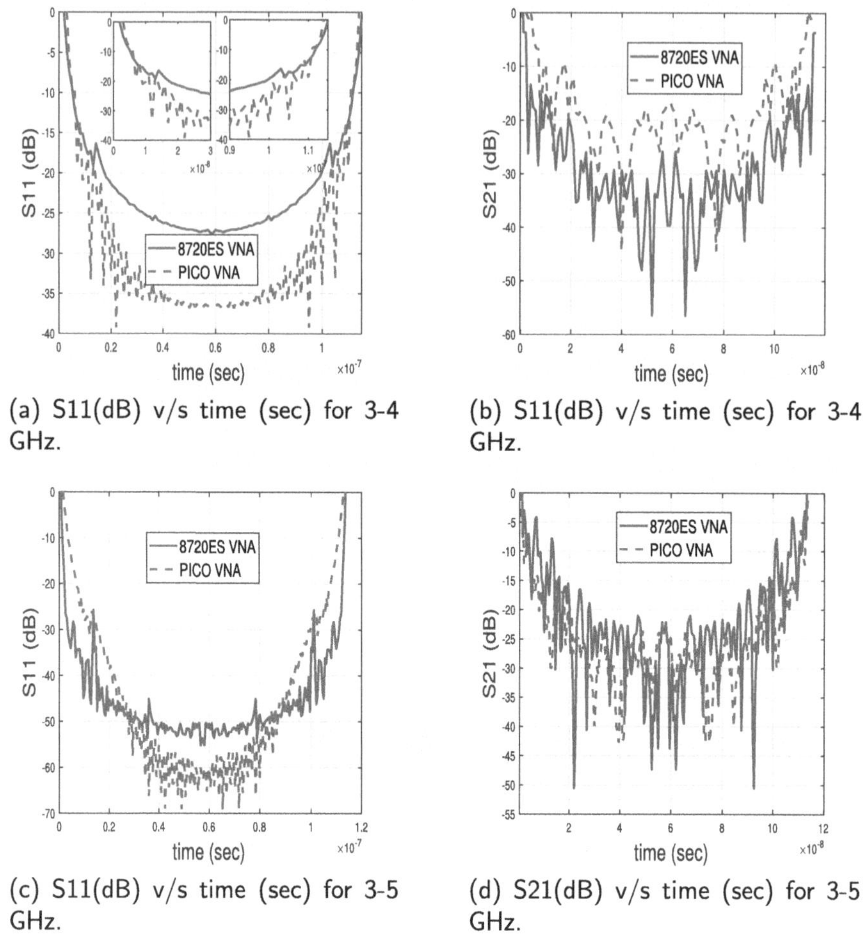

(a) S11(dB) v/s time (sec) for 3-4 GHz.

(b) S11(dB) v/s time (sec) for 3-4 GHz.

(c) S11(dB) v/s time (sec) for 3-5 GHz.

(d) S21(dB) v/s time (sec) for 3-5 GHz.

Fig. 5. Comparison of antenna response v/s time for in-body measurements.

S11 is found at 3607.5 MHZ with −28.57 dB. Apart from this peak, the antenna response correlates well for both VNAs. Similarly, the S21 v/s frequency plot is shown in Fig. 4(b) some difference in results is found at 3–7 GHZ band but overall, both VNAs have S21 well below −50 dB level. The antenna response for capsule antenna (antenna 3) is shown in Fig. 4(c). It can be visualized from Fig. 4(c) that the response obtained from both the VNAs is very similar with identical peaks in S22.

Further, the time domain analysis with in-body measurements is presented in Fig. 5. The results are plotted by taking IFFT of antenna response from 3 GHz to 4 GHz for Fig. 5(a) and (b) whereas 3 GHz to 5 GHz band is taken for Fig. 5(c) and (d). It can be visualized from Fig. 5(a) and (c) that the time domain response of 9720ES VNA is almost flat whereas PICO VNA shows more variations. This may result in the availability of more information content in the signal but can also be caused as a result of noise and error in measurements. The plot of S21 plots v/s time for both the VNAs is shown in Fig. 5(b) and (d) wherein it can be seen that S21 results from both VNAs show a similar trend with 3–5 GHz results overlapping at all time values.

5 Conclusion

A comparative analysis of two commercially available VNAs (8720ES S-parameter Network Analyzer by Agilent Technologies and PicoVNA 108 by PICO Technology) is presented in this paper. The suitability of these two VNAs for biomedical monitoring applications is tested based on their parametric properties such as size, accuracy, power consumption, resolution, etc. It is observed from numerous on-body and in-body trials that the performance of relatively cheaper PICO VNA 108 is at par with 8720ES VNA. The 8720ES VNA has a higher ground in terms of larger frequency range of operation, lower temperature drift, higher resolution and lower phase noise. On the other hand, the PICO VNA has better performance in terms of trace noise, sweep time and overall size/weight. The in-body and on-body measurements showcase that both VNAs perform at par with other standard VNAs. In future, an analytical framework will be developed for a more thorough analysis based on advanced statistical features of the signal captured by the VNA.

Acknowledgment. This work was supported by the University of Oulu Emerging Program Project, 6G-enabled sustainable society (6GESS) program: 6GESS6 and 6GBRIDGE - Next generation healthcare and wearable diagnostics utilizing 6G project (11146 /31 /2022). The authors thank INDFICORE (India-Finland cooperation on 6G) under the 6G Flagship group at the University of Oulu, Finland for providing valuable discussions.

References

1. Anritsu: Calculating VNA measurement accuracy. https://www.microwavejournal.com/ext/resources/BGDownload
2. Hamdi, A., Nahali, A., Harrabi, M., Brahem, R.: Optimized design and performance analysis of wearable antenna sensors for wireless body area network applications. J. Inf. Telecommun. **7**(2), 155–175 (2023)
3. Hayden, L.: VNA error model conversion for n-port calibration comparison. In: 2007 69th ARFTG Conference, pp. 1–10 (2007)
4. Kissi, C., Särestöniemi, M., Pomalaza-Raez, C., Sonkki, M., Srifi, M.N.: Low-UWB directive antenna for wireless capsule endoscopy localization. In: 13th EAI International Conference on Body Area Networks 13, pp. 431–442. Springer (2020)
5. Lewandowski, A., Williams, D.F., Hale, P.D., Wang, J.C.M., Dienstfrey, A.: Covariance-based vector-network-analyzer uncertainty analysis for time- and frequency-domain measurements. IEEE Trans. Microw. Theory Tech. **58**(7), 1877–1886 (2010)

6. Lin, M., Zhang, Y.: Covariance-matrix-based uncertainty analysis for NVNA measurements. IEEE Trans. Instrum. Meas. **61**(1), 93–102 (2012)
7. Särestöniemi, M., et al.: Realistic 3D phantoms for validation of microwave sensing in health monitoring applications. Sensors **24**(6), 1975 (2024)
8. Särestöniemi, M., Singh, D., von und zu Fraunberg, M., Myllylä, T.: Microwave technique for linear skull fracture detection—simulation and experimental study using realistic human head models. Biosensors **14**(9), 434 (2024)
9. Särestöniemi, M., Singh, D., Heredia, C., Nikkinen, J., von und zu Fraunberg, M., Myllylä, T.: Digital twins for development of microwave-based brain tumor detection. In: Nordic Conference on Digital Health and Wireless Solutions, pp. 240–254. Springer (2024)
10. Shang, J., Yu, Y.: An ultrawideband capsule antenna for biomedical applications. IEEE Antennas Wirel. Propag. Lett. **18**(12), 2548–2551 (2019)
11. Shang, X., et al.: Interlaboratory comparison of dielectric measurements from microwave to terahertz frequencies using VNA-based and optical-based methods. IEEE Trans. Microwave Theory Tech. 1–12 (2024)
12. Singh, D., et al.: Preliminary studies on mm-wave radar for vital sign monitoring of driver in vehicular environment. In: Nordic Conference on Digital Health and Wireless Solutions, pp. 480–493. Springer (2024)
13. Singh, D., Vihriälä, E., Särestöniemi, M., Myllylä, T.: Microwave technique based noninvasive monitoring of intracranial pressure using realistic phantom models. In: Nordic Conference on Digital Health and Wireless Solutions, pp. 413–425. Springer (2024)
14. Stumper, U., Schrader, T.: Influence of different configurations of nonideal calibration standards on vector network analyzer performance. IEEE Trans. Instrum. Meas. **61**(7), 2034–2041 (2012)
15. 8720ES S-parameter Network Analyzer, 50 MHz to 20 GHz. https://www.keysight.com/us/en/product/8720ES/sparameter-network-analyzer.html
16. PicoVNA 100 Series. https://www.picotech.com/download/datasheets/picovna-vector-network-analyzer-data-sheet.pdf
17. PicoVNA 5 User's Guide. https://www.picotech.com/download/manuals/picovna-vector-network-analyser-picovna-5-users-guide.pdf
18. Wang, M., Zhao, Y., Loh, T.H., Xu, Q., Zhou, Y.: Efficient uncertainty evaluation of vector network analyser measurements using two-tier Bayesian analysis and Monte Carlo method. In: 12th European Conference on Antennas and Propagation (EuCAP 2018), pp. 1–5 (2018)

Leveraging Deep Learning for Real-Time Object Detection in Campus Surveillance

S. Sudharsan[1], P. Arun Eswar[1], P. Sasi Kumar[1](✉), P. Arulmozhivarman[2], and S. Maheswari[3]

[1] School of Electronics Engineering, Vellore Institute of Technology, Vellore 632014, Tamil Nadu, India
sudharsan.s2023c@vitsudent.ac.in, aruneswar.p2023@vitstudent.ac.in, sasikumar.p@vit.ac.in

[2] Centre for Clean Environment, and Office of Academic Research, Vellore Institute of Technology, Vellore 632014, Tamil Nadu, India
parulmozhivarman@vit.ac.in

[3] School of Computer Science and Engineering, Vellore Institute of Technology, Chennai 600127, Tamil Nadu, India
maheswari.s@vit.ac.in

Abstract. A machine learning technique called "deep learning" teaches computers to do tasks more efficiently. For some tasks, artificial intelligence matches human intelligence. Neural networks are trained to accomplish this. In computer vision object detection and classification are the two effective tasks. Object detection is divided into two stages: one for single-stage detection and another for two-stage detection is one of the primary tasks of deep learning. In this research, we developed a real-time object detection system that can identify pedestrians and cars on our university campus, enabling the use of surveillance and monitoring. This is accomplished by combining a Raspberry Pi module hardware interface with the state-of-the-art "You Only Look Once" (YOLO Version 8) algorithm, which is a single-stage detector, to produce an effective real-time performance with an output result efficiency of 98.4%.

Keywords: YOLO · Object detection · Neural Network · Raspberry Pi · Computer Vision · Deep Learning

1 Introduction

The algorithm known as "YOLO," is used for object detection in image processing tasks. Its purpose is to identify and categorize items within picture or video frames. YOLO's primary advantage over other object detection techniques is its capacity to process the full image in a single forward neural network pass. Using numerous passes and region recommendations in traditional object detection algorithms can be computationally costly. In contrast, the YOLO algorithm bounds the box around the image creates a grid out of the image, and concurrently according to the label and class of the

K. Atul et al. (Eds.): BodyNets 2024, LNICST 666, pp. 415–428, 2026.
https://doi.org/10.1007/978-3-032-16099-7_33

dataset. For real-time applications like video analysis and driverless cars, this makes it extremely effective. Each bounding box is defined with its coordinate's axis represented as (x, y) for the box's top-left corner and its width and height (w, h). YOLO uses these bounding boxes to predict and detect objects within the frame, allowing for efficient and accurate object detection. In computer vision, object identification using convolutional neural networks (CNNs) is a job where a neural network is trained to recognize and find objects in images. Because CNNs can automatically extract hierarchical characteristics from the input data, they are very well suited for this kind of work. During training, the CNN is fed with labeled training data containing images and corresponding bounding box annotations. The network learns to adjust its parameters (weights and biases) to minimize the difference between its predictions and the ground truth annotations. Popular architectures for object detection using Convolutional Neural Networks involving Single Stage Detectors, Faster Region-Convolutional Neural Networks, and YOLO. These architectures often incorporate additional components like anchor boxes, region proposals, and non-maximum suppression to improve accuracy and speed. YOLOv8, the most recent iteration of the YOLO model, is suitable for tasks like instance segmentation, object detection, and image classification. YOLOv8's increased speed and accuracy over earlier iterations are two of its main characteristics. It uses a deeper and bigger neural network architecture that was trained on a large dataset to do this. Detection, segmentation, classification, and key point detection are among the several tasks that YOLOv8 can perform. There are several goals and use cases for each of these jobs. You can select the right task for your computer vision application by knowing how these tasks differ from one another.

2 Literature Review

Object detection in the autonomous vehicles has been a challenging task in the emerging technology. In this sector Pasricha, S (2022) has proposed a comprehensive state of the art in the object detection algorithms and states the open challenges in object detection. Shankhdhar, A (2022) on the title of Deep Learning Techniques for Image Recognition and Object Detection discussed on the depth of the object recognition. Tiwari (2023) represents a web app-based ML/DL model that performs traffic surveillance and detection with high accuracy and efficiency. Kamath (2021) In this research, they have used Efficient, again a single stage detector which holds a greater detection phase has an integer quantization technique to perform real-time object detection on a Raspberry Pi using the popular Efficient Det backbone. Diwan,T (2020), they proposed a real time object detection with the yolo architecture and reached a good accuracy of about 95% and also discussed the challenges in the real time successor. Chaturvedi (2023) proposed the algorithm that works for identifying the peoples violating the traffic rule such as triple riders, not wearing helmets inside the university campus.They implemented the yolo v8 architecture and achieved a good accuracy on the real time performance manifesting on the topic of Detection of traffic rule violations in university campuses using deep learning model. Another helpful research on the topic of Real-Time Theft Detection Using YOLOv5 Object Detection Model involved in detecting and tracking of objects with the real time camera feeds proposed by Varun, S (2023). On the research topic of

Object detection in high-resolution optical image based on deep learning technique, this work produced a high-quality dataset for object detection based on the high-resolution remote sensing images of the Triple SAT. Li, H (2022). LI, H (2023), he proposed a model based on the helmet detection, The algorithm he proposed was YOLO -PL based on the architecture of YOLO-v4, which is a tiny single stage detector model used for real time inference.

3 Methodology of Object Detection

The subtasks that makeup object detection are localization, which locates an item in an image (or video frame), and classification, which gives an object a class such as "Person", "Van", "Bike", and "car".

3.1 Two-Stage Detection

When detecting objects, two-stage detectors are classified as Faster R-CNN and Region-based Fully Convolutional Network. Although RFCN operates slowly, it detects things with a high order of precision when compared to other approaches, such as remote sensing photos. However, because of the tiny size of the objects, the positive and negative samples are not balanced. The process starts with the creation of region suggestions, or possible areas where objects may be found. In the second step, these suggestions are further developed and categorized. This two-step process makes it possible to analyse the picture more thoroughly, which facilitates accurate item categorization and exact location [1]. The great precision of two-stage detectors is one of their main advantages. Robust detection performance is achieved by allowing for a more thorough inspection of the picture through distinct area proposals and classification steps. Additionally, because of its careful region proposal procedure, two-stage detectors frequently perform well in situations with tiny objects or overlapping occurrences. The output from single-stage detectors is expressed as a bounding box for the suggested region, whereas the two-stage detectors exhibit superior performance, providing high probability zones only for item detection in the image.

3.2 Single-Stage Detector

YOLO (You Only Look Once) YOLO is a neural network that predicts class probabilities and bounding boxes. In [2] study has proposed a method to implement object detection based on video proximity detection, using the YOLO (Version 2) model, copy move attack in passive blind videos, proposed an automatic detection of counterfeited objects in the video has a 0.99 confidence score, for performing a real-time [3] object detection (DCNN), Deep Convolutional Neural network. In [4] study proposes object detection in autonomous vehicles and has classified various stages of YOLO. The research of [5] YOLO (Version 5) implementation is used for real-time tool detection in smart manufacturing techniques. This proposed work implemented a YOLO Version 8 model for detecting the objects on the university campus. As it proposes a state-of-the-art model. Anchor-free detection is specific for YOLO (Version 8). Anchor-free detection works concerning the reference of the image. An object class with the appropriate size and aspect ratio may be obtained by utilizing anchor boxes, which are a predefined collection of boxes with specified heights and widths. It is based on the size of the image used for the training model. 2) Single shot detector (SSD): It predicts both the classes and the border boxes directly from feature maps in a single pass without the need for a specialized area proposal network [6]. The primary distinction between YOLO and SSD architectures is that the YOLO architecture has two completely linked layers, while SSD employs many convolutional layers of different resolutions [7]. Several further layers, often referred to as extra layers, are built on top of the underlying networks of single-shot detectors and come after them eventually. With its real-time capability, the YOLO transformed object detection and is considered one of the more ideas in single-stage detectors. This operates by first splitting the input photos into a grid and then calculating the prediction for each grid cell, which contains the class probability and bounding box coordinates (Fig. 1).

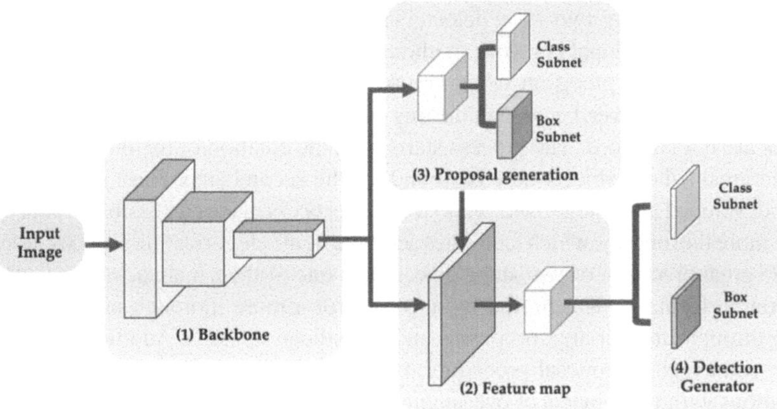

Fig. 1. This Figure represents the Two Stage detector flow from the data input to the output of the image class.

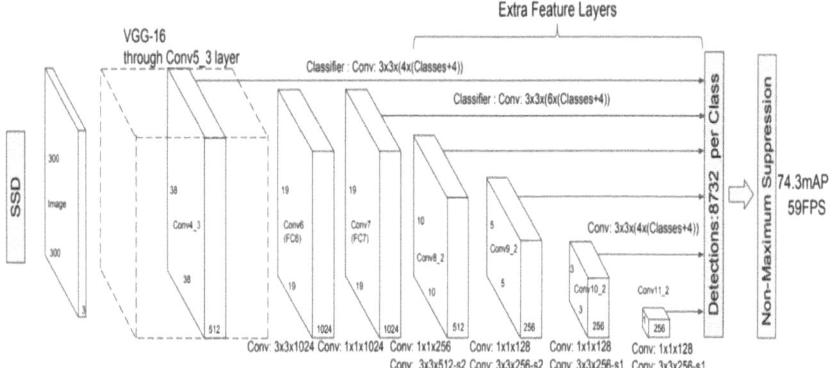

Fig. 2. This Figure represents that YOLO is one of the single-stage detector mechanisms under this SSD flow, which is a single-stage detector flow from the data input to the result of this image class.

4 Yolo V8 Architecture

YOLO Version 8 architecture combines elements of the Restnet-50 and Darknet-53 systems. They are YOLO Version 8 architecture that combines elements of the Restnet-50 and Darknet-53 systems. They are intended to detect things efficiently and are composed of several residual connections and additional convolutional layers. To increase the model's accuracy, it additionally includes spatial pyramid pooling. YOLO Version 8 is built on the framework of YOLO Version 5, and it features various architectural and developer experience enhancements, as well as a single framework for training models to conduct object detection. YOLO Version 8 has specific techniques for detecting the objects. Anchor-based detection and anchor-free detection. Anchor-based detection is used to detect the objects by their bounding boxes with the aid of predefined anchor boxes. Anchor-free detection is used to identify the objects without the support of anchor boxes [8]. The output structure of the You Only Look Once model's feature mapping is intended to forecast the probability of the class, the confidence interval, and the bounding box coordinates. Because of its ability to recognize many objects in the neural network model, YOLO outperforms other convolutional approaches in terms of object identification process performance when done end-to-end [9].

4.1 Anchor Box Detection

A significant issue with object detection was fixed via anchor boxes. A grid cell containing the middle of the item is assigned to it before anchor boxes. It is difficult to build bounding boxes and assign objects to different classes if two objects have the same center point. Consider anchor boxes as prefabricated forms. Assume for the moment that we have Anchor Box 1 and Anchor Box 2. Assigning the anchor box to the class will include looking through the list of anchor boxes to see which has the Largest overlap, or IoU, with the ground truth bounding box. Anchor Box 1 is helpful for figures that are horizontally extended, like horses, while Anchor Box 2 is good for figures that are vertically elongated [4] (Fig. 3).

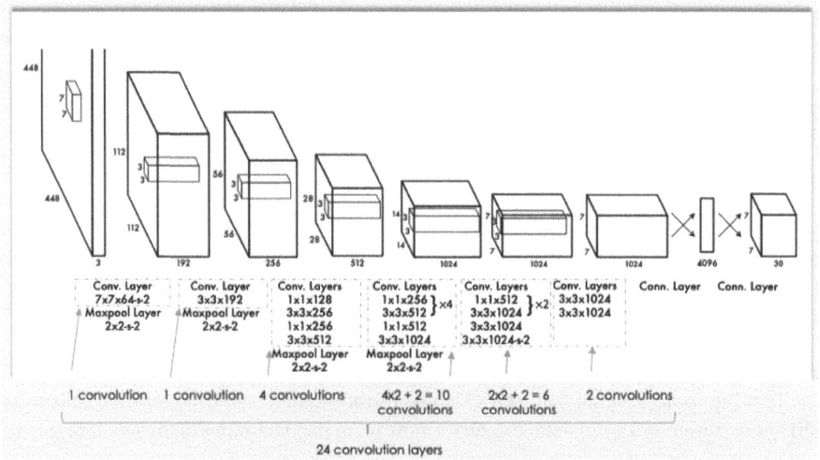

Fig. 3. This Figure represents the YOLO Architecture it has overall 24 convolutional layers, four max-pooling layers, and two fully connected layers.

4.2 Mosaic Data Augmentation

YOLO Version 8 performs several picture augmentations on training sets. Mosaic data augmentation is one example of such augmentation. A straight-forward augmentation method called mosaic data augmentation involves stitching four separate photos together and feeding the resulting input into the model [10]. This enables the model to learn the real objects in partial occlusion and at various locations. The network's fully connected layers forecast the output probabilities and coordinates, whereas the network's first convolutional layers gather particulars from the object. The Google LeNet algorithm for image classification is based on a model for this network design. 24 convolutional layers make up our network, and then there are 2 completely linked layers. We develop 1 x 1 reduction layers accompanied by 3 × 3 convolutional layers, familiar to Lin et al., in place of the inception modules used by GoogleNet [11]. In Fig. 2, the whole network is displayed. We indulge in developing a specific functionality that aims to detect the speed of object detection. A neural network used by Fast YOLO has nine convolutional layers as opposed to 24 and fewer filters in each layer. All the testing and training parameters are identical for the YOLO and Fast YOLO algorithms other than the model size [12].

5 Proposed Flow

The process of detecting objects involves training the dataset using software that selects the most suitable model for the data. The Computer Vision Annotation Tool It is utilized to train the model by creating bounding boxes around objects in the images and assigning defined classes to them. Then, it moves the software results to the Raspberry Pi for the detection process in the backend software (Table 1 and Fig. 4).

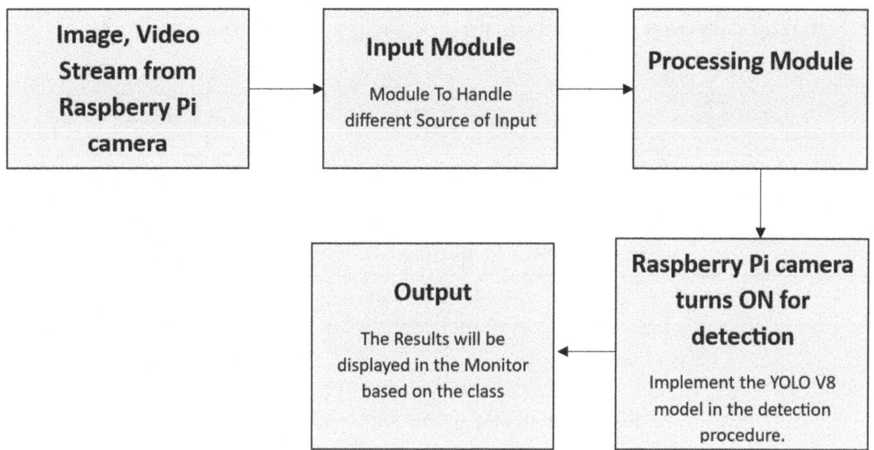

Fig. 4. Methodology for Hardware setup

Table 1. Description of dataset

Dataset	Images
Train	1500
Validate	740
Test	280

The table is about the dataset collected manually for the detection phase and how the data are split into the Train and Test Phase.

5.1 Model Selection

The system uses YOLO Version 8 for its excellent performance in real-time object detection tasks. We conducted a comparative analysis of YOLO Version 8, YOLO Version 7, and Faster R-CNN, evaluating metrics such as accuracy (ACC), precision (PR), recall (RE), and frame rate (FR). The dataset comprises annotated photos and videos featuring people, bikes, and cars on a university campus. Rotation, scaling, and flipping are examples of data augmentation techniques that were used to improve the model's accuracy inside the university campus (Fig. 5).

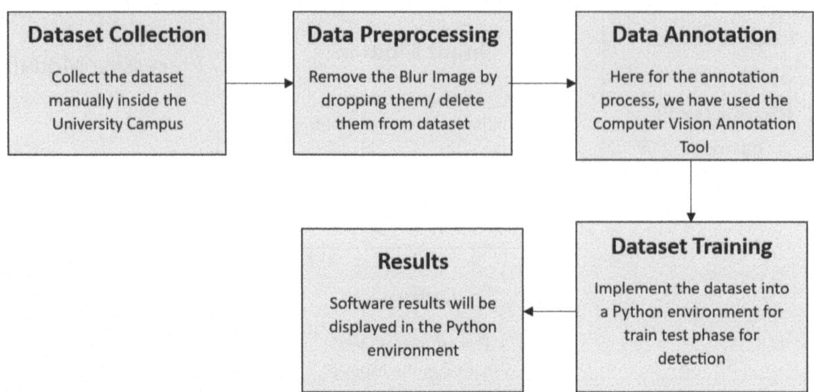

Fig. 5. Methodology for Software Process

5.2 Training, Testing, and Validation

The YOLO Version 8 had been trained on a 70-percent split of the enhanced dataset. The training procedure was tuned for real-time inference, taking into account both speed and accurate detection. Following that, 10% of the dataset was separated for the model's testing phase. The remaining 20% of the data was utilized as a validation set for evaluating model performance. The precision of the bounding box predictions was evaluated using performance metrics such as the Intersection over Union (IoU).

5.3 Integration with Raspberry Pi Module

Hardware integration involves connecting the Raspberry Pi and camera module to a desktop computer for developing the detection phase script and uploading the software dataset in the Raspberry Pi. Where every aspect of the software will be integrated with the Raspberry module during the detection phase.

5.4 Hyper Parameter Tuning and Video Processing

This process involves tuning the learning rate, batch size, and regularization techniques to ensure stable training and optimal performance of the YOLO Version 8 model. In this phase, the video will detect the object using the bounding box which has been trained using the YOLO algorithm and if the object lies within the frame, it detects the object class, if not so then it again checks for the next frame.

5.5 Detection Phase

This phase will involve acquiring the results that have been received through the monitor feed as output, where the class will be recognized on the display by a training process that will operate in the background and provide the result in the display.

6 Result

The dataset was Pre-trained with the YOLO Version 8 model for object detection over 100 epochs and 0.184 h of training time. The optimal and final weights will be detected. Various YOLO models for object detection utilizing deep learning models were compared to other object detection methods versions of (YOLOV7, YOLOV5, YOLO V3), and YOLOV8 outperformed them in terms of accuracy, speed, and efficiency. YOLOV5 features more loss functions when compared to the proposed model. We achieved a 90% detection rate with a model trained for approximately 100 epochs in YOLO Version 8 (Table 2).

Table 2. Performance value of Validation test

Class	Box(Precision)	Recall	mAP50	mAP50–90
ALL	0.992	0.956	0.994	0.842
Car	1	0.96	0.992	0.864
Person	0.975	1	0.995	0.78
Bike	1	0.907	0.995	0.882

The Dataset was collected manually for the Training, Testing, and Validation in the Software Process and the performance value for the object detection in the Validation process (Table 3).

Table 3. Comparison with Various Version YOLO Algorithms

Model(mAP Value in Percentage)	ALL	Person	Car	Bike
YOLO V3	0.6524	0.6835	0.5879	0.66
YOLO V5	0.7325	0.6282	0.6986	0.6125
YOLO V7	0.8051	0.7743	0.7102	0.7225
YOLO V8	0.9944	0.992	0.995	0.995

7 Evaluation Metrics

7.1 Mean Average Precision

The mean average precision gives the average precision value of each class. It determines the object class labels from the prediction. The confusion model matrix is based on the parameters used True Positive, False Positive, True Negative, False Negative. It determines how much the object is precise.

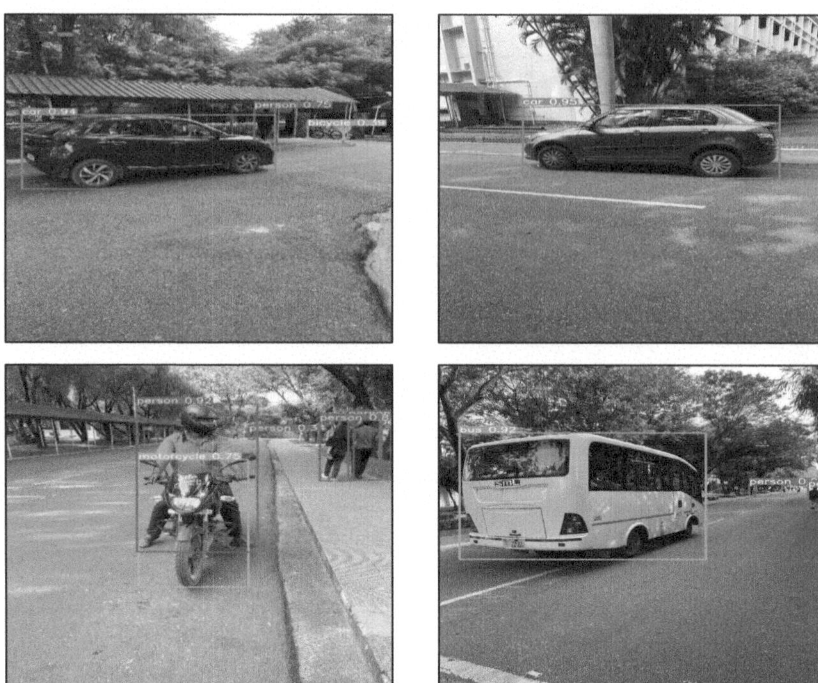

Fig. 6. These output images are predicted with the trained YOLOv8n model.

7.2 Correlation Matrix

A confusion matrix provides a matrix form of the prediction summary. It represents the percentage of each of each class's predictions that were correct and incorrect. It aids in comprehending the classes that the model confuses for other classes. In the custom dataset, we have obtained the correlation values from minus 1 (-1) to plus (Tables 4 and 5).

Table 4. DWT Statistical Features and Formulas

Feature	Formula	Description
Mean	$\mu = \frac{1}{N}\sum_{i=1}^{N} x_i$ x_i: DWT coefficient	The average value of the coefficients
Variance	$\sigma^2 = \frac{1}{N-1}\sum_{i=1}^{N}(x_i - \mu)^2$ x_i: DWT coefficient, μ: Mean	Measure of the spread of coefficients
Standard Deviation	$\sigma = \sqrt{\frac{1}{N-1}\sum_{i=1}^{N}(x_i - \mu)^2}$ x_i: DWT coefficient, μ: Mean	The square root of the variance

Table 5. Correlation Matrix

Data	All	Car	Bike	Person
All	0.99200	0.536660	0.783399	0.558499
Person	0.558499	0.830000	0.638501	1
Car	0.536660	0.96650	0.7586	0.830000
Bike	0.783399	0.7586	1	0.638501

1 (+1), which denotes the dataset's exact percentage of the input. A statistical tool called a confusion matrix is used to assess the linear direction of two variables and outputs the results in a matrix format with three numerical representations of 1, − 1, and 0. The degree to which the data and pictures are perfectly connected is denoted by the value 1. The parameters in the model that the negative class accurately predicts are determined by the number − 1. The value of 0 indicates that it has no relationship to the data. There are 4 main quadrants in the confusion matrix for determining how much the dataset matches our predictions and it gives values based on 4 quadrants they are: True Positive, True Negative False Positive, and False Negative. In Fig. 6 the confusion matrix values for the dataset (Fig. 7).

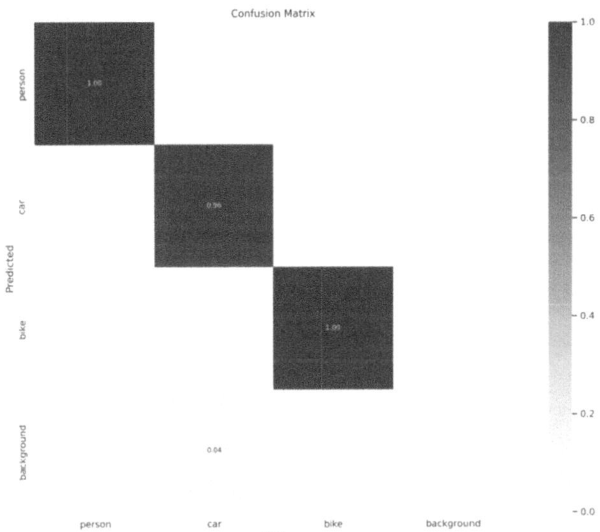

Fig. 7. This is the Correlation matrix obtained for the Object detection. The matrix is a table in which every cell contains a correlation coefficient, where 1 is considered a strong relationship between variables, 0 a neutral relationship, and − 1 a not strong relationship.

7.3 Precision Recall Curve

This curve states that a decision of a threshold is based on the desirable value of precision and recall. If the value is higher than our model it gives the more related results for our model.

$$P = \frac{TP}{TP + FP} \tag{2}$$

$$R = \frac{TP}{TP + FN} \tag{3}$$

7.4 Precision Confidence Curve

The precision-confidence curve is a visual representation of the relationship between precision and confidence threshold in object detection at the university campus using the YOLOv8 model. It plots the precision value at different confidence thresholds. Starting from a high confidence threshold, the precision will be relatively high because only confident predictions are considered valid. Where, (Figs. 8 and 9)

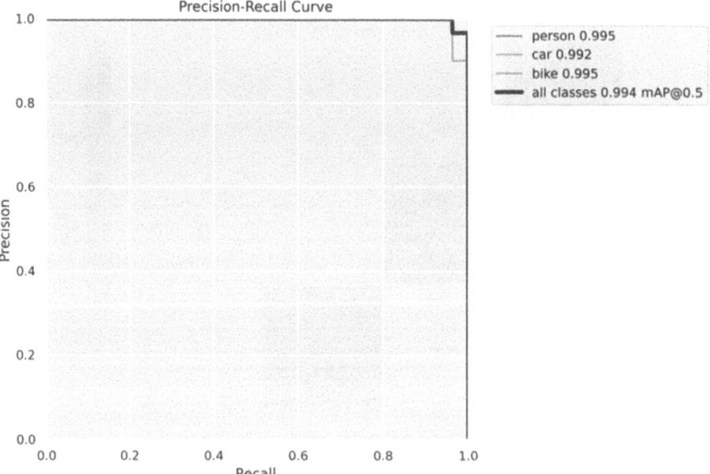

Fig. 8. This Precision-Recall curve states that shows the trade-off between precision and recall for different thresholds The high area under the curve represents both high recall and high precision, where high precision relates to a low false positive rate, and high recall relates to a low false negative rate at the threshold of 0.994

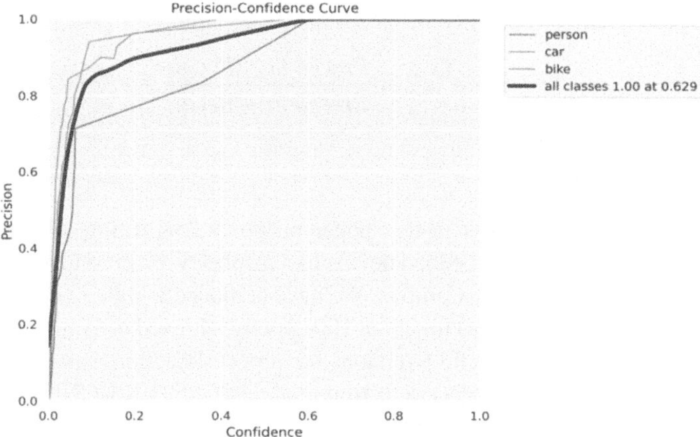

Fig. 9. This is a Precision confidence curve obtained for Object detection. A precision score of 1.00 signifies that the model made no false-positive predictions at the confidence threshold of 0.649.

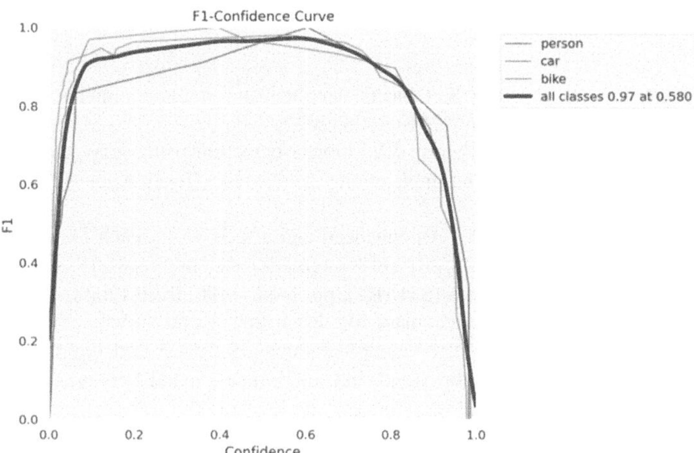

Fig. 10. This is the F1 confidence curve for object detection. The F1 score is the harmonic mean of precision and recall, providing a balanced assessment of a model's performance while considering both false positives and false negatives. The F1 score is 0.97 at the interval of 0.580, indicating high model accuracy.

7.5 F1 Confidence Curve

The model value range is 0 to 1, and the F1 score aids in the analysis of a weighted average of the precision and recall values for the specified model. The objective of the F1 score is to accurately categorize events as positive or negative. It is a measure of a model's accuracy that accounts for both precision and recall. Recall is the percentage of actual positive instances that were accurately anticipated, whereas precision represents the percentage of predicted positive instances that were genuinely positive (Fig. 10).

$$F1\,Score = 2 \times \frac{Precision \times Recall}{Precision + Recall} \tag{4}$$

8 Conclusion

The final part of the conclusion in this paper proposes a real-time object detection deployed on the edge cutting embedded device like raspberry-pi 4 module with a YOLO v8 algorithm inside a University Campus. We have achieved a higher accuracy of 94% detection rate with a model trained for about 100 epochs achieved in a minimum run time inference. Various models of YOLO versions for object detection using deep learning model while comparing other object detection methods(FASTER RCNN) and versions of (YOLOV7, YOLOV5), and YOLOV8 outscores in terms of accuracy, speed, and efficiency. YOLOV5 has more loss functions while comparing the proposed model. The future scope enhancements involve SMS alerts and mail notifications. A wide variety of datasets including Camera Calibration, for further accuracy and frame speed high-speed controller (Jetson Nano) can be used.

References

1. Balasubramaniam, A., Pasricha, S.: Object detection in autonomous vehicles: Status and open challenges. arXiv preprint arXiv:2201.07706 (2022)
2. Diwan, T., Anirudh, G., Tembhurne, J.V.: Object detection using yolo: challenges, architectural successors, datasets and applications. Multimedia Tools Appl. **82**(6), 9243–9275 (2023)
3. Agrawal, N.K., Shankhdhar, A.: An enhanced and effective approach for object detection using deep learning techniques. In: 2022 11th International Conference on System Modeling & Advancement in Research Trends (SMART), pp. 1482–1486. IEEE (2022)
4. Tiwari, R., Rumaney, A.H., Saravanan, M.: Real-time traffic surveillance and detection using deep learning and computer vision techniques. In: 2023 2nd International Conference on Vision Towards Emerging Trends in Communication and Networking Technologies (ViTECoN), pp. 1–6. IEEE (2023)
5. Kamath, V., Renuka, A.: Performance analysis of the pre-trained efficientdet for real-time object detection on raspberry pi. In: 2021 International Conference on Circuits, Controls and Communications (CCUBE), pp. 1–6. IEEE (2021)
6. Bhatti, M.T., Khan, M.G., Aslam, M., Fiaz, M.J.: Weapon detection in real-time CCTV videos using deep learning. IEEE Access **9**, 34366–34382 (2021)
7. Chaturvedi, P., Lavingia, K., Raval, G.: Detection of traffic rule violation in university campus using deep learning model. Int. J. Syst. Assur. Eng. Manag. **14**(6), 2527–2545 (2023)
8. Zendehdel, N., Chen, H., Leu, M.C.: Real-time tool detection in smart manufacturing using you-only-look-once (yolo) v5. Manufact. Lett. **35**, 1052–1059 (2023)
9. Varun, S., Bhuvanesh, V.: Real-time theft detection using yolov5 object detection model. In: 2023 3rd International Conference on Innovative Sustainable Computational Technologies (CISCT), pp. 1–5. IEEE (2023)
10. Qi, W.: Object detection in high-resolution optical image based on deep learning technique. Nat. Hazards Res. **2**(4), 384–392 (2022)
11. Li, H., Wu, D., Zhang, W., Xiao, C.: Yolo-pl: helmet wearing detection algorithm based on improved yolov4. Digit. Signal Process. 104283 (2023)
12. Yin, Y., Li, H., Fu, W.: Faster-yolo: an accurate and faster object detection method. Digit. Signal Process. **102**, 102756 (2020)

Next-Gen Microwave Sensing for Brain Monitoring: Fusion of Machine Learning and Digital Twin Technology

Daljeet Singh[1,2(✉)], Sarthak Acharya[3], Rajkujmar Saini[4], Hem Dutt Joshi[5], Mariella Säreståniemi[1,2,6], and Teemu Myllylä[1,2,7,8]

[1] Research Unit of Health Sciences and Technology, Faculty of Medicine, University of Oulu, Oulu, Finland
{daljeet.singh,mariella.sarestoniemi,teemu.myllyla}@oulu.fi
[2] Infotech Oulu, University of Oulu, Oulu, Finland
[3] M3S Research Unit, ITEE, University of Oulu, Oulu, Finland
sartak.acharya@oulu.fi
[4] Department of Computer Science, Electrical and Space Engineering, Luleå University of Technology, Luleå, Sweden
rajkumar.saini@ltu.se
[5] Department of Electronics and Communication Engineering, Thapar Institute of Engineering and Technology, Patiala, Punjab, India
hemdutt.joshi@thapar.edu
[6] Centre for Wireless Communications, Faculty of Information Technology and Electrical Engineering, University of Oulu, Oulu, Finland
[7] Medical Research Center, Oulu, Finland
[8] Optoelectronics and Measurements, Faculty of Information Technology and Electrical Engineering, University of Oulu, Oulu, Finland

Abstract. Integration of multiple technologies amid Industry 5.0 is observed in most of the engineering application. However, Machine Learning (ML) and Digital Twin Technology (DTT) play a major role in data acquisition, processing, data analytics and decision making process of almost every automated system. Due to the gigantic amount of data generated in healthcare and medicine applications, manual analysis of this data becomes very cumbersome and time consuming. Therefore, ML, artificial intelligence (AI), data science, DTT and Cyber Physical Systems (CPSs) emerge as powerful tools for efficient, accurate, automated and fast processing of this medical data including 1D, 2D signals as well as multidimensional images. This paper presents an overview and comparative analysis of machine learning algorithms and tools utilized for brain monitoring applications especially focusing on microwave techniques. A systematic review and meta analysis based on PRISMA approach is presented and analyzed. A brief outline of ML algorithms utilized for different applications focusing on brain temperature measurement, stroke detection, and Intracranial Pressure (ICP) measurement are elaborated along with ML tools for microwave imaging.

Keywords: Artificial intelligence · brain monitoring · deep learning · microwave · digital twin · Wearable Antenna

K. Atul et al. (Eds.): BodyNets 2024, LNICST 666, pp. 429–440, 2026.
https://doi.org/10.1007/978-3-032-16099-7_34

1 Introduction

The healthcare industry is always espousing the latest technologies to serve the global populace, whether it be continuous monitoring of chronic illness, providing healthcare access to remote locations, or real-time data measurement and management [24,29]. We are surrounded by microwaves around which our lives revolve. Microwaves have found their place in healthcare in both diagnostic and therapeutic applications. Microwaves are utilized for non-invasive diagnosis of stroke, tumor, stones, and other medical conditions as well as for monitoring vital signs such as heart rate and breathing rate [45]. It is also used extensively in hyperthermia and thermal ablation treatments. Some of the key applications in healthcare originated from microwaves include: i) ambient assisted living environments for healthcare using integrated sensing and communication (ISAC) [30,46], ii) advanced wireless brain-computer interaction (BCI) for remote patient monitoring by expanding the realms of communication from traditional voice and video to other human senses including touch, smell, and taste, [22,48] iii) smart infrastructure for healthcare using machine-centric communication, wireless body area networks, (WBANs), cloud, fog, & edge computing tailored into the thread of AI resulting in Internet of Medical Things (IoMT) [33], iv) diverse body-centric communication with smart sensors and extended reality [11]. Apart from these applications, microwaves can easily penetrate through human body without any harmful effects and are used extensively in the study and diagnosis of biological tissues in form of wearable radio frequency (RF) systems.

When compared to its rivals, the use of microwaves in healthcare offers several advantageous features such as i) safety due to the use of a non-ionizing electromagnetic (EM) field as compared to Computer Tomography (CT) and nuclear imaging, ii) higher penetration depth compared to optical modalities which can be controlled using suitable frequency band and adaptive sensitivity and specificity, iii) mobility of equipment due to low power small size transducers and transceivers as compared to positron emission tomography (PET) and magnetic resonance imaging (MRI), iv) ease of application due to non-invasive nature and possibility to be used from a distance (wireless measurements from bedside without requirements of moving the patient), v) fast signal acquisition for time-critical applications, v) lower cost of equipment and usage, etc. [39,40]. These benefits make microwaves an ideal solution for in vitro wireless sensing and imaging applications. Further, microwaves also aid in transferring data and power wirelessly to and from the implant and wearable devices [47].

Machine learning (ML) is emerging as a powerful tool to boost manufacturing, productivity, and precision in every sector of the economy [12]. Healthcare sector is also taking maximal advantage of ML and Artificial Intelligence (AI) for various applications such as patient monitoring, drug discovery, hospital administration, and most importantly medical data analysis [15]. ML has huge potential for brain monitoring and diagnosis of artifacts in related biological phenomena. AI along with ML plays a key role in analyzing massive complex image datasets from multimodal measurements. Feature extraction, supervised and unsupervised learning, classification, prediction using regression models, computerized quantitative evaluation etc. [5].

This paper presents an in-depth analysis of microwave aided brain monitoring systems with special emphasis on ML algorithms and tools for brain monitoring applications. Several key modalities utilized for brain monitoring are discussed along with their advantages and drawbacks. Three main applications: brain temperature estimation, stroke diagnosis and Intracranial Pressure (ICP) measurement are taken into consideration. The rest of the paper is organized as follows: the brain anatomy and different modalities are presented in Sect. 2. Machine learning for brain monitoring along with key applications are presented in Sect. 3. Section 4 holds the concluding remarks of the paper.

2 Brain Anatomy and Modalities for Brain Monitoring

The complexity of brain composition and its sensitivity towards environmental factors poses a great challenge in its study. The human brain is very prone to infections caused by in-vivo procedures and measurements. Thus microwave-based systems for in-vitro sensing from the skin have proved to be very suitable for the study and analysis of brain heath and related phenomena [41]. A streamlined version of brain anatomy representing different parts of the human brain is shown in Fig. 1. The invasive methods for brain monitoring includes insertion of catheter, probe or implantable transducers inside the skin and/or skull of the subject. These methods are shown in Fig. 1. Transcranial acoustic (TCA), Otic, measurement of Optic nerve sheath diameter, Near-infrared spectroscopy (NIRS), imaging methods such as MRI, Computer Tomography (CT), Ultrasound, infrared imaging, Electroencephalogram (EEG) and microwave are primarily non-invasive methods utilized for brain monitoring. The popular modalities utilized for brain monitoring including both invasive and non-invasive methods are also shown in Figs. 1 and 2.

3 Integration of Emerging Fields in Brain Monitoring

The amalgamation of the emerging technologies are the modern pillar in almost every discipline since the last decade, as major applications are becoming multidisciplinary in nature [1]. Efficient data acquisition, monitoring, faster processing at the edge nodes, predictive analytics, optimal decision making and etc., are the key requirements of next generation sensing applications. Some of the key technological drivers in WBANs are IoT, CPS, ML, AI, DTT and communication technologies [49].

3.1 Digital Twin Technology

Industry 4.0 era has introduced many technologies and approaches for smarter research and developments, of which DTT is considered as one of the most

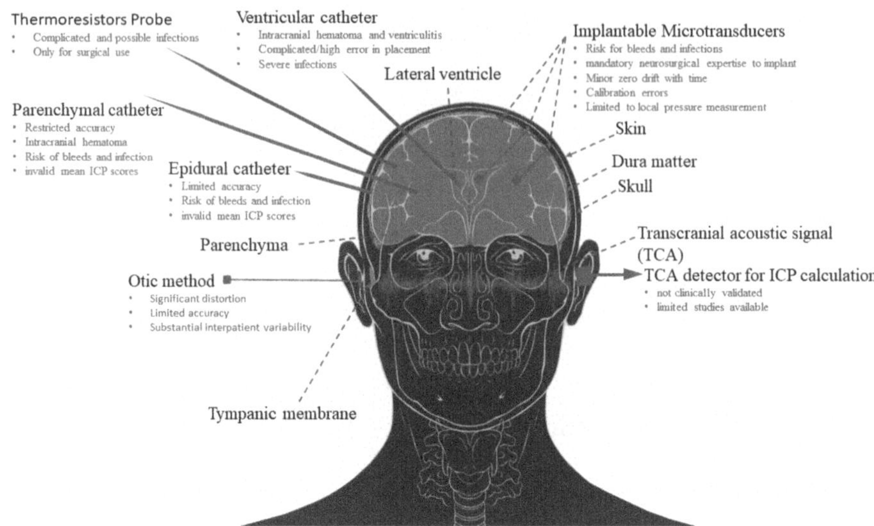

Fig. 1. Brain anatomy and its monitoring: Part 1.

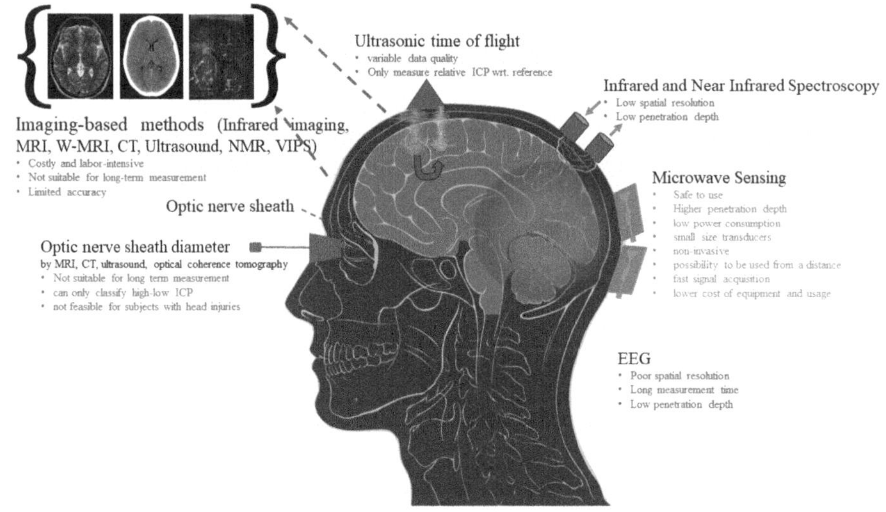

Fig. 2. Brain anatomy and its monitoring: Part 2.

evolving paradigm in various sectors. Digital Twins (DTs) are the high-fidelity digital replica of any real-world/physical assets, which is synchronised in real-time with their counterparts via sensors [2]. In one of the recent work [4], a DT architecture, using the concepts of 5G/6G communication, is proposed for future healthcare applications. In the realm of integrated sensing & communication (ISAC), the digital twin networks (DTNs) are focused over conventional simulators for testing and validation of future BANs [20]. However, DTs use the technical corners of different technologies such as IoT, AI and ML (indicated in Fig. 3), to train and update models for WBAN applications [49]. An overview of AI and ML-based inclusions in WBANs are outlined in the following section.

3.2 Machine Learning and AI

Figure 3 shows a typical block diagram of data flow in a typical ML based classification or prediction system. The first step includes data acquisition from different modalities. These modalities can be from, for example, multiple antennas in a microwave based system or even from different sources such as microwave antennas, MRI images, CT scans etc. in a multimodal measurement setup. The data acquired from these modalities is then fed to a pre-processing block wherein different types of filtering and normalization operations are applied on data depending on its data type and source to make it suitable for further analysis. It is to be noted that typically, the complete dataset is divided into training, valuation and testing datasets in this stage. Further, feature extraction block provides key features from the data that primarily represent its characteristics. The next step include training the ML model and optimizing its parameters using feedback system in which loss (difference of actual and predicted value) is used to train the model in supervised learning. Finally, classification or prediction is applied on the testing dataset to check its efficiency towards unknown data so that the ML model can be utilized for real-life applications. The three main application of brain monitoring using microwaves are presented in the following subsections.

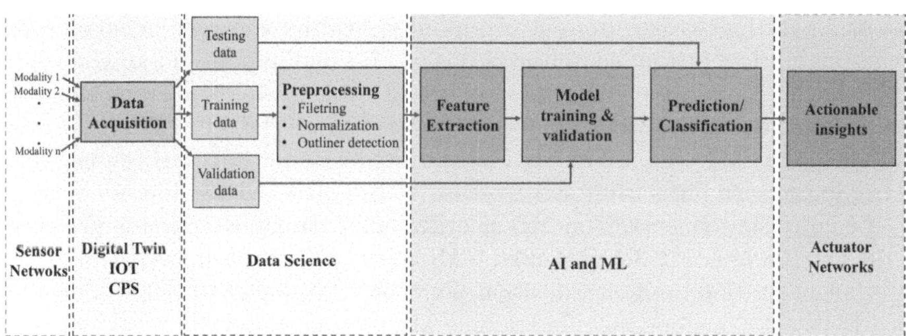

Fig. 3. Block diagram depicting data flow in a typical ML based classification or prediction system.

4 Targeted Applications

4.1 Brain Temperature Estimation

A variety of methods are proposed in the literature for brain temperature measurement including both invasive and non-invasive. The invasive Probe-based methods involve thermoresistors being implanted inside the skull which is accurate but only feasible in a surgical environment (as shown in Fig. 1). The temperature measurement by these methods is also limited to the implanted area and cannot be used to measure thermal imbalance. These probes are made of gold or platinum and covered by a polyimide glass substrate [16,34]. The non-invasive methods include microwaves, Magnetic resonance imaging (MRI), Computed Tomography (CT) scan etc.

Kazemi et al. [18] presented a comparative analysis of various ML models for temperature compensation in microwave based systems. Decision tree, random forest, SVM, k-nearest neighbors (KNN) algorithms are compared in this analysis. Authors in [9] developed a Random forest and SVM based classification system for cold pain perception from microwave radiations. The use of deep learning (DL) is emphasized in [50] to tackle challenges associated with hypothermia treatments. Khan in [21] proposed a DL method for thermal imaging and temperature analysis. A more comprehensive analysis of data mining techniques and ML algorithms in Microwave Radiometry (MWR) is presented in [23].

4.2 Stroke Diagnosis

In the last decade, advancements in endovascular therapy (EVT) have proved to be very effective for treating stroke patients. Though successful, EVT is a very time-dependent procedure and is only available at very few medical centers. Therefore, early detection of stroke condition and type is of utmost importance for a patient suffering from either hemorrhagic or ischemic stroke [7]. The process of separating strokes from stroke mimics, healthy controls, or large vessel occlusions (LVOs) further complicates this process and imposes major challenges in the diagnosis and timely treatment of actual stroke cases. Numerous technologies are reported in the literature for stroke diagnosis [17]. Out of these, portable technologies include the use of EEG [8], Infrared-scanner [37], ultrasound, volumetric impedance phase shift spectroscopy (VIPS) [19], NIRS, and microwaves.

A comprehensive survey on ML algorithms for stroke detection is presented in [10,13]. Roohi et al. [38] presented a Ml approach for automated stroke diagnosis, segmentation, and classification. Further, Mariano et al. [28] proposed a linearized scattering operator for training ML models efficiently. A Ml model for hemorrhage stroke detection is presented in [32]. Additionally, Singh et al. presented a comparative analysis of different ML algorithms utilized in microwave based stroke diagnosis [44].

Table 1. State of the art ML algorithms used in different brain monitoring applications

No.	Year	Ref	Technique	phantom/dataet	Application
1	2004	[5]	evolutionary algorithm and stochastic optimization	kidney, lever and muscle phantoms	Tumor detection by imaging
2	2018	[12]	K-Means Clusteringand Support Vector Machine	dataset of 600 samples at 10, 25 and 40 dB SNR	Stroke Localization and Classification
3	2022	[15]	deep learning-based YOLOv5 object detection model	400 RMW image samples from microwave head imaging system	detection of brain abnormalities
4	2022	[26]	convolutional neural network (CNN)	meta analysis	esophageal cancer (EC) diagnosis
5	2022	[29]	DeepHealth algorithm	digital mammography screens from 109000 distinct women from BreastScreen WA, Western Australia biennial population screening programme	cancer detection
6	2021	[27]	Convolutional Neural Network (CNN) and Long-Short Term Memory (LSTM)	480 3D skull models using NextEngine 3D laser machine	skull damage detection
7	2021	[25]	Feature Pyramid Network (FPN)	1922 image dataset from Union Hospital of Fujian Medical University	Skull fracture detection
8	2023	[3]	deep neural network (DNN)	2414 numerical simulations	bone fracture diagnosis

4.3 Intracranial Pressure (ICP) Measurement

Alexander Monro was the first to present a hypothesis on intracranial pressure (ICP) which was followed by experiments performed by Kellie. The landmark work in the form of MonroKellie doctrine attracted the research and medical fraternity to study the phenomena related to ICP and its measurements [35]. The human brain is surrounded by a rigid bone structure that maintains a constant pressure inside the skull by optimizing the volume of its contents. The intracranial section in humans comprises three main parts i.e. parenchyma of the central nervous system (CNS), cerebrospinal fluid (CSF), and blood, each with consistent volumes for maintaining specific ICP [36]. The measurement of ICP is usually performed in three cases. The first and most common case is TBI which causes ICP change due to brain edema, infra-tentorial mass lesions, contusional injuries, and vascular engorgement. In such cases, ICP measurement is utilized for mortality forecasting and assessment of functional outcomes in the near future [14]. The second case is for non-TBI patients who require neuro-intensive observation, especially in situations of subarachnoid hemorrhage and bleeding in the spontaneous intracerebral area. Further, patients suffering from hypertensive encephalopathy and severe liver or kidney failure also come under this category. Finally, the third case includes patients with CSF instability or when CSF flow is obstructed, and intracranial hypertension [43,48].

Miyagawa et al. [31] presented a ML method for predicting increased ICP. Further, in a similar study, Schweingruber et al. [42] proposed recurrent machine learning model for ICP measurements. The use of ML in prediction of elevated ICP during traumatic brain injury (TBI) is presented in [6]. Thereafter, Ye et al. also studied the effect of TBI and its relation with ICP using ML models in [51]. A comparative analysis of different ML algorithms used in different brain monitoring applications is presented in Table 1. It can be visualized from Table 1 that all of these studies use a large dataset for training and tasting the ML models which is a key parameter for success of any ML system.

5 Concluding Remarks

Microwaves has enormous potential in non-invasive brain monitoring applications due to its various advantageous features. However, the full potential of microwaves can only be achieved using efficient data analysis in form of AI and ML. A comprehensive analysis has been presented in this paper on different ML algorithms proposed in literature. Three key applications of microwave for brain monitoring are analyzed in detail i.e. brain temperature estimation, stroke diagnosis and ICP measurement wherein the ML algorithms utilized in related studies are highlighted. In order to make these ML models suitable for clinical applications in future, real-time data analysis, threat detection, data safety and secrecy, scalability and flexibility of ML models to handle data, and integration of ML models with existing technologies are required. Finally, Strong standardization and regulatory compliance are also required for ethical use of ML in healthcare applications.

References

1. Acharya, S., et al.: Interoperability challenges and opportunities in vehicle-in-the-loop testings: insights from nuve lab's hybrid setup. In: 65th International Conference of Scandinavian Simulation Society, SIMS 2024, and Second SIMS EUROSIM Conference on Modelling and Simulation, SIMS EUROSIM 2024 (2024)
2. Acharya, S., Wintercorn, O., Tripathy, A., Hanif, M., Van Deventer, J., Päivärinta, T.: Twins interoperability through service oriented architecture: a use-case of industry 4.0. In: Proceedings of the Annual Symposium of Computer Science 2023 co-located with The International Conference on Evaluation and Assessment in Software Engineering (EASE 2023). R. Piskac c/o Redaktion Sun SITE, Informatik V, RWTH Aachen (2023)
3. Beyraghi, S., et al.: Microwave bone fracture diagnosis using deep neural network. Sci. Rep. **13**(1), 16957 (2023)
4. Brahmi, R., Boujnah, N., Ejbali, R.: Elaboration of innovative digital twin models for healthcare monitoring with 6G functionalities. IEEE Access (2024)
5. Caorsi, S., Massa, A., Pastorino, M., Rosani, A.: Microwave medical imaging: potentialities and limitations of a stochastic optimization technique. IEEE Trans. Microw. Theory Tech. **52**(8), 1909–1916 (2004)
6. Chen, W., Cockrell, C., Ward, K.R., Najarian, K.: Intracranial pressure level prediction in traumatic brain injury by extracting features from multiple sources and using machine learning methods. In: 2010 IEEE International Conference on Bioinformatics and Biomedicine (BIBM), pp. 510–515. IEEE (2010)
7. Fhager, A., McKelvey, T., Persson, M.: Stroke detection using a broadband microwave antenna system. In: Proceedings of the Fourth European Conference on Antennas and Propagation, pp. 1–3. IEEE (2010)
8. Foreman, B., Claassen, J.: Quantitative EEG for the detection of brain ischemia. Crit. Care **16**(2), 1–9 (2012)
9. Geng, D., Yang, D., Cai, M., Hao, W.: Evaluation of acute tonic cold pain from microwave transcranial transmission signals using multi-entropy machine learning approach. IEEE Access **8**, 2780–2791 (2020)
10. Gopalakrishnan, K., et al.: Applications of microwaves in medicine leveraging artificial intelligence: future perspectives. Electronics **12**(5), 1101 (2023)
11. Gravina, R., Fortino, G.: Wearable body sensor networks: state-of-the-art and research directions. IEEE Sens. J. **21**(11), 12511–12522 (2020)
12. Guo, L., Abbosh, A.: Stroke localization and classification using microwave tomography with k-means clustering and support vector machine. Bioelectromagnetics **39**(4), 312–324 (2018)
13. Guo, L., Alqadami, A.S., Abbosh, A.: Stroke diagnosis using microwave techniques: review of systems and algorithms. IEEE J. Electromagnet. RF Microwaves Med. Biol. **7**(2), 122–135 (2022)
14. Harary, M., Dolmans, R.G., Gormley, W.B.: Intracranial pressure monitoring–review and avenues for development. Sensors **18**(2), 465 (2018)
15. Hossain, A., Islam, M.T., Almutairi, A.F.: A deep learning model to classify and detect brain abnormalities in portable microwave based imaging system. Sci. Rep. **12**(1), 6319 (2022)
16. Izhar, U., Piyathilaka, L., Preethichandra, D.: Sensors for brain temperature measurement and monitoring-a review. Neurosci. Inform. **2**(4), 100106 (2022)
17. Karthik, R., Menaka, R., Johnson, A., Anand, S.: Neuroimaging and deep learning for brain stroke detection-a review of recent advancements and future prospects. Comput. Methods Programs Biomed. **197**, 105728 (2020)

18. Kazemi, N., Abdolrazzaghi, M., Musilek, P.: Comparative analysis of machine learning techniques for temperature compensation in microwave sensors. IEEE Trans. Microw. Theory Tech. **69**(9), 4223–4236 (2021)
19. Kellner, C.P., Sauvageau, E., Snyder, K.V., Fargen, K.M., Arthur, A.S., Turner, R.D., Alexandrov, A.V.: The vital study and overall pooled analysis with the VIPS non-invasive stroke detection device. J. Neurointerventional Surg. **10**(11), 1079–1084 (2018)
20. Khaldi, R., Lehmann, A., Ghita, B., Trick, U.: Future bans-DTN applications and requirements. In: Mobilkommunikation; 28. ITG-Fachtagung, pp. 70–75. VDE (2024)
21. Khan, T.: An intelligent microwave oven with thermal imaging and temperature recommendation using deep learning. Appl. Syst. Innov. **3**(1), 13 (2020)
22. Lee, S., Shin, Y., Woo, S., Kim, K., Lee, H.N.: Review of wireless brain-computer interface systems. Brain-Computer Interface Systems-Recent Progress and Future Prospects, pp. 215–238 (2013)
23. Levshinskii, V., Galazis, C., Ovchinnikov, L., Vesnin, S., Losev, A., Goryanin, I.: Application of data mining and machine learning in microwave radiometry (MWR). In: Biomedical Engineering Systems and Technologies: 12th International Joint Conference, BIOSTEC 2019, Prague, Czech Republic, 22–24 February 2019, Revised Selected Papers 12, pp. 265–288. Springer (2020)
24. Li, C., Tofighi, M.R., Schreurs, D., Horng, T.S.J.: Principles and Applications of RF/Microwave in Healthcare and Biosensing. Academic Press (2016)
25. Liu, G., Wu, Q., Yuan, G., Wu, X.: Skull fracture detection method based on improved feature pyramid network. In: 2021 International Conference on Electronic Information Engineering and Computer Science (EIECS), pp. 756–762. IEEE (2021)
26. Ma, H., Wang, L., Chen, Y., Tian, L.: Convolutional neural network-based artificial intelligence for the diagnosis of early esophageal cancer based on endoscopic images: a meta-analysis. Saudi J. Gastroenterol. **28**(5), 332–340 (2022)
27. Mangrulkar, A., Rane, S.B., Sunnapwar, V.: Automated skull damage detection from assembled skull model using computer vision and machine learning. Int. J. Inf. Technol. **13**, 1785–1790 (2021)
28. Mariano, V., Tobon Vasquez, J.A., Casu, M.R., Vipiana, F.: Brain stroke classification via machine learning algorithms trained with a linearized scattering operator. Diagnostics **13**(1), 23 (2022)
29. Marinovich, M.L., et al.: Artificial intelligence (AI) to enhance breast cancer screening: protocol for population-based cohort study of cancer detection. BMJ Open **12**(1), e054005 (2022)
30. Memon, M., Wagner, S.R., Pedersen, C.F., Beevi, F.H.A., Hansen, F.O.: Ambient assisted living healthcare frameworks, platforms, standards, and quality attributes. Sensors **14**(3), 4312–4341 (2014)
31. Miyagawa, T., Sasaki, M., Yamaura, A.: Intracranial pressure based decision making: prediction of suspected increased intracranial pressure with machine learning. PLoS ONE **15**(10), e0240845 (2020)
32. Ojaroudi, M., Bila, S., Salimitorkamani, M.: A novel machine learning approach of hemorrhage stroke detection in differential microwave head imaging system. In: 2020 European Conference on Antennas and Propagation (2020)
33. Pattnaik, S.K., et al.: Future wireless communication technology towards 6G IoT: an application-based analysis of IoT in real-time location monitoring of employees inside underground mines by using BLE. Sensors **22**(9), 3438 (2022)

34. Poole, S., Stephenson, J.: Body temperature regulation and thermoneutrality in rats. Q. J. Exp. Physiol. Cognate Med. Sci. Transl. Integr. **62**(2), 143–149 (1977)
35. Rabelo, N.N., et al.: The historic evolution of intracranial pressure and cerebrospinal fluid pulse pressure concepts: two centuries of challenges. Surg. Neurol. Int. **12** (2021)
36. Raboel, P., Bartek, J., Andresen, M., Bellander, B., Romner, B., et al.: Intracranial pressure monitoring: invasive versus non-invasive methods—a review. Critical Care Res. Pract. **2012** (2012)
37. Robertson, C.S., et al.: Clinical evaluation of a portable near-infrared device for detection of traumatic intracranial hematomas. J. Neurotrauma **27**(9), 1597–1604 (2010)
38. Roohi, M., Mazloum, J., Pourmina, M.A., Ghalamkari, B.: Machine learning approaches for automated stroke detection, segmentation, and classification in microwave brain imaging systems. Prog. Electromagnet. Res. C **116**, 193–205 (2021)
39. Särestöniemi, M., Singh, D., Dessai, R., Heredia, C., Myllymäki, S., Myllylä, T.: Realistic 3D phantoms for validation of microwave sensing in health monitoring applications. Sensors **24**(6), 1975 (2024)
40. Särestöniemi, M., Singh, D., Heredia, C., Nikkinen, J., von und zu Fraunberg, M., Myllylä, T.: Digital twins for development of microwave-based brain tumor detection. In: Nordic Conference on Digital Health and Wireless Solutions, pp. 240–254. Springer (2024)
41. Särestöniemi, M., Singh, D., Reponen, J., Myllylä, T.: Tailored 3D breast models for development of microwave based breast tumor screening. Finnish J. eHealth eWelfare **16**(1), 23–34 (2024)
42. Schweingruber, N., et al.: A recurrent machine learning model predicts intracranial hypertension in neurointensive care patients. Brain **145**(8), 2910–2919 (2022)
43. da Silva Filho, R.C.M., de Mello Santa Maria, P.E.: Intracranial pressure: Invasive methods of monitoring. Neurocritical Care for Neurosurgeons: Principles and Applications, pp. 45–56 (2021)
44. Singh, A., et al.: Microwave antenna-assisted machine learning: a paradigm shift in non-invasive brain hemorrhage detection. IEEE Access (2024)
45. Singh, D., et al.: Preliminary studies on mm-wave radar for vital sign monitoring of driver in vehicular environment. In: Nordic Conference on Digital Health and Wireless Solutions, pp. 480–493. Springer (2024)
46. Singh, D., et al.: Generalized adaptive spreading modulation: a novel waveform for integrated sensing and communication oriented vehicular applications. IEEE Internet Things J. (2024)
47. Singh, D., Ouamri, M.A., Alzaidi, M.S., Alharbi, T.E., Ghoneim, S.S.: Performance analysis of wireless power transfer enabled dual hop relay system under generalised fading scenarios. IEEE Access **10**, 114364–114373 (2022)
48. Singh, D., Vihriälä, E., Särestöniemi, M., Myllylä, T.: Microwave technique based noninvasive monitoring of intracranial pressure using realistic phantom models. In: Nordic Conference on Digital Health and Wireless Solutions, pp. 413–425. Springer (2024)
49. Yadav, M., Shoran, P., Saxena, E., Bijalwan, A., Bijalwan, J.G.: IoTs-based wearable health monitoring through wireless body area networks. In: Healthcare Industry Assessment: Analyzing Risks, Security, and Reliability, pp. 231–254. Springer (2024)

50. Yago Ruiz, Á., Cavagnaro, M., Crocco, L.: Hyperthermia treatment monitoring via deep learning enhanced microwave imaging: a numerical assessment. Cancers **15**(6), 1717 (2023)
51. Ye, G., Balasubramanian, V., Li, J.K., Kaya, M.: Machine learning-based continuous intracranial pressure prediction for traumatic injury patients. IEEE J. Transl. Eng. Health Med. **10**, 1–8 (2022)

S-Transform Based Method for Gait Analysis in Children Suffering from Cerebral Palsy

Arpit Omar[1], Harshit Rathore[1], Pyari Mohan Pradhan[1(✉)], Satyabrata Aich[2], Prateek Kumar Panda[3], Indar Kumar Sharawat[3], and Osama Neyaz[3]

[1] Indian Institute of Technology, Roorkee, Roorkee, India
pmpradhan@ece.iitr.ac.in
[2] Wellmatix Co. Ltd., Busan, South Korea
[3] All India Institute of Medical Sciences, Rishikesh, Rishikesh, India

Abstract. Children with cerebral palsy (CP) face a higher health risk due to imbalance and gait variability. The spatiotemporal gait parameters can be estimated using data collected from inertial measurement units (IMUs) containing accelerometer and gyroscope sensors. The existing algorithms for gait analysis using data collected from IMUs provide many false initial contact/final contact (IC/FC) points. This paper proposes an S-transform based method for detecting IC/FC points in continuous inertial data collected using IMU from children suffering from CP. This study provides a comprehensive comparative analysis of the spatiotemporal gait parameters of children affected by CP. The performance of the proposed method is compared with that of three existing state-of-the-art methods. The algorithms are evaluated using single IMU data from twenty-five children affected by CP and ten children without CP. Among the three competing algorithms, one method only estimates temporal parameters, whereas the other two provide spatiotemporal parameters. The accuracy of the proposed S-transform based method in calculating spatiotemporal parameters is the highest among the competing algorithms. Therefore, the proposed S-transform-based approach could be a better candidate for reducing the false IC/FC points during gait analysis of children suffering from CP.

Keywords: accelerometer · spatiotemporal gait parameters · gait algorithms · cerebral palsy · IC/FC points · IMU

1 Introduction

In the last decade, the use of wearable sensors for analyzing human movement for gait analysis has increased significantly. Among the various types of sensors used for gait analysis, accelerometers, and gyroscopes have emerged as prominent choices due to their ability to capture detailed movement dynamics. The

K. Atul et al. (Eds.): BodyNets 2024, LNICST 666, pp. 441–456, 2026.
https://doi.org/10.1007/978-3-032-16099-7_35

sensors are integrated into wearable devices like smartwatches, fitness trackers, and inertial measurement units (IMUs) [22]. Gait analysis focuses on the systematic study of how individuals walk or run. It plays a pivotal role in various fields, including biomechanics, rehabilitation [31], sports science, and assistive technology. Modern gait analysis techniques include optical motion capture systems, force platforms, IMUs, and pressure-sensitive mats. These systems enable clinicians to precisely capture detailed kinematic, kinetic, and spatiotemporal gait parameters.

The ground reaction force plates and camera-based systems are the most widely used techniques for performing gait analysis in lab environments in hospitals and clinics. However, these devices are very costly and unsuitable for use outside the laboratories. The development of wearable sensors offered a low-cost alternative that could be used outside a laboratory's restrictive environment. The latest ecosystem of wearable sensors comprises insole sensors that measure pressure, goniometers at joints, body-worn accelerometers with pressure sensors inside shoes, and inertial sensors (accelerometer and/or gyroscopes) around the thigh/foot. Every wearable device has benefits and drawbacks specific to the type of sensor being used. These devices can be attached to different body parts, such as the feet, shins, or waist, to capture detailed information about gait dynamics. Due to their simple algorithms, the consumer sector commonly uses insole pressure sensors. Their usefulness is restricted as the sensors usually need to be changed after a few uses. On the contrary, with the introduction of wearable technology in the consumer market, inertial-based systems have shown notable advancements. This category includes hybrid systems that integrate accelerometers and gyroscopes as they need little power and are inexpensive. IMUs allow for continuous monitoring and assessment of gait patterns in a natural environment, providing a more comprehensive understanding of locomotion than traditional laboratory-based methods. Gyroscopes provide orientation and angular velocity data, a valuable addition to accelerometer-based systems.

Finding the step length of children suffering from cerebral palsy is a complex task that can be approached in various ways, depending on where the sensor is positioned. Most algorithms assume that the sensor is firmly attached to the body, either near the Center Of Mass (COM), along the spine, or distributed along the leg [24]. These placements are especially effective for navigation as they directly correlate with the human's walking cycle. With body-fixed sensors, existing step-length models can be categorized into biomechanical and parametric models. Biomechanical models usually place the sensor at the COM and treat the leg as an inverse pendulum [8], using a geometric relationship between the COM's vertical displacement and step length. Other geometric-based models are also proposed in [9]. On the other hand, the parametric model calculates step length using step frequency and accelerometer data variance, either in combination or separately [18]. The method introduced by Zijlstra and Hof [35] analyzes the gait of various groups, including adults [17], children, and Parkinson's disease patients [4]. A detailed literature review motivates a comparative analysis of the existing techniques in terms of sensitivity, false detection rate (FDR), and accuracy of spatiotemporal gait parameters.

The contributions of this paper are as follows:

- This paper proposes a S-transform based approach for gait analysis for children suffering from cerebral palsy.
- The hardware prototypes are designed and compared in a hospital environment.
- The proposed approach estimates the spatiotemporal gait parameters using accelerometer and gyroscope signals using a single IMU attached to the L5 vertebra of children.
- The data collected using the developed prototype includes both cases *i.e.* data for control as well as children suffering from cerebral palsy.
- A comparative analysis of spatiotemporal gait parameters obtained from the proposed method and two other state-of-the-art methods is carried out.

2 Literature Review

Gait analysis algorithms have been extensively applied in clinical settings to assess and monitor patients with neurological and musculoskeletal disorders. Mazure *et al.* [1] have explored the use of multiple correspondence analysis (MCA) to classify and understand gait patterns in patients with cerebral palsy. Ferrari *et al.* [5] have introduced a gait analysis system leveraging zero-velocity updates and Kalman filtering. This system uses inertial sensors attached to shoes to estimate real-time gait parameters like stride length, gait speed, and cadence. The Kalman filter enhances estimation accuracy by effectively handling sensor noise and variances in gait dynamics.

Grimmer *et al.* [7] have used angular velocity data from lower limb segments to identify different phases of gait. The stance and swing phase during walking are estimated by analyzing the direction and magnitude of these velocities. Liu *et al.* [11] have performed a literature survey on gait analysis using wearable devices. This research indicates that the wearable devices can accurately track daily activities for control and mobility affected persons suffering from Parkinson's disease and cerebral palsy. This study also discusses the integration of data analysis algorithms for gait assessment. Lora-Castro *et al.* [12] have proposed an algorithm to enhance the accuracy and reliability of identifying specific gait events, such as heel strikes and toe-offs in children suffering from cerebral palsy. Ghoussayni's algorithm is used for gait analysis in children with bilateral spastic cerebral palsy, showing effectiveness at a speed of 0.5 m/s. Rezvanian and Lockhart [16] have developed a real-time system for detecting freezing of gait (FOG) in patients with Parkinson's disease. It uses data collected from wireless accelerometers which are attached to the patient's body to continuously monitor the movement. The wavelet transform is applied on the accelerometer data to analyze both time and frequency domain features, allowing for the identification of FOG with high accuracy.

IMUs consisting of accelerometers and gyroscopes [19] have emerged as a promising wearable sensor technology for analyzing gait. The primary challenge in using IMUs for gait analysis is the accurate fusion of sensor data. Algorithms, including the Kalman filter and complementary filter, combine accelerometer, gyroscope, and magnetometer data to estimate orientation and linear acceleration accurately [18]. Slijepcevi *et al.* [20] have explored machine learning techniques for classifying and analyzing gait patterns in children suffering from cerebral palsy, focusing on the most effective subsets of 3D gait analysis data for classification. Ruoyu Zhi [32] has described an approach integrating a complementary filter to minimize accelerometer drift. This method enhances the reliability of 3D orientation and displacement measurements, making it suitable for applications requiring precise tracking and positioning.

Peak detection is essential for identifying initial contact (IC) and final contact (FC) required for gait analysis. Various methods for the detection of IC and FC have been proposed in the literature, including the derivative method [15], local maximum method [28], curve fitting method [30], and wavelet transform-based method [25,29]. In the continuous wavelet transform (CWT) based method, the IC/FC detection algorithm [3] identifies the peaks or valleys in the coefficient data. Zhang *et al.* [25] have proposed a method that improves IC/FC detection accuracy by incorporating information about peaks, valleys, and zero-crossings within the CWT coefficient data. Many gait analysis algorithms use peak detection [10] or thresholding as well as frequency analysis techniques [33]. Additionally, researchers have started investigating more advanced machine learning models like Bayes classifiers [13], Markov models [6], and neural networks for gait event detection. Robust rules-based algorithms can provide high accuracy and are well-suited for real-time gait analysis. Trojaniello *et al.* [26] have discussed the sensitivity and specificity of five distinct algorithms in calculating gait parameters. These methods use accelerometer data from a single IMU placed on the hip to measure key gait events like stride duration and gait cycle time. This study shows single-sensor setups for reliable gait analysis, offering a robust and sensitive solution for clinical and research applications. Zhou *et al.* [34] have developed an algorithm to evaluate gait improvements in post-stroke patients undergoing rehabilitation, demonstrating significant enhancements in gait symmetry and stability.

3 System Design

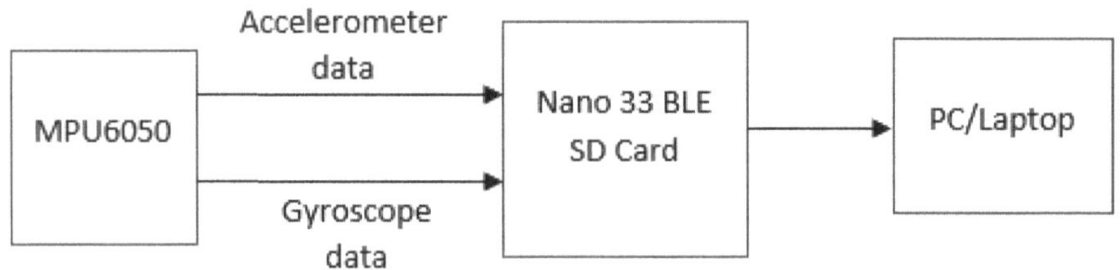

Fig. 1. Block diagram showing hardware components and process of data flow in the proposed study

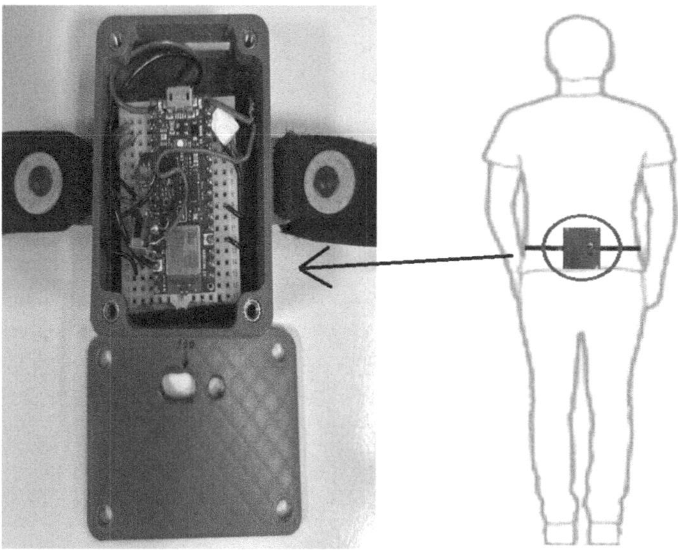

Fig. 2. Experimental Setup: Hardware prototype of wearable gait device and device was located in L5 vertebra

3.1 Data Collection and Hardware

Twenty-five children suffering from cerebral palsy and ten control children participated in this study carried out at AIIMS Rishikesh. The participants are between 3 to 13 years old.

This study uses a lightweight (69 g), compact IMU (5.8 cm × 4.4 cm × 4.8 cm) equipped with an accelerometer and gyroscope (MPU 6050) and a microcontroller (Arduino Nano 33 BLE). Figure 1 shows the hardware components and the methodology used for data processing. The accelerometer and gyroscope sense the acceleration and orientation data and save it to an SD card. Figure 2 shows the prototype of the wearable device used in this study. The data is recorded at a sampling frequency of 100 Hz. The prototype is attached to the L5 vertebra with its z-axis oriented vertically.

3.2 Signal Model

The signal can be modeled as the sum of sensed data and noise terms.

$$\mathrm{s}[k] = \begin{bmatrix} \mathrm{s}_a[k] \\ \mathrm{s}_\omega[k] \end{bmatrix} = \begin{bmatrix} a[k] \\ \omega[k] \end{bmatrix} + \begin{bmatrix} \eta_a[k] \\ \eta_\omega[k] \end{bmatrix} \tag{1}$$

where $k \in \mathbb{N}$ denotes the time index of the sensed data with a sampling frequency $f_s = \frac{1}{T_s}$. In this study, $f_s = 100\,\text{Hz}$. $\mathbf{s}_a \in \mathbb{R}^3$ denotes the sum of accelerometer data $a[k]$ and corresponding noise $\eta_a[k]$. $\mathbf{s}_\omega \in \mathbb{R}^3$ denotes the sum of gyroscope data $s[k]$ and corresponding noise $\eta_\omega[k]$.

3.3 Pre-processing

Pre-processing of the raw data is essential for accurate detection of gait parameters. Since the frequency of human gait is below 6 Hz, high-frequency components are removed. This is accomplished using a low pass 4th order Butterworth filter, with a 15 Hz cut-off frequency. The filtered accelerometer and gyroscope data are represented by $\tilde{\mathbf{s}}_a[k]$ and $\tilde{\mathbf{s}}_\omega[k]$.

When the sensor is not attached to the body, the orientation of the sensor continuously changes and cannot be determined easily. Consequently, the initial orientation of the prototype is uncertain. Hence, rather than focusing on individual elements of the accelerometer and gyroscope data vectors, the emphasis is on analyzing the norm of the filtered components. The norm of the filtered accelerometer and gyroscope data are as follows:

$$\tilde{\mathrm{s}}_{norm}[k] = \begin{bmatrix} \tilde{\mathrm{s}}^a_{norm}[k] \\ \tilde{\mathrm{s}}^\omega_{norm}[k] \end{bmatrix} \tag{2}$$

where

$$\tilde{\mathrm{s}}^a_{norm}[k] = \parallel \tilde{\mathrm{s}}^a[k] \parallel = \sqrt{\tilde{a}^2_x[k] + \tilde{a}^2_y[k] + \tilde{a}^2_z[k]} \tag{3}$$

$$\tilde{\mathrm{s}}^\omega_{norm}[k] = \parallel \tilde{\mathrm{s}}^\omega[k] \parallel = \sqrt{\tilde{\omega}^2_x[k] + \tilde{\omega}^2_y[k] + \tilde{\omega}^2_z[k]} \tag{4}$$

4 Methodology for Gait Analysis

4.1 Correction of Sensor Misalignment and Gravitational Offset

When the wearable is attached to the L5 vertebra of the children, its orientation can change due to attachment errors or variations in body shape. Moreover, gravity exerts force along one of the axes. The participants were asked to stand still for a few seconds to address gravity and attachment errors to record data in one position. Thereafter, the mean of the data that the sensor captures on each axis is subtracted from the corresponding data to remove alignment errors and offsets. The approach used for converting the tri-axial data into a Cartesian coordinate system using trigonometry has been described in [3].

4.2 Detection of IC and FC Points

Three existing methods to detect IC and FC points in the corrected data are discussed below. Considering the limitations of the existing approaches, an S-transform based method for IC and FC detection is proposed.

CWT-Based Method [3]**:** The CWT is a powerful signal processing technique used to find gait parameters by analyzing the time-frequency characteristics of signals. This method recognizes minima and maxima points in CWT coefficients, resulting in IC and FC points. The inverse pendulum model is used to calculate the spatial parameters of gait. The step length and stride length are computed as

$$\text{step length} = k\sqrt{2mn - n^2} \tag{5}$$

$$\text{stride length} = 2 * \text{step length} \tag{6}$$

where m is the height of IMU from the ground, k is a constant, and n represents the deviation in the height of IMU when double integration of the acceleration along the z-axis between two consecutive IC events is carried out.

Angular Velocity-Based Method: In this method, noisy angular data is processed using a low-pass filter, to remove high-frequency noise while retaining meaningful gait patterns. This helps to smooth the data and reduces the impact of transient fluctuations. After that IC/FC points are detected using filtered gyroscope data [7]. Positive peaks in the angular data correspond to mid-swing events, with the negative peak preceding mid-swing indicating IC and the negative peak following mid-swing indicating FC. The step and stride lengths are evaluated by double-integration of the acceleration along the x-axis.

AHRS-Based Method [2]**:** In this method, the IMU orientation is calculated using the Attitude and Heading Reference System (AHRS) developed by Madgwick. Using quaternion representation, the AHRS provides a distinct measurement of the orientation of the body segment where the sensor is attached. The rotated acceleration is computed using quaternion and raw data, yielding acceleration components relative to the earth's reference system. IC and FC are detected based on the thresholding of the accelerometer data [32]. A threshold is set to differentiate between stance and swing phases. The stance and swing phases are identified as the duration for which the acceleration is below and above the threshold, respectively.

Proposed Method: The S-transform provides precise time-frequency localization and is useful in detecting and identifying IC and FC points. It uses a variable-length window to analyze the signal at different frequencies, thereby enhancing the accuracy of relevant gait parameters in a non-stationary signal. Figure 3 shows the block diagram of the proposed approach for S-transform based detection of IC and FC points. The valleys and peaks in the S-transform coefficients are identified as IC and FC points. When the S-transform is applied to the velocity data, the detected valley points are recognized as IC points. Further, the S-transform is again applied to the previously calculated S-transform coefficients, and the detected peaks are recognized as FC points. The inverse pendulum model is used to calculate the step length and stride length.

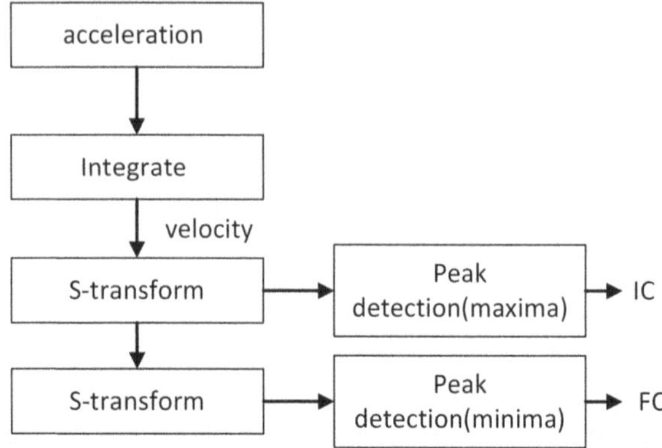

Fig. 3. Block diagram of proposed S-transform based method for detection of IC and FC

4.3 Drift Correction Using ZUPT Algorithm

Drift correction [21] aims to adjust or remove systematic errors or biases that can cause the accelerometer data to deviate from its actual values over time. The Zero Velocity Update (ZUPT) technique is widely used for drift correction because it uses the periodic stationary phases of the foot during walking, providing regular and reliable "zero-velocity" reference points. Unlike methods that require external sensors like GPS [14], which are unsuitable for indoors, or magnetometers, which are vulnerable to interference, and machine learning-based drift correction [27] requires a large dataset, high computational power, and may not generalize well across diverse gait patterns, ZUPT only relies on IMU data, making it versatile across environments. The ZUPT algorithm is applied during the stance phase of walking when the foot is in contact with the ground. During the detection of IC and FC points, the algorithm resets the velocity to zero. This correction helps to mitigate accumulated errors in the IMU data, improving the accuracy of position and velocity estimates. By frequently resetting the velocity to zero during each step, the algorithm effectively reduces drift errors inherent in the inertial sensors, enhancing the overall reliability of the gait analysis.

5 Performance Assessment, Experimental Results and Analysis

To address the issue of missing data in certain methods, the following steps are taken to complete the dataset for statistical analysis.

1. When some values of IC/FC events were missing, and gait parameters were not calculated, then missing values are replaced with the mean of the available values of those parameters.
2. If all values of IC/FC events were missing, then all missing values were filled with the worst value found in other participants.

By assuming worst-case values, the method becomes more sensitive to errors, which can help prevent false assumptions about gait parameters. However, using worst-case values can also impact the statistical validity of the findings. Approaches may introduce a conservative bias, leading to overestimated error rates or underestimated performance in typical scenarios. This could change the overall results, such as mean and standard deviation, and result in higher variability, as these extreme values can excessively influence the data distribution.

The normality test is performed to compare the mean and standard deviation of the spatiotemporal gait parameters obtained using the four methods. The Friedman test is a non-normal distribution that detects differences when the same data is used multiple times for different methods. This test is used to compare the estimates of spatiotemporal gait parameters.

The discrepancies between the estimated values of the spatiotemporal gait parameters for control children (p) and the standard values of children (p_t) [23] of the same age are determined for each method based on the data collected through a single IMU. The error is calculated for each parameter estimated by the four methods using the following formula:

$$E = p - p_t \tag{7}$$

$$E\% = \frac{|p - p_t|}{|p_t|} \times 100 \tag{8}$$

The estimated spatiotemporal gait parameters for control children are further examined for each method. Figures 4 and 5 show spatial and temporal gait parameters for control children, respectively. The x-axis represents the method, and the y-axis represents the error in the respective gait parameter. The figures show the variability in gait parameters based on the IC and FC detection methods. The error in gait parameters estimated by the proposed S-transform based method is smaller than those of the other competing methods. The S-transform based method could detect the IC and FC points more accurately than the three competing algorithms. The Friedman test showed that the differences observed in the step length and stride length among the methods were not statistically significant as the critical value (5.991 with p = 0.05) is greater than the Friedman statistic for the degree of freedom is equal to 2. However, in the temporal parameters (stride, step, and stance), there was a significant difference among the methods.

The tables present a comparative analysis of several methods for estimating gait parameters in children affected by cerebral palsy. Table 1 presents the mean and standard deviation of estimated spatial gait parameters *i.e.* step length, stride length, velocity, and cadence, while Table 2 summarizes the mean and standard deviation of estimated temporal gait parameters *i.e.* stance time, stride time, stance and swing phase. The AHRS-based method estimates only temporal gait parameters. Notably, the angular velocity-based method uses the gyroscope signal to estimate the physical characteristics of gait. In Table 1, the proposed method estimates the highest mean values for step length, stride length, and cadence compared to the other methods. However, it also reveals comparatively

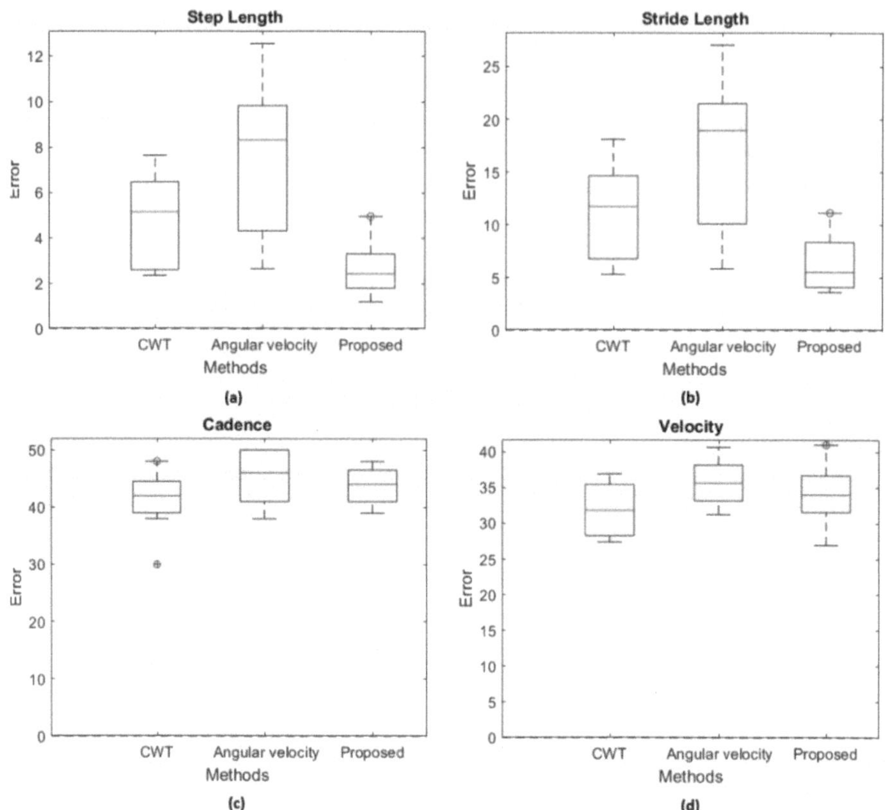

Fig. 4. Error in estimated spatial gait parameters (a) Step length (cm)(b) Stride length (cm) (c) Cadence (steps/min) (d) Velocity (cm/sec) for control children. All data are reported as minimum, first quartile (FQ), median, third quartile (TQ), and maximum values. Errors above $FQ1 + 1.5(TQ3 + FQ)$ or below $FQ - 1.5(TQ - FQ)$ are identified as outliers and are depicted with circles.

high standard deviations for these parameters (11.63 cm for step length and 19.59 cm for stride length), indicating the highest measurement variability. This variation might indicate that the proposed approach is more sensitive to individual variations in gait. Although the CWT-based method offers more consistent data, it may be less sensitive to small changes in gait because of its moderate mean values and lower standard deviations. The Angular velocity-based method shows lower means and moderate standard deviations.

In Table 2, the proposed method demonstrates higher mean values for stride time, stance time, and swing phase compared to state-of-the-art methods, along with relatively larger standard deviations (1.45 s for stride time), suggesting greater variability in gait patterns. Both the CWT-based and Angular velocity-based methods display similar mean values for stride and stance times but with lower standard deviations, indicating less detailed data. The AHRS-based

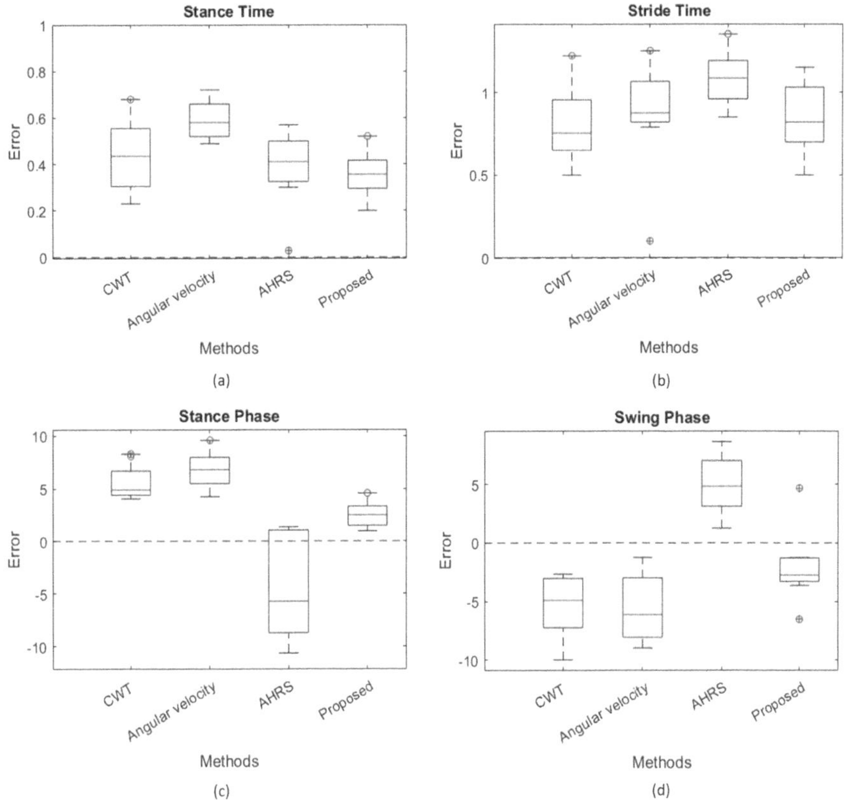

Fig. 5. Error in estimated temporal gait parameters (a) Stance time (sec) (b) Stride time (sec) (c) Stance phase (%) (d) Swing phase (%) for control children. All data are reported as min., first quartile (FQ), median, third quartile (TQ), and max. values. Errors above $FQ+1.5(TQ+FQ)$ or below $FQ-1.5(TQ-FQ)$ are identified as outliers and are depicted with circles.

method shows a different trend, with the lowest mean stance phase and a higher standard deviation, suggesting reduced consistency.

There is a trade-off between time and frequency resolution in CWT. The estimated gait parameters using the CWT-based method are sensitive to the choice of mother wavelet and scale. The angular velocity-based method detects false IC and FC events in some cases where gyroscope data is too noisy. The AHRS-based method is inaccurate as it is based on thresholding. The S-transform is a suitable choice for estimating gait parameters as it captures both high and low-frequency components of the signal with the added benefit of time localization information.

The tables provide a detailed comparison of spatial and temporal gait parameters of control children using various gait analysis methods. Table 3 focuses on spatial gait parameters (step length, stride length, cadence, and velocity). Table 4

Table 1. Mean and standard deviation of spatial gait parameters of children suffering from cerebral palsy

Methods	Step length		Stride length		Cadence		Velocity	
	mean	std	mean	std	mean	std	mean	std
CWT-based method	40.01	5.89	81.27	12.96	65	12	41.44	4.06
Angular velocity-based method	33.56	9.68	70.90	5.67	170	21	80.85	4.72
Proposed method	52.3	11.63	101.49	19.59	80	13	42.65	8.63

Table 2. Mean and standard deviation of temporal gait parameters of children suffering from cerebral palsy

Methods	Stride time		Stance time		Stance phase		Swing phase	
	mean	std	mean	std	mean	std	mean	std
CWT-based method	2.95	0.58	1.86	0.25	63.05	4.8	36.01	3.85
Angular velocity-based method	2.90	0.42	1.59	0.49	54.67	11.8	45.17	15.18
AHRS-based method	3.18	0.38	1.61	0.27	50.73	6.23	49.37	9.89
Proposed method	3.55	1.45	1.97	0.35	55.49	12.9	44.50	17.9

focuses on temporal gait parameters (stride time, stance time, stance phase, and swing phase), and Table 5 on the error percentage for temporal gait parameters.

Table 3 presents the mean and standard deviation of spatial gait parameters measured using three methods. The Angular velocity-based method shows high mean values for step length and stride length, and it also has relatively high standard deviations (3.79 cm for stride length), indicating greater variability in the measurements. This high mean suggests that the method captures larger steps or strides due to noisy gyroscope data. The mean value of cadence and velocity is low because of the large stride time. The CWT-based method shows moderate step and stride length and high cadence (68 steps/min) with lower variability, indicating consistent measurements. The proposed method estimates a lower mean for step and stride lengths but maintains relatively low standard deviations, indicating consistent and more accurate parameters.

Table 4 shows the mean and standard deviation of temporal gait parameters such as stride time, stance time, stance phase, and swing phase. The Angular velocity-based method estimates the mean stride time and stance time with moderate standard deviations, suggesting variability in temporal gait phases that reflect inconsistencies in time intervals. The AHRS-based method has a high stance and swing phase mean with a high standard deviation (4.02 % and 3.01%, respectively) due to thresholding. The CWT-based method has the lowest stride and stance time with a lower standard deviation, indicating the lowest variability. The proposed method provides more balanced mean values across all parameters with moderate standard deviations, suggesting that it estimates a consistent range of temporal gait characteristics with moderate variability.

Table 3. Mean and standard deviation of spatial gait parameters of control children

Methods	Step length		Stride length		Cadence		Velocity	
	mean	std	mean	std	mean	std	mean	std
CWT-based method	65.25	2.5	133.50	2.58	68	6	73.08	4.47
Angular velocity-based method	68.52	3.25	140.2	3.79	62	7	68.15	6.96
Proposed method	62.25	1.56	126.15	1.98	66	4	70.23	5.05

Table 4. Mean and standard deviation of temporal gait parameters of control children

Methods	Stride time		Stance time		Stance phase		Swing phase	
	mean	std	mean	std	mean	std	mean	std
CWT-based method	1.85	0.5	1.20	0.45	64.86	3.85	35.15	2.5
Angular velocity-based method	2.01	0.75	1.34	0.85	66.63	2.75	33.37	1.59
AHRS-based method	2.11	1.02	1.15	0.89	54.50	4.02	45.49	3.01
Proposed method	1.91	0.3	1.20	0.26	62.82	2.69	37.17	1.86

Table 5. Error (%) of spatiotemporal gait parameters of control children

Methods	Step length	Stride length	Cadence	Velocity	Stride time	Stance time	Stance phase	Swing phase
CWT-based method	8.75	11.25	38.18	30.4	68.5	60	8.1	12.1
Angular velocity-based method	14.2	16.83	42.52	35.09	82.27	78.6	11.05	16.57
AHRS-based method	-	-	-	-	91.81	53.333	9.16	13.72
Proposed method	3.75	5.12	40.00	33.11	73.63	60.00	4.7	7.07

Table 5 demonstrates the error percentages of spatiotemporal gait parameters measured by different methods compared to a reference standard. The proposed method generally shows lower error percentages in spatial gait parameters, such as step and stride length, indicating higher accuracy in measuring these parameters. In contrast, the Angular velocity-based method has higher errors in stance time and stance phase, cadence, and velocity, which means that this approach leads to significant inaccuracies when recording gyroscopic data. The AHRS-based method also shows the highest errors in stride and stance time but lower errors in stance and swing phase because stride and stance time are very inaccurate, but the ratio of stance time to stride time defined as stance phase is lower. So, this method does not reliably capture dynamic changes in gait. The CWT-based method shows a balanced error profile but with higher errors in step and stride length, stride time, and stance time, which could indicate that it provides consistent measurements but does not always align closely with actual gait values. The proposed method offers lower standard deviations and provides more consistent and accurate measurements due to better filtering and more robust algorithms that account for noise and fluctuations in gait data.

The proposed method exhibits higher variability in gait parameters suffering from cerebral palsy due to the fact that the participating children are not walking in a straight path, resulting in inconsistent data collection across trials. This non-linear path introduces variations in sensor readings, as changes in direction can alter the recorded angular velocity and acceleration, making it challenging to identify consistent gait cycles. Additionally, the method lacks sensor fusion approaches, which could integrate data from multiple sensor types—such as accelerometers, gyroscopes, and magnetometers—to provide a more stable and accurate estimate of gait parameters. Sensor fusion often compensates for individual sensor limitations by balancing noise and drift across different data sources, leading to more reliable and consistent results.

6 Conclusion

The existing algorithms for gait analysis suffer from a high rate of false detection of IC and FC points when the data collected from a single IMU is used. This paper proposes an S-transform-based method for detecting IC and FC points. This paper also demonstrates a prototype for collecting accelerometer and gyroscope data for gait analysis outside the laboratory environment. A single IMU and a microcontroller are used to collect and store the data in real-time. The spatiotemporal gait parameters estimated using the three state-of-the-art techniques and the proposes method are compared. The estimated spatiotemporal gait parameters for control children have been compared with the standard values.

In the future, machine learning methods can be incorporated to classify patients suffering from cerebral palsy and control patients based on the estimated spatiotemporal gait parameters. Advances in wearable technology, such as improved sensor accuracy, battery life, etc., will facilitate longer and more precise data collection, thereby improving gait analysis outcomes.

Acknowledgement. The authors would like to acknowledge the funding received from iHUB DivyaSampark IIT Roorkee, under the project grant code iHUB-2240-ECD, to carry out this research work.

References

1. Bonnefoy-Mazure, A., Sagawa, Y., Lascombes, P., De Coulon, G., Armand, S.: Identification of gait patterns in individuals with cerebral palsy using multiple correspondence analysis. Res. Dev. Disabil. **34**(9), 2684–2693 (2013)
2. Chang, C.W., Yan, J.L., Chang, C.N., Wen, K.A.: IMU-based real time four type gait analysis and classification and circuit implementation. In: 2022 IEEE Sensors, pp. 1–4 (2022)
3. Din, S., et al.: Instrumented gait assessment with a single wearable: an introductory tutorial. F1000 Res. **5** (2016)

4. Esser, P., Dawes, H., Collett, J., Feltham, M.G., Howells, K.: Validity and inter-rater reliability of inertial gait measurements in Parkinson's disease: a pilot study. J. Neurosci. Methods **205**(1), 177–181 (2012)
5. Ferrari, A., Ginis, P., Hardegger, M., Casamassima, F., Rocchi, L., Chiari, L.: A mobile Kalman-filter based solution for the real-time estimation of spatio-temporal gait parameters. IEEE Trans. Neural Syst. Rehabil. Eng. **24**(7), 764–773 (2016)
6. Ghassemi, N.H., et al.: Segmentation of gait sequences in sensor-based movement analysis: a comparison of methods in Parkinson's disease. Sensors **18** (2018)
7. Grimmer, M., Schmidt, K., Duarte, J., Neuner, L., Koginov, G., Riener, R.: Stance and swing detection based on the angular velocity of lower limb segments during walking. Front. Neurorobot. **13**, 1–15 (2019)
8. Jahn, J., Batzer, U., Seitz, J., Patino-Studencka, L., Gutiérrez Boronat, J.: Comparison and evaluation of acceleration based step length estimators for handheld devices. In: 2010 International Conference on Indoor Positioning and Indoor Navigation, pp. 1–6 (2010)
9. Kim, J.W., Jang, H.J., Hwang, D.H., Park, C.: A step, stride and heading determination for the pedestrian navigation system. J. Glob. Positioning Syst. **01** (2004)
10. Ledoux, E.D.: Inertial sensing for gait event detection and transfemoral prosthesis control strategy. IEEE Trans. Biomed. Eng. **65**(12), 2704–2712 (2018)
11. Liu, X., et al.: Wearable devices for gait analysis in intelligent healthcare. Front. Comput. Sci. **3** (2021)
12. Lora-Castro, S., Alvarado-Rodríguez, F., Vélez-Pérez, H.: Gait event detection algorithm for spastic cerebral palsy. In: 2023 IEEE EMBS R9 Conference, p. 1 (2023)
13. Martinez-Hernandez, U., Dehghani, A.: Adaptive Bayesian inference system for recognition of walking activities and prediction of gait events using wearable sensors. Neural Netw. Off. J. Int. Neural Netw. Soc. **102**, 107–119 (2018)
14. Nilsson, J.O., Skog, I., Händel, P., Hari, K.: Foot-mounted ins for everybody - an open-source embedded implementation. In: Proceedings of the 2012 IEEE/ION Position, Location and Navigation Symposium, pp. 140–145 (2012)
15. O'Haver, T.C.: An introduction to signal processing in chemical measurement. J. Chem. Educ. **68**(6), A147 (1991)
16. Rezvanian, S., Lockhart, T.E.: Towards real-time detection of freezing of gait using wavelet transform on wireless accelerometer data. Sensors **16**(4) (2016)
17. Senden, R., Grimm, B., Heyligers, I., Savelberg, H., Meijer, K.: Acceleration-based gait test for healthy subjects: reliability and reference data. Gait Posture **30**(2), 192–196 (2009)
18. Shin, S.H., Park, C.G., Kim, J.W., Hong, H.S., Lee, J.M.: Adaptive step length estimation algorithm using low-cost mems inertial sensors. In: 2007 IEEE Sensors Applications Symposium, pp. 1–5 (2007)
19. Shull, P.B., Jirattigalachote, W., Hunt, M.A., Cutkosky, M.R., Delp, S.L.: Quantified self and human movement: a review on the clinical impact of wearable sensing and feedback for gait analysis and intervention. Gait Posture **40**(1), 11–19 (2014)
20. Slijepcevic, D., Zeppelzauer, M., Unglaube, F., Kranzl, A., Breiteneder, C., Horsak, B.: Explainable machine learning in human gait analysis: a study on children with cerebral palsy. IEEE Access **11**, 65906–65923 (2023)
21. Suresh, R.P., Sridhar, V., Pramod, J., Talasila, V.: Zero velocity potential update (zupt) as a correction technique. In: 2018 3rd International Conference on Internet of Things: Smart Innovation and Usages (IoT-SIU), pp. 1–8 (2018)
22. Tao, W., Liu, T., Zheng, R., Feng, H.: Gait analysis using wearable sensors. Sensors **12**(2), 2255–2283 (2012)

23. Thevenon, A., et al.: Collection of normative data for spatial and temporal gait parameters in a sample of French children aged between 6 and 12. Ann. Phys. Rehabil. Med. **58**(3), 139–144 (2015)
24. Tien, I., Glaser, S.D., Bajcsy, R., Goodin, D.S., Aminoff, M.J.: Results of using a wireless inertial measuring system to quantify gait motions in control subjects. IEEE Trans. Inf Technol. Biomed. **14**(4), 904–915 (2010)
25. Tong, X., et al.: Multiscale peak detection in wavelet space. Analyst **140** (2015)
26. Trojaniello, D., Cereatti, A., Della Croce, U.: Accuracy, sensitivity and robustness of five different methods for the estimation of gait temporal parameters using a single inertial sensor mounted on the lower trunk. Gait Posture **40** (2014)
27. Wang, J., Shu, J., Li, Z., Tong, R.K.Y.: Combating sensor drift with an LSTM neural network enhanced by autoencoder preprocessing. In: 2023 IEEE SENSORS, pp. 1–4 (2023)
28. Yang, C., He, Z., Yu, W.: Comparison of public peak detection algorithms for MALDI mass spectrometry data analysis. BMC Bioinform. **10**, 4 (2009)
29. Yang, G., Dai, J., Liu, X., Chen, M., Wu, X.: Spectral feature extraction based on continuous wavelet transform and image segmentation for peak detection. Anal. Methods **12** (2019)
30. Yu, Y.J., et al.: Chemometric strategy for automatic chromatographic peak detection and background drift correction in chromatographic data. J. Chromatogr. A **1359**, 262–270 (2014)
31. Zhao, H., et al.: Analysis and evaluation of hemiplegic gait based on wearable sensor network. Inf. Fusion **90**, 382–391 (2023)
32. Zhi, R.: A drift eliminated attitude & position estimation algorithm in 3D. Graduate College Dissertations and Theses (2016)
33. Zhou, H., et al.: Towards real-time detection of gait events on different terrains using time-frequency analysis and peak heuristics algorithm. Sensors **16**(10) (2016)
34. Zhou, L., et al.: Validation of an IMU gait analysis algorithm for gait monitoring in daily life situations. In: 2020 42nd Annual International Conference of the IEEE Engineering in Medicine & Biology Society (EMBC), pp. 4229–4232 (2020)
35. Zijlstra, W., Hof, A.L.: Assessment of spatio-temporal gait parameters from trunk accelerations during human walking. Gait Posture **18**(2), 1–10 (2003)

Signal Processing and Sensors

A Metasurface-Based Dual Band Stop Filter with High Angular Stability for ISM Band Applications

Soham Banerjee[1], Arjab Sengupta[1], Vishnu Kumar Mishra[2], Gobinda Sen[1], Sayan Sarkar[1], Ardhendu Kundu[1], and Somak Bhattacharyya[2(✉)]

[1] Institute of Engineering and Management, Gurukul, Y-12, Block-EP, Sector-V, Salt Lake Electronics Complex, Kolkata 700091, West Bengal, India

[2] Indian Institute of Technology (BHU), Varanasi 221005, Uttar Pradesh, India
somakbhattacharyya.ece@iitbhu.ac.in

Abstract. The proposed work introduces a metasurface-based dual band stop filter having very high attenuation; thus making it suitable for wearable biomedical applications. The use of jeans substrate makes the structure perfectly wearable and suitable for biomedical applications. Each unit cell in the proposed structure comprises of an outer metallic strip and inner novel double dumbbell shaped resonators. Each unit cell has a dimension of $0.24\lambda_0 \times 0.24\lambda_0$ with a thickness of $0.002\lambda_0$ making it quite small and size efficient. The first stop band from this design is realized at exactly 2.45 GHz while the second stop band is achieved at 5.74 GHz with an attenuation greater than 30 dB at both the bands. To comprehend the reflection and transmission phenomena better, the surface current distribution on the patches is also examined. The study of the electric field distributions at the two bands reveals the roles of the patches used in the unit cell design. The structure has also been found to be angularly stable up to 75^0 incidence.

Keywords: Metasurface · band stop filter · wearable · Industrial · Scientific · Medical (ISM) band

1 Introduction

Over the last few decades, left-handed metamaterial structures have gathered a lot of interest from the scholarly community because of their numerous uses since Vaselago first proposed the idea in 1968 [1] and later Pendry put it into practice [2, 3]. Periodic structures that meet the effective homogeneity limit for incident waves and have artificial electromagnetic properties that are not available in nature are known as metamaterials [4]. An expanding number of engineering electromagnetics applications have been posed by these metamaterial structures, such as passive component design, the creation of antennas, and gain enhancement in electrically tiny antennas (ESAs). Furthermore, multifunctional antennas (MFAs) for smart radio systems, polarization-converting

K. Atul et al. (Eds.): BodyNets 2024, LNICST 666, pp. 459–466, 2026.
https://doi.org/10.1007/978-3-032-16099-7_36

structures, and ultra-thin absorption structures are all developed using metamaterials [4–9]. They are also essential for the development of cognitive and multifunctional radio antennas too [10–12]. Two-dimensional metamaterials, also known as metasurfaces, are widely used because of their ultra-thin feature.

Spatial filters are mostly used to allow some frequencies while rejecting others. Typically, band stop filters have a patch-type construction because of their equivalent inductance and capacitance effect. Different shapes of metallic patches provide different distinct resonance behaviors. Nowadays, metasurfaces are increasingly reported as filters instead of traditional ones due to their compact and superior performance [13]. In [14], a conventional stopband FSS filter was designed on a bulky structure. The structure is quite large and gives only one band stop with two pass bands. Moreover, the angular stability of the structure is quite low and it is stable up to just 20 degrees as found out from the design results. In [15–20], a few research works demonstrated these types of filters with extremely low return losses. On the other hand, wearable band stop filters, which is found to have great potential for use in biological applications, are not well explored by the researchers and hence has a huge scope of possibility for further research.

In this work, a flexible jeans substrate is used to create a small, low-profile, high attenuation, sharp roll off band stop filter based on metasurface structure intended for wearable applications. The unit cell of the suggested metasurface structure is made up of two metallic patches with distinct shapes. First, a metallic square pattern with extra metallic strip pointing towards center around outside which has been later loaded with dumbbell like patch at the center. With two separate ISM stop bands having center frequencies of 2.45 GHz and 5.74 GHz, the design exhibits good angular stability. For these bands, the insertion loss is greater than 30 dB. The proposed filter exhibits two stop bands with -10 dB bandwidths of 0.23 GHz and 0.99 GHz at the ISM bands with center frequencies at 2.45 GHz and 5.74 GHz, respectively. The suggested filter shows encouraging application potential in biomedical fields.

2 Unit Cell Design

The unit cell of the proposed structure consists of an outer rectangular metallic strip with four metallic strips protruding inside from the centre of each side and a novel dumbbell shaped patch at the centre. The substrate used is jeans offering a permittivity of 1.7 and a loss tangent 0.025 [21]. The top and the isometric views of the unit cell are shown in Fig. 1(a) and Fig. 1(b), respectively. All the optimized dimensions used in the unit cell are mentioned in the caption of Fig. 1. The use of jeans as substrate makes the structure flexible in nature and hence suitable for various biomedical wearable applications. Ansys HFSS 2019v2 has been used for the design and simulation of the proposed structure.

I. Design Methodology:

The proposed unit cell structure has been evolved from the basic square ring patch in three steps as illustrated in Fig. 2 while the respective responses are shown in Fig. 3. In step 1, a single band stop response at 3.4 GHz is obtained. By addition of four rectangular stubs at the centre of the patch in step 2, the structure exhibits a band stop response at a lower frequency due to the loading of additional current path. The final structure in step 3 is obtained by cascading with another centre-connected cross dumbbell shape resonator to realize a dual band stop response at the ISM bands.

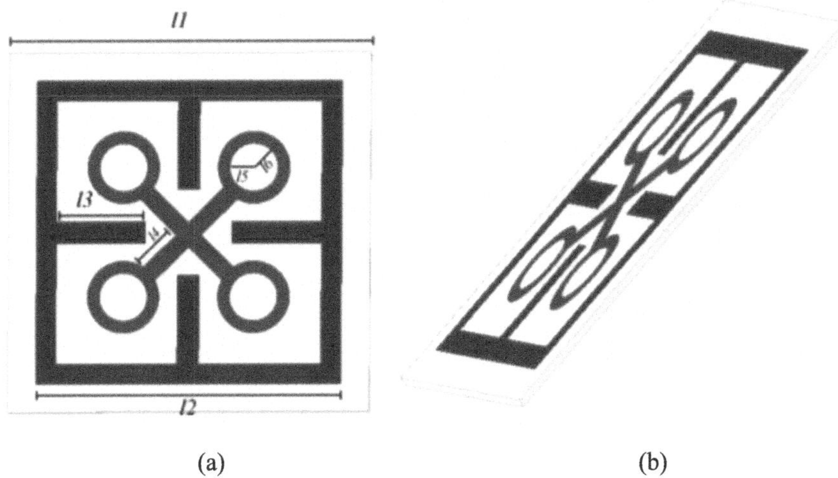

Fig. 1. (a) Top view and (b) isometric view of the unit cell of the proposed band stop filter (Dimensions (in mm): *l1* = *28, l2* = *27, l3* = *3.85, l4* = *1.42, l5* = *5, l6* = *4*).

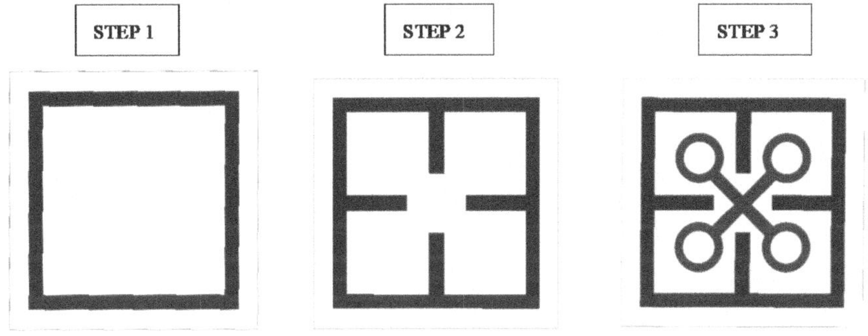

Fig. 2. Evolution steps of the proposed structure.

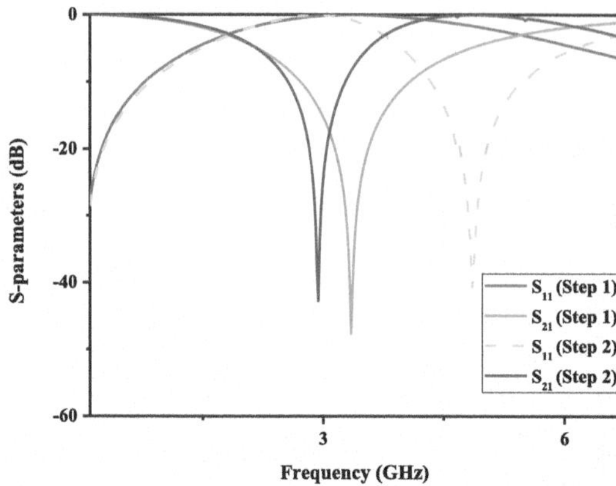

Fig. 3. Simulated S-parameters of the steps in the evolution described in Fig. 2.

3 Results and Discussions

The simulated reflection and transmission coefficients of the proposed filter as obtained in step 3 is illustrated in Fig. 4. After the addition of the dumbbell shaped metallic patch at the centre, the second stop band appears at 5.74 GHz. The insertion loss at both these frequencies are found to be greater than 30 dB; thereby confirming the stopband performance.

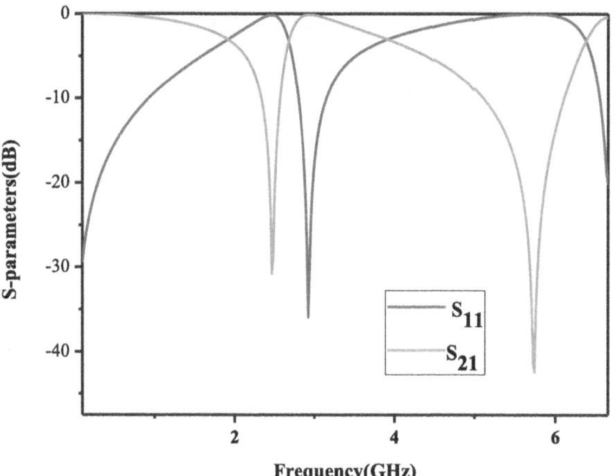

Fig. 4. Simulated transmission and reflection coefficients of the proposed band stop filter.

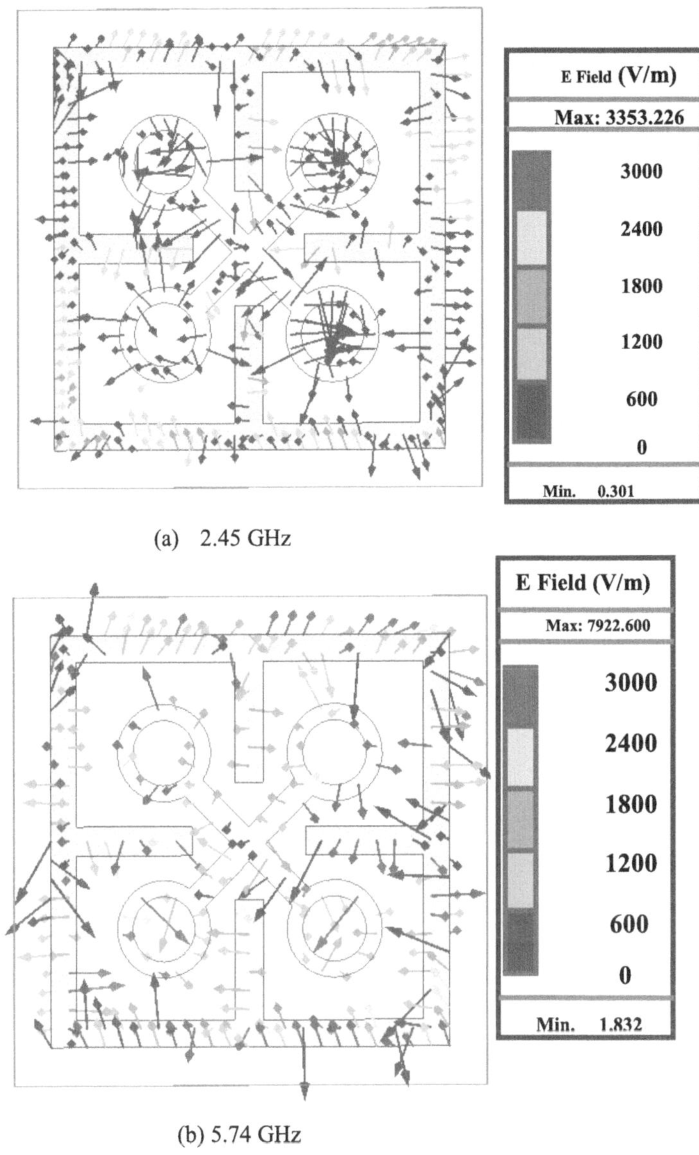

Fig. 5. E-field distribution on the metasurface patch at (a) 2.45 and (b) 5.74 GHz.

The analysis of the electric field distributions on the unit cell of the suggested filter in the corresponding stop bands of 2.45 GHz and 5.74 GHz has been carried out in Figs. 5(a) and (b), respectively. At 2.45 GHz, the electric field is mostly concentrated on the outer patch as evident form Fig. 5(a), whereas at 5.74 GHz it is mostly on the inner patch as seen clearly from Fig. 5(b).

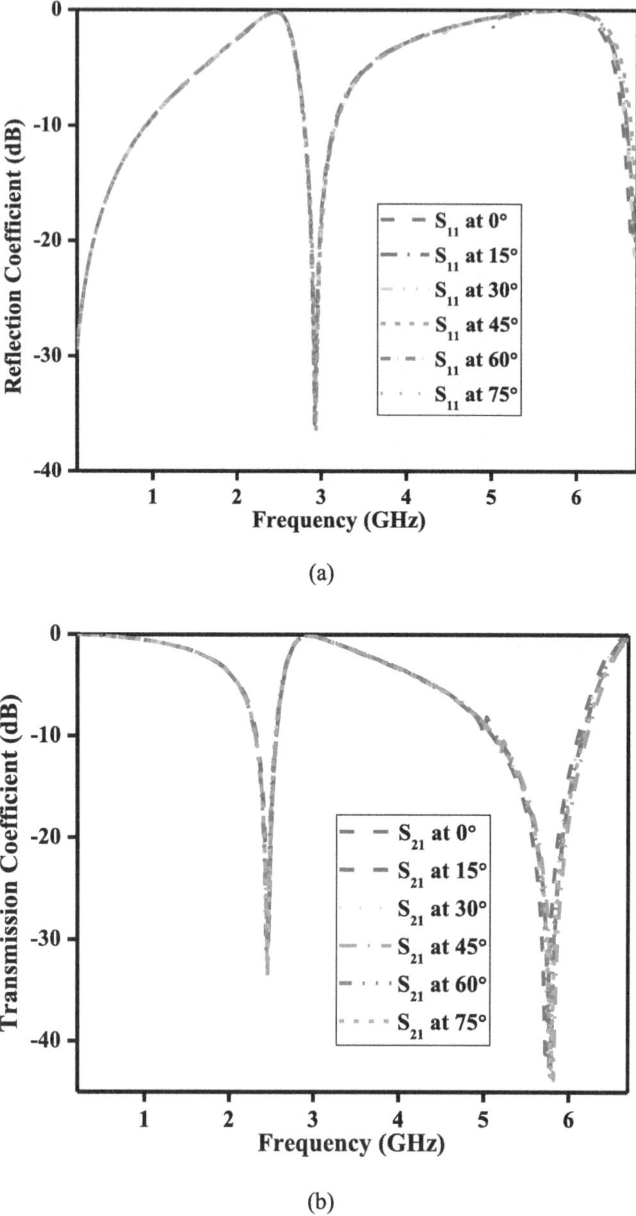

Fig. 6. Angular stability of device in terms of (a) reflection and (b) transmission coefficients.

The angular stability of the proposed design with reflection coefficient (S_{11}) and transmission coefficient (S_{21}) are illustrated in Figs. 6(a) and 6(b), respectively. From both the figures, it can be observed that the proposed design performances do not alter with change in incident angles up to 75^0 and hence the design offers highly angular stability.

Table 1. Comparison of the proposed work with previous stopband filters

Reference no	Stop Band Frequencies (GHz)	Insertion Loss (dB)	Dimension (λ_0^3)
[15]	3.2, 5.2, 5.8	16, 22.1, 23.5	0.3 × 0.18 × 0.017
[16]	5 to 6	12, 15	0.47 × 0.28 × 0.008
[17]	3.91, 4.47, 5.2, 6.32	8.5, 7, 12, 10	0.46 × 0.39 × 0.010
[18]	2.5 to 3.8	40	0.11 × 0.06 × 0.007
[19]	5.8, 6.8, 5.6/7.4	32, 34, 42	0.35 × 0.28 × 0.010
[20]	2.44, 3.65	26.93, 24.06	0.32 × 0.32 × 0.013
This work	**2.45, 5.74**	**34.25, 42.50**	**0.24** × **0.24** × **0.002**

The performance of the proposed structure has been compared with a few stop band metasurface structures reported as listed in Table 1. It can be observed that the proposed structure with wearable feature offers dual stopband responses at ISM bands maintaining compactness.

4 Conclusion

The proposed wearable filter exhibits dual band stop responses with centre frequencies at 2.45 GHz and 5.74 GHz, both of which are ISM bands. The substrate jeans being a wearable material makes the filter highly suitable for biomedical applications. Moreover, the high angular stability of the filter makes it more suitable for wide range of bio-medical applications by acting as electromagnetic interference shield to reduce the harmful radiations mostly in the unlicensed bands.

References

1. Vaselgo, V.: The electrodynamics of substances with simultaneously negative values of μ and ε. Soviet Phys. Uspekhi **10**(4), 509–514 (1968)
2. Pendry, J.B., Holden, A.J., Stewart, W.J., Youngs, I.: Extremely low frequency plasmons in metallic mesostructure. Phys. Rev. Lett. **76**(25), 4773–4776 (1996)
3. Pendry, J.B., Holden, A.J., Robbins, D.J., Stewart, W.J.: Magnetism from conductors and enhanced nonlinear phenomena. IEEE Trans. Micr. Theory. Tech **47**(11), 2075–2084 (1999)
4. Bhattacharya, S., Saha, C., Siddiquiand, J.Y.: High frequency applications of metamaterials and metasurfaces. In: 2019 IEEE Recent Advances in Geoscience and Remote Sensing: Technologies, Standards and Applications (TENGARSS), Kochi, India, pp. 96–99 (2019)
5. Chu, L.J.: Physical limitations on omni-directional antennas. J. Appl. Phys. **19**, 1163–1175 (1948)
6. McLean, J.S.: A re-examination of the fundamental limits on the radiation Q of electrically small antennas. IEEE Trans. Antennas Propag. **44**(5), 672 (1996)
7. Ziolkowski, R.W., Erentok, A.: Metamaterial-based efficient electrically small antennas. IEEE Trans. Antennas Propag. **54**(7), 2113–2130 (2006)
8. Zhu, H., Cheung, S.W., Yuk, T.I.: Enhancing antenna boresight gain using a small metasurface lens. IEEE Antennas Wireless Propag. Mag. **10**, 35–44 (2016)

9. Kannan, K., George, E., Surendran, K.P., Saha, C.: Boresight gain enhancement of a dielectric resonator antenna using a metasurface lens. In: 2017 IEEE International Conference on Antenna Innovations Modern Technologies for Ground Aircraft and Satellite Applications (iAIM), pp. 1–3 (2017)
10. Mitola, J.: Cognitive radio: an integrated agent architecture for software defined radio. Ph.D. dissertation (2000)
11. Shaik, L.A., Saha, C., Antar, Y.M., Siddiqui, J.Y.: An antenna advance for cognitive radio. IEEE Antennas Propag. Mag. **1045**(9243/18) (2018)
12. Saha, C., Siddiqui, J.Y., Antar, Y.M.M.: Multifunctional ultrawideband antennas: trends. In: Techniques and Applications. CRC Press (2019)
13. Aseri, K., Yadav, S., Sharma, M.M.: A compact frequency selective surface based band-stop filter for WLAN applications. In: 2015 Fifth International Conference on Communication Systems and Network Technologies, pp. 328–332. IEEE (2015)
14. Dhegaya, S., Tanwar, L.: Design of dual band pass and band stop frequency selective surface: for wireless communication. In: 2022 Trends in Electrical, Electronics, Computer Engineering Conference (TEECCON). IEEE (2022). https://doi.org/10.1109/TEECCON54414.2022.9854824
15. Fertas, K., Ghanem, F., Challal, M., Aksas, R.: Design and development of compact reconfigurable tri-stopband band stop filter using hexagonal metamaterial cells for wireless applications. Prog. Electromagnet. Res. M **80**, 93102 (2019)
16. Fertas, K., Ghanem, F., Challal, M.: Design and implementation of a novel tri-band bandstop filter based on hexagonal metamaterials split ring resonators. In: The International Conference on Electrical Engineering-Boumerdes (ICEE-B), Boumerdes, Algeria, October 29 31 (2017)
17. Asci, C., Sadeqi, A., Wang, W., Nejad, H.R., Sonkusale, S.: Design and implementation tunable quad-band filter utilizing split-ring resonators at microwave frequencies. Sci. Rep. **10**, 1050 (2020). https://doi.org/10.1038/s41598-020-57773-6
18. Boubakar, H., Abri, M., Benaissa, M.: Electronically reconfigurable HM-SIW band pass filter based on new CSRR design using PIN diode. J. Inform. Math. Sci. **13**(1), 5969 (2021)
19. Boubakar, H., Abri, M., Benaissa, M.: Design of complementary hexagonal metamaterial based HMSIW band pass lter and reconfigurable SIW filter using PIN diodes. Adv. Electromagnet. (AEM) **10**(2) (2021)
20. Chavda, K.D., Sarvaiya, A.K.: Development of reconfigurable band stop filter using metamaterial for WLAN application. In: 2022 PhotonIcs & Electromagnetics Research Symposium (PIERS), Hangzhou, China, 25–27 April
21. Ghodake, A.P., Sale, H.B., Hogade, B.: Effect of ground plane dimensions on the performance of wearable jeans antenna. In: 2022 IEEE Conference on Interdisciplinary Approaches in Technology and Management for Social Innovation (IATMSI), Gwalior, India, pp. 1–4 (2022). https://doi.org/10.1109/IATMSI56455.2022.10119293

Basic Hand Movement Classification Using Q Factor Based Wavelet Scattering Transform

Gowri Krishnan[1(✉)], Anurag Nishad[1], and Abhay Upadhyay[2]

[1] BITS Pilani, KK Birla Goa Campus, Goa, India
{p20230419,anuragn}@goa.bits-pilani.ac.in
[2] Indian Institute of Information Technology, Kota, Kota, Rajasthan, India

Abstract. This paper conducted a study on the classification of basic hand movement from the two-channel surface Electromyogram (sEMG) data acquired from the upper limb. For classification, the scattering coefficients are obtained from sEMG signals by applying wavelet scattering transform with different quality (Q) factors. The statistical features namely mean value, summation, root mean square value, variance, maximum value, kurtosis, and skewness were computed from the scattering coefficients. The features were ranked using the ReliefF algorithm and classified using different machine learning algorithms to determine the most accurate classifier model. A comparative study of the performance of different classifiers in terms of accuracy has been done in this study. The proposed method has been applied to the sEMG data obtained from five subjects. The simulation results show that the average classification accuracy achieved by the proposed method is 93.4%.

Keywords: surface Electromyogram signals · Scattering wavelet transforms · Tunable Q-factor wavelet transform · Scattering coefficients · Statistical features · ReliefF algorithm · Machine learning

1 Introduction

The upper limbs are a versatile and crucial part of the human anatomy, supporting a wide range of physical, sensory, and cognitive functions. Their importance extends to daily life, work, communication, and creative expression. The loss of a hand can also lead to physical discomfort, including phantom limb sensations or pain [1]. A few hundred years ago individuals with hand amputations were often relegated to using hook prostheses, which offered limited functionality and were associated with considerable social stigma [2]. However, in today's society, a hand amputee can expect a replacement that replicates the functions of a normal hand and looks extremely lifelike [2]. The development of prosthetics for the upper limb continues to evolve, driven by materials and technology

Supported by the Cross-Disciplinary Research Framework (CDRF) grant by BITS Pilani University.

K. Atul et al. (Eds.): BodyNets 2024, LNICST 666, pp. 467–480, 2026.
https://doi.org/10.1007/978-3-032-16099-7_37

advancements. These devices play a crucial role in improving the quality of life for individuals who have experienced upper limb loss. The modern prosthetic hand has been engineered to closely replicate the natural limb in both appearance and functionality [3]. In general, prosthetic devices could be body-powered, pneumatic-powered, or electric-powered [4]. Myoelectric prosthetics use electromyographic (EMG) signals generated by the user's remaining muscles to control the movements of the prosthetic limb. The EMG signals are collected and processed to study the coordination of hand movements for the activation of different muscles in the upper limb. The EMG signal is composed of the action potentials from groups of muscle fibers organized into functional units called motor units (MUs) [2]. This signal can be detected with sensors placed on the skin's surface or with needle or wire sensors introduced into the muscle tissue [2]. Advanced myoelectric systems allow for more intuitive and natural control of the prosthetic hand and fingers. Research is ongoing to incorporate sensory feedback into prosthetic limbs [2]. This includes technologies that provide users with a sense of touch, pressure, or temperature, enhancing their ability to interact with the environment. Advancements in technology have brought exciting new areas of research and development known as the Wireless Body Area Networks (WBANs). This comprises of a network of intelligent, low-power micro and nano-technology sensors and actuators that can be positioned on the body, implanted within the body, or even introduced into the bloodstream, providing timely data [5]. This also helps avoid costly and frequent visits to the hospitals [5]. The most recent standardization of Wireless Body Area Networks (WBANs), IEEE 802.15.6 [6], seeks to establish a global standard for low-power, short-range (within the human body), and highly reliable wireless communication around the human body. A WBAN consists of a network of sensor nodes that can sample, process, and communicate various information with each other [7]. WBANs have the potential to significantly advance various fields, including the development of prosthetic arms [8]. The transition from wired to wireless technology in prosthetic arms will reduce wear and tear while enhancing the arm's range of motion and degrees of freedom [8]. Many communication protocols can be used for wireless data transfer and the selection of a specific communication technology depends on the final application requirements and the precise definition of throughput and latency specifications [9]. This can also be integrated with the Internet of Things in Healthcare (IoTH), offering a more efficient method for data collection and storage. This approach facilitates handling large datasets with ease, enhancing data management capabilities in healthcare applications.

In recent advances, the integration of machine learning and deep learning in prosthetics contributes to adaptive control systems. These systems can learn and adapt to the user's preferences and movements over time. Typically, trained experts detect the onset and offset events in surface electromyographic (sEMG) signals through visual inspection [10]. However, while developing upper limb prosthesis, there is no time to inspect sEMG signals visually and decide the hand movement [11]. Due to this, machine learning and deep learning have shown their effectiveness in interpreting sEMG signals for various applications [12], including gesture classification [13], muscle fatigue detection [14] and EMG pattern [15]. Machine learning and artificial neural networks have become very popular in biomedical signal processing for real time hand gesture recognition [16].

The above mentioned algorithms for hand movement classification are based on sEMG signals. For a hand movement, the contraction in muscle causes spikes and oscillatory components in the sEMG signals. This bring us the motivation to develop a signal processing method which can trace the oscillatory and transients components in the sEMG signals corresponding to different hand movement. Based on the developed method, and an algorithm can be design to classify hand movements. To achieve this objective, a novel quality (Q) factor based wavelet scattering transform is proposed in this paper. The variation in Q factor can be used to analyze different oscillatory components in the sEMG signal [17]. The paper is arranged as follows: Sect. 2 includes the methodology explaining the proposed Q factor-based wavelet scattering transform, feature extraction and ranking, and classification. Section 3 explains the results and discussion of the simulation work and, finally, Sect. 4 includes the conclusion and future works.

2 Methodology

This section discusses the proposed algorithm in the following sub-sections. Figure 1 shows the different blocks of the proposed method.

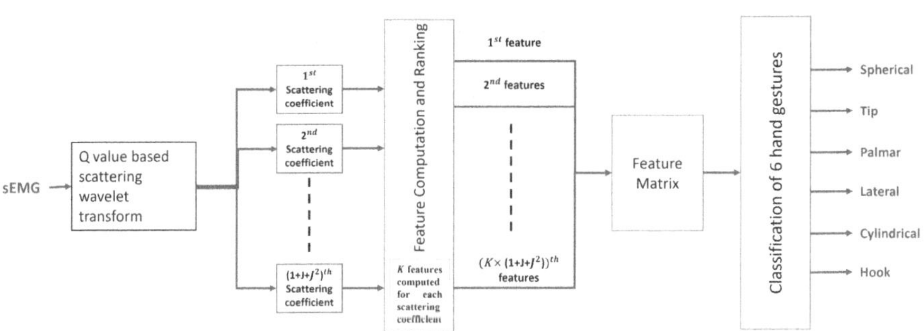

Fig. 1. Block representation of the 6 hand gesture classification using Q factor based wavelet scattering transform.

2.1 Data Set

In the proposed method, the input sEMG signals are obtained from the basic hand movement dataset [18]. The database includes the sEMG signals corresponding to 6 hand movements using Delsys' EMG System. The signals were acquired from 5 subjects (3 females and 2 male subjects). The subjects performed 6 basic hand movements: Spherical, Tip, Palmar, Lateral, Cylindrical,

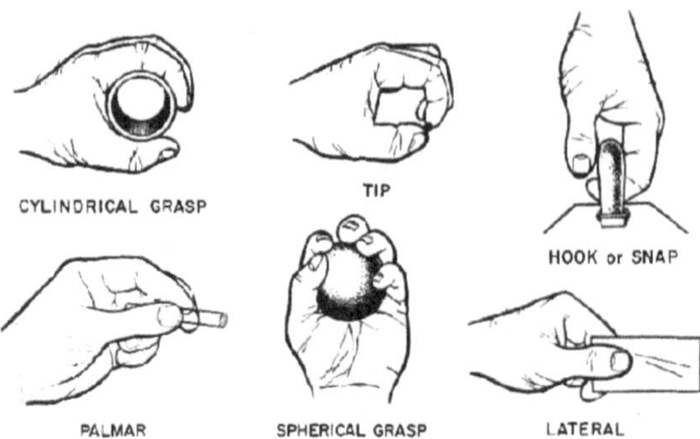

Fig. 2. Six basic hand grasp gestures [19]

and Hook. Each movement was repeated 30 times. Figure 2 shows the 6 different hand movements performed by the subjects. Each movement was captured using a two-channel data acquisition system, and thus there will be two sets of data for each movement.

2.2 Q-Factor Based Wavelet Scattering Transform

In this step, the proposed Q-factor based wavelet scattering transform has been applied on sEMG signals. A wavelet scattering transform is computed through a series of wavelet transforms followed by modulus non-linearity [20]. Its computational framework resembles that of a deep convolutional neural network [21], but it does not require any learning process. The transform generates time-averaged coefficients, offering valuable signal invariants over potentially extended time scales [20]. The proposed Q-based wavelet scattering transform depends on the scaling factor, Q, the level of decomposition (J) and the redundancy (R). The decomposition level J decides the number of subbands produced which will be J+1. There will be J number of high-frequency bands and one low-frequency band.

Figure 3 shows each decomposition level of the wavelet scattering transform. $x(n)$ is the input signal and $\Phi(n)$ is the scaling function which is the $(J+1)^{th}$ subband. In Fig. 3 there are three levels of decomposition (L) and each layer has J^l wavelet coefficients (where l ranges from 0 to L). The structure of the Q based scattering transform is shown in Fig. 3. For L = 0 the fist scattering coefficient $S_{01}(n) = x(n) * \Phi(n)$. At L = 1 the $x(n)$ is convolved with $\varphi_{\lambda^{1j}}(n)$ $(1 \leq j \leq J)$ [22], where $\varphi_{\lambda^{1j}}(n)$ represents wavelet corresponding to j^{th} subband. The modulus of this convolution is again convolved with the scale factor $\Phi(n)$ to produce scattering coefficient $S_{i1}(n)$ to $S_{iJ}(n)$. Similarly at L = 2, $S_{2(j' \times j'')}(n) = ||x(n) * \varphi_{\lambda_{1j'}}(n)|| * \varphi_{\lambda_{2j''}}(n)| * \Phi(n)$ where $1 \leq j^{'}, j^{''} \leq J$ [22]. In Fig. 3 the symbol $| * |$ represents a convolution operation followed by a modulus operation and symbol $*$ represents convolution operation. The structure of Q based scattering transform as shown in Fig. 3 consist of convolution, modulus, and cascading

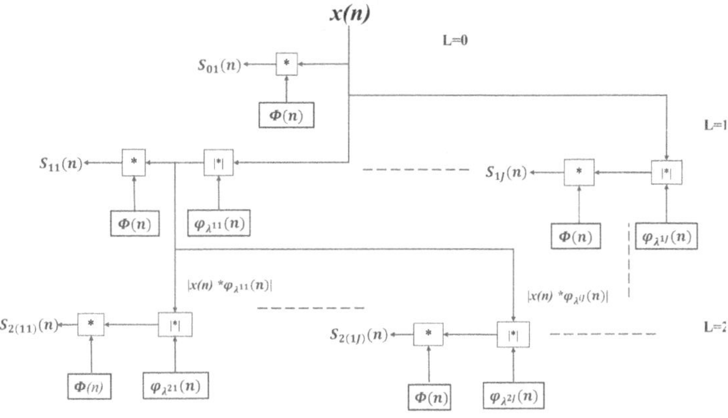

Fig. 3. Decomposition levels of the wavelet scattering transform depicting the computation of wavelet coefficients. This figure shows a three-level decomposition (L) of the signal $x(n)$.

of modulus of convolution [21]. Here, $S_{01}(n) = x(n) * \Phi(n)$ removes all the high frequencies and these high-frequency components (ψ_λ (λ being the center frequency of the signal)) are retrieved by modulus transform $|x(n) * \varphi_{\lambda^{ij}}(n)|$ [22], where j varies from 1 to J and, i ranges from 0 to L. This contributes to the next decomposition layer. The first layer will produce $J+1$ coefficients, $S_{iJ}(n) = |x(n) * \varphi_{\lambda^{ij}}(n)| * \Phi(n)$ and it is the first-order scattering coefficients.

In this study, we have varied the quality (Q) factor to vary the mother wavelet's oscillatory nature to help capture the signal's different oscillatory components. We have opted for a Tunable Q-factor wavelet transform (TQWT). In TQWT the Q can be varied to change the amount of oscillation in the scaling function. This also results in the change of the bandwidth of subband $J+1$ [cite selesnick's TQWT paper]. In frequency domain, the subband $J+1$ is low pass filter which captures the low frequency information of the signal $x(n)$ [17]. Here, along with the Q-factor, the J was also tuned to study the effect of bandwidth of sub-band $J+1$, and number of sub-bands. The R should be set such that the transition bands of the frequency responses will not be relatively narrow and the time-domain response (wavelet) is well localized [23]. For this, the R is set not close to unity [23]. The Q-factor contributes to the oscillatory nature of the wavelet. Varying the Q-factors will help capture different oscillatory epochs of the input signal.

2.3 Feature Extraction and Ranking

As shown in Fig. 1, after producing the coefficients, the K number of features can be computed from each scattering coefficient. For this work, we computed 7 distinct features in terms of mean value, summation, root mean square value, variance, maximum value, kurtosis, and skewness from each scattering coefficient. The Q factor was varied from 1, 2, 3, 4, 5, 10, and 20, and correspondingly the J values were varied from 3, 5, and 7. Since we have used a three-layer decomposition and for each decomposition, the Q and J values were varied therefore depending on the J value, each decomposition will produce the corresponding number of coefficients. The number of coefficients will be equal to $(1+J+J^2)\times K$. Since J was selected as 3, 5, and 7, and k was 7, the total number of features was 91, 217, and 399 respectively. To rank the features, we used the ReliefF algorithm [23]. ReliefF algorithm randomly selects an instance from one of the classes in the database and identifies the k nearest neighboring (KNN) instances [24]. The KNN instances within the same class are referred to as Near Hits, while the k nearest neighbors from different classes are called Near Misses [25]. The number of ranked features were varied from 1 to the maximum number of features in the feature matrix. For each variation the model was trained with its best model (model with maximum accuracy for validation) and the accuracy for that model was recorded. The feature matrices for the five subjects were computed and uploaded to the Matlab "Classifier" app. The classifier app classifies each hand gesture into the corresponding classes. The hand gestures are classified as class 0 for cylindrical movement, class 1 for hook movement, class 2 for lateral movement, class 3 for palmar movement, class 4 for spherical movement, and class 5 for tip movement.

2.4 Classifier Model Accuracy

In the final block (from Fig. 1) the extracted features were utilized to determine the precision of the validation of each classifier model in the Classifier application in MATLAB. In the Classifier application, the cross-validation fold (k) was set to 10 for this study.

In this study, the classifiers based on tree, discriminant analysis, naive bayes, support vector machine, nearest neighbor, ensemble, are tested taht are available in the classifier application of MATLAB. The classification accuracy as the performance evaluation parameter is used in this study. The most accurate training model was selected for each dataset to study the variations in this accuracy with a change in the number of ranked features selected.

3 Result and Discussion

The Tables 1, 2, 3, 4, and 5 show the validation accuracy and the corresponding classifier training model concerning different variations in Q and J values for each dataset. For the dataset of first female subject (here onward referred to as Female 1), the study shows that the **Subspace KNN** model produced the most accurate validation (**91.7%**) for the Q and J values of 2 and 7 respectively. For the dataset of second female subject (here onward referred to as Female 2), the results show that the **Subspace KNN** model produced the most accurate validation (**87.2%**) for the Q and J values of 4 and 5 respectively. Similarly, the **Quadratic SVM** model produced the most accurate validation (**94.4%**) for the Q and J values of 2 and 5 respectively for the dataset of 3rd female subject (here onward referred to as Female 3). For the dataset of 1st male subject (here onward referred to as Male 1), the study shows that the **Quadratic SVM** model produced the most accurate validation (**92.8**%) for the Q and J values of 1(and 3) and 5 (and 7) respectively. For the dataset of the 2nd male subject (here onward referred to as Male 2), the **Subspace KNN** model produced the most accurate validation (**96.4**%) for the Q and J values of 3 and 7 respectively.

Table 1. Performance of different classifier models for female_1 dataset. The Subspace KNN produced the most accurate validation at 91.7%.

Female 1	Q						
J	1	2	3	4	5	10	20
3	85.3% Medium Neural Network	85.0% Subspace Discriminant	82.2% Subspace Discriminant	80.0% Linear Discriminant	77.2% Boosted Trees	74.2% Bagged Trees	71.4% Boosted Trees
5	88.6% Subspace Discriminant	87.8% Subspace KNN	82.5% Bagged Trees	83.9% Bagged Trees	82.2% Bagged Trees	78.3% Bagged Trees	73.6% Bagged Trees
7	86.9% Subspace KNN	**91.7% Subspace KNN**	85.6% Boosted Trees	85.6% Boosted Trees	80.0% Subspace KNN	75.3% Bagged Trees	71.7% Bagged Trees

For each of these models corresponding to each dataset, the change in accuracy was studied by varying the number of ranked features. The graph in Fig. 4 shows the variation in the accuracy of each model with respect to varying the number of ranked features used for training the model. It was observed that as the number of ranked features increased from 1 to its maximum number, the model's accuracy increased drastically to a certain point and then became almost constant. The accuracy was shown to be very low when only the most significant features (first 1 to 10 features after ranking) were selected. Using all features did not necessarily yield maximum accuracy. The accuracy of the model can be increased by selecting different ranked features. For the Female 1 dataset, the maximum accuracy of validation obtained was **91.8**%, when the number of ranked features selected were 362, 371, and 387 out of a total of 399 features. In the case of the Female 2 dataset, the maximum accuracy of validation obtained was **89.7**%, when the number of ranked features selected was 383, 107 and 110 out of a total of 217 features. In the Female 3 dataset, the maximum accuracy of validation was increased from 94.4% (for all the 217 features selected) to **94.7**% when the number of ranked features selected were 141, 142, 150, 151, 152, 153, 157, and 180 out of a total of 217 features. There was an increase in accuracy from 92.8% to **93.9**% for the Male 1 data set when selecting 149 to 153 ranked features. For computational ease, J was taken to be 5 and Q as 1. The accuracy

Table 2. Performance of different classifier models for female_2 dataset. Most accurate validation of 87.2% was produced by the subspace KNN.

Female 2	Q						
J	1	2	3	4	5	10	20
3	82.8% Subspace Discriminant	86.4% Efficient Logistic Regression	85.8% Subspace Discriminant	84.7% Bagged Trees	86.1% Subspace Discriminant	84.7% Quadratic SVM	82.2% Boosted Trees
5	84.4% Subspace KNN	86.1% Subspace KNN	85.3% Subspace KNN	**87.2% Subspace KNN**	86.7% Subspace KNN	81.9% Subspace Discriminant	77.5% Bagged Trees
7	86.9% Cubic SVM	86.1% Subspace KNN	85.3% Quadratic SVM	85.6% Subspace KNN	86.7% Quadratic SVM	84.4% Bagged Trees	77.8% Bagged Trees

Table 3. Performance of different classifier models for female_3. Quadratic SVM showed the best validation accuracy of 94.4%.

Female 3	Q						
J	1	2	3	4	5	10	20
3	93.1% Efficient Logistic Regression	88.9% Cubic SVM	86.1% Subspace Discriminant	84.2% Linear SVM	83.1% Bagged Trees	84.7% Boosted Trees	85.3% Quadratic SVM
5	93.3% Quadratic SVM	**94.4% Quadratic SVM**	86.7% Bagged Trees	84.7% Quadratic SVM	83.6% Cubic SVM	83.6% Bagged Trees	83.9% Bagged Trees
7	92.5% Subspace KNN	94.2% Quadratic SVM	92.8% Bagged Trees	85.0% Quadratic SVM	84.7% Quadratic SVM	82.5% Quadratic SVM	82.5% Bagged Trees

improved to **96.7**% for the Male 2 data as well for a selected number of ranked features.

The Fig. 5 shows the confusion matrices for each of the datasets having the maximum accuracy corresponding to the Q and J values. The matrix shows the classifier model's True Positive Rate (TPR) and False Negative Rate (FNR). The TPR measures the sensitivity of the model and shows how well the model correctly identifies positive cases, and the FNR indicates the percentage of positive cases that were incorrectly classified [26]. As an example, Fig. 5, (a) shows the confusion matrix for the Female 1 dataset for subspace KNN and here Class 0 (Cylindrical hand gesture) was classified as class 0 with an accuracy of 90.0%

Table 4. Performance of different classifier models for Male_1. 92.8% validation accuracy was produced by Quadratic SVM model.

Male 1	Q						
J	1	2	3	4	5	10	20
3	91.1% Cubic SVM	90.0% Cubic SVM	89.4% Cubic SVM	88.3% Bagged Trees	85.0% Bagged Trees	79.7% Quadratic SVM	79.2% Boosted Trees
5	**92.8% Quadratic SVM**	92.2% Quadratic SVM	91.4% Cubic SVM	85.0% Bagged Trees	86.4% Bagged Trees	78.3% Boosted Trees	80.3% Boosted Trees
7	92.1% Quadratic SVM	91.3% Cubic SVM	**92.8% Quadratic SVM**	88.1% Subspace Discriminant	88.1% Boosted Trees	84.7% Bagged Trees	78.3% Bagged Trees

Table 5. Performance of different classifier models for Male_2. A validation accuracy of 96.4% was produced by Subspace KNN model.

Male 2	Q						
J	1	2	3	4	5	10	20
3	95.0% Cubic SVM	93.3% Quadratic SVM	93.1% Subspace Discriminant	90.0% Linear Discriminant	88.9% Quadratic SVM	83.9% Wide Neural Network	76.1% Bagged Trees
5	95.3% Subspace Discriminant	95.8% Subspace KNN	93.9% Cubic SVM	92.5% Subspace Discriminant	89.7% Subspace Discriminant	85.8% Subspace Discriminant	76.1% Bagged Trees
7	95.6% Cubic SVM	95.3% Wide Neural Network	**96.4% Subspace KNN**	93.1% Subspace Discriminant	90.6% Subspace Discriminant	84.4% Subspace Discriminant	83.6% Bagged Trees

as shown by the TPR value. 10.0% of class 0 were misclassified as shown by the FNR. Similarly, the sensitivity of all the models are shown in the TPR and FNR matrix in Fig. 5. The accuracy of the model depends on how precisely the model matches the predicted class to the true class. Similarly, the TPR and FNR corresponding to different hand movements for each subject is shown in Fig. 5 Due to FNR, some classes are not predicted with 100 % accuracy.

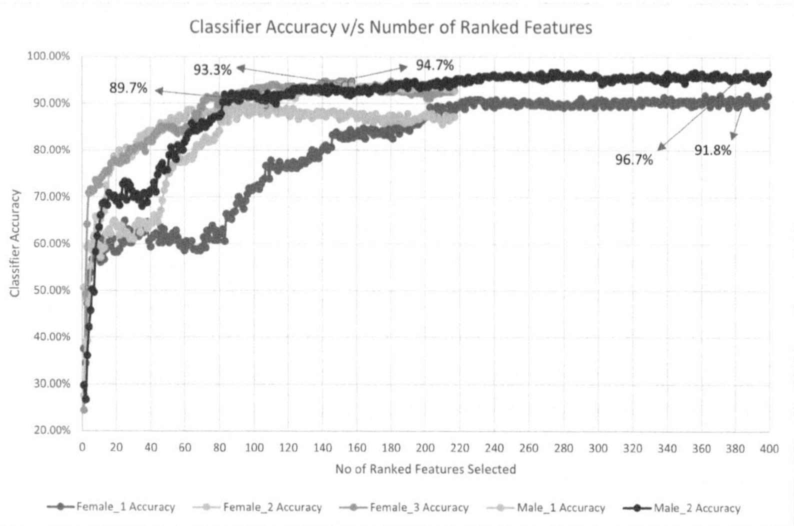

Fig. 4. The number of ranked features was varied from 1 to the maximum features and the accuracy of the classifier model was observed.

3.1 Computational Complexity

Assuming that the computational time to generate wavelets is the same as that of TQWT, the computational cost for a radix-2 TQWT of a N-point sequence is $O(rN\log_2 N)$ [23], where r is the redundancy and N is the length of the signal. In this method, we have chosen three levels of decomposition. Following a similar computational pattern as in [17], if the average time for convolution of the signal "$x(n)$" with the scaling factor is C, then for the first level the computational time is C. For the second level of decomposition, the convolution is performed twice and continued for all the J values. In this way, the computational complexity becomes $2 \times J \times C$. From the second level of decomposition, the $J \times J$ coefficients are produced. For the third level of decomposition, the convolution is performed three times and continued for all the J values. Thus, the computational complexity becomes $3 \times J^2 \times C$. The computational complexity for obtaining the feature matrix will be $O(rN\log_2 N)+(C+(2\times J\times C)+(3\times J^2\times C))$. On an average each feature extraction will take T_f time and therefore the total time taken for feature computation is $T_f \times K \times (1 + J + J^2)$. Assuming the computational complexity for the classification is T_c, the total computational complexity of the method is $(O(rN\log_2 N) + (C + (2 \times J \times C) + (3 \times J^2 \times C))) + (T_f \times K \times (1 + J + J^2)) + T_c$. The computational complexity is dependent on the J values. As we increase the value of J, the computational complexity also increases.

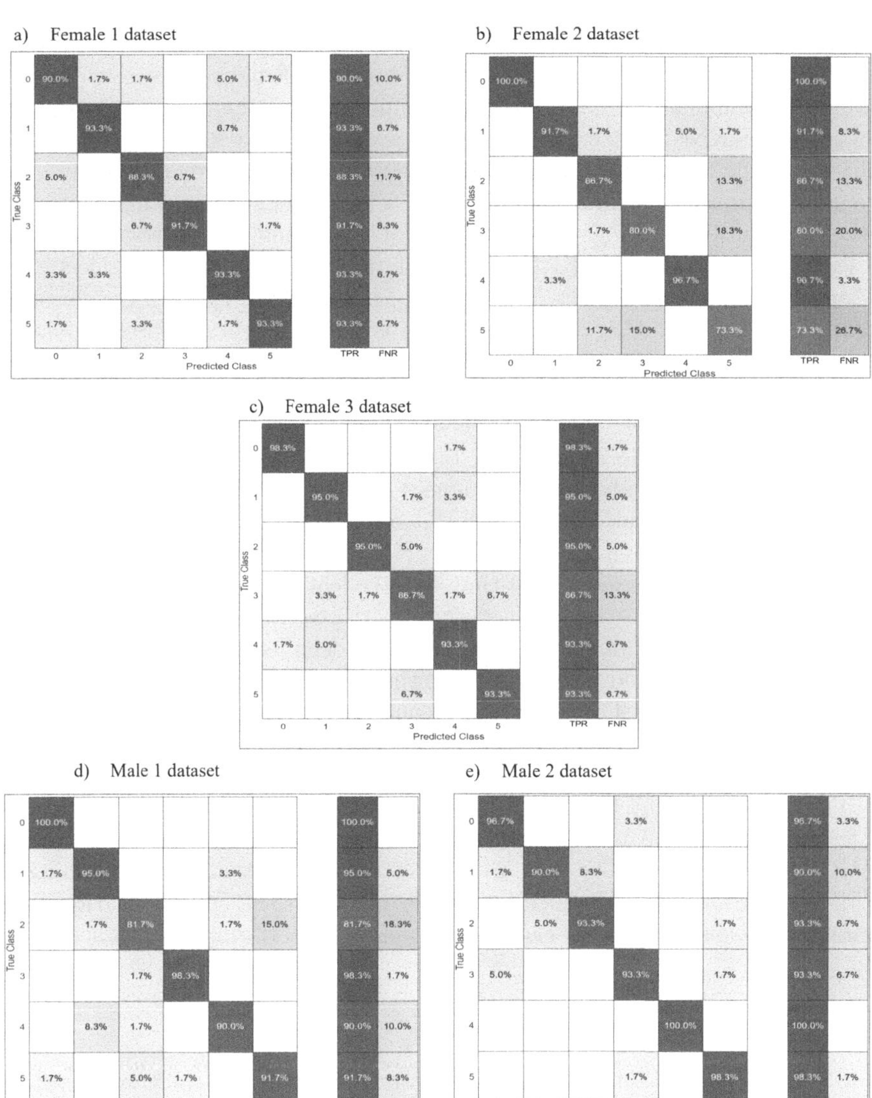

Fig. 5. Confusion matrices for all datasets with maximum accuracy, showing the TPR and FNR.

4 Conclusion and Future Works

In this study, we propose the Q based scattering transform in which the Q factor is varied in the wavelet scattering transform to explore the changes in the oscillatory nature of the scaling function $\phi(n)$. The variation in the scaling function has an impact on low frequency information extracted from signal from which features are computed. With this tunable Q factor and scaling coefficients, the efficacy of various machine learning classifiers in interpreting sEMG signals from different subjects was studied. The research demonstrates that specific parameter combinations yield the highest validation accuracies for each dataset. The Subspace KNN model consistently outperformed other classifiers for certain subjects, while the Quadratic SVM model excelled for others. The accuracy of the models improved significantly with the selection of specific ranked features, rather than utilizing all available features. This finding demonstrates that not all features contribute equally to model performance, and a targeted selection of the most informative features can improve accuracy. The average classification accuracy when considering all the features was 92.5%, which increased to 93.36% when using selected ranked features.

In addition, the study underscores the cost effectiveness of using a two-channel data acquisition system. This approach simplifies the hardware setup and reduces costs while maintaining high performance [17]. Two-channel systems are less expensive and easier to manage compared to multi-channel systems, making them a practical choice for sEMG signal acquisition without sacrificing accuracy. Future research could further explore the integration of WBANs with prosthetic devices, leveraging real-time data collection and analysis to improve the functionality of prosthetics and user experience. In addition, incorporating advanced machine learning techniques, such as deep learning models and reinforcement learning, could further improve the adaptability and accuracy of prosthetic control systems. This integration could lead to prosthetics that not only mimic natural limb movements more closely but also provide real-time feedback and adaptation, significantly improving the user's quality of life.

The study concludes that both the choice of classifier and the careful selection of features are crucial to optimizing the accuracy of the interpretation of the sEMG signal. It highlights the importance of personalized model training in sEMG signal analysis, where tailoring the model to the specific features and characteristics of the data set can lead to significant performance improvements.

References

1. Stephens-Fripp, B., Alici, G., Mutlu, R.: A review of non-invasive sensory feedback methods for transradial prosthetic hands. IEEE Access **6**, 6878–6899 (2018)
2. Clement, R.G.E., Bugler, K.E., Oliver, C.W.: Bionic prosthetic hands: a review of present technology and future aspirations. Surgeon **9**(6), 336–340 (2011)
3. Allin, S., Eckel, E., Markham, H., Brewer, B.R.: Recent trends in the development and evaluation of assistive robotic manipulation devices. Phys. Med. Rehabil. Clin. **21**(1), 59–77 (2010)
4. De Luca, C.J., Adam, A., Wotiz, R., Gilmore, L.D., Nawab, S.H.: Decomposition of surface EMG signals. J. Neurophysiol. **96**(3), 1646–1657 (2006)
5. Movassaghi, S., Abolhasan, M., Lipman, J., Smith, D., Jamalipour, A.: Wireless body area networks: a survey. IEEE Commun. Surv. Tutor. **16**(3), 1658–1686 (2014)
6. Astrin, A.: IEEE standard for local and metropolitan area networks part 15.6: Wireless body area networks. IEEE Std 802.15.6 (2012)

7. Otto, C., Milenkovic, A., Sanders, C., Jovanov, E.: System architecture of a wireless body area sensor network for ubiquitous health monitoring. J. Mob. Multimedia **1**(4), 307–326 (2005)
8. Saleh, A., et al.: A wireless body area network architecture for a prosthetic arm. In: 2015 7th International Congress on Ultra Modern Telecommunications and Control Systems and Workshops (ICUMT), pp. 275–280. IEEE (2015)
9. Brunelli, D., Farella, E., Giovanelli, D., Milosevic, B., Minakov, I.: Design considerations for wireless acquisition of multichannel sEMG signals in prosthetic hand control. IEEE Sens. J. **16**(23), 8338–8347 (2016)
10. Tenan, M.S., Tweedell, A.J., Haynes, C.A.: Analysis of statistical and standard algorithms for detecting muscle onset with surface electromyography. PLoS ONE **12**(5), e0177312 (2017)
11. Selvan, S.E., Allexandre, D., Amato, U., Yue, G.H.: Unsupervised stochastic strategies for robust detection of muscle activation onsets in surface electromyogram. IEEE Trans. Neural Syst. Rehabil. Eng. **26**(6), 1279–1291 (2018)
12. Faust, O., Hagiwara, Y., Hong, T.J., Lih, O.S., Acharya, U.R.: Deep learning for healthcare applications based on physiological signals: a review. Comput. Methods Programs Biomed. **161**, 1–13 (2018)
13. Lee, K.H., Min, J.Y., Byun, S.: Electromyogram-based classification of hand and finger gestures using artificial neural networks. Sensors **22**(1), 225 (2021)
14. Wang, J., Sun, S., Sun, Y.: A muscle fatigue classification model based on LSTM and improved wavelet packet threshold. Sensors **21**(19), 6369 (2021)
15. Phinyomark, A., Scheme, E.: EMG pattern recognition in the era of big data and deep learning. Big Data Cogn. Comput. **2**(3), 21 (2018)
16. Jaramillo-Yánez, A., Benalcázar, M.E., Mena-Maldonado, E.: Real-time hand gesture recognition using surface electromyography and machine learning: a systematic literature review. Sensors **20**(9), 2467 (2020)
17. Pachori, R.B., Nishad, A.: Cross-terms reduction in the Wigner-Ville distribution using tunable-Q wavelet transform. Signal Process. **120**, 288–304 (2016)
18. Sapsanis, C., Tzes, A., Georgoulas, G.: sEMG for Basic Hand movements. UCI Machine Learning Repository (2014). https://doi.org/10.24432/C5TK53
19. Akben, S.B.: Low-cost and easy-to-use grasp classification, using a simple 2-channel surface electromyography (sEMG). Biomed. Res. **28**(2), 577–582 (2017)
20. Mallat, S.: Group invariant scattering. Commun. Pure Appl. Math. **65**(10), 1331–1398 (2012)
21. Andén, J., Mallat, S.: Deep scattering spectrum. IEEE Trans. Signal Process. **62**(16), 4114–4128 (2014). https://doi.org/10.1109/TSP.2014.2326991
22. LeCun, Y., Kavukcuoglu, K., Farabet, C.: Convolutional networks and applications in vision. In: Proceedings of 2010 IEEE International Symposium on Circuits and Systems, pp. 253–256. IEEE (2010)
23. Selesnick, I.W.: Wavelet transform with tunable Q-factor. IEEE Trans. Signal Process. **59**(8), 3560–3575 (2011)
24. Benazzouz, A., Guilal, R., Amirouche, F., Hadj Slimane, Z.E.: EMG feature selection for diagnosis of neuromuscular disorders. In: 2019 International Conference on Networking and Advanced Systems (ICNAS), Annaba, Algeria, pp. 1–5 (2019). https://doi.org/10.1109/ICNAS.2019.8807862.

25. Robnik-Šikonja, M., Kononenko, I.: Theoretical and empirical analysis of ReliefF and RReliefF. Mach. Learn. **53**, 23–69 (2003)
26. Jadhav, A.S.: A novel weighted TPR-TNR measure to assess performance of the classifiers. Expert Syst. Appl. **152**, 113391 (2020)
27. Nishad, A., Upadhyay, A., Pachori, R.B., Acharya, U.R.: Automated classification of hand movements using tunable-Q wavelet transform based filter-bank with surface electromyogram signals. Futur. Gener. Comput. Syst. **93**, 96–110 (2019)

Channel Selection Strategy for Early Prediction of Epileptic Seizure Event for Wearable EEG Sensors

Teena Jangid(✉) and A. D. Darji

Sardar Vallabhbhai National Institute of Technology (SVNIT), Surat, India
d23ec005@svnit.ac.in, add@eced.svnit.ac.in

Abstract. Electroencephalogram (EEG) contains important physiological information that can reflect the activity of human brain so that it is useful for epileptic seizure detection and epilepsy diagnosis. In this paper, we develop a novel unified framework for real-time monitoring of EEG for epileptic seizure prediction with minimum number of electrodes for wearable application without any prior knowledge. This research work uses Principal Component Analysis (PCA) for ranking the highest contribution of channels during seizure period to reduce the number of EEG scalp electrodes. CHB-MIT data has average 23 channels for each patient, but obtained results of our study show that average five to six channels are enough to get good sensitivity with less False Prediction Rate (FPR) per hour. In this research work, different channels combinations in the term of accuracy, sensitivity and FPR/hr have been analyzed and the result obtained 92.73% sensitivity and 0.073 FPR/hr for only 10 channels.

Keywords: Short-time Fourier transform (STFT) · Spectrogram · Power spectral density (PSD) · Electroencephalogram (EEG) · Intracranial EEG (iEEG) · Stereotaxic-EEG (sEEG) · Channel selection · Principal Component Analysis (PCA) · Electrode reduction

1 Introduction

According to the World Health Organization (WHO) survey till Feb 2024, around 50 million people worldwide are facing the epilepsy seizure problems [1]. It is becoming one of the most common neurological diseases globally and it is estimated that if this disease properly diagnosed and treated, almost up to 70% people who suffering with this neurological disease could live seizure-free. An epileptic seizure is nothing but synchronous neuronal brain activity with transient occurrence of symptoms, it's short trigger of involuntary movement. Globally, an estimated 5 million people are diagnosed with epilepsy each year [1]. Therefor, it is very necessary to track every activity of brain signal of patient who are suffering from epileptic disease in order to predict the seizures so that injuries due to loss of consciousness can be avoided and the treatment quality can be improved. Many underlying disease can lead to epilepsy, the cause of the

K. Atul et al. (Eds.): BodyNets 2024, LNICST 666, pp. 481–494, 2026.
https://doi.org/10.1007/978-3-032-16099-7_38

disease is still unknown in about 50% of cases globally [1]. Irrespective pf reasons early prediction of epilepsy seizure is very much required for better severity of treatment.

An electroencephalogram (EEG) signal is a recording of the electrical activity produced by millions of cortical neurons of the brain. If the EEG signals are recorded from intracranial electrodes, it is known as *intracranial EEG (iEEG)*. If the EEG signal recorded by putting the electrodes on the scalp it is known as scalp EEG or *stereotaxic-EEG*(sEEG). As EEG signal is non-stationary signal which means the frequency of the signal ranges from 0.1 Hz to over 100 Hz and varies with time. According the range of frequency bands the state of brain can be categorized. These EEG brain waves represent the behavior of human activities such as sleeping, comma, asleep, relaxed, meditation, excitement etc. EEG signal contains a wide range of artifacts, including external medical artifacts, cardiac artifacts, muscular artifacts, and retinal artifacts [8]. Each EEG signal is the voltage difference between two scalp electrodes which is refer as one channel. EEG technician uses up-to 256 electrodes [2] for the clinical activity. If patient experiences the seizure very frequently then to avoid critical situation real-time monitoring of EEG signal is essential. It is tedious to wear large number of electrodes on scalp continuously. On the other hand, neurologists can usually specify partial channels which is relevant to seizure type for each patient. There are two different types of seizures, based on location from where it starts in the brain. Under these two categories, there are many different types of epilepsy activity. According to the National Institute of Neurological Disorders and Stroke, doctors have discovered more than 30 different types of seizures.

However, a large amount of the feature matrix may increase the computational complexity, and may not be feasible for the wearable device due to the constraint of low computational power. Thus, the aim of this work is to propose a novel and patient specific approach to reduce the number of electrodes require for seizure prediction and to reduce the computational load of the-feature classification. In this paper, following issues are addressed.

1. To investigate EEG electrodes selection approach based on the PCA.
2. To present an efficient signal processing technique using spectrogram for each channel on five frequency bands for feature extraction in time-frequency domain and to select the channel based on the contribution of the electrode with principle component during seizure period.
3. Compute power spectral density for selected channels which are closely related to effective region of subject brain.
4. Use the Machine learning based benchmark classification algorithm to report various analysis parameters and to validate the hypothesis.
5. To compare the result obtained with reported similar research work.

The paper is organized as follows: Sect. 2 explores related work and Sect. 3 illustrates proposed method and dataset used. The results with discussion is covered in Sect. 4 and the Sect. 5 presents conclusion with future scope.

2 Related Work

Epilepsy seizure prediction has been a subject of interest because of its potential to boost patient outcomes by allowing treatment at the earliest time possible. One of the biggest components in building the models of seizure predictions is with the right choice of the channels of the EEG. The current literature review focuses on the issue of channel selection techniques and their implications for seizure prediction.

Coşgun et al. (2021) [7] prove that not all EEG channels are equally valuable to predict seizure. This study offers a way of choosing a set of informative channels which increases the signal-to-noise ratio and increases prediction quality. This study presents the patient specific technique to select the channels based on the variance difference between preictal and interictal clips. Several criteria for channel selection have been put forward with a view to enhance seizure prediction. Wang et al. (2022) [15] discussed a patient specific approach with a channel increment strategy together with 1-D convolutional neural networks for seizure prediction based on intracranial EEG data. Besides enhancing the prediction accuracy, the method enhances computational efficiency. The study pays much attention to the kind of channels that capture different features of the seizure activity; this improves the interpretability and effectiveness of the model. All electrodes of EEG brain signal are not relevant for seizure prediction and detection as it is dependent on type of seizure. [11]. Some researchers already have used channel selection approaches to reduce the number of channel set for efficient seizure prediction [3,14]. Das et al. [9] represent the principle component analysis based method based channel selection method and selected 5 channels, achieving an average accuracy of 72.92%, with a sensitivity of 88.55% on the CHB-MIT Daatset.

3 Proposed Method

3.1 Dataset

The CHB-MIT EEG recordings are provided by the Massachusetts Institute of Technology (MIT) USA, which is an open-source EEG database collected at the Children's Hospital Boston [10]. This database consists of the EEG recording of 23 patients (18 females and 5 males) with intractable seizures. Recording hours are not same for all subjects, and vary person to person. Mostly it contains one hour recording clip but for subject 4 it is 2 to 4 h recording clips. The age of the subjects ranges from 1.5 to 22 years. All the EEG wave signals are sampled at 256 Hz using the international 1020 system of EEG electrode positions. The database consists of 916 h of continuous scalp EEG and contains 157 seizure events. Majorly recording contains 23 electrodes for recording but some files contain 24 or 26 electrodes. Most of the EEG signal recorded continuously but some of the recording interrupted in between and there is a gape between recording files. If we think in the term of real-time application the type of seizure, seizure event period and pre-ictal period is not same for all the subjects, so by focusing on these variations, some constraints are fixed to select the group of some subjects which confine our study to one direction.

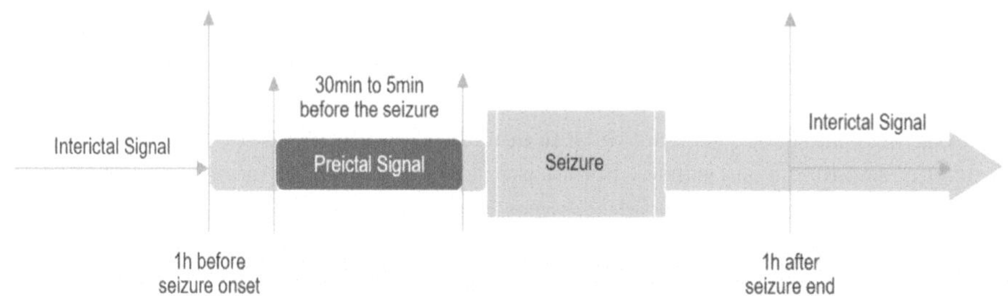

Fig. 1. Epileptic seizure phases.

In the case of seizure prediction, the seizure occurrence period (SOP) is defined as the period during which a seizure event is expected to arise and the seizure prediction hour is the period from an alert buzzer to beginning of the SOP [12]. Preictal period is defined as the sum of SOP and seizure prediction horizon (SPH) together. According to the previous research work, there is no fixed standard value of SOP and SPH were considered because they vary person to person and also depend on artifacts and physical activity of subject etc. [4]. Figure 1 represents the different phases of seizure signal. For this study, the subject with continuous recording without interruption and who carry atleats 23 channels is selected. The preictal time is selected as 5-min - 30 min (continuous availability) before seizure onset for prediction with condition as subject should be in normal state atleast for 1 h before next seizure. If the gape duration between two seizure is less than an hour then, the interictal period from that period is not possible to extract because of the overlapping of postictal of previous seizure and preictal of next seizure. Interictal signal extracted one hour before and after the seizure event. In this case, the seizure with previous seizure is merged and only the onset of first seizure is used. Twelve subjects are selected for this study as given in Table 1 from CHB-MIT dataset based on the conditions.

3.2 System Architecture

This section discusses the proposed system architecture presented by Fig. 2 which consists many steps like preprocessing the raw signal, feature learning with multi channel, ranking the channels, selection of highly dominants channels for seizure period, classification on different group of channels. As shown in Fig. 3, it has been noticed that "T8-P8" is duplicated as channel 15 and channel 23. Figure 3 represents the sharp difference between seizure signal (right side of blue line) and seizure free (left side of blue line) signal. The signal with 10 s window size which contains 2560 samples (sampling frequency = 256) is segmented in preprocessing

Table 1. Selected dataset for this study from open CHB-MIT datset

Case	Gender	Age	Seizure type	Brain location	No. of Seizure	Duration of No. of recording
chb01	F	11	SP, CP	Frontal	7	40:33:08
chb03	F	14	SP, CP	Frontal	7	38:00:06
chb05	F	07	CP, GTC	Frontal	5	39:00:10
chb07	F	14.5	SP, CP, GTC	Temporal	3	67:03:08
chb08	M	3.5	SP, CP, GTC	Frontal	5	20:00:23
chb09	F	10	CP, GTC	Tempotal/Occipital	4	67:52:18
chb10	M	3	SP, CP, GTC	Temporal	7	50:01:24
chb17	F	12	SP, CP, GTC	Temporal	3	21:00:24
chb18	F	18	SP, CP	Frontal	6	35:38:05
chb20	F	6	SP, CP, GTC	Temporal/Parietal	8	27:36:06
chb21	F	13	SP, CP	Temporal/Parietal	4	32:49:49
chb22	F	9	-	Temporal	3	31:00:11
chb23	F	6	-	Temporal	7(*5)	26:33:30

**:- No. of seizures after merging.*

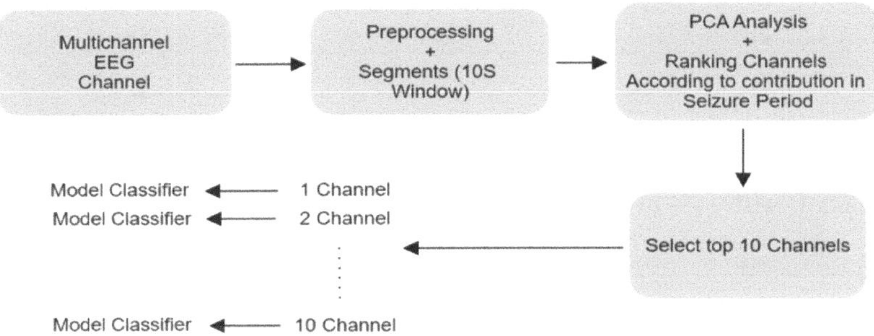

Fig. 2. System Architecture

and labeled the segment as discussed in previous section. Preictal segment labled as 1 and interictal segment labeled as 0. Since the interictal and preictal intervals are highly unbalanced 50% overlapping with sliding window for preictal interval is used to generate extra preictal segments as shown in Fig. 4 and non-overlapping sliding window for interictal interval. Table 3 gives full information about the interictal clips and preictal clips of each subject

Different cerebral rhythms of brain waves are classified based on their range of frequency which is shown in Table 2 so the time-frequency features from the scalp EEG wave signals are captured. Figure 5 shows the frequency spectra of interictal and preictal sEEGs recorded by the 23-channel seizure advisory system in subject 1 (chb01). It can be noticed that, for both interictal and preictal sEEGs, a significant amount of brain wave information is concentrated in the low-frequency band (less than 50 Hz), where there is no much relevant information in the high-frequency band (greater than 50 Hz).

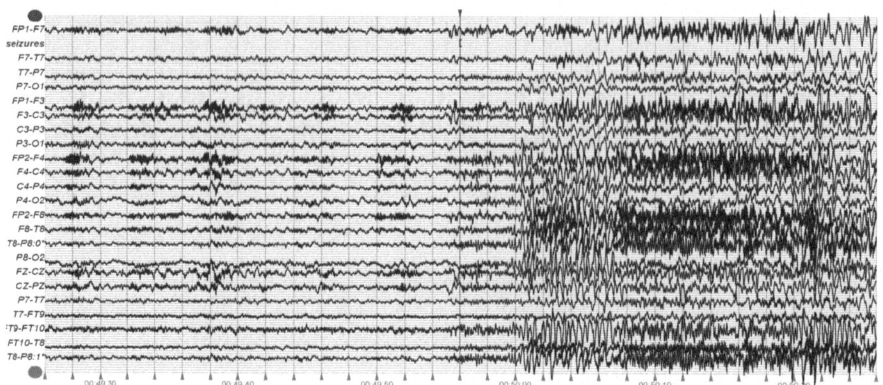

Fig. 3. EEG recording example of subject 1

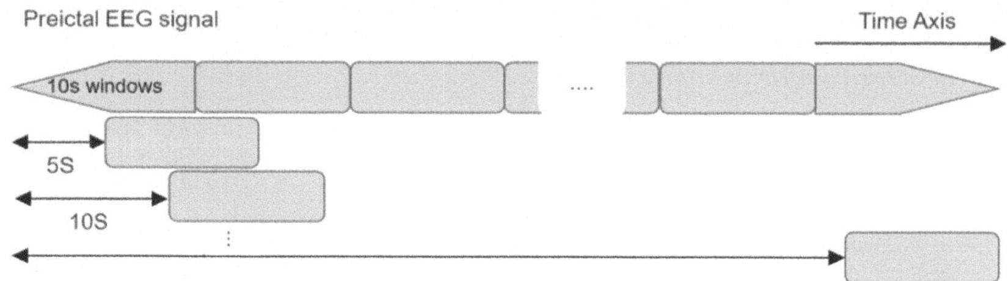

Fig. 4. Overlapped sampling technique to generate extra preictal segments by sliding a 10 s window with 50% overlapping along the time axis.

In this study, the Short Time Fourier Transform (STFT) is used to obtain a time - frequency representation of each scalp EEG segment. First interictal and preictal intervals partitioned into shorter segments of equal sample length and then the Fourier transform is computed for each individual segment per channel for time-frequency parameter computation. As EEG is non-stationary signal, the power spectral is a function of time and frequency. Figure 6 shows the three-dimensional spectrogram of a 10 - min preictal scalp EEG signal clip which is evident that the signal power of EEG signal decays along the frequency axis.

The power spectrogram $P(t, \omega)$ is given by:

$$P(t, \omega) = |\text{STFT}\{x(t)\}(t, \omega)|^2 \tag{1}$$

where:

- $\text{STFT}\{x(t)\}(t, \omega)$ is the Short-Time Fourier Transform of the signal $x(t)$ at time t and frequency ω.
- $|\cdot|$ denotes the magnitude of the complex number.
- Squaring the magnitude yields the power.

Table 2. Rhythms of distinct frequency ranges:

S.No	Wave	Frequency Band	Brain State	Location
1	Deltawave (δ)	0.5 Hz–4 Hz (slowest)	Deeep sleep, Dreaming, mental Comma state	Everywhere
2	Thetawaves (θ)	4 Hz–8 Hz	Creative thought, stress, Deep Meditaion, Drowsiness	Temporal and partial
3	Alphawaves (α)	8 Hz–12 Hz	Calm Mental states, Relaxation, Restful	Occipital and Parietal
3	betawaves (β)	12 Hz–30 Hz	Busy active mind, attention, coordination	Parietal and frontal
4	Gamamwaves(γ)	greater than 30 Hz	Motor functions, problem solving, concentration, multitasking work	Occipitalheight

In this research, channels are selected by PCA due to the fact that the PCA is dimensionality reduction technique which transforms original features into a new set of features called principal components. The principal components are linear combinations of the original features. These principal components are ordered by the amount of variance as explained in the data, so the first few components usually capture most of the information. The variance graph as shown in Fig. 7 visually represents how much of the total variance in the dataset is captured by each principal component. Enough components (from 4–8 components varying per subject) have been selected to explain a significant amount 95% of variance, and the remaining components can be discarded to reduce dimensionality without losing significant information. These new features are not directly interpretable in terms of the original feature names but capture the most variance in the data. To understand which original features contribute most to the principal components, one has to look at the loading of the PCA components. Each principal component is a weighted combination of the original features. The weights (loading) indicate the contribution of each original feature to the principal component. According to the contribution of each feature for principal component ranking of channels is done. After channel selection the power spectral density of each segment per selected channel is considered as input data for the binary classification.

PCA involves the following steps: Data Centering, Covariance Matrix, Eigen Decomposition, Projection, Feature loadings etc. For each channel x_j, the contribution to a specific principal component PC_i is given by the absolute value $|w_{ij}|$ of its loading score. To evaluate the total importance of each channel across all selected components the sum of the absolute loading scores over the chosen k components is taken. So, if we select k components out of n the channel contribution c_j for channel x_j is:

$$c_j = \sum_{i=1}^{k} |w_{ij}|$$

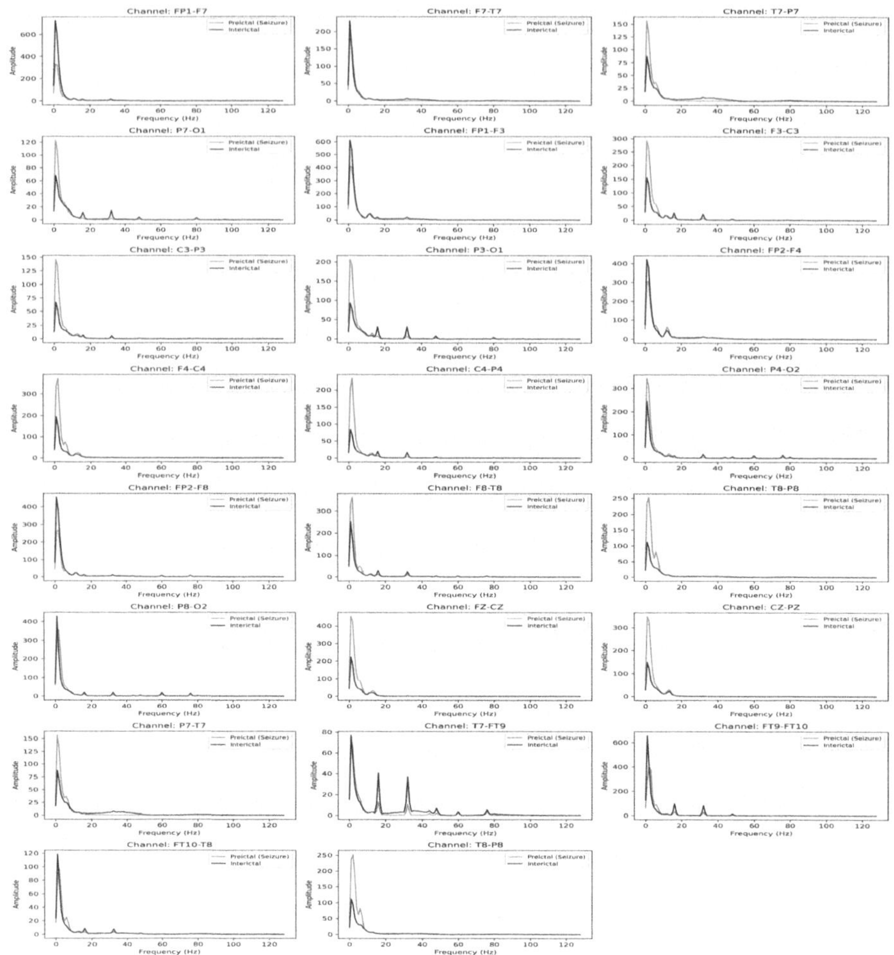

Fig. 5. Frequency spectra of preictal (red) and interictal (blue) sclap-EEG signals collected by the 23 scalp electrodes (channels) of the seizure advisory system in Subject 1. (Color figure online)

where:

- w_{ij} is the loading score for channel x_j in component PC_i.
- k is the number of principal components chosen to explain a certain percentage of the variance.

3.3 ML Based Classifier

The SVM classifier is used to classify events as either epileptic or non-seizure. SVM is a model of supervised learning in artificial intelligence usually utilized

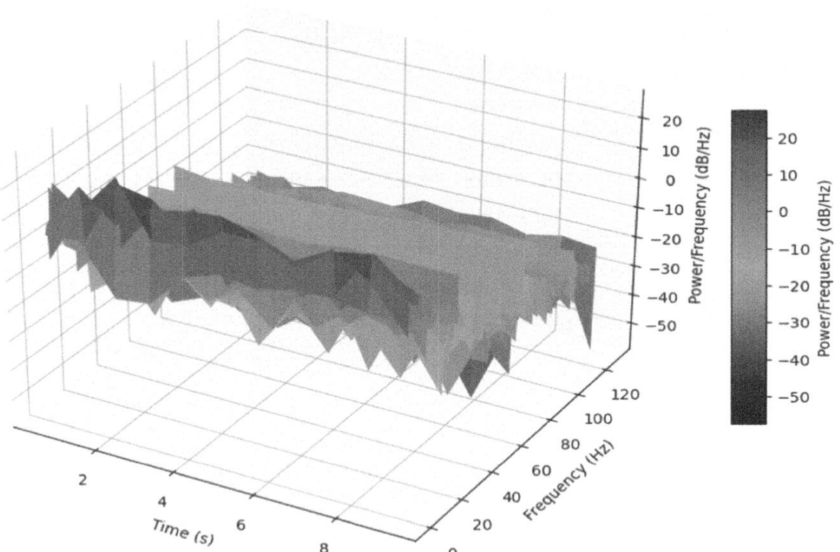

Fig. 6. 3D Spectrogram of a 10-min preictal sEEG segment.

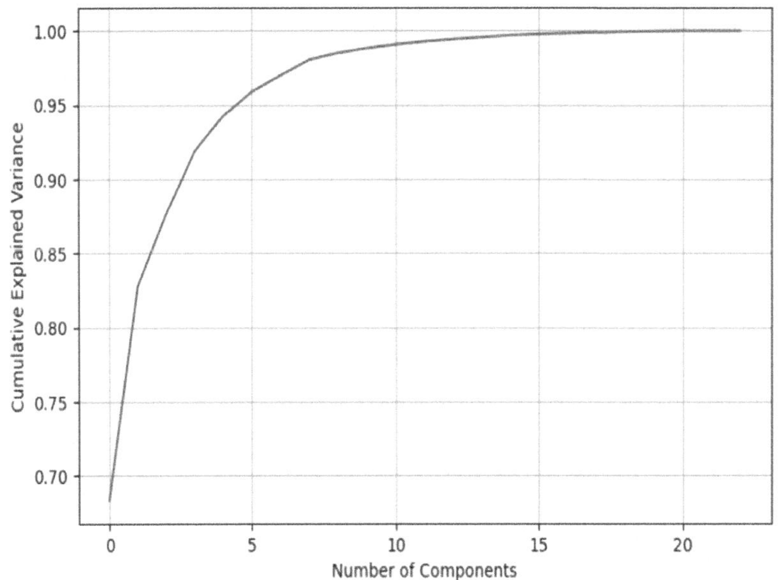

Fig. 7. Explained Variance by PCA Components for subject 1

Table 3. Description of the dataset use for this study and selected channels using PCA

Subject	Recording hr	30 min preictal		Selected channels by PCA interictal
chb01	40:33:08	12929	32257	8, 6, 15, 21, 5, 9, 17, 0, 14, 4
chb03	38:00:06	11160	12939	6, 19, 8, 21, 5, 13, 8, 7, 22, 0, 1
chb05	39:00:10	11082	48964	19, 1, 9, 5, 6, 17, 18, 16, 7, 10
chb07	67:03:08	3004	20885	10, 17, 4, 16, 6, 22, 0, 11, 21, 13, 3
chb08	20:00:23	884	5402	22, 15, 21, 0, 1, 12, 17, 8, 3, 6, 13
chb09	67:52:18	7440	20981	10, 3, 13, 19, 12, 8, 21, 16, 22, 5
chb10	50:01:24	12962	12984	6, 9, 3, 11, 0, 3, 7, 1, 22, 18, 13
chb17	21:00:24	5666	6480	19, 9, 11, 10, 0, 22, 16, 15, 3, 5, 17
chb18	35:38:05	11673	32403	19, 17, 14, 9, 10, 8, 13, 2, 18, 16
chb20	27:36:06	8291	11412	3, 16, 21, 17, 19, 10, 7, 22, 9, 13, 12
chb21	32:49:49	7364	10439	3, 21, 15, 14, 6, 2, 18, 17, 13, 19
chb22	31:00:11	5577	10081	21, 3, 11, 5, 12, 19, 16, 7, 8, 10, 4
chb23	31:00:11	6334	11985	17, 5, 15, 16, 22, 19, 8, 6, 14, 11

*Note: 'FP1-F7'-**0**, 'F7-T7'-**1**, 'T7-P7'-**2**, 'P7-O1'-**3**, 'FP1-F3'-**4**, 'F3-C3'-**5**, 'C3-P3'-**6**, 'P3-O1'-**7**, 'FP2-F4'-**8**, 'F4-C4'-**9**, 'C4-P4'-**10**, 'P4-O2'-**11**, 'FP2-F8'-**12**, 'F8-T8'-**13**, 'T8-P8'-**14**, 'P8-O2'-**15**, 'FZ-CZ'-**16**, 'CZ-PZ'-**17**, 'P7-T7'-**18**, 'T7-FT9'-**19**, 'FT9-FT10'-**21**, 'FT10-T8'-**22**.*

for recognition of patterns, categorization and regression modeling. It was previously employed as an outstanding performance predictor in numerous prior research [13]. The RBF-SVM is employed rather than an linear-SVM to get better accuracy with lower number of EEG channels. Hype-parameter tuning is employed for the other parameters (c and γ).

The equation for the SVM classifier is given by:

$$f(x) = \text{sign}(w^T x + b) \tag{2}$$

The optimization objective of SVM is to minimize:

$$\frac{1}{2}\|w\|^2 \tag{3}$$

subject to

$$y_i(w^T x_i + b) \geq 1, \quad for\, all\, i \tag{4}$$

4 Results and Discussion

This research work focuses on segment based analysis without any post processing. Four parameters are used for the analysis of the effectiveness of proposed epilepsy diagnosis method: correctness (ACC), specialization (SPE) sensitivities (SEN) for each patient.

$$Accuracy = \frac{TP + TN}{TP + TN + FP + FN} \tag{5}$$

$$Precision = \frac{TP}{TP + FP} \tag{6}$$

$$Recall = \frac{TP}{TP + FN} \tag{7}$$

$$FPR = \frac{FP}{FP + TN} \tag{8}$$

The proposed method is evaluated based on CHB-MIT dataset. The comparison is assessed by metrics such as number of channels, type of features, accuracy, sensitivity, specificity and FPR. In the experiments, Anaconda Navigator 3.5.2.0 and Python 3.10 are used to simulate the brain waves using computer with intel core i7 processor, and 16 GB of RAM and Windows 10 (64-bit) operating system. Table 4, represents the accuracy, sensitivity and FPR of selected channels. The result clearly shows the impact of the number of channels for early seizure prediction. As the number of channel increases the result increases gradually but then gets almost saturated. Figure 8 represents the average analysis of parameters for each channel. The graph clearly shows that the accuracy, sensitivity and FPR/Hr get saturated at average number of channels (5–6) (Table 5).

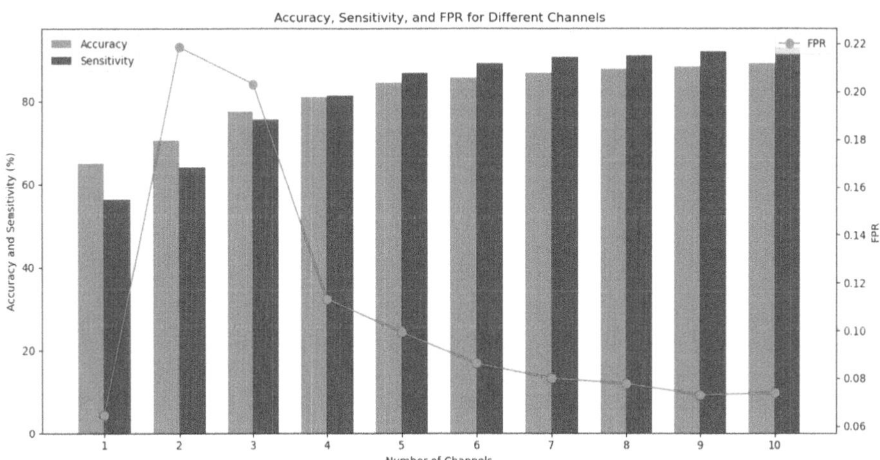

Fig. 8. Accuracy, Sensitivity, and FPR for Different Channels.

Table 4. Results of segment-based performance assessment on CHB-MIT EEG data for top 10 channels

sub id		No. Of Channels									
		1	2	3	4	5	6	7	8	9	10
chb01	Acc	52	66	77	80	84	86	86	87	87	87
	Sen	51	69	87	87	90	92	94	94	95	95
	FPR(1/H)	0.04	0.13	0.10	0.08	0.08	0.06	0.06	0.06	0.06	0.06
chb03	Acc	57	65	72	75	77	79	80	81	83	83
	Sen	59	67	77	82	85	86	88	89	90	92
	FPR (1/H)	0.05	0.15	0.12	0.10	0.10	0.09	0.09	0.09	0.08	0.08
chb05	Acc	88	88	90	91	92	93	94	94	95	96
	Sen	33	36	43	49	58	64	69	69	75	77
	FPR (1/H)	0.02	0.0003	0.0003	0.0002	0.0002	0.0002	0.0002	0.0001	0.0001	0.0001
chb07	Acc	99	99	99	100	100	100	100	100	100	100
	Sen	58	64	88	100	100	100	100	96	96	96
	FPR (1/H)	0.0003	0.0007	0.0002	0.0002	0.0002	0.0002	0.0002	0.0001	0.0001	0.0001
chb08	Acc	89	93	98	100	100	100	100	100	100	100
	Sen	85	96	100	100	100	100	100	100	100	100
	FPR(1/H)	0.005	0.08	0.08	0.03	0.00	0.00	0.00	0.00	0.00	0.00
chb09	Acc	69	76	81	84	85	85	87	88	88	89
	Sen	66	71	81	87	91	93	94	96	96	97
	FPR(1/H)	0.0054	0.19	0.16	0.13	0.12	0.11	0.11	0.10	0.10	0.10
chb10	Acc	52	56	60	63	72	76	79	80	82	83
	Sen	51	57	60	63	72	76	79	80	82	83
	FPR(1/H)	0.05	0.12	0.12	0.10	0.09	0.08	0.08	0.07	0.07	0.07
chb17	Acc	59	62	73	81	85	88	88	90	91	91
	Sen	60	63	79	85	90	92	94	95	95	95
	FPR(1/H)	0.18	0.29	0.28	0.24	0.17	0.15	0.12	0.12	0.11	0.10
chb18	Acc	65	71	78	81	84	84	85	86	85	87
	Sen	58	63	71	83	87	89	89	91	90	92
	FPR(1/H)	0.05	0.12	0.10	0.09	0.08	0.07	0.060.06	0.06	0.06	0.06
chb20	Acc	55	59	76	83	87	88	89	90	92	92
	Sen	54	60	78	87	92	93	94	95	96	96
	FPR(1/H)	0.08	0.06	0.19	0.18	0.12	0.09	0.07	0.07	0.06	0.05
chb21	Acc	52	63	67	72	76	78	78	79	79	81
	Sen	52	64	73	77	84	88	88	88	89	91
	FPR(1/H)	0.05	0.24	0.19	0.19	0.17	0.16	0.16	0.16	0.16	0.16
chb22	Acc	54	64	73	75	79	70	80	82	83	84
	Sen	52	65	77	81	85	88	92	91	91	91
	FPR(1/H)	0.19	0.27	0.24	0.20	0.19	0.17	0.17	0.17	0.17	0.15
chb23	Acc	53	54	64	67	77	84	82	83	83	84
	Sen	54	57	67	71	84	88	86	87	89	90
	FPR(1/H)	0.12	0.26	0.27	0.22	0.20	0.16	0.12	0.12	0.11	0.13
Avg	Acc	64.92	70.46	77.53	80.92	84.46	85.46	86.76	87.69	88.30	89
	Sen	56.38	64	75.61	81.23	86.61	89.07	90.53	90.84	91.84	92.76
	FPR	0.064	0.218	0.203	0.113	0.099	0.086	0.080	0.077	0.07	0.073

Table 5. Existing channel selection approaches vs. our approach

Ref.	#Patient	Selection Method	Channels	Acc	Sen	FPR/h
[9]	23	PCA based channels selection and Variational Mode Decomposition	5	79.92	88.55	NR
[6]	10	Ranking based on PCA and combination testing	18	86.7	NR	NR
[5]	23	Randon forest Ranking	3	NR	80.87	2.5/h
[3]	23	Neural network with attention mechanism mechanism	2	71.91	78.90	0.35
Our approach	13	Ranking based on contribution o n PCA component and top 1 to 10 channels testing	1–10	avg 85% to 89%	89% to 92.76%	0.07 to 0.08

5 Conclusion

In this study, we present the patient specific approach for seizure prediction with minimum number of EEG channels. Since the seizure event has dependencies on number of channels the proposed approach analyzes the various parameters of seizure detection based on different number of channels combinations. The proposed method achieves average 92.76% sensitivity and 0.07 FPR/h with 10 channels. According to the Table 4, it is proved that the proposed approach uses only six channels to predict epileptic seizures without loosing any accuracy and the same as evident from Fig. 8. By reducing the number of electrodes, the prediction time as well as computation complexity has been reduced significantly. Less number of electrodes beneficial for the design of low power wearable EEG system for the real-time monitoring and prediction. As future work, the performance can be improved by adding more time frequency features and required EEG channels can be further reduced.

Acknowledgment. The research work is supported by Chip to Startup (C2S) project sponsored by Ministry of Electronics and Information Technology (MeitY), New Delhi, India.

References

1. World health organization (WHO). Epilepsy fact sheet (2020). https://www.who.int/news-room/fact-sheets/detail/epilepsy. Accessed 09 July 2018
2. Acharya, J.N., Hani, A.J., Cheek, J., Thirumala, P.D., Tsuchida, T.N.: American clinical neurophysiology society guideline 2: guidelines for standard electrode position nomenclature. J. Clin. Neurophysiol.: Off. Publ. Am. Electroencephalogr. Soc. **33 4**, 308–11 (2016). https://api.semanticscholar.org/CorpusID:23136047
3. Affes, A., Mdhaffar, A., Triki, C., Jmaiel, M., Freisleben, B.: Personalized attention-based EEG channel selection for epileptic seizure prediction. Expert Syst. Appl. **206**, 117733 (2022). https://doi.org/10.1016/j.eswa.2022.117733, https://www.sciencedirect.com/science/article/pii/S0957417422010144
4. Alaei, H.S., Mohammad, A.K., Gorji, A.: Optimal selection of sop and SPH using fuzzy inference system for on-line epileptic seizure prediction based on eeg phase synchronization. Aust. Phys. Eng. Sci. Med. **42**(4), 1049–1068 (2019). https://www.proquest.com/scholarly-journals/optimal-selection-sop-sph-using-fuzzy-inference/docview/2325192245/se-2. Copyright - Australasian Physical Engineering Sciences in Medicine is a copyright of Springer (2019). All Rights Reserved; Last updated - 2023-11-19

5. Birjandtalab, J., Baran Pouyan, M., Cogan, D., Nourani, M., Harvey, J.: Automated seizure detection using limited-channel EEG and non-linear dimension reduction. Comput. Biol. Med. **82**, 49–58 (2017). https://doi.org/10.1016/j.compbiomed.2017.01.011, https://www.sciencedirect.com/science/article/pii/S0010482517300185
6. Chakrabarti, S., Swetapadma, A., Pattnaik, P.K.: A channel selection method for epileptic EEG signals. Adv. Intell. Syst. Comput. (2018). https://api.semanticscholar.org/CorpusID:69632804
7. Coşgun, E., Çelebi, A., Güllü, M.K.: A channel selection method for epilepsy seizure prediction. In: 2021 International Conference on INnovations in Intelligent SysTems and Applications (INISTA), pp. 1–5 (2021). https://doi.org/10.1109/INISTA52262.2021.9548583
8. Costa, G., Teixeira, C., Pinto, M.: Comparison between epileptic seizure prediction and forecasting based on machine learning. Sci. Rep. (2024)
9. Das, P., Manikandan, M.S., Ramkumar, B.: Detection of epileptic seizure event in EEG signals using variational mode decomposition and mode spectral entropy. In: 2018 IEEE 13th International Conference on Industrial and Information Systems (ICIIS), pp. 42–47 (2018). https://doi.org/10.1109/ICIINFS.2018.8721426
10. Goldberger, A.L., et al.: PhysioBank, PhysioToolkit, and PhysioNet: components of a new research resource for complex physiologic signals. Circulation (2000)
11. Jana, R., Mukherjee, I.: Deep learning based efficient epileptic seizure prediction with EEG channel optimization. Biomed. Signal Process. Control **68**, 102767 (2021). https://doi.org/10.1016/j.bspc.2021.102767
12. Li, C., Deng, Z., Song, R., Liu, X., Qian, R., Chen, X.: EEG-based seizure prediction via model uncertainty learning. IEEE Trans. Neural Syst. Rehabil. Eng. **31**, 180–191 (2022). https://api.semanticscholar.org/CorpusID:253184182
13. Raghu, S., Sriraam, N., Temel, Y., Rao, S.V., Hegde, A.S., Kubben, P.L.: Performance evaluation of DWT based sigmoid entropy in time and frequency domains for automated detection of epileptic seizures using SVM classifier. Comput. Biol. Med. **110**, 127–143 (2019). https://doi.org/10.1016/j.compbiomed.2019.05.016, https://www.sciencedirect.com/science/article/pii/S0010482519301726
14. Romney, A., Manian, V.: Optimizing seizure prediction from reduced scalp EEG channels based on spectral features and MAML. IEEE Access **9**, 164348–164357 (2021). https://doi.org/10.1109/ACCESS.2021.3134166
15. Wang, X., Zhang, C., Kärkkäinen, T., Chang, Z., Cong, F.: Channel increment strategy-based 1D convolutional neural networks for seizure prediction using intracranial EEG. IEEE Trans. Neural Syst. Rehabil. Eng. **31**, 316–325 (2023). https://doi.org/10.1109/TNSRE.2022.3222095

Design and Development of Flexible Tactile Sensor Based Force Myography Device

Sanjeet Kumar Maddheshiya[1](✉), Parikshith Chavakula[1], Priya Ranjan Muduli[2], Neeraj Sharma[1], and Deepesh Kumar[1]

[1] School of Biomedical Engineering, Indian Institute of Technology (BHU) Varanasi, Varanasi, India
sanjeetkmaddheshiya.rs.bme23@itbhu.ac.in

[2] Department of Electronics Engineering, Indian Institute of Technology (BHU) Varanasi, Varanasi, India

Abstract. Wearable technologies have revolutionized muscle activity monitoring, offering significant advances in fields such as prosthetics, rehabilitation, and human-computer interaction. While Electromyography (EMG) has been a staple in capturing muscle signals, it comes with limitations like precise electrode placement, noise susceptibility, and user discomfort. Force Myography (FMG) emerges as a promising alternative, using pressure variations on the skin to detect muscle movements. This study introduces a novel flexible tactile sensor array, integrated into an armband for FMG applications, aimed at improving muscle signal monitoring. The sensor array was fabricated using piezoresistive materials, specifically Velostat, which offers flexibility and durability. Eight customized sensors were arranged in an armband structure, capturing forearm muscle movements and translating them into electrical signals. The developed FMG armband was tested for hand gesture recognition in five healthy participants, achieving an average classification accuracy of 96.34% ± 2.5% using the Random Forest classifier. This work demonstrates the potential of flexible FMG-based wearable devices, providing an accurate, cost-effective, and user-friendly alternative to traditional methods. It paves the way for applications in neurorehabilitation and human-computer interaction.

Keywords: Hand gesture classification · Force myography · FSR Armband · Piezoresistive · Tactile sensor

1 Introduction

Wearable technologies are now commonly utilized to monitor muscle activities and record movement-related metrics [1, 2]. Accurate detection and interpretation of muscle activity signal can lead to significant advancement in prosthetics, physical rehabilitation, and human-computer interaction [3, 4]. Traditionally, Electromyography (EMG) has been the primary method for capturing muscle signals [5]. However, EMG has limitations, including the need for precise electrode placement, susceptibility to noise, and

K. Atul et al. (Eds.): BodyNets 2024, LNICST 666, pp. 495–504, 2026.
https://doi.org/10.1007/978-3-032-16099-7_39

discomfort during extended use [6]. In contrast, Force Myography (FMG) offers a less invasive and more user-friendly alternative by detecting changes in muscle volume and stiffness through pressure variations on the skin [7]. FMG has demonstrated effectiveness in various applications, such as prosthetic control [8]. Rehabilitation [9, 10], and gesture recognition [11], making it a robust option for muscle signal monitoring. FMG, in particular, does not necessitate considerable skin preparation or specialized electrode positioning, nor does it necessitate specialist knowledge for optimal deployment [12]. Other benefits include greater signal stability over time for static gestures, resistance to external electrical interference and sweating, simpler signal processing compared to EMG datasets, and cost-effectiveness [13]. These issues are critical for deploying FMG-based wearable devices in the general population.

Recently, FMG has gained traction due to its simplicity and reliability. Studies have shown that FMG can be particularly effective in prosthetic control, where accurate gesture recognition is essential [14]. Despite its advantages, a significant challenge in FMG systems lies in designing sensors that can accurately capture muscle movements while ensuring user comfort [15]. Traditional FMG devices often rely on rigid sensors, which can limit comfort and restrict the range of detectable muscle movement [16]. This limitation has led to increased interest in developing flexible, durable, and sensitive sensors that can conform to the body's natural contours without sacrificing accuracy.

Flexible sensors, especially fabric-based piezoresistive sensors, have shown great promise in addressing these challenges [17]. These sensors offer flexibility, lightweight construction, and the ability to conform to complex body shapes, making them ideal for wearable applications [18]. While previous studies have explored the use of fabric sensors in various fields, such as healthcare monitoring and soft robotics, their application in FMG is still relatively new [19].

The objective of this research is to design and develop a flexible tactile sensor array using fabric-based piezoresistive materials, integrated into an armband for FMG applications. The primary goal is to demonstrate that a customized, flexible tactile sensor can accurately capture forearm muscle movements and that these signals can be used to classify different hand gestures using machine learning techniques [20]. This work not only contributes to the advancement of FMG technology but also offers valuable insights into the potential applications of flexible tactile sensors in wearable electronics and human-machine interaction.

2 Materials and Methods

In this study, a non-invasive, wearable FMG band has been designed and its applicability for hand gesture recognition in rehabilitation has been tested. The following sections detail the design and experimental procedure adopted in this study.

2.1 Design of a Force Sensitive Resistor

In this study, a fabric-based piezoresistive tactile sensor was developed to be used as a force-sensitive resistor (FSR). The piezorestive material's resistance has inverse relationship with the applied pressure and therefore can be utilized to develop tactile sensor. The piezoresistive tactile sensor is made up of a force-sensitive material known as Velostat, which is a composite polymer material formed of a carbon-impregnated polyethylene [21]. Velostat is created by converting dielectric polyethylene into an electrically conductive composite material by embedding carbon powder, making it part of the piezoresistive material family. This versatile material is widely used, particularly in the development of flexible sensors, which are highly sought after in biomedical and mechatronic applications [22]. As shown in Fig. 1(a), the fabrication process involves layering velostat between the conductive fabric. The conductive fabric is made up by combining different fibers, such as cotton or nylon, and conductive metals, such as copper, silver, and stainless steel. To safeguard the circuitry, a stretch cotton layer is fused at both the top and bottom of the sensor. When pressure is applied to the sensing unit the piezoresistive material deforms and alters the resistance, which is then used to characterize the applied pressure.

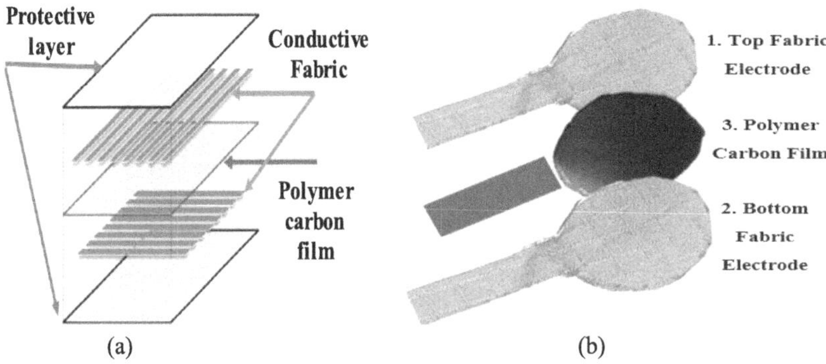

Fig. 1. (a) Schematic of fabric-based FSR sensor design (b) prototype of FSR sensor developed

2.2 Design of Force-Myography (FMG) Arm Band

The FSR sensor developed in the previous section is then used to create an armband for the FMG analysis of forearm muscles. For this, we interconnected eight customized FSR sensors in an armband structure as shown in Fig. 2(a) to transform muscular pressure into electrical impulses. FSRs operate based on the idea that resistance decreases as applied force or pressure increases. When FSRs are directly attached to the human body, there is a chance that the incongruous pressure from the muscle contraction stiffness or the incorrect bending of the FSR will cause unintended outputs and/or damage to the FSR. As a result, each FSR sensor was given a unique casing (Fig. 2(b)) to prevent bending and get rid of the inconsistent muscle contraction pressures. The main purpose of the FSR casing, which was made up of a chassis, was to convey the muscle contraction force from the forearm to the customized FSR sensor. The armband has a slider part whose bottom end slid inside the casing's chassis, while the top end, measuring 40 × 22 mm, is in direct contact with the subject's skin. A 1.2 mm thick, custom-built, little circular step with a diameter of 18 mm was integrated into the upper section. The purpose of this phase was to evenly distribute the muscle power onto the FSR sensor's sensing area. Each FSR sensor with casing in armband measured 42 × 22 × 9.8 mm in size. Polylactic acid (PLA) was used in the 3D printing of the casings' chassis and slider. Figure 2(b) depicts the 3D-printed FSR casing and Fig. 2(c) shows the FSR placed inside the casing (Fig. 4).

Finally, the 35 cm long loop portion of the Velcro strap in the armband had eight customized FSR sensor casings fastened to it. The Velcro strap's hook part was positioned at the bottom of the casing, which made it easier to tighten the casing and helped to modify where the sensor was placed on the strap.

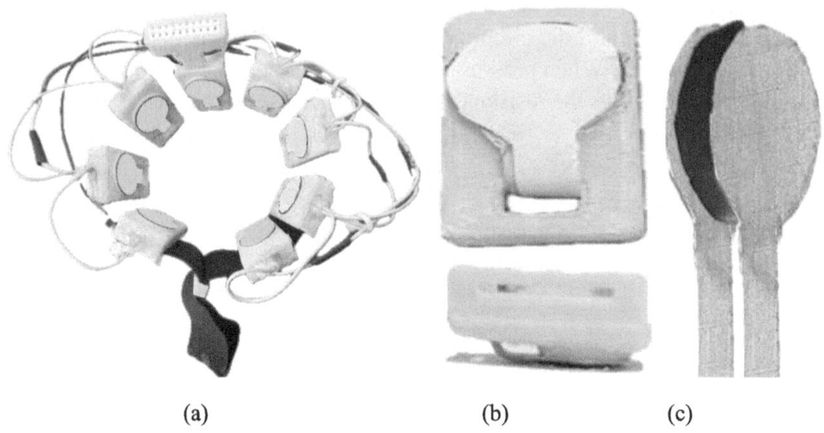

(a) (b) (c)

Fig. 2. (a) FSR armband (b) casing of FSR sensor (c) Designed FSR sensor unitsensor.

2.3 FMG Data Acquisition Systems

Signals from the arm band's FSRs were extracted using the buffered voltage divider circuit as shown in Fig. 3(a). The voltage divider circuit was connected to one of the FSR's two terminals, while the other terminal was connected to a 5V DC source. The force-to-voltage conversion equation for the FSR sensor is given by.

$$V_{out} = \frac{R_m}{R_m + R_{FSR}} \times V_{in} \tag{1}$$

where V_{in} is the input voltage, R_{FSR} is the resistance of the FSR sensor, and R_m is the ground resistor (the value of R_m selected for this study was 10 kΩ). (Punetha et al., 2023).

The voltage divider circuit's signals were digitalized using an Arduino Mega board that had a 16 MHz ATmega2560 CPU and a 10-bit analog-to-digital converter (ADC). The schematic of the data acquisition from the FMG band is shown in the following Fig. 3(b). Using this DAQ system, the FSR sensor data was sampled at a rate of 10 Hz.

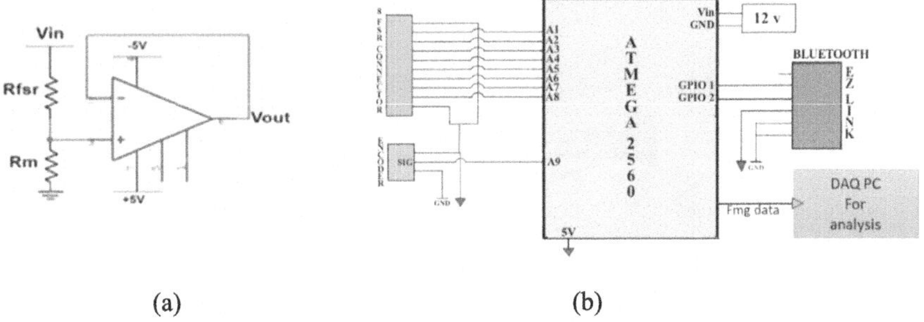

(a) (b)

Fig. 3. (a) Buffered voltage divider circuit for FSR (b) The schematic of the data acquisition system for the FSR armband.

2.4 Sensor Calibration and Measurement Protocol

To evaluate the sensor's performance, a testing apparatus was designed. this device allowed for the application of a known static load (ranging from 0.01 kg to 1 kg) onto a small base directly over the sensor area. During each load application, the sensor's output voltage was recorded.

2.5 Data Collection and Experimental Protocol

To evaluate the performance of the armband for force myography application, we designed a hand gesture recognition experiment. In this experiment, the participants needed to wear the armband on their dominant forearm and perform specific hand gestures. The hand gestures were (1) Hand Close (2) Hand Open (3) Precision Grasp (4) Supination (5) pronation.

For this study, we recruited five healthy participants. Each participant wore the customized FSR armband on their dominant forearm and performed above mentioned series of pre-programmed hand gestures causing various muscular contractions. The participants' characteristics is shown in Table 1. The participants were physically active and free of diabetes or any other skin-related conditions. After receiving both oral and theoretical explanations regarding the experiment, each subject completed an informed permission form prior to participation.

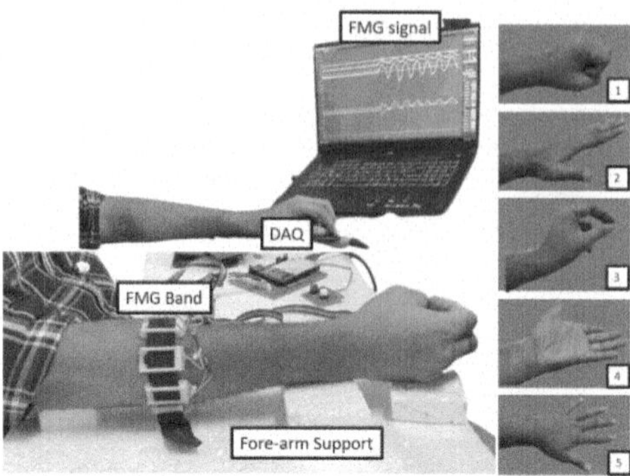

Fig. 4. Experimental setup for FMG recording for hand gesture recognition.

2.6 Feature Extraction and Classification

To analyze the FMG data, we extracted six key statistical features from the preprocessed signals of each of the 8 FMG band channels. These features include mean, median, RMS (Root Mean Square), standard deviation (SD), kurtosis, and skewness. Each feature provides unique insights into the FMG signals, aiding in classification. The mean represents the signal's central tendency, while the median, which is robust against outliers, reflects the data's central location. RMS captures the signal's magnitude, and SD indicates the variability around the mean. Kurtosis measures the tail heaviness, with higher values suggesting more outliers, and skewness assesses asymmetry, revealing potential biases in measurement.

Once the features were extracted, the feature matrix was fed to the classifier for hand gesture classification. Among various classical machine learning algorithms, the Random Forest algorithm was employed for this purpose [23]. Random Forests (RF) construct multiple decision trees during the training process, aggregating their predictions to enhance accuracy and robustness, thus providing a reliable approach for classification tasks.

To evaluate classifier performance, the data was split into 80% training and 20% testing sets, collected from all subjects. The confusion matrix, a table describing classifier performance, was used to assess true positive, true negative, false positive, and false negative rates. Additionally, accuracy metrics were derived from this split, providing a comprehensive assessment of each classification algorithm's effectiveness.

3 Result and Discussions

3.1 Custom-Built Sensor Calibration Curve

As discussed in Sect. 2.4, calibration of the developed FSR sensor was performed by placing a static load ranging from 0.01 kg to 1 kg and recording the sensor's response. Figure 5 shows the calibration curve (load vs. output voltage) of the developed sensor, presented for five different values of pull-up resistors. The curves demonstrate that the customized FSR sensor exhibited high sensitivity to pressure variations, with a linear response for a 10 kΩ pull-up resistor in the range of 0.01 kg to 1 kg (0.1–10 N).

The force sensors fabricated from velostat and conductive fabric exhibited a close to linear relationship between applied force and output voltage. Notably, the sensor displayed a higher sensitivity, which could be optimized by incorporating a resistor with a value of less than 10kΩ in the voltage divider circuit to achieve stable readings.

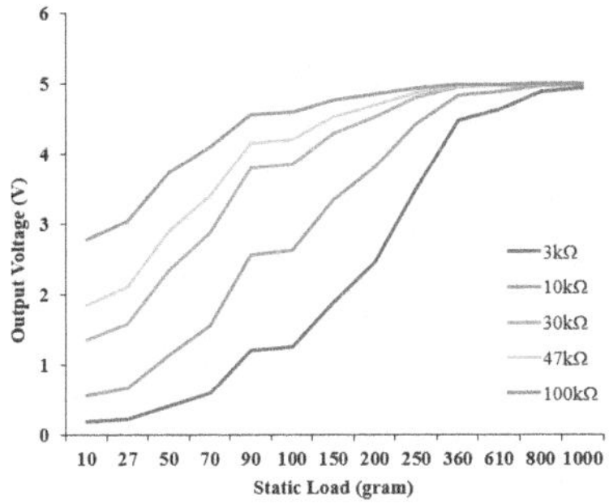

Fig. 5. Load vs output voltage curve of the developed FSR sensor

3.2 Pattern of Recorded FMG

The FMG band, comprising eight sensors, was rigorously tested for signal stability and effectiveness in capturing FMG signals. Preliminary assessments revealed high repeatability in the sensor's output across various hand gestures, including hand open, hand close, precision grip, supination, and pronation of the forearm. This consistency was crucial in ensuring reliable data collection from multiple subjects. The signal patterns for different gestures are depicted below in Fig. 6.

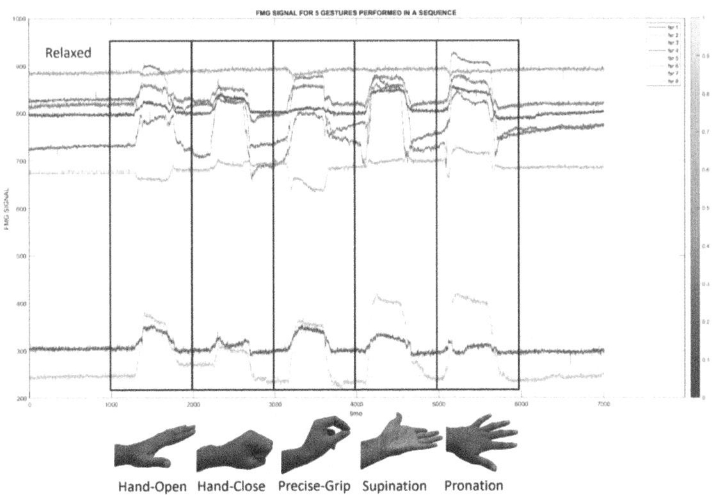

Fig. 6. FMG signals acquired for various gestures

3.3 Hand Gesture Classification

The results of hand gesture classification are presented here. Multiclass classification (6 hand gesture classes) was performed using the Random Forest classifier. A holdout approach was adopted for classification, with 80% of the collected data used for training and the remaining 20% for testing. Five-fold cross-validation was applied to eliminate bias in the training and testing data.

Figure 7 shows the confusion matrix obtained by the classifier. In the confusion matrix shown, the rows represent the actual gestures, and the columns represent the predicted gestures. The diagonal entries indicate the proportion of correctly classified gestures, while the off-diagonal entries represent the proportion of misclassified gestures. Using the Random Forest classifier, we were able to achieve an average classification accuracy of 96.34% ± 2.5%. This result underscores the potential of the developed custom-built FSR armband sensors for hand gesture recognition applicable to neurorehabilitation applications.

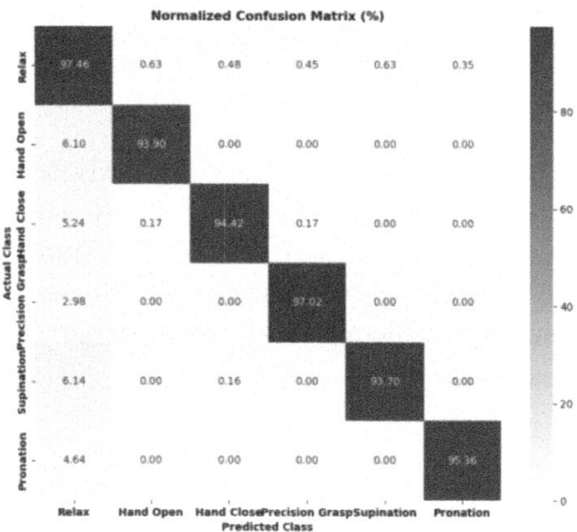

Fig. 7. Confusion matrix and classification performance of hand gesture recognition

4 Conclusion and Future Work

In this study, a novel design and development of a flexible tactile sensor array integrated into an armband for FMG applications was proposed. The focus was on creating a customized, fabric-based piezoresistive sensor capable of accurately capturing forearm muscle movements. These bespoke sensors not only matched the accuracy and linearity of commercial counterparts but also significantly reduced costs, offering an accessible alternative. The force-myography armband, equipped with eight such sensors, underwent rigorous calibration and testing, with five healthy volunteers performing six distinct hand and forearm gestures. Using Random Forest-based machine learning models, the study achieved impressive hand gesture classification accuracy of 96.34% ± 2.5%.

This study highlights the significant potential of flexible FMG-based sensor arrays, emphasizing their adaptability for wearable technologies in prosthetics, rehabilitation, and human-computer interaction. The development of cost-effective, personalized sensors could bridge the gap between technology and human movement, offering new opportunities for individuals. However, the study has some limitations, including the need to improve the sensing range and sensitivity by optimizing the piezoresistive material. Additionally, the experiment was conducted with a small sample of participants and focused on simple hand gestures. Future research could expand the participant pool to include individuals with upper limb movement disorders and explore more complex hand gestures to further assess the capabilities of the FMG armband.

Acknowledgment. The authors would like to express their gratitude to the Department of Biotechnology (DBT) for supporting this research through funding.

References

1. Filippeschi, A., Schmitz, N., Miezal, M., Bleser, G., Ruffaldi, E., Stricker, D.: Survey of motion tracking methods based on inertial sensors: a focus on upper limb human motion. Sensors **17**(6), 1257 (2017). https://doi.org/10.3390/s17061257
2. Punetha, D., Kumar, A., Pandey, S.K., Chakrabarti, S.: Wearable piezoelectric nanogenerator-based hazardous gas monitoring gadget for self-powered ammonia early warning. In: Kymissis, I., List-Kratochvil, E.J., Inal, S. (eds.) Organic and Hybrid Sensors and Bioelectronics XVI, p. 28. SPIE (2023). https://doi.org/10.1117/12.2678555
3. Cesqui, B., Tropea, P., Micera, S., Krebs, H.I.: EMG-based pattern recognition approach in post stroke robot-aided rehabilitation: a feasibility study. J. Neuroeng. Rehabil. **10**, 75 (2013). https://doi.org/10.1186/1743-0003-10-75
4. Al Rumon, M.A., et al.: ElboSense: a novel capacitive strain sensor for textile-based elbow movement monitoring. In: 2023 IEEE 19th International Conference on Body Sensor Networks (BSN), pp. 1–4. IEEE, Boston (2023). https://doi.org/10.1109/BSN58485.2023.10433120
5. Raez, M.B.I., Hussain, M.S., Mohd-Yasin, F.: Techniques of EMG signal analysis: detection, processing, classification and applications. Biol. Proced. Online **8**, 11–35 (2006). https://doi.org/10.1251/bpo115
6. Boyer, M., Bouyer, L., Roy, J.-S., Campeau-Lecours, A.: Reducing noise, artifacts and interference in single-channel EMG signals: a review. Sensors **23**(6), 2927 (2023). https://doi.org/10.3390/s23062927
7. Delva, M.L., Lajoie, K., Khoshnam, M., Menon, C.: Wrist-worn wearables based on force myography: on the significance of user anthropometry. Biomed. Eng. Online **19**(1), 46 (2020). https://doi.org/10.1186/s12938-020-00789-w
8. Gharibo, J.S., Naish, M.D.: Multi-modal prosthesis control using sEMG, FMG and IMU sensors. In: Annual International Conference on IEEE Engineering in Medicine and Biology Society, vol. 2022, pp. 2983–2987 (2022). https://doi.org/10.1109/EMBC48229.2022.9871586
9. Sadarangani, G.P., Jiang, X., Simpson, L.A., Eng, J.J., Menon, C.: Force myography for monitoring grasping in individuals with stroke with mild to moderate upper-extremity impairments: a preliminary investigation in a controlled environment. Front. Bioeng. Biotechnol. **5**, 42 (2017). https://doi.org/10.3389/fbioe.2017.00042
10. Kumar, D., Goyal, Y., Nair, S., Chauhan, A., Lahiri, U.: Design of a physiologically informed virtual reality based interactive platform for individuals with upper limb impairment. In: The 23rd IEEE International Symposium on Robot and Human Interactive Communication, pp. 112–117. IEEE, Edinburgh (2014). https://doi.org/10.1109/ROMAN.2014.6926239

11. Jiang, X., Merhi, L.-K., Xiao, Z.G., Menon, C.: Exploration of force myography and surface electromyography in hand gesture classification. Med. Eng. Phys. **41**, 63–73 (2017). https://doi.org/10.1016/j.medengphy.2017.01.015
12. Castellini, C., et al.: Proceedings of the first workshop on peripheral machine interfaces: going beyond traditional surface electromyography. Front. Neurorobotics **8**, 22 (2014). https://doi.org/10.3389/fnbot.2014.00022
13. Jiang, S., Gao, Q., Liu, H., Shull, P.B.: A novel, co-located EMG-FMG-sensing wearable armband for hand gesture recognition. Sens. Actuat. Phys. **301**, 111738 (2020). https://doi.org/10.1016/j.sna.2019.111738
14. Ahmadizadeh, C., Pousett, B., Menon, C.: Investigation of channel selection for gesture classification for prosthesis control using force myography: a case study. Front. Bioeng. Biotechnol. **7**, 331 (2019). https://doi.org/10.3389/fbioe.2019.00331
15. Xiao, Z.G., Menon, C.: A review of force myography research and development. Sensors **19**(20), 4557 (2019). https://doi.org/10.3390/s19204557
16. Wang, H., Zuo, S., Cerezo-Sánchez, M., Arekhloo, N.G., Nazarpour, K., Heidari, H.: Wearable super-resolution muscle-machine interfacing. Front. Neurosci. **16**, 1020546 (2022). https://doi.org/10.3389/fnins.2022.1020546
17. Yin, Y., Guo, C., Li, H., Yang, H., Xiong, F., Chen, D.: The progress of research into flexible sensors in the field of smart wearables. Sensors **22**(14), 5089 (2022). https://doi.org/10.3390/s22145089
18. Liu, Y., Wang, H., Zhao, W., Zhang, M., Qin, H., Xie, Y.: Flexible, stretchable sensors for wearable health monitoring: sensing mechanisms, materials, fabrication strategies and features. Sensors **18**(2), 645 (2018). https://doi.org/10.3390/s18020645
19. Alvarez, J.T., et al.: Toward soft wearable strain sensors for muscle activity monitoring. IEEE Trans. Neural Syst. Rehabil. Eng. Publ. IEEE Eng. Med. Biol. Soc. **30**, 2198–2206 (2022). https://doi.org/10.1109/TNSRE.2022.3196501
20. Pyun, K.R., et al.; Machine-learned wearable sensors for real-time hand-motion recognition: toward practical applications. Natl. Sci. Rev. **11**(2), nwad298 (2024). https://doi.org/10.1093/nsr/nwad298
21. Lee, K.T., Chee, P.S., Lim, E.H., Kam, Y.H.: Data glove with integrated polyethylene-carbon composite-based strain sensor for virtual reality applications. Chem. Eng. Technol. **46**(12), 2480–2486 (2023). https://doi.org/10.1002/ceat.202200569
22. Dzedzickis, A., et al.: Polyethylene-carbon composite (Velostat®) based tactile sensor. Polymers **12**(12), 2905 (2020). https://doi.org/10.3390/polym12122905
23. Shi, H., Jiang, X., Dai, C., Chen, W.: EMG-based multi-user hand gesture classification via unsupervised transfer learning using unknown calibration gestures. IEEE Trans. Neural Syst. Rehabil. Eng. **32**, 1119–1131 (2024). https://doi.org/10.1109/TNSRE.2024.3372002

Design of a Flexible Metasurface-Based Dual Bandpass Filter in ISM and IoT Bands Towards Wearable Applications

Arjab Sengupta[1(✉)], Soham Banerjee[1], Vishnu Kumar Mishra[2], Gobinda Sen[1], Sayan Sarkar[1], Ardhendu Kundu[1], and Somak Bhattacharyya[2]

[1] Department of Electronics and Communication Engineering, Institute of Engineering and Management, Gurukul, Block-EP, Sector-V, Salt Lake Electronics Complex, Kolkata Y-12700 091, West Bengal, India
Arjab.Sengupta2022@iem.edu.in

[2] Electronics Engineering Department, Indian Institute of Technology (BHU), Varanasi 221 005, Uttar Pradesh, India

Abstract. This work presents a single layered metasurface (MS)-based slot type dual bandpass wearable filter with low insertion loss and sharp roll off performances. The substrate material selected is jeans, having a relative permittivity of 1.68; thereby making the design wearable in nature. The proposed structure's unit cell comprises mainly three shapes of slots viz., a rectangular ring, a square and a dumbbell-shaped. The filter exhibits two transmission peaks at 2.45 GHz and 4.7 GHz, respectively and hence is well suited for biomedical applications at the ISM and IoT bands. Furthermore, the proposed filter also has a good stop band in between the transmission bands and hence can be useful for wearable applications. The 3-dB transmission bandwidths of the wearable filter have been computed as 1.21 GHz and 0.86 GHz respectively. The electric field distributions at the transmission peaks are studied to understand the roles of the various slots in the final design. The angular stability of the proposed filter is also analyzed under incident angle variation to find its potential use in various wearable applications.

Keywords: Metasurface · Dual bandpass filter · Wearable spatial filter · Slot type FSS

1 Introduction

The use of 2-D metamaterials, also known as metasurfaces (MSs), have been instrumental in improving the electromagnetic phenomena of devices operating over a broad range of frequencies [1–3]. The manipulation of electromagnetic (EM) properties of the devices has helped researchers significantly in finding applications over a wide range viz., filters, antenna, polarization converters, absorbers, cloaking [4–8]. MS filters are nowadays being increasingly preferred over other types of conventional filters due to the compact,

K. Atul et al. (Eds.): BodyNets 2024, LNICST 666, pp. 505–512, 2026.
https://doi.org/10.1007/978-3-032-16099-7_40

angularly stable and low-profile features, making them mounted on any transceivers system. Further, the use of conductive textiles as substrates is also becoming popular, due to the growing usages in wearable devices such as sensors, relays, etc. [9]-[10].

Various MS-based filtering structures have been explored recently in the microwave frequency range. Gil *et. al* [11] had earlier provided a study on the combination of many metasurface filters, using resonating transmission lines. Depending upon the structural orientation to the polarization state of the incident EM wave, planar self-complementary metasurfaces have also been used as bandstop or bandpass filters [12]. Qu *et al.* [13] proposed a frequency selective surface (FSS) for providing a bandpass response at 2.4 GHz. In some works, transmission line approach has been employed for achieving wide-band bandpass filters [14]. A large number of metasurface-based filters have come into existence, including both metallic screen printing as well as printing on bulk electric [13, 15–18]; thereby limiting the filter's flexibility. Moreover, MS-based filters have faced challenges in attaining optimal performances by maintaining a good angular stability and flexibility simultaneously [10]; hence limiting their wide range of applications. MSs potentially use the interaction of surface waves across gaps and dielectric spaces [19], where the surface currents can lead (or lag) depending upon the individual resonating elements, which can be spatially changed as and when desired. This phenomenon enables to tune wavefronts while passing through a metasurface, thereby opening up a wide range of solutions [20]. To achieve such results, a large number of research works have been done and tested for designing bandpass filters in the radio frequency domain [21–25].

This article presents a low-profile, low loss, high roll off MS-based dual band spatial filter having passbands centered at 2.45 GHz and 4.7 GHz; thereby finding a wide range of wearable applications in the IoT and ISM bands. The design geometry has been kept concise and simple, having an outer rectangular ring-shaped slot, a pair of dumbbell-shaped slots and a total of six square slots on both the inner side of the rectangular ring. The corresponding insertion losses observed at the 2.45 GHz and 4.7 GHz are less than 0.5 dB; thus, providing negligible attenuation and hence is well suited for spatial filter applications. In addition, a wide stopband has also been realized at 4 GHz with a high roll-off feature; resulting in a good separation between the transmission bands. All the designs and analyses are performed with high frequency simulator ANSYS HFSS v2023.

This article is arranged in number of sections, Sect. 1 discusses about the background of the conducted research. In Sect. 2, the proposed structure's design methodology is demonstrated and in the next section, the results along with the experimental analyses, are given. Finally in the conclusion part, the novelty of the wearable filter is highlighted with potential applications.

2 Design Methodology

Figs. 1(a) and 1(b) show the top and perspective views of the unit cell geometry of the proposed dual band wearable spatial filter. The unit cell of the proposed structure has dimensions of 30 mm × 30 mm and is designed on a 0.5 mm thick jeans substrate (relative permittivity of 1.68, loss tangent = 0.02) [26] which makes the structure flexible; thereby making it wearable in nature. The metallic patch is made of copper, having a thickness of 35-micron. The unit cell of the proposed filter is geometrically simple and is made by cutting distinct slots (white colored in Fig. 1) from the copper sheet (light blue colored in Fig. 1). The design comprises of a rectangular ring slot combined with a pair of dumbbell shaped slots at the center and 3 smaller square slots on each side of the unit cell to make the filter functional at the desired frequencies. The optimized geometrical dimensions of the structure are mentioned in the caption of Fig. 1. All the design modelling and simulations under periodic boundary conditions of the proposed filter are obtained with ANSYS HFSS 2023 v2.

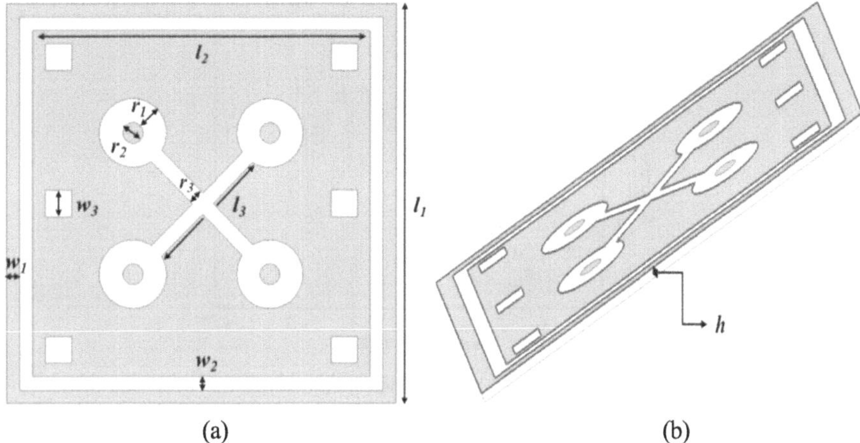

Fig. 1. (a) Top and (b) perspective views of the proposed metasurface-based bandpass filter for wearable applications. (Dimensions: *l1* = 30 mm, *l2* = 27 mm, *l3* = 12 mm, *w1* = 1.5 mm, *w2* = 1 mm, *w3* = 2 mm, *r1* = 2.48 mm, *r2* = 0.8 mm, *r3* = 1.1 mm, *h* (thickness) = 0.5 mm).

3 Results and Discussion

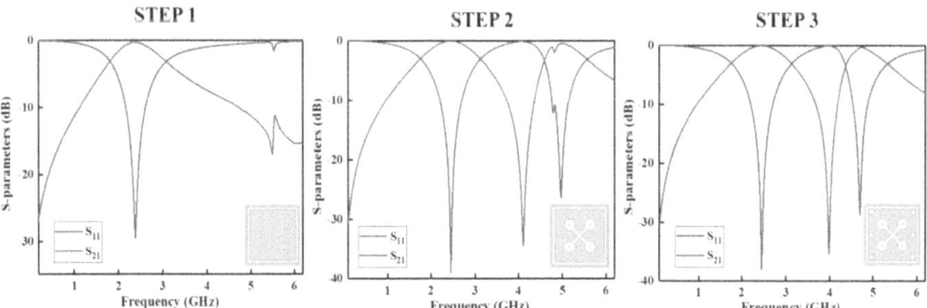

Fig. 2. Evolution of the proposed structure of the unit cell in multiple steps.

The illustrations in Fig. 2 provide the design evolution of the proposed MS-based structure and their corresponding responses. There are majorly three steps involved in the design. Initially, an outer rectangular ring shape slot is cut out from the metallic sheet (Step 1). This results in the formation of a single bandpass window having a center frequency at 2.4 GHz with an insertion loss of 0.22 dB. In the second step, a pair of dumbbell shaped slots are etched out, giving rise to an uneven dual bandpass response having center frequencies at 2.4 GHz and 4.7 GHz together with low insertion losses. Finally, in step 3, three square slots have been etched out on each side of the dumbbell shaped slots. This incorporation resulted in a dual band pass response at 2.45 GHz and 4.7 GHz having extremely low insertion loss values of 0.08 dB and 0.34 dB and high return loss values of 37.29 dB and 28.21 dB, as depicted in Fig. 3 clearly.

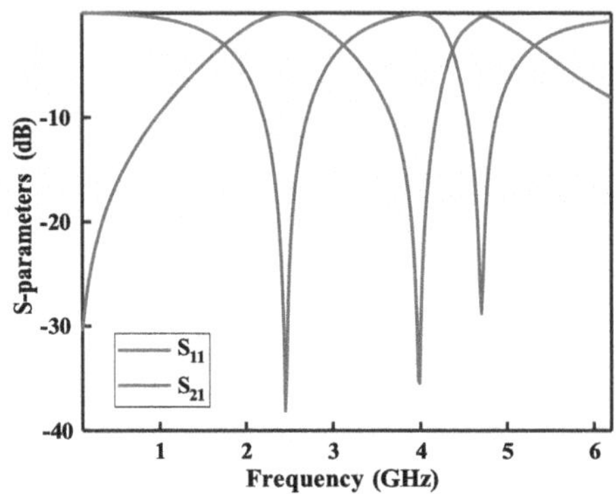

Fig. 3. Depiction of reflection and transmission parameters of the proposed filter

The frequency responses of the reflection and transmission coefficients of the final unit cell under periodic boundary conditions have been shown in Fig. 3, which elaborates a dual pass band response at 2.45 GHz and 4.7 GHz along with one band stop response at 4 GHz. The respective insertion losses of 0.08 dB and 0.34 dB are observed at the frequencies 2.45 GHz and 4.7 GHz, respectively. The 1-dB bandwidths are computed as 0.55 GHz and 0.77 GHz at 2.45 GHz and 4.7 GHz respectively while the respective 3-dB bandwidths are 1.21 GHz and 0.86 GHz at the two bands.

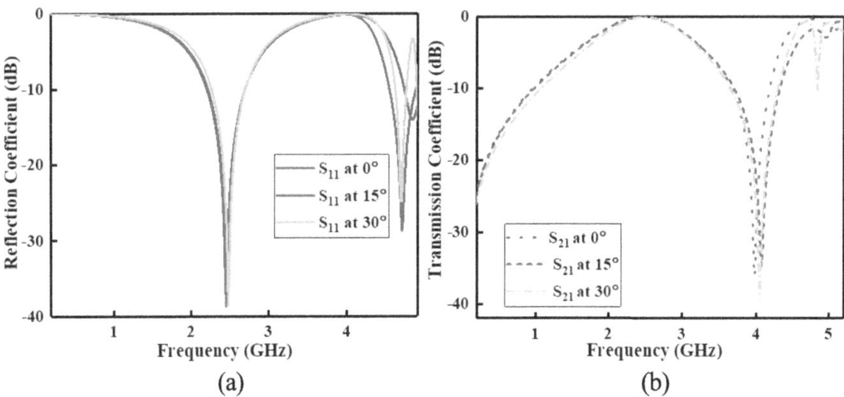

Fig. 4. Frequency responses of (a) reflection and (b) transmission coefficients under oblique incidence.

The angular stability of the proposed structure has been studied with respect to different incident angles of the EM waves. Fig. 4(a) depicts the variation of the reflection coefficient with the changes in incident angle whereas, Fig. 4(b) illustrates the same for the transmission coefficient. It has been noticed that the proposed structure has been found to be stable for incident angles of up to 30°. Further, a strong attenuation of 35.51 dB has been achieved at 4 GHz; thereby strongly rejecting the satellite communication frequency band.

The electric field distributions of the proposed filter have also been studied and observed at the passband frequencies, i.e., 2.45 GHz and 4.7 GHz in Fig. 5(a) and Fig. 5(b), respectively. It is noted from Fig. 5 that the electric fields are found to be maximum at around the outer and inner slots respectively at 2.45 GHz and 4.7 GHz, thereby highlighting their roles in yielding the dual passband response.

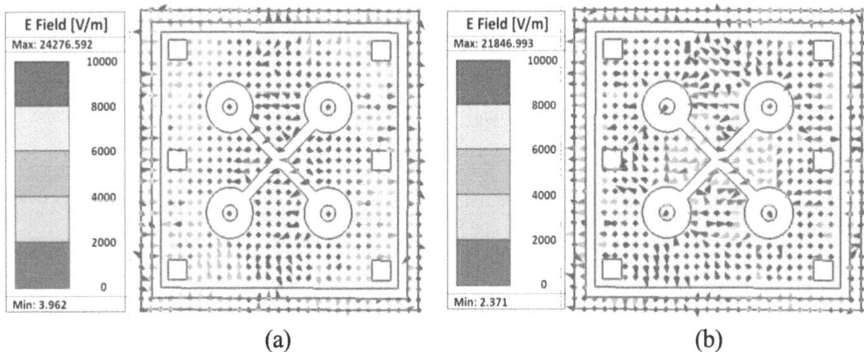

Fig. 5. Electric field distributions on the unit cell of the structure at the two transmission peaks viz., (a) 2.45 GHz and (b) 4.7 GHz.

The performance of the proposed design structure has been compared with some of the existing works listed in Table I and emphasizes the superiority of the proposed work in terms of efficient behavior and multiband performances suitable for both ISM and IoT bands maintaining compactness and ultra-thin feature. Moreover, the use of jeans substrate makes the structure flexible in nature making it suitable for various wearable applications (Table 1).

Table 1. Comparison of proposed design with existing bandpass filters

Reference No	No. of bands	Frequencies (GHz)	Unit cell size (λ0)	Thickness (mm)	-3 dB BW (*Δf/fo*)
[27]	1	6.78	0.018 × 0.018	0.76	43%
[28]	1	330	0.207 × 0.207	0.188	32%
[16]	1	10.4	0.276 × 0.276	0.964	32%
[29]	1	10.3	0.26 × 0.26	2.6	87%
[30]	1	405	0.353 × 0.353	0.261	27%
This Work	2	2.45, 4.7	0.25 × 0.25	0.535	49.29%, 17.84%

4 Conclusion

This work presents a low profile, compact and flexible spatial bandpass filter with simple slot type geometry for simultaneous applications in both the ISM and IoT bands. The choice of jeans as a substrate makes the structure flexible and thus enhances the wearable nature of the filter. Achieving a 1-dB bandwidths of 0.55 GHz and 0.77 GHz and 3-dB bandwidths of 1.21 GHz and 0.86 GHz at 2.45 GHz and 4.7 GHz respectively, the filter shows performances with very low insertion loss (below 0.5 dB) and sharp roll-off; thereby making it suitable for wearable purposes. The dual bandpass responses at both the ISM and IoT frequencies makes the filter suitable for applications in fields like point-to-point communications and satellite communications along with being used for various bio-medical purposes.

References

1. Holloway, C.L., Kuester, E.F., Gordon, J.A., O'Hara, J., Booth, J., Smith, D.R.: An overview of the theory and applications of metasurfaces: the two-dimensional equivalents of metamaterials. IEEE Antennas Propag. Mag. **54**(2), 10–35 (2012). https://doi.org/10.1109/MAP.2012.6230714
2. Bhattacharyya, S.: Metamaterials and metasurfaces for high-frequency applications. In: Photonics, Plasmonics and Information Optics, pp. 31–65. CRC Press (2021)
3. Li, A., Singh, S., Sievenpiper, D.: Metasurfaces and their applications. Nanophotonics **7**(6), 989–1011 (2018)

4. Yang, B., Li, Q., Jia, M., Xiao, S., Zhou, L.: Terahertz metasurface for flexible band-pass filter. In: 2018 International Applied Computational Electromagnetics Society Symposium-China (ACES), pp. 1–2. IEEE (2018)
5. Orazbayev, B., Mohammadi Estakhri, N., Beruete, M., Alù, A.: Metasurface-based ultrathin carpet cloak. In: 2016 10th European Conference on Antennas and Propagation (EuCAP), pp. 1–3. IEEE (2016)
6. Paul, A., Nilotpal, S.B., Dwivedi, S.: Design and mathematical analysis of a metasurface-based THz bandpass filter with an equivalent circuit model. Appl. Opt. **60**(22), 6429–6437 (2021)
7. Munaga, P., Bhattacharyya, S., Ghosh, S., Srivastava, K.V.: An ultra-thin compact polarization-independent hexa-band metamaterial absorber. Appl. Phys. A **124**, 1–12 (2018)
8. Samantaray, D., Bhattacharyya, S.: A metasurface based gain enhanced dual band patch antenna using SRRs with defected ground structure. Radio Sci. **56**(2), 1–13 (2021)
9. Tennant, A., Hurley, W., Dias, T.: Experimental knitted, textile frequency selective surfaces. Electron. Lett. **48**(22), 1386–1388 (2012)
10. Brzeziński, S., Rybicki, T., Malinowska, G., Karbownik, I., Rybicki, E., Szugajew, L.: Effectiveness of shielding electromagnetic radiation, and assumptions for designing the multi-layer structures of textile shielding materials. Fibres Text. Eastern Eur. **1**(72), 60–65 (2009)
11. Gil, M., Bonache, J., Martin, F.: Metamaterial filters: a review. Metamaterials **2**(4), 186–197 (2008)
12. Ortiz, J.D., Baena, J.D., Losada, V., Medina, F., Marques, R., Araque Quijano, J.L.: Self-complementary metasurface for designing narrow band pass/stop filters. IEEE Microwave Wirel. Comp. Lett. **23**(6), 291–293 (2013)
13. Qu, M., Li, B., Sun, S., Li, S.: Angularly stable bandpass frequency selective surface based on metasurface. IEEE Access **8**, 41684–41689 (2020)
14. Sánchez-Soriano, M.Á., Quendo, C.: Systematic design of wideband bandpass filters based on short-circuited stubs and λ/2 transmission lines. IEEE Microwave Wirel. Comp. Lett. **31**(7), 849–852 (2021). https://doi.org/10.1109/LMWC.2021.3076924
15. Cao, Y.F., Zhang, X.Y., Xue, Q.: Compact shared-aperture dual-band dualpolarized array using filtering slot antenna and dual-function metasurface. IEEE Trans. Antennas Propag. **70**(2), 1120–1131 (2021)
16. Lalbakhsh, A., Afzal, M.U., Esselle, K.P., Smith, S.L.: All-metal wideband frequency-selective surface bandpass filter for TE and TM polarizations. IEEE Trans. Antennas Propag. **70**(4), 2790–2800 (2022)
17. Huang, W., Luo, X., Lu, Y., Hu, F., Li, G.: Ultra-broad-band terahertz bandpass filter with dynamically tunable attenuation based on a graphene– metal hybrid metasurface. Appl. Opt. **60**(22), 6366–6370 (2021)
18. Guo, J., Chen, Y., Yang, D., Ma, B., Liu, S., Pan, J.: Design of a circuit-free filtering metasurface antenna using characteristic mode analysis. IEEE Trans. Antennas Propag. **70**(12), 12322–12327 (2022)
19. Eleftheriades, G.V., Balmain, K.G.: Negative-Refraction Metamaterials: Fundamental Principles and Applications. Wiley (2005)
20. Asgari, S., Fabritius, T.: Equivalent circuit model of graphene chiral multi-band metadevice absorber composed of U-shaped resonator array. Opt. Express **28**(26), 39850–39867 (2020)
21. Collin, R.E.: Foundations for Microwave Engineering. Wiley (2007)
22. Orfanidis, S.J.: Electromagnetic waves and antennas (2002)
23. Hesham, M., Abdellatif, S.O.: Compact bandpass filter based on split ring resonators. In: 2019 International Conference on Innovative Trends in Computer Engineering (ITCE), pp. 301–303. IEEE (2019)

24. Hong, Y.-P., Hwang, I.-J., Yun, D.-J., Lee, D.-J., Lee, I.-H.: Design of single-layer metasurface filter by conformational space annealing algorithm for 5G mm- wave communications. IEEE Access **9**, 29764–29774 (2021)
25. Li, T., Chen, Z.N.: Metasurface-based shared-aperture 5G *S* -/ *K* -band antenna using characteristic mode analysis. IEEE Trans. Antennas Propag. **66**(12), 6742–6750 (2018)
26. Khan, H., et al.: Design and analysis of a wearable monopole antenna on jeans substrate for RFID applications. In: IJ Wireless and Microwave Technologies, MECS, pp. 24–35 (2016)
27. Noor, A., Koziel, S.: Dual-Polarized Wideband Bandpass Metasurface-Based Filter. IEEE Antennas Wirel. Propag. Lett. (2023)
28. Pirrone, D., et al.: Metasurface-based filters for high data rate THz wireless communication: Experimental validation of a 14 Gbps OOK and 104 Gbps QAM-16 wireless link in the 300 GHz band. IEEE Trans. Wireless Commun. **21**(10), 8688–8697 (2022)
29. Anwar, R.S., Wei, Y., Mao, L., Ning, H.: Miniaturised frequency selective surface based on fractal arrays with square slots for enhanced bandwidth. IET Microwaves Antennas Propag. **13**(11), 1811–1819 (2019)
30. Sun, D., Qi, L., Liu, Z.: Terahertz broadband filter and electromagnetically induced transparency structure with complementary metasurface. Results Phys. **16**, 102887 (2020)

Development of CNT Based Smart Fabric Sensor for Monitoring Muscle Movement

J. Emmanuel Rajapandian[1], Sabhareesh Prabhuraj[1], V. Pradeep[1], J. M. Subashini[1,2], Hiroya Ikeda[3], and Pandiyarasan Veluswamy[1,4(✉)]

[1] SMart and Innovative Laboratory for Energy Devices (SMILE), Indian Institute of Information Technology Design and Manufacturing (IIITDM), Kancheepuram, Chennai 600127, India
pandiyarasan@iiitdm.ac.in

[2] School of Interdisciplinary Design and Innovation (SIDI), Indian Institute of Information Technology Design and Manufacturing (IIITDM) Kancheepuram, Chennai 600 127, India

[3] Research Institute of Electronics, Shizuoka University, Hamamatsu, Japan

[4] Department of Electronics and Communication Engineering, Indian Institute of Information Technology Design and Manufacturing (IIITDM), Kancheepuram, Chennai 600127, India

Abstract. Smart textile materials have huge applications on wearable physiological monitoring devices. Monitoring of muscular stretch and bending is important for sports and geriatric people due to their continuous physical activities and due to age factors their muscles become weak which leads to muscular disorders. In this research, a carbon nanotube (CNT) based smart fabric is developed for monitoring the bending activities of the hand with respect to wrist moment in different angles of bending. The conductive fabric is developed from cotton fabric, coated with multi-walled carbon nanotube (MWCNT) synthesis using a hydrothermal process. The developed material acts as a sensor which is placed along with the glove near the wrist. The sensor resistance is tested in four different zones. The sensor converts the bending angle stimuli into voltage, such that the various zones within the range of motion of the wrist are comprehended by the algorithm. The range of resistance was monitored with the aid of a serial monitor. The results show resistance values exceeding 190 Ω for the Green Zone; a range of 182–190 Ω for the Yellow Zone; 174–182 Ω for the Red Zone; and resistance values dipping below 174 Ω for extension beyond 51o, where 1000 Ω was used as the known resistance of the circuit.

Keywords: Flexible sensor · carbon nanotube · wrist monitoring · wearable device

---

Supported by organization x.

K. Atul et al. (Eds.): BodyNets 2024, LNICST 666, pp. 513–522, 2026.
https://doi.org/10.1007/978-3-032-16099-7_41

1 Introduction

1.1 A Subsection Sample

The technological development and increasing demand of wearable electronics has made the development of flexible sensors that can monitor various physical parameters like human activities, joint movements and fitness monitoring. One such application is monitoring of joint movement which is more important for sports and geriatric people. Smart textile materials are used in different application in development of flexible sensor. The smart textile material are made of conductive fibers that act as an active sensor to monitor the physical movement occurring in the joint muscles with respect to the bending actions. Electromyography (EMG) is the standard technique for monitoring of muscle activity, where a pair of electrodes are placed on the specific location in human body and the signals are detected [1]. Most commonly needle type of electrodes are used which creates pain to the user when place onto the surface of the skin. Mechanomyographic is another technique for monitoring muscle activity using vibration transducer or piezoelectric crystal contact sensor where the contraction muscle movement is detected [2]. The conventional devices for monitoring of joint movements are developed based on metals and semiconductors that are rigid in nature though some of them are used in wearable applications as electrode [3]. The advantages of using the textile material as conductive substrate are due to its flexibility, stretchability, deformability and highly comfort to the user [4]. There are three types of joints present in human body which are immovable, semi-movable and freely movable. The freely movable joints are called as synovial joints. These synovial joints are classified into six different types namely pivot, hinge, saddle, plane, condyloid and balt-and-socket joint. In this the condyloid joint (joint between radius and carpal bones of wrist) is one of the highly usable joints by human [5,6] shown in Fig. 1. Scientifically, the joint movement occurs through the contraction and relaxation of the muscles and the contractile force related to the change of muscle length at the joint location [7]. With different joint angles, motions and postures, the magnitude of muscle length changes during each contraction. The strength and the health condition of the muscles can be determined by the force generated by the muscles with respect to the joint and angle and postures at different activity levels [8]. To measure the joints condition different tracking techniques are used based on joint angle, joint motion, range of motion (ROM) and skeletal tracking [9].

Smart sensing fabric integrated with garments provides parallel feedback on self-rehabilitation, physical training, and intelligent prosthetics [10]. The Carbon nanotube (CNT) based fabric sensor has been developed by a researcher to monitor the temperature and strain sensing performance, where the CNT fabric sensor is integrated with stretchable fabric and made as a chest band to be worn around the chest for sensing [11]. In a research flexible sensor has been developed in CNT forests onto a poly-dimethyl siloxane (PDMS), where the device can be attached to human body parts, and the strain generated in the particular region is monitored corresponding to a detachable electrical resistance variation [12]. A super stretchable and highly sensitive capacitive strain sensor has been

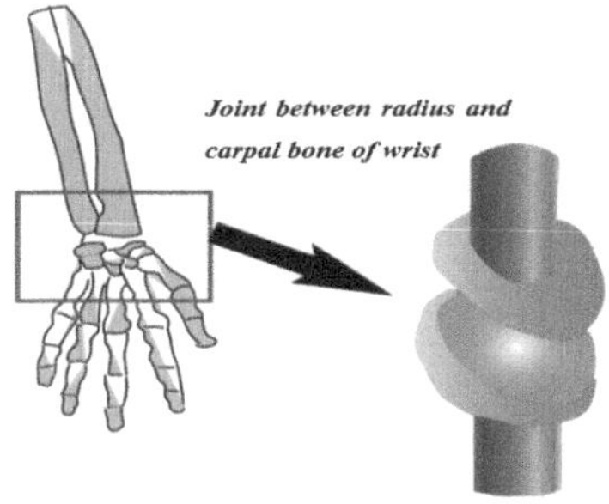

Fig. 1. Illustration of Condyloid joint.

made [13] with CNT CNT-based electrode where the sensor has a fast signal response time of approximately 8ms and also good mechanical deformation. A smart fabric sensor developed by a researcher using a single-walled carbon nanotube (SWCNT) filled with the binary polymer of polyvinylidene fluoride/ poly (3, 4-ethylene dioxythiophene) – poly (styrene sulfonate), used to detect the bending angle, where the sensor response at stable range from 0–120o of angle [14]. Carbon nano materials such as CNTs, have been used in a wide range of sensing applications due to their excellent mechanical property and high electrical conductivity [15]. Thus in this paper, we developed a carbon nanotube (CNT) coated fabric sensor to monitor wrist movement. The CNT sensor shows good electrical conductivity which helps to sense the change in movement of the wrist, where it helps to record the real-time joint activity. The fabricated sensor is connected to an Arduino Uno R3 to measure the change in voltage with respect to time. The conditional code written in the Arduino backend will convert the values accordingly and then display the zone according to the change in the position of the wrist. Figure 2 represents the schematic illustration of the working system.

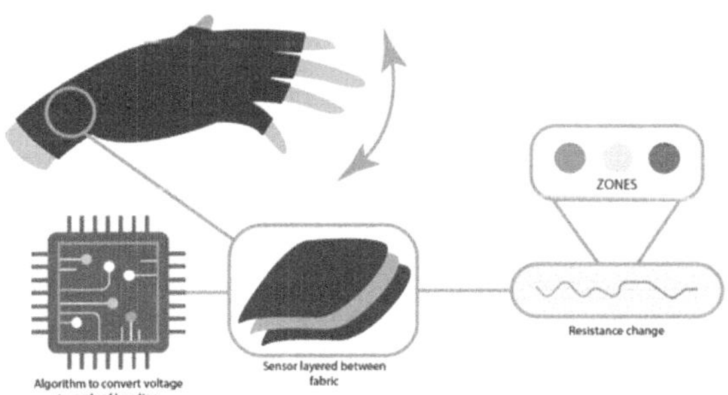

Fig. 2. Schematic representation of system

2 Fabrication of Sensors

2.1 Material

The fabrication of the proposed sensor requires three key components. Multiwalled Carbon Nanotube (MWCNT) powder (sourced from Ad Nano Technologies, Karnataka, India). Liquid Ethanolamine (2-aminoethanol) of Analytical Reagent (AR) grade was bought from Research-Lab Fine Chem Industries, Maharashtra, India. A clean sample of non-dyed cotton fabric was used as the cellulose substrate for the sensor.

2.2 Methodology

The cotton fabric of 5×10 cm is taken scoured in alkaline water and dried for 12 h to remove the impurities that are present in the fabrics. A 0.1 v/V solution of ethanolamine in deionized water is prepared in a beaker and the fabric is dipped into the solution, with a clip being used to position the fabric appropriately. The beaker is then placed on a magnetic stirrer and the solution is stirred for 2 h at a constant speed of 500 rpm. A yellow discoloration of the fabric sample is observed. The fabric is then dried for 60 min under a temperature of 80 °C. A 0.0025 w/V suspension of acidified MWCNT powder in deionized water is then prepared and sonicated for 60 min at an ambient room temperature of 32 °C. The mixture is sonicated to ensure a uniform spread of MWCNT particles in the solvent and prevent cluster formation. The dried fabric is now dipped into the CNT suspension in the ultrasonic sonicator for 2 more hours. A uniform coating of black MWCNT particles is observed on the surface of the cotton substrate. The final step involves drying the sample in a hot air oven for 60 min at 100oC. Figure 3 explains the step-by-step synthesis process.

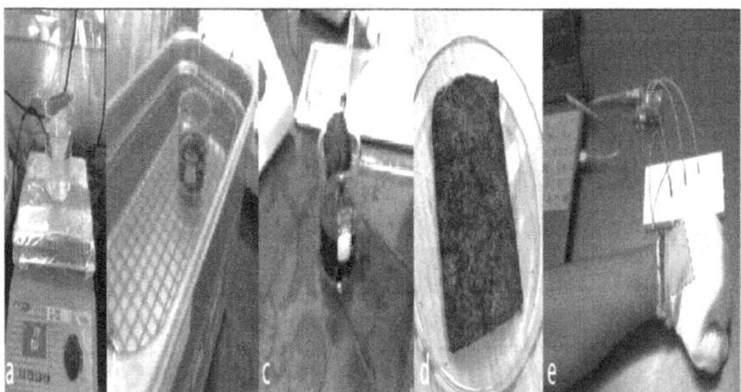

Fig. 3. Synthesis process of CNT fabric sensor a) Fabric is dipped in the solution consisting of ethanolamine b) Sonication of MWCNT powder c) Dipping of fabric into MWCNT d) Dried sample coated with MWCNT

The presence of primary and secondary hydroxy groups in cellulose results in a large network of intra and intermolecular hydrogen bonding, which can be utilized to better the adherence of multi-walled carbon nanotubes onto its surface. MWCNTs due to their excellent conductive properties are an ideal choice for coating onto the cellulose substrate, but due to Vander Waals interactions within itself, tend to form clusters when in a suspension. Therefore, to achieve the desired levels of adherence and spread, slightly acidified MWCNT is made to condense with ethanolamine to form a functionalized molecule. Figure 4 represents the reaction between cellulose treated with ethanolamine and MWCNT during sonication and drying processes. The amino group in the molecule aids in the formation of additional hydrogen bonds with the cellulose and also imparts antimicrobial properties to the sensor itself. A hurdle of adherence and durability in the previous sensors is thus alleviated through this fabrication process.

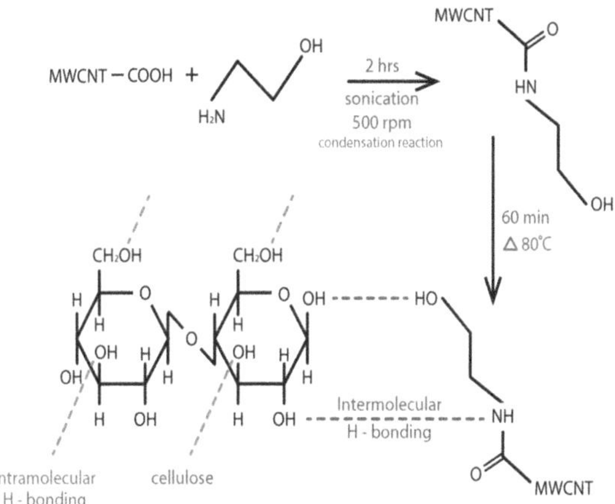

Fig. 4. Reaction between cellulose treated with ethanolamine and MWCNT during sonication and drying processes

3 Anthropometry Study

The study was made to find the correct position for the placement of the sensor. Figure 5 shows the different views of products designed according to the bending motion with the integration of the sensor module. The human wrist has two degrees of freedom of motion, namely extension-flexion and radial-ulnar deviations. The fabricated sensor can detect changes in the angle of bending. The human body has a natural range of motion (ROM). Movement within the proper ROM promotes blood circulation and flexibility which could lead to more comfort and higher productivity. Despite the need to promote motion, users should try to avoid repetitive movements and certain extremes in their ROM over long periods.

Considering the two-dimensional movement of the wrist perpendicular to the forearm axis, the range of motion associated with the movement is classified into

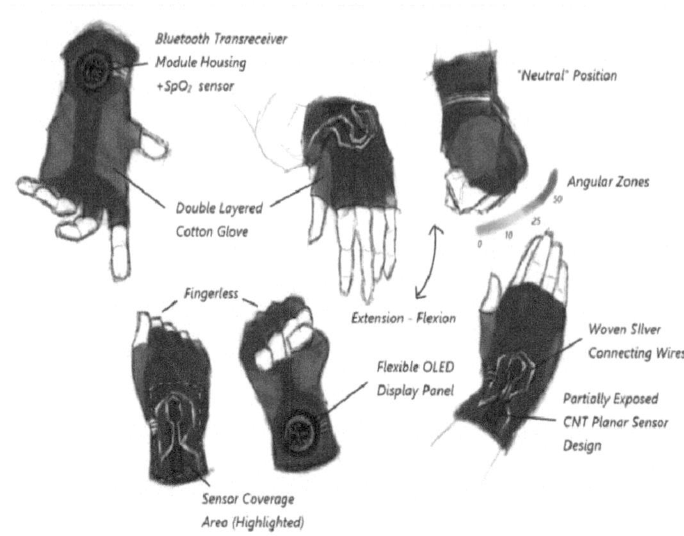

Fig. 5. Illustration of Product Design

four zones based on the angle of bending shown in Fig. 6. For an average human male aged 20, the equilibrium/neutral position of the wrist corresponds to 0–10°, the Green Zone; 11–25° pertains to an admissible Yellow Region; extremities of wrist flexion of 26–50° correspond to a cautious Red Zone; angles exceeding 51° classified as the impermissible Beyond Red Zone. Repetitive actions performed in the red zone and beyond carry potential risk of injuries, and can be determined by the number of times the joint goes beyond the comfort zone - which is within the capacity of the fabricated sensor.

4 Sensor Validation and Inference

The electrical conductivity of the sensor was measured by a digital multimeter. Response of the sensor to wrist bending is used to determine the number of times the wrist joint goes beyond the comfort zone, and this application serves to demonstrate the capability of the sensor to record real-time joint activity. The fabricated sensor is connected to an Arduino Uno R3 to measure raw output data as voltage readings with respect to time. One terminal of the sensor was connected to a fixed power output pin rated at 5 V and the other end was connected to the analog input pin a0 of the Arduino as shown in Fig. 7. A resistor of known resistance is connected between the a0 and ground pins. The input measured by the analog pin corresponds to the potential difference across the known resistance. A conditional code then equates the current across the sensor with the current flowing through the resistor in accordance with Kirchhoff's

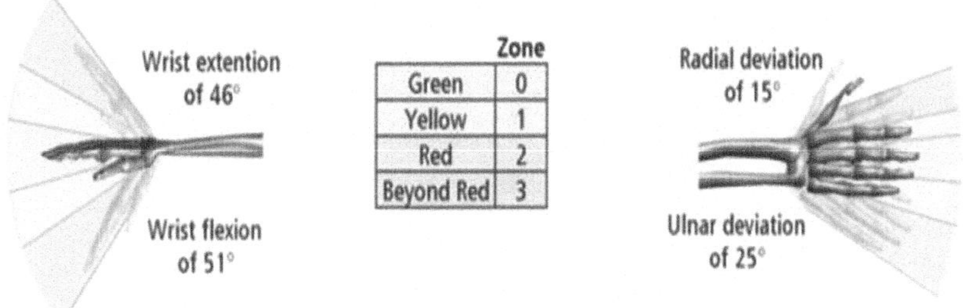

Fig. 6. Performance angle with respect to different zones

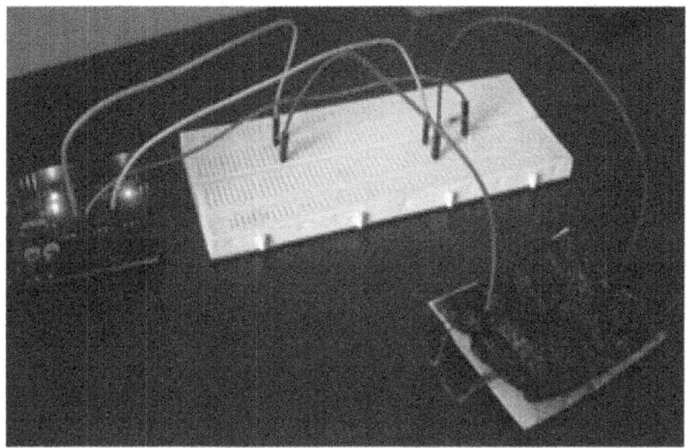

Fig. 7. Testing of fabric sensor

Circuit Law, which yields the resistance of the sensor. This resistance output is plotted with respect to time and the variation observed.

For the purpose of testing, the sensor was fastened to the wrist at the target joint by sandwiching it between two non-conductive spandex gloves as shown in Fig. 8. The sensor is fastened in such a way that it is held without any lateral slippage while bending. Metal clips were connected on two opposing ends of the sensor to serve as electrodes for connection with the Arduino. The test is preceded by first calibrating the sensor with a particular value at the neutral position of the wrist. Then the sensor was bent at various angles pertaining to the different zones of wrist motion and the resistance variation was plotted continuously. A serial plotter helps visualize the response of the sensor to the bending stimulus shown in Fig. 10. The range of resistance for each two dimensional zone was monitored with the aid of a serial monitor for both extension and flexion of the wrist. The results showed in Fig. 9 where the resistance values exceeding 190 Ω for the Green Zone; a range of 182–190 Ω for the Yellow Zone; 174–182 Ω corresponding to the Red Zone; and resistance values dipping below 174 Ω for extension beyond 51o (Beyond Red Region). Figure 11 shows the graphical representation of resistance respect to time. While scanning the results, it was found that this particular sensor sample exhibited better behaviour when the known resistance was chosen to be 1000 Ω.

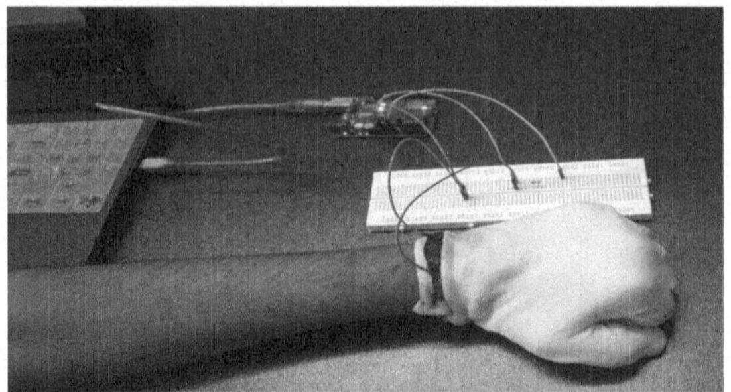

Fig. 8. Testing of fabric sensor

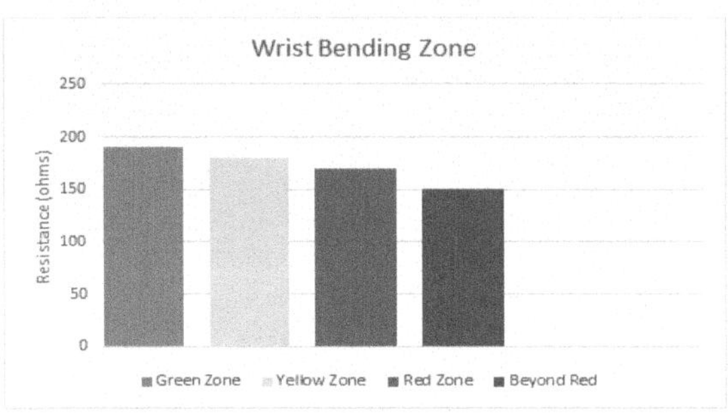

Fig. 9. Calibrated zones and the corresponding resistance

```
COM3
- Beyond Red Zone
Analog reading = 144.13
 - Beyond Red Zone
Analog reading = 144.13
 - Beyond Red Zone
Analog reading = 145.41
 - Beyond Red Zone
Analog reading = 145.41
 - Beyond Red Zone
Analog reading = 141.58
 - Beyond Red Zone
```

```
COM3
- Red Zone
Analog reading = 177.01
 - Red Zone
Analog reading = 179.72
 - Red Zone
Analog reading = 172.97
 - Beyond Red Zone
Analog reading = 177.01
 - Red Zone
Analog reading = 177.01
 - Red Zone
```

```
COM3
- Yellow Zone
Analog reading = 186.56
 - Yellow Zone
Analog reading = 187.94
 - Yellow Zone
Analog reading = 187.94
 - Yellow Zone
Analog reading = 187.94
 - Yellow Zone
Analog reading = 189.31
 - Yellow Zone
```

```
COM3
Analog reading = 197.66
 - Green Zone
Analog reading = 197.66
 - Green Zone
Analog reading = 197.66
 - Green Zone
Analog reading = 196.26
 - Green Zone
Analog reading = 196.26
 - Green Zone
```

Fig. 10. Zonal resistance values as seen in the serial monitor

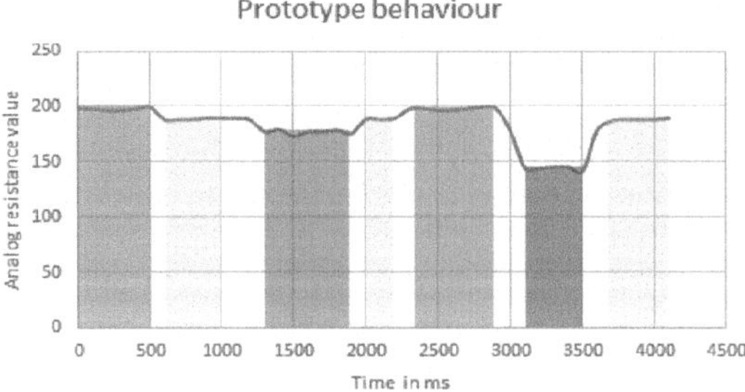

Fig. 11. Sensor behavior with respect to resistance and time

5 Conclusion

An analysis of the behaviour of the fabric sensor led to the conclusion that the sample is sensitive to surface deformation and is able to detect minute changes in joint posture. Changing resistance can be ascribed to the formation and breaking of new contact points among embedded CNT nanofibers on the substrate when subjected to bending. Variation in electrical resistance was found consistent and predictable for distinct zonal angles over multiple cycles, hence indicating that the sensor is able to retain its electromechanical properties for extended periods of usage. The invariance of its properties can be attributed to the strong hydrogen bonding between the conductive CNT and the cellulose substrate, which helps the sensor resist external agents of erosion to a satisfactory degree. This types of fabric sensor has the potential to make a sizable impact in real-time data monitoring activities in medical and athletic fields. Further optimization of the form, function, and fabrication procedure of the sensor may allow it to be scaled appropriately to meet the demands of accuracy in these applications while proving commercially profitable.

References

1. Moritani, T., Yoshitake, Y.: The use of electromyography in applied physiology. J. Electromyogr. Kinesiol. **8**, 363–381 (1998)
2. Orizio, C., Gobbo, M., Diemont, B., Esposito, F., Veicsteinas, A.: The surface mechanomyogram as a tool to describe the influence of fatigue on biceps brachii motor unit activation strategy. Historical basis and novel evidence. Eur. J. Appl. Physiol. **90**, 326–333 (2003)
3. Kim, K.K., et al.: Highly sensitive and stretchable multidimensional strain sensor with prestrained anisotropic metal nanowire percolation networks. Nano Lett. **15**, 5240–5247 (2015)
4. Li, L., Fan, T., Hu, R., Liu, Y., Lu, M.: Surface micro-dissolution process for embedding carbon nanotubes on cotton fabric as a conductive textile. Cellulose **24**, 1121–1128 (2017)
5. Mow, V.C., Lai, W.M.: Recent developments in synovial joint biomechanics. SIAM Rev. **22**, 275–317 (1980)
6. Hui, A.Y., McCarty, W.J., Masuda, K., Firestein, G.S., Sah, R.L.: A systems biology approach to synovial joint lubrication in health, injury, and disease. Wiley Interdiscip. Rev. Syst. Biol. Med. **4**, 15–37 (2012)
7. Bergmann, T., Peterson, D.: Chiropractic technique: chapter 2 joint anatomy and basic biomechanics. In: Chiropractic Technique, pp. 11–34. Elsevier/Mosby, Amsterdam (2010)
8. Ha, M., Han, D.: The relationship between knee joint angle and knee flexor and extensor muscle strength. J. Phys. Ther. Sci. **29**, 662–664 (2017)
9. Faisal, A.I., Majumder, S., Mondal, T., Cowan, D., Naseh, S., Deen, M.J.: Monitoring methods of human body joints: state-of-the-art and research challenges. Sens. (Basel) **19**(11), 2629 (2019). https://doi.org/10.3390/s19112629
10. Polygerinos, P., Wang, Z., Galloway, K.C., Wood, R.J., Walsh, C.J.: Soft robotic glove for combined assistance and at-home rehabilitation. Robot. Auton. Syst. **73**, 135–143 (2015)

11. Wang, L., Loh, K.J.: Wearable carbon nanotube-based fabric sensors for monitoring human physiological performance. Smart Mater. Struct. **26**(5), 055018 (2017)
12. Yamada, T., et al.: A stretchable carbon nanotube strain sensor for human-motion detection. Nat. Nanotechnol. **6**, 296–301 (2011)
13. Hu, X., et al.: A super-stretchable and highly sensitive carbon nanotube capacitive strain sensor for wearable applications and soft robotics. Adv. Mater. Technol. **7**(3), 2100769 (2022)
14. Aziz, S., Chang, S.H.: Smart-fabric sensor composed of single-walled carbon nanotubes containing binary polymer composites for health monitoring. Compos. Sci. Technol. **163**, 1–9 (2018)
15. Brook, I., Tchoudakov, R., Suckeveriene, R.Y., Narkis, M.: Electro-mechanical sensors based on conductive hybrid nanocomposites. Polym. Adv. Technol. **26**(7), 889–897 (2015)

EEG Signal Analysis for Seizure Detection with Hierarchical Clustering

V. Nageshwar(✉), Vikram Raj Samanta, Kakarla Divya Santhosxshi, and Koukuntla Satish Chandra

Department of EIE, VNR VJIET, Hyderabad, India
nageshwar_v@vnrvjiet.in

Abstract. The neurological condition known as epilepsy, which is marked by recurring seizures, presents considerable obstacles to prompt diagnosis and treatment. We investigate the effectiveness of hierarchical clustering (HC) as a feature extraction technique for pre-processing electroencephalogram (EEG) signals using data from publicly accessible datasets. Preictal and ictal state-balanced samples are included in the dataset, enabling reliable model training and assessment. The performance of hierarchical clustering as a pre-processing technique for a biological signal like EEG is evaluated by training couple of models and obtaining the evaluation metrics from them and finally all the metrics are compared together.

Keywords: Hierarchical Clustering · CNN Model · SVM Classifier · MLP Model · Dendrogram · Clusters

1 Introduction

The neurological condition known as epilepsy is typified by recurring seizures, which are bursts of aberrant brain activity. Tremors, seizures, and even unconsciousness are some of the symptoms that these aberrant electrical discharges might cause. To effectively treat and manage epilepsy, seizures must be detected early and accurately. A non-invasive method for measuring brain electrical activity is electroencephalography (EEG). EEG is a useful instrument for recording the quick changes in electrical activity that take place during seizures because of its high temporal resolution. Historically, skilled neurologists have used eye inspection in conjunction with EEG data to diagnose seizures. This method is subjective, labor-intensive, and error prone.

Recent advancements in machine learning and signal processing have opened doors for developing automated seizure detection systems. These systems aim to analyze EEG recordings and automatically identify seizure events. Supervised learning techniques, which require labelled data for training, have been widely employed for this purpose. However, acquiring large amounts of labelled EEG data can be challenging due to privacy concerns and the expertise required for accurate labelling. This research explores the potential of hierarchical clustering (HC) as an unsupervised pre-processing step for EEG analysis in seizure detection. HC is a data mining technique that groups similar

K. Atul et al. (Eds.): BodyNets 2024, LNICST 666, pp. 523–536, 2026.
https://doi.org/10.1007/978-3-032-16099-7_42

data points, potentially revealing hidden structures within the data. By applying HC to EEG recordings, we aim to identify inherent groupings that may be indicative of normal brain activity and seizure-related activity.

This paper utilizes the publicly available CHB-MIT dataset, a well-established resource for EEG seizure research. Since the CHB-MIT data is preprocessed and labelled, it allows us to focus on the effectiveness of HC in extracting features relevant to seizure classification. Following HC, feature extraction techniques are applied to the resulting clusters to generate informative representations suitable for further analysis. The investigation of unsupervised learning techniques for seizure identification in EEG signals is furthered by this work. We measure how well HC performs in locating seizure-related patterns in the data and how it affects classification accuracy. The results of this investigation will be given and examined about current seizure detection techniques, emphasizing the possible advantages of using HC as a pre-processing tool to increase the accuracy of seizure classification.

2 Objectives

The aim is to prove that hierarchical clustering (HC) is a suitable choice for applying signal analysis and seizure detection on CHB MIT Data Set. Get features from HC-formed clusters in common data. Then standardize them and merge with them. Train and assess the CNN model, CNN + SVM, and MLP model to track which model works better in seizure detection and the purpose of HC in the EEG analysis is to verify its role in seizure monitoring and the ability whether it is an adequate, good, or outstanding method.

3 Related Works

Many studies have contributed to innovative approaches and methods in the field of EEG signal analysis and detection of epilepsies. This section reviews related work and explores the various strategies researchers are using to improve the accuracy and efficiency of seizure detection using EEG data. Each article provides unique insights and methods that will significantly contribute to the evolving landscape of medical signal processing and deep learning applications. First, (2) examined the accumulation of EEG signals in arm and leg motor and imagined motor tasks. Their research focused on EEG data preprocessing, including denoising and spectral density analysis, followed by the application of five clustering algorithms to identify motor and fictive motor tasks. Their results highlighted the effectiveness of hierarchical clustering (HC) for arm fictive motor tasks and the spectral clustering algorithm for both leg motor tasks.

Then in (3) they developed a deep learning model and linked it to behavioral medicine knowledge, focusing on combining classification results, identifying significant frequency patterns, and highlighting signal waveforms that contribute to ictal predictions. Their method showed successful generalization of interpatient variability and achieved a high F1 score for seizure detection. After that, in the paper (4) they designed a cross-validated CNN structure and achieved high accuracy, sensitivity and specificity in seizure detection. Their study highlighted the simplicity and efficiency of the CNN-based recognition system and suggested future research directions for further improvement. In (5), they used entropic properties and their classifier, which achieved high classification accuracy between healthy seizures, healthy seizures, and seizures.

Finally, (6) discussed the need to develop new methods to extract diagnostic information from EEG recordings of epileptic patients, with a focus on childhood insufficiency epilepsy (CAE). They proposed a method based on wavelet coherence (WC) and hierarchical clustering (HC) to estimate the density of EEG network connections. Their approach involved analyzing WC behavior over time, determining a WC-based difference index, and using HC to correlate electrode array changes and brain state changes during seizures.

4 Methodology

CHB-MIT dataset, which is a well-balanced dataset suitable for seizure detection using deep learning techniques. The dataset comes from (1), which provides a reliable basis for our research. Although the Bonn dataset is also popular among researchers, the CHB-MIT dataset stands out due to its larger size and availability in a convenient ".csv" format. Data preprocessing involved extracting data points from the edf files, ensuring that equal amounts of preictal and ictal files were extracted. The first step involved standardizing the data set to normalize the data distribution, thus ensuring a consistent and reliable analysis. The dataset being so large, subsampling was performed to reduce computational complexity while retaining important information. This project's suggested technique entails a number of crucial elements. The CHB MIT dataset is used first. Owing to the enormity of the dataset, a more manageable subset of 30,000 samples is produced using subsampling. After that, the subsampled data is normalized to guarantee consistency in scale throughout the features. The standardized subsampled data are subjected to Ward's method of hierarchical clustering (HC), which yields clustered data with extracted cluster characteristics. To create a composite dataset, these cluster properties are reintegrated into the subsampled data. Three distinct models are trained using this pooled set of data. After training the three models on the clustered data, we then verify the model performance on the preprocessed data and make inferences about Hierarchical Clustering as a preprocessing method (Fig. 1).

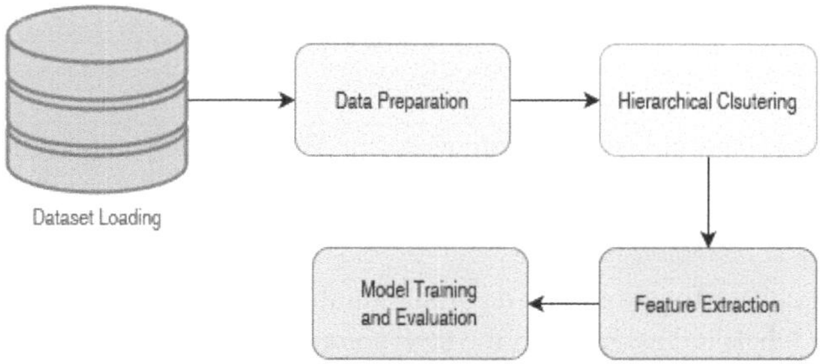

Fig. 1. Block Diagram

Data Preprocessing

- We start by removing the target column ('Outcome') from our dataset, as it represents the class labels and should be separated from the input features.
- Next, we standardize the input characteristics. Machine learning models perform better when the characteristics mean is 0 and the standard deviation is 1. This is achieved by standardization.
- We perform subsampling to reduce computational complexity while preserving essential information. We randomly sample 30,000 data points from the dataset and standardize the subsampled data.

Hierarchical Clustering

After preprocessing the data, we perform hierarchical clustering to identify patterns and structures within the standardized and subsampled data.

- We use the linkage function from SciPy to perform hierarchical clustering based on the ward method and Euclidean distance metric.
- The Ward method, minimizes the variance when merging clusters. This method is effective for identifying compact and well-separated clusters, making it suitable for our seizure detection analysis.
- We opt for the Euclidean distance metric, which calculates the straight-line distance between two data points in a multidimensional space.
- This metric is widely used and suitable for continuous data like EEG signals, providing a reliable measure of similarity or dissimilarity between data points.
- The hierarchical clustering results are visualized using a dendrogram, which is a tree-like diagram illustrating the clustering hierarchy.
- The dendrogram displays the merging of clusters at different distances, allowing us to interpret the clustering structure and identify optimal cluster configurations.
- The dendrogram provides insights into the hierarchical relationships between data points and helps determine the optimal number of clusters for our analysis.
- We analyze the statistics of the generated clusters, including the distribution of data points within each cluster and the distribution of outcome labels (ictal vs. pre-ictal) within each cluster.
- This analysis offers valuable insights into the characteristics and distribution of data points, aiding in the interpretation and further analysis of the clustering results (Fig. 2).

Understanding the Dendrogram

After performing hierarchical clustering using the Ward method and Euclidean distance metric, we generate a dendrogram to visualize the clustering hierarchy and gain insights into the clustering structure.

- Using the f cluster function with a certain number of clusters (number of clusters = 10), cluster labels are assigned to the data points.
- The cluster labels are then analyzed to determine the data points in each cluster and the distribution of outcome markers (ictal vs. pre-ictal) within each cluster.

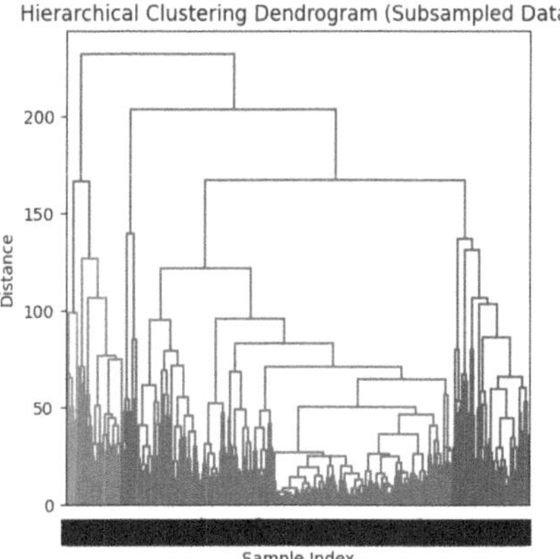

Fig. 2. Hierarchical Clustering Dendrogram

- The dendrogram illustrates the merging of clusters at different distances, allowing us to observe the hierarchical relationships between data points and clusters.
- We calculate the number of data points in each unique cluster label (unique clusters) and present the distribution of data points across clusters.
- Additionally, we analyze the distribution of outcome labels (0 for pre-ictal and 1 for ictal) within each cluster to understand how seizure-related data points are grouped within the clustering structure.
- The distribution of outcome labels (0 and 1) within each cluster is visualized and analyzed to identify patterns or trends in how seizure-related data points are clustered together.
- This analysis provides insights into the clustering effectiveness in distinguishing between pre-ictal and ictal data points within different clusters.

Feature Extraction

After understanding the dendrogram and ensuring Hierarchical clustering was performed properly, we extracted additional features from the data by incorporating cluster information into the dataset.

- We start by setting a threshold value 't' to define the clustering distance threshold. This threshold determines the proximity at which data points are grouped into clusters based on their distances in the hierarchical clustering dendrogram.
- Using the clustering distance threshold 't', we assign cluster labels to each data point using the f cluster function. These cluster identifiers classify data points into different groups based on their hierarchical proximity to clusters.
- To incorporate cluster information into our dataset, we convert the cluster labels into one-hot encoded values using the to-categorical function.
- One-hot encoding transforms categorical data (such as cluster labels) into binary format, where each cluster label becomes a binary feature indicating the presence or absence of that cluster for each data point.

- The one-hot encoded cluster labels are then considered as cluster features. These cluster features represent the clustering patterns identified during hierarchical clustering. Each cluster feature corresponds to a specific cluster identified in the dataset.
- We combine the cluster features with the previously standardized and subsampled data. This integration enhances the dataset by adding cluster-related information, allowing machine learning models to leverage clustering patterns for improved analysis and prediction.
- Cluster features capture additional structural information about the dataset, revealing underlying patterns and relationships that may not be evident from individual features alone.

Relevance of Cluster Features

- Hierarchical clustering groups similar data points into clusters based on their voltage values across all channels. This helps in identifying distinct patterns or clusters of data points that exhibit similar characteristics in terms of EEG signals.
- The cluster features, being binary (0 or 1), serve as additional features that complement the original voltage values across channels.
- By including cluster features alongside the raw voltage data, you create a more comprehensive and nuanced representation of the EEG signals, capturing both the individual channel information and the clustering-based patterns.
- Machine learning models trained on datasets with cluster features often demonstrate improved discriminative power.
- The cluster features provide supplementary information that can help the model differentiate between different EEG patterns, such as distinguishing between seizure and non-seizure activities.
- Hierarchical clustering and subsequent creation of cluster features can also aid in reducing the dimensionality of the dataset.
- Instead of working with raw voltage data from all channels, the cluster features condense and summarize key information, making it more manageable for modelling and analysis.
- The model can learn to recognize not just individual channel voltages but also higher-level patterns that may span multiple channels and time points, enhancing its ability to detect seizures accurately.

Model Training and Evaluation

After extracting cluster-based features and preparing the dataset, we proceed to train machine learning models to identify scenes and evaluate their performance.

- We train a CNN model using the combined features obtained from the hierarchical clustering and extraction process.
- After prediction using the trained CNN model, a confusion matrix is derived after model prediction.
- Following that, we extract the features from the CNN model which becomes the input for the SVM classifier and similarly, we make a confusion matrix and determine the metrics.

- "Table 1" is the CNN model summary and detailed representation of the layers used in the model.
- Finally, the models are compared with each other based on their metrics.
- "Table 2" is the MLP model summary, and a detailed representation of the layers used in the model.

Table 1. CNN Model Details

Layer(type)	Output Shape	Param
conv1d-58 (Conv1D)	(None, 1877, 32)	128
max-pooling1d-58 (MaxPooling1D)	(None, 938, 32)	0
conv1d-59 (Conv1D)	(None, 936, 32)	3104
max-pooling1d-59 (MaxPooling1D)	(None, 468, 32)	0
flatten-27 (Flatten)	(None, 14976)	0
dense-86 (Dense)	(None, 512)	7668224
dropout-28 (Dropout)	(None, 512)	0
dense-87 (Dense)	(None, 1)	513

Table 2. MLP Model Details

Layer(type)	Output Shape	Param
flatten-28 (Flatten)	(None, 1879)	0
dense-88 (Dense)	(None, 128)	240640
dropout-29 (Dropout)	(None, 128)	0
dense-89(Dense)	(None, 64)	8256
dense-90(Dense)	(None, 64)	4160
dense-91(Dense)	(None, 32)	2080
dense-92 (Dense)	(None, 1)	33

5 Result and Discussion

The following section presents the results obtained from training and evaluating the CNN, Support SVM classifier on CNN-extracted features, and MLP models for EEG analysis in seizure detection. The discussion delves into the performance metrics, confusion matrices, and comparative analysis of these models, highlighting their strengths and limitations. The 30,000 samples include around 15,018 samples which are ictal and around 14,982 samples are preictal, which will act as the benchmark and evaluation of the confusion matrices obtained from the models.

Convolutional Neural Network (CNN) Model

Through a thorough analysis of the confusion matrix, the effectiveness of the CNN model in classifying EEG data for seizure detection is determined "Fig. 3" represents the confusion matrix of true and false metrics after model prediction.

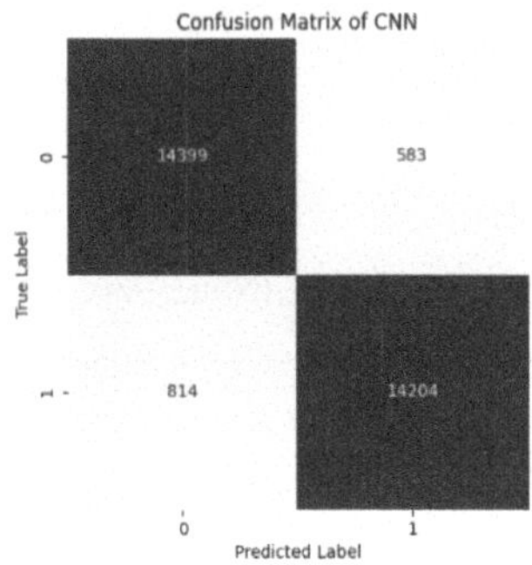

Fig. 3. CNN Model Confusion Matrix

To properly evaluate the CNN model with the Hierarchical Clustered data, the evaluation metrics are calculated from the confusion matrix and displayed in "Table 3".

Table 3. CNN Model Evaluation Metrics

Accuracy	Precision	Sensitivity	F1-Score
95.3433%	96.0573%	94.5798%	95.3129%

Examining the fluctuations in loss and accuracy metrics during training and validation provides valuable insights into the model's learning dynamics and generalization capability.

The comparison between training and validation accuracy in "Fig. 4" is a crucial aspect of evaluating the performance of our Convolutional Neural Network (CNN) model. Training accuracy measures the model's ability to correctly predict outcomes on the training data it has seen during training. Validation accuracy measures the effectiveness of how the model generalizes to new, unknown samples, showing its capacity to produce accurate predictions.

It is possible to obtain insights into the model's learning process, possible overfitting or underfitting problems, and overall efficacy in producing accurate predictions on new data instances by examining the trends and discrepancies between these two-accuracy metrics.

To evaluate the effectiveness and capacity for generalization of our CNN model, we must first look at the training versus validation loss in "Fig. 5". During the training

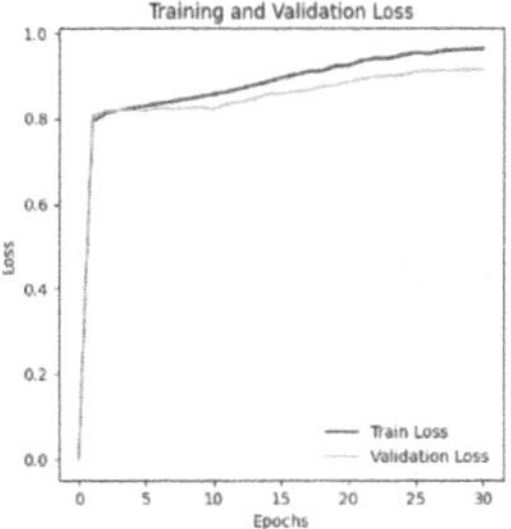

Fig. 4. CNN Model Train Vs Validation Accuracy

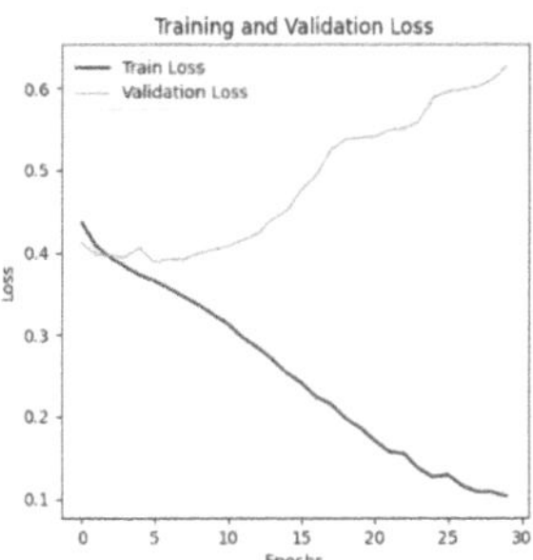

Fig. 5. CNN Model Train Vs Validation Loss

phase, the difference between the actual targets and the expected output of the model is represented by the training loss. As an assessment of how effectively the model generalizes to new data, the validation loss, evaluates the model's performance on a different validation set that it was not exposed to during training. We can spot possible problems like overfitting or underfitting by comparing the patterns and sizes of the training and validation losses.

Support Vector Machine (SVM) Classifier on CNN-Extracted Features
After evaluating the CNN model's performance, we explore the effectiveness of utilizing features extracted from the CNN model and give it as the input to the SVM classifier. This hybrid approach aims to leverage the strengths of both CNN-based feature extraction and SVM classification for improved seizure detection (Fig. 6).

However, based on "Table 3" and "Table 4", there is no significant improvement between the CNN model and the SVM classifier applied to the CNN model.

Multi-Layer Perceptron (MLP) Model
After splitting the data, occurrences of each class (ictal and pre-ictal) in the validation set are carefully counted and displayed. This segmentation allowed us to assess how well the MLP model performs in distinguishing between ictal (seizure) and pre-ictal (non-seizure) states, providing valuable insights into its classification accuracy and predictive capabilities. The 30,000 samples are now split, where the data used to make the confusion matrix, has a sample size of 6000 and from that around 3008 samples are ictal and 2992

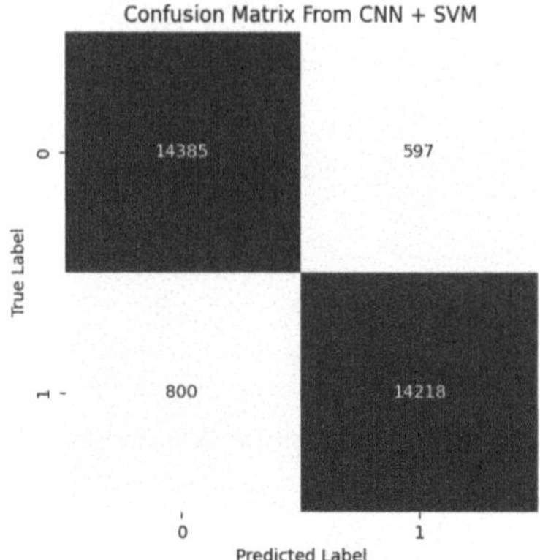

Fig. 6. SVM Classifier Confusion Matrix

Table 4. SVM Classifier Evaluation Metrics

Accuracy	Precision	Sensitivity	F1-Score
95.3433%	95.9703%	94.6731%	95.3173%

samples are pre-ictal. "Fig. 7" shows the metrics obtained from the confusion matrix of the MLP model obtained from the 6000 samples (Table 5).

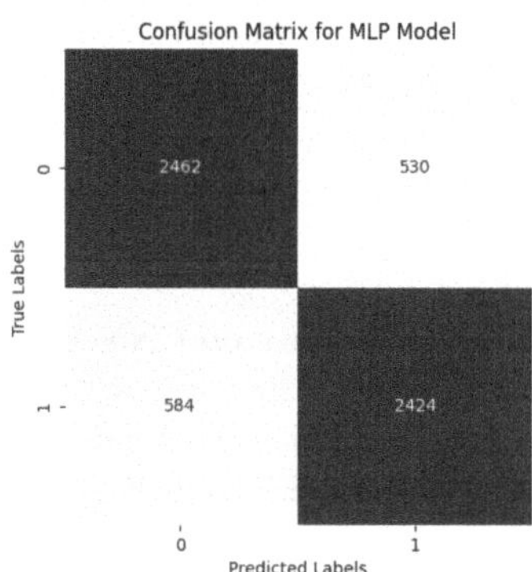

Fig. 7. MLP Model Confusion Matrix

Table 5. MLP Model Evaluation Metrics

Accuracy	Precision	Sensitivity	F1-Score
81.4333%	82.0582%	80.5851%	81.315%

The comparison between training and validation accuracy in "Fig. 8" is a pivotal aspect in evaluating the performance of our Multi-Layer Perceptron (MLP) model. Training accuracy assesses the model's proficiency in accurately predicting outcomes on the training dataset it was exposed to during training sessions. Conversely, validation accuracy measures the model's generalization capability, indicating how effectively it can make accurate predictions on new, unseen data samples.

An important part of evaluating the performance of our MLP model is to compare the training and validation losses in "Fig. 9". Smaller values indicate a better fit. Training loss is about the model fitting the training data and validation loss is about making correct predictions.

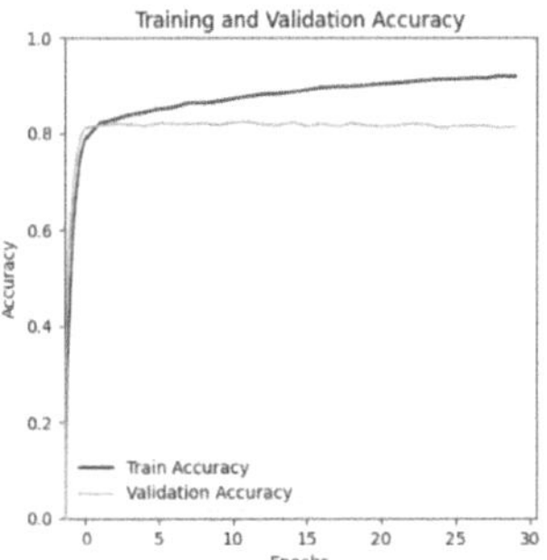

Fig. 8. MLP Model Train Vs Validation Accuracy

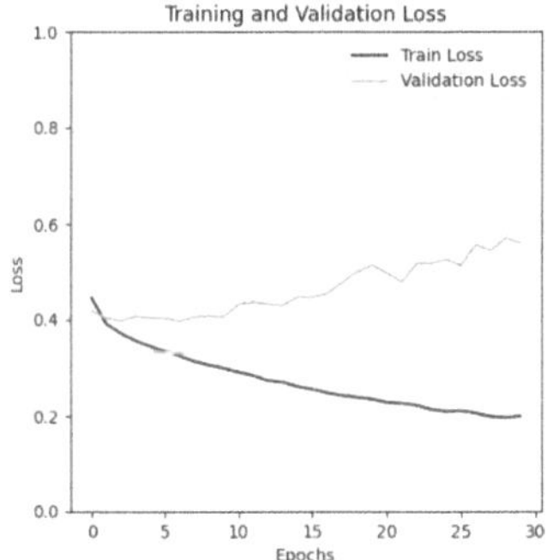

Fig. 9. MLP Model Train Vs Validation Accuracy

Overall Model Comparison

Here, all the metrics obtained after training the models are presented, like "Fig. 10" that shows the graph of comparison of all the models.

Along with the individual metrics in figures below. "Fig. 11" represents the Accuracy, Sensitivity and F1 Score plots, which clearly shows that the CNN and CNN + SVM performing better than MLP and being almost similar (Table 6).

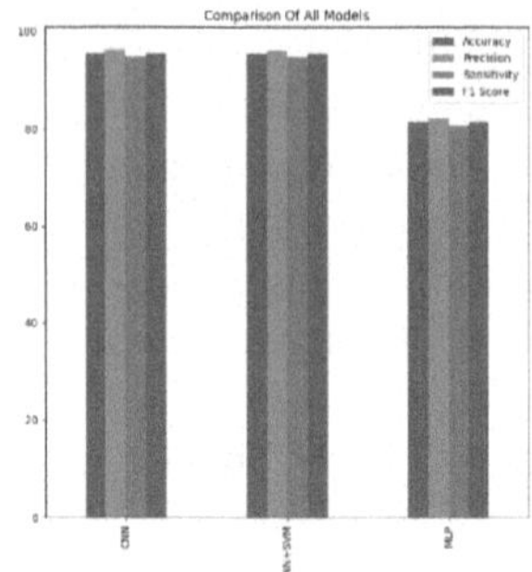

Fig. 10. Comparison of All Models

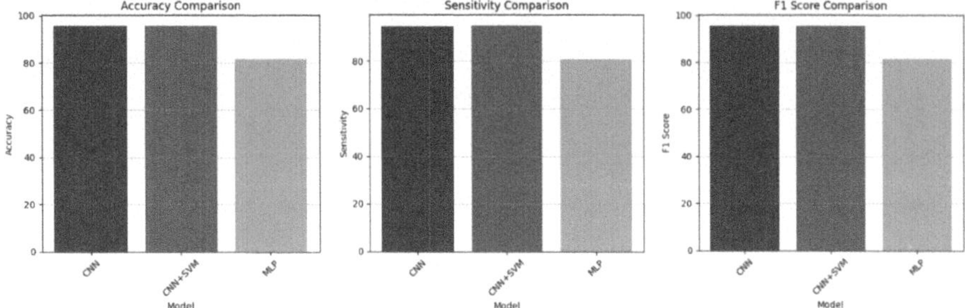

Fig. 11. Comparison of Accuracies, Sensitivities and F1 Score

Table 6. Comparison with Existing Techniques

Ref	Methodology	Results
(16)	Prep Pipeline, temporal mean CNN, LTSM	Accuracy 94% Sensitivity 93.8%
(17)	Spike detection, average filter	Accuracy 92%
18)	Current Maxima, Segment Matching Homogeneity	Accuracy 92.66%
(19)	Shannon entropy, ANOVA test Hidden Markov Model	Accuracy 95% (Ictal vs Preictal)
Proposed Work	Hierarchical Clustering CNN + SVM	Accuracy 95.34%, Sensitivity 94.67%

6 Conclusion

Although we recognized that more advanced techniques could produce better outcomes, our assessment sought to give a broad picture of how well HC performed when combined with current models.

With 80.59% recall (sensitivity) and 82.06% precision, the Multi-Layer Perceptron (MLP) classifier produced an accuracy of 81.43% and an F1 score of 81.32%. This model, which was the least successful of the three examined, represented a balanced compromise between recall and precision. By comparison, the Convolutional Neural Network (CNN) model performed better, with an F1 score of 95.31% and 95.34% accuracy, 96.06% precision, and 94.58% recall. With 95.34% accuracy, 96.97% precision, and 94.67% recall, the Support Vector Machine (SVM) classifier likewise showed commensurate efficacy, as seen by its 95.32% F1 score. Additionally, the CNN model with SVM performed marginally better than the CNN model alone, highlighting the need of utilizing complementing models to improve classification accuracy.

Even while our research may not present revolutionary developments in seizure detection techniques, it offers insightful information about the usefulness of HC in the pre-processing of EEG data for better seizure classification.

Acknowledgment. We would like to thank all the members who helped us directly or indirectly.

References

1. Deepa, B., Ramesh, K.: Preprocessed CHB-MIT Scalp EEG Database. IEEE Dataport, 22 May 2021. https://doi.org/10.21227/awcw-mn88
2. Asanza, V., Pelaez, E., Loayza, F.: EEG signal clustering for motor and imaginary motor tasks on hands and feet, October 2017. https://doi.org/10.1109/etcm.2017.8247451
3. Gabeff, V., et al.: Interpreting deep learning models for epileptic seizure detection on EEG signals (2021). https://doi.org/10.1016/j.artmed.2021.102084
4. Abiyev, R.H., Arslan, M., Idoko, J.B., Sekeroglu, B., Ilhan, A.: Identification of epileptic EEG signals using convolutional neural networks, June 2020. https://doi.org/10.3390/app10124089
5. Dash, D.P., Kolekar, M.H.: Hidden Markov model based epileptic seizure detection using tunable Q wavelet transform (2020). https://doi.org/10.7555/jbr.34.20190006
6. Ieracitano, C., Duun-Henriksen, J., Mammone, N., Foresta, F.L., Morabito, F.C.: Wavelet coherence-based clustering of EEG signals to estimate the brain connectivity in absence epileptic patients (2017). https://doi.org/10.1109/ijcnn.2017.7966002
7. Guess, M.J., Wilson, S.B.: Introduction to hierarchical clustering (2002). https://doi.org/10.1097/00004691-200203000-00005
8. Mert, A., Akan, A.: Hilbert-huang transform based hierarchical clustering for EEG denoising, p. 1, September 2013
9. Safayari, A., Bolhasani, H.: Depression diagnosis by deep learning using EEG signals: a systematic review (2021). https://doi.org/10.1016/j.medntd.2021.100102
10. Statsenko, Y., et al.: Automatic detection and classification of epileptic seizures from EEG data: finding optimal acquisition settings and testing interpretable machine learning approach (2023). https://doi.org/10.3390/biomedicines11092370
11. Jia, M., et al.: Efficient graph convolutional networks for seizure prediction using scalp EEG (2022). https://doi.org/10.3389/fnins.2022.967116
12. Lasefr, Z., Ayyalasomayajula, S.S.V.N.R., Elleithy, K.: Epilepsy seizure detection using EEG signals (2017). https://doi.org/10.1109/uemcon.2017.8249018
13. Gunawan, P.I., Kurube, C.M.F., Noviandi, R., Samosir, S.M.: Electroencephalography patterns in children with first unprovoked. Seizure (2021). https://doi.org/10.21203/rs.3.rs-955347/v1
14. Jaafar, S.T., Mohammadi, M.: Epileptic seizure detection using deep learning approach (2019). https://doi.org/10.21928/uhdjst.v3n2y2019.pp41-50

15. Xie, D., Toutant, D., Ng, M.: Residual seizure rate of intermittent inpatient EEG compared to a continuous EEG model (2023). https://doi.org/10.1017/cjn.2023.241
16. Aslam, M., et al.: Classification of EEG signals for prediction of epileptic seizures (2022). https://doi.org/10.3390/app12147251
17. Slimen, I.B., Boubchir, L., Seddik, H.: Epileptic seizure prediction based on EEG spikes detection of ictal preictal states (2020). https://doi.org/10.7555/jbr.34.20190097
18. Das, K., Daschakladar, D., Roy, P.P., Chatterjee, A., Saha, S.: Epileptic seizure prediction by the detection of seizure waveform from the pre-ictal phase of EEG signal (2020). https://doi.org/10.1016/j.bspc.2019.101720
19. Dash, D.P., Kolekar, M.H.: Epileptic seizure detection based on EEG signal analysis using hierarchy based Hidden Markov Model (2017). https://doi.org/10.1109/icacci.2017.8125991

Estimation of the Instantaneous Frequency of Mono-components in Non-stationary Signals Using Wavelet Transform with Dynamic Q Values

Amaya Rose Abraham[1(✉)], Anurag Nishad[1], and Abhay Upadhyay[2]

[1] BITS Pilani, K K Birla Goa Campus, Sancoale, India
{p20230023,anuragan}@goa.bits-pilani.ac.in

[2] Indian Institute of Information Technology Kota, Kota, Rajasthan, India

Abstract. The non-stationary signals are the signals with statistical properties that change with time. The spectral properties of the non-stationary signals can be analyzed by estimating the instantaneous frequency (IF). The separation of the individual mono-components from the multi-component signal is essential for the IF estimation. In this paper, we propose a methodology for the separation of the mono-components from a multi-component non-stationary signal based on a dynamic Q-value-based wavelet transform (DQVWT) method. The windowing of the time domain signal with a moving Gaussian function and the separation of components using an array of tunable Q wavelet transform (TQWT) blocks results in the mono-component separation followed by the IF computation. The proposed methodology is applied to signals that consist of linearly frequency modulated (LFM) mono-components and non-LFM (NLFM) mono-components. The IF estimation by the proposed method is compared with the existing TQWT-based filter bank (TQWT-FB) method and the Fourier Bessel/time order method. The proposed method has been applied to estimate the IF of the fundamental frequency component of the speech signal. The performance is analyzed in terms of mean square error (MSE) and the proposed method has shown better performance than the other compared methods.

Keywords: Dynamic Q value based wavelet transform · Non-stationary signals · Mono-components · Instantaneous frequency

1 Introduction

The non-stationary signal analysis is an advanced signal processing field with enormous applications. The statistical properties of non-stationary signals vary with time [1]. The physiological signals like speech signals, electroencephalogram (EEG) signals, and electrocardiogram (ECG) signals are some common examples of non-stationary signals [2,3]. The multi-component non-stationary signals

K. Atul et al. (Eds.): BodyNets 2024, LNICST 666, pp. 537–549, 2026.
https://doi.org/10.1007/978-3-032-16099-7_43

contain multiple mono-components and their separation is important for the instantaneous frequency (IF) estimation. As an example, the speech signal is a non-stationary signal that is generated by the excitation of the vocal tract system [4]. In the voiced region, speech signals consist of a fundamental frequency component (FFC) and its harmonics. The estimation of IF of FFC can be used for emotion estimation in wireless body area network [5]. To estimate the IF of mono-components present in a signal, they are separated using different signal decomposition methods.

There are several existing methods for the decomposition of a multi-component non-stationary signal to extract mono-components [6]. The common signal decomposition methods are empirical mode decomposition (EMD) [7], empirical wavelet transform (EWT) [8], variational mode decomposition (VMD) [9], Fourier Bessel [10], time order [6] and tunable quality (Q) wavelet transform based filter bank (TQWT-FB) [11] methods. In literature, EMD decomposes the signal into intrinsic mode functions (IMF) [7]. The operation is by shifting process and extracts the non-stationary part from the input signal. The lack of mathematical theory limits the EMD method [7]. The EWT method is an adaptive method that depends on the frequency spectrum of the signal [8]. EWT is a signal-dependent decomposition method and detects the boundaries in the signal spectrum [8]. The VMD method is a decomposition method with concurrent mode extraction based on their center frequencies [9]. The separation of the narrow band components from the multi-component non-stationary signal using intrinsic mode functions (IMF) is used in VMD method [9]. The Fourier Bessel method uses spectral analysis with Fourier Bessel coefficients and the components are separated based on these coefficients [10]. If the components of composite signals are separated in the frequency domain, the separate reconstruction of each component can be done with the Fourier Bessel coefficients using a range of coefficients [10]. The Fourier Bessel method effectively works only if the components are separated in frequency domain [10]. The time order method work effectively with the components being well separated in the time-frequency domain but overlapped frequency domain [10]. The segmentation and windowing of the input signals and then the calculation of Fourier Bessel coefficients results in the separation of components in the time order method [10]. The TQWT-FB method is a discrete WT with tunable parameters like Q for oscillatory signals and decomposing into constant bandwidth sub-bands. The multiple wavelets with different Q values are available in the filter bank for the analysis of different oscillatory components present in the signal [11]. Once the mono-components are separated, their IF can be estimated by computing the derivative of the phase angle [3,12].

In this paper, we propose a dynamic Q- value based wavelet transform (DQVWT) method for the separation of mono-components from multi-component non-stationary signals. The signal is windowed by a Gaussian function followed by the boundary detection in the spectrum to locate the components in the spectrum. Then the input parameters of TQWT like Q, r and J are computed dynamically to separate such components. The separated components are then accumulated to generate mono-components of the signal. Once the mono-components are obtained, their IF is computed. The performance of the proposed methodology is compared with Fourier Bessel, the time order method, and TQWT-FB method in terms of mean square error (MSE).

The paper is arranged as follows: Sect. 2 is the overview of TQWT and Sect. 3 details the proposed methodology. Section 4 discusses the simulation results. Finally, Sect. 5 concludes the paper.

2 Overview of TQWT

The TQWT is a discrete WT used for the analysis of oscillatory signals with tunable parameters. The value of Q in TQWT is changeable in accordance with the oscillatory behavior of the signal [13]. The Q is the ratio of the center frequency to the bandwidth of a wavelet sub-band [13]. The Q can be expressed as:

$$Q = \frac{f_c}{BW} \tag{1}$$

where, f_c is the center frequency and BW is the bandwidth of a wavelet sub-band.

The parameters for TQWT are quality factor Q, redundancy r and decomposition level J. The r decides the localization of the wavelet in the time domain. The J is the number of decomposition levels and decides the number of sub-bands [13]. The variation in the value of Q results in the variations in the oscillations in the wavelets [13].

The TQWT is composed of two channel filter banks which are cascaded. The two-channel filter bank is formed by the low pass channel and high pass channel and the output of the low pass channel is fed to the next two-channel filter bank [13]. The outputs are scaled by the scaling factors L_s and H_s, low pass and high pass, respectively [13]. The TQWT parameters can be expressed in terms of L_s and H_s as:

$$Q = \frac{f_c}{BW} = \frac{2 - H_s}{H_s} \tag{2}$$

$$r = \frac{H_s}{1 - L_s} \tag{3}$$

For perfect reconstruction $L_s + H_s > 1$ has to be satisfied. TQWT decomposes the signal into total $J + 1$ sub-bands [13]. The flexibility of the parameters makes TQWT as a useful tool for the analysis of non-stationary signals.

3 Proposed Method for IF Estimation

The proposed method is based on DQVWT for the separation of mono-components from a non-stationary multi-component signal and the estimation of the IF of separated mono-components. The block diagram of the proposed method is shown in Fig. 1. The block diagram consists of seven blocks which are the window block, Gaussian window block, cut-off frequency computation block, TQWT parameters computation block, the array of TQWT blocks, mono-component generation block, and finally P IF computation blocks if P mono-components are detected. Each block is explained below:

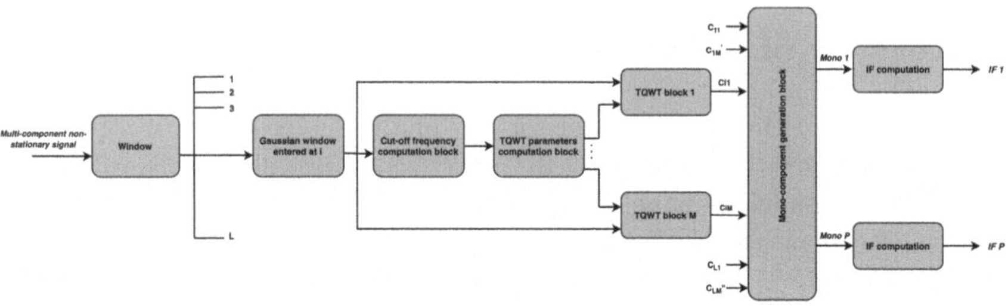

Fig. 1. Block diagram of the proposed methodology for the IF estimation of mono-components.

The first block in the block diagram is a window function block. The multi-component non-stationary input signal consists of L samples and is fed to the window block in which the window $W_{win}(n)$ is defined as:

$$W_{win}(n) = \begin{cases} G_{nor}(m_{w_1}, s_{w_t}) & 1 \leq \text{n} \leq m_{w_1} \\ 1 & m_{w_1} + 1 \leq \text{n} \leq m_{w_2} \\ G_{nor}(m_{w_2}, s_{w_t}) & m_{w_2} + 1 \leq \text{n} \leq L \end{cases} \tag{4}$$

G_{nor} is the normalized Gaussian function of length L. The m_{w_1} or m_{w_2} are the mean and s_{w_t} is the standard deviation. The window $W_{win}(n)$ truncates the signal smoothly at its starting and ending samples. Because of $W_{win}(n)$, the signal spectrum does not disperse in the frequency domain if the signal spectrum is analyzed by considering only starting or ending samples. The components present in the signal at the starting and ending samples are easily distinguishable.

Followed by the window block, in the next block, the signal is windowed by a Gaussian function centered at i, where $1 \leq i \leq L$. The standard deviation of the Gaussian function is set to s_{w_t}. Then the Gaussian windowed signal is passed to the cut-off frequency computation block. In this block, different components present in the Gaussian windowed signal are separated in the frequency domain by the boundary detection method suggested in EWT method [8].

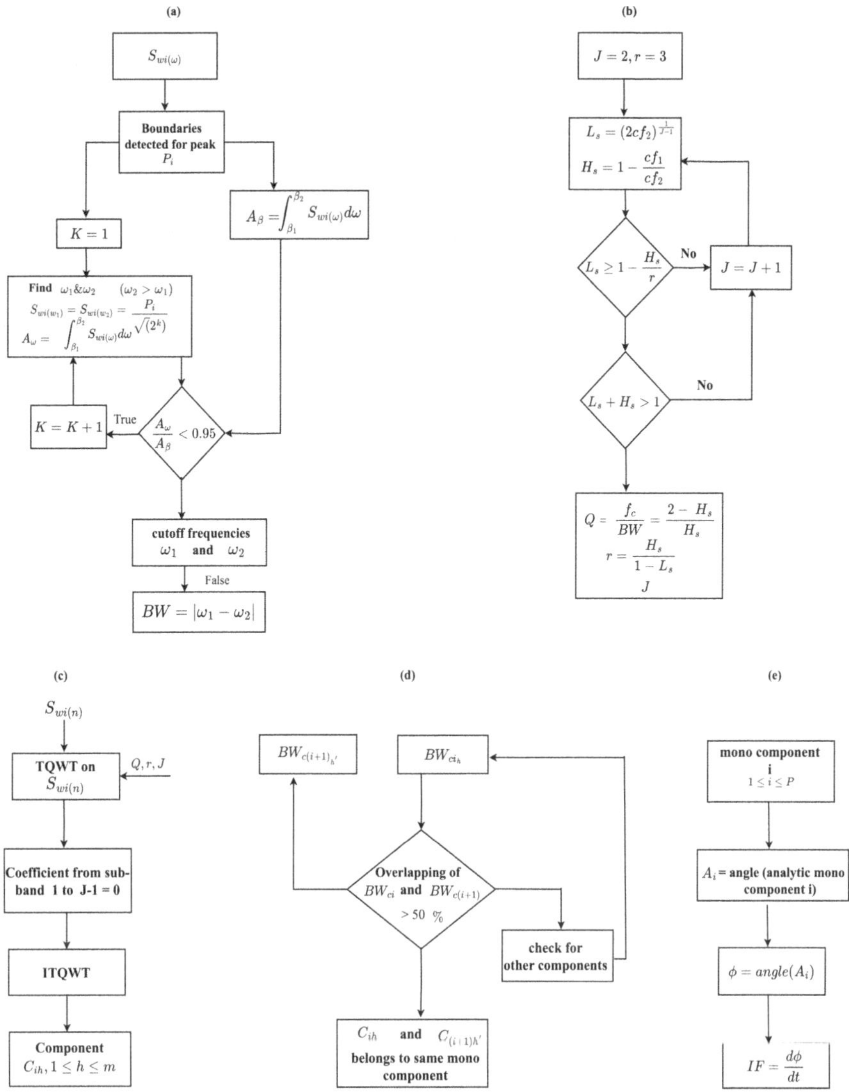

Fig. 2. Flowchart of different blocks (a) Boundary detection block (b) TQWT parameters computation block (c) TQWT array block (d) Mono-component generation block (e) IF computation block

The next block is cut-off frequency computation block and the operation is shown in the Fig. 2(a). To detect the actual bandwidth of a component, separated after boundary detection, the peak magnitude (P_i) of the component in the spectrum is detected and the peak exists between two detected boundaries β_1 and β_2. Using detected peak two frequencies ω_1 and ω_2 are computed for which the magnitude of the spectrum $S_{wi}(w)$ at w_1 and w_1 is $S_{wi}(w_1) = S_{wi}(w_2) =$

$\frac{P_i}{\sqrt{2^k}}$ at k = 1. A_β is the area covered in the spectrum between β_1 and β_2 and A_ω the area covered between ω_1 and ω_2. If the ratio of $\frac{A_\omega}{A_\beta} < 0.95$, then the new value of ω_1 and ω_2 is computed by incrementing k by 1. The minimum value of ω_1 and ω_2 are considered to be cutoff frequencies for which $\frac{A_\omega}{A_\beta} \geq 0.95$. The difference between the cutoff frequencies results in the bandwidth of the component.

Using the bandwidth computed by the cut-off frequency computation block the TQWT parameters namely Q, r, and J, are computed in the next block and the same is shown in Fig. 2(b). Initially, the decomposition level $J = 2$ and redundancy $r = 3$ are set and the scaling factors L_s and H_s are computed. Let's say cf_1 and cf_2 are the computed cut-off frequencies where $cf_2 > cf_1$. The $L_s = (2cf_2)^{\frac{1}{J-1}}$ and $H_s = 1 - \frac{cf_1}{cf_2}$ are computed. Then their relation according to (3) is checked. If the relation is not satisfied, then the value of J is incremented by 1. This process is repeated until the relation $L_s \geq 1 - \frac{H_s}{r}$ is satisfied. Once this relation is satisfied, the value of J is increased until the perfect reconstruction condition in TQWT is satisfied. From the final value of L_s and H_s the Q and r are computed from (2) and (3). The value of J to compute the final value of L_s and H_s is considered as its final value. In this process, the TQWT parameters are computed for the mth component where $1 \leq m \leq M$. Here, let's say that M is the number of components separated by boundaries at the ith iteration.

After the computation of TQWT parameters, an array of TQWT blocks are present. The combined operations TQWT and inverse TQWT are performed using the array of TQWT blocks. After applying TQWT process all coefficients are set to zero for the ITQWT (ITQWT) operation except J^{th} sub-band coefficient. The total number of blocks of TQWT is M. In Fig. 1, it is assumed that the M, M' and M'' components are obtained for i, $i = 1$ and $i = L$, receptively. The C_{iM} represents the Mth component obtained at i^{th} iteration. The overall process is represented in Fig. 2 (c).

The components generated by the array of TQWT blocks pass to the mono-component generation block. In this block, if the bandwidth of the components BW_{ci_h} and $BW_{ci_{h'}'}$ belonging to i^{th} and $(i+1)^{th}$ iteration overlaps by more than fifty percent, then they are considered to be part of the same mono-components. This process is shown in Fig. 2 (d). The addition of such components generates the mono-component. Once the mono-components are obtained, they are converted to an analytic signal. The IF computation process is represented in Fig. 2 (e). The IF is estimated by computing the derivative of the phase of analytic signal [12].

4 Simulation Results

The proposed methodology DQVWT estimates the IFs of mono-components of non-stationary multi-component signals. The DQVWT is applied on two synthetic signals and on one speech signal for whose mono-components exhibit different characteristics in the time-frequency (T-F) plane. The performance of the proposed method and other compared methods in terms of mean square error

(MSE) under different noisy conditions in which the signal is corrupted by additive white Gaussian noise (AWGN) at 0 dB signal-to-noise ratio (SNR), 10 dB SNR and ∞ dB SNR are discussed below. In proposed method the values of the m_{w_1} and m_{w_2} are 30 and 470 respectively. The standard deviation is set to 15 and the length of the window $W_{win}(n)$ is 500. The signals which are used in the proposed methodology for the simulation are as follows:

Signal 1 ($S_1(n)$): The first signal contains two linearly frequency-modulated (LFM) mono-components. The mono-components are overlapped in the time domain and frequency domain. The signal can be mathematically expressed as:

$$S_1(n) = \cos((\frac{185}{300000})\pi n^2 + \frac{6}{10}n) + \cos(\frac{9443}{1000000}n^2 + \frac{178}{100}n) \quad (5)$$

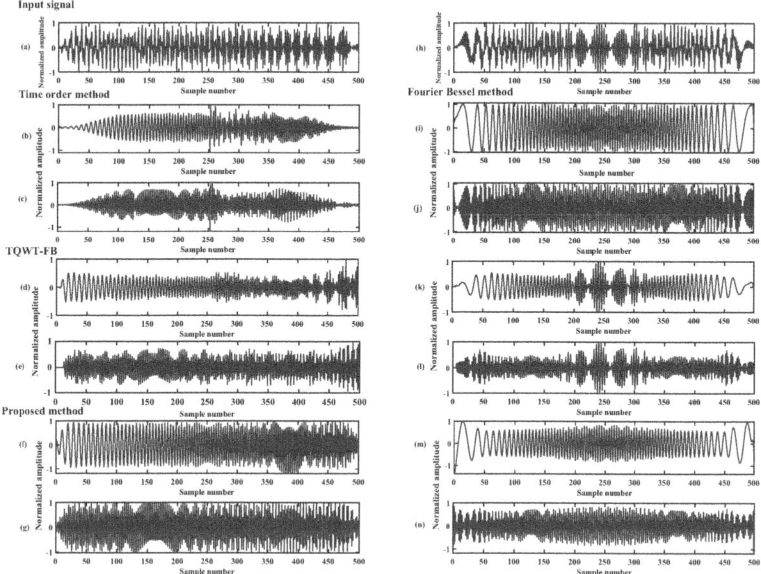

Fig. 3. At ∞ dB SNR, the signal (a) $S_1(n)$ (b) The first mono-component of $S_1(n)$ (c) Second mono-component of $S_1(n)$ obtained by the time order method of signal. (d) The first mono-component of $S_1(n)$ (e) Second mono-component of $S_1(n)$ obtained by the TQWT-FB method of signal. (f) The first mono-component of $S_1(n)$ (g) Second mono-component of $S_1(n)$ obtained by the proposed method of signal. The signal (h) $S_2(n)$ (i) The first mono-component of $S_2(n)$ (j) Second mono-component of $S_2(n)$ obtained by the Fourier Bessel method of signal. (k) The first mono-component of $S_2(n)$ (l) The second mono-component of $S_2(n)$ obtained by the TQWT-FB of signal. (m) The first mono-component of $S_2(n)$ (n) The second mono-component of $S_2(n)$ obtained by the proposed method of signal.

Signal 2 ($S_2(n)$): The second signal contains two non-LFM (NLFM) mono-components. The mono-components are non-overlapped in the frequency domain. The signal is given by:

$$S_2(n) = \cos(\frac{365}{100}) + 300\cos(\frac{5\pi n}{2560}) + \cos((\frac{-3}{10}n) - 300\cos(\frac{5\pi n}{2560})) \tag{6}$$

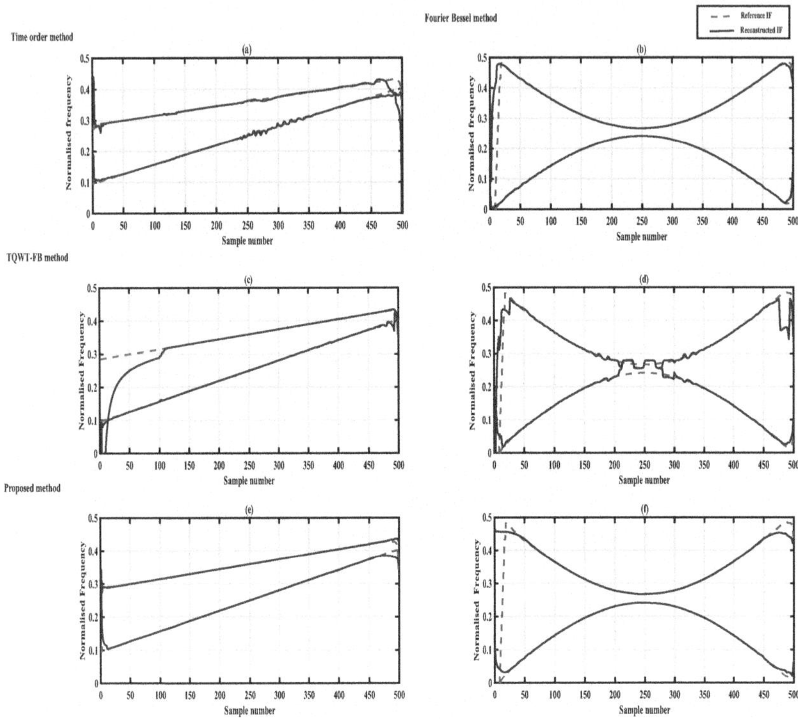

Fig. 4. IF of mono-components of (a) $S_1(n)$ by time order method (b) $S_2(n)$ computed by Fourier Bessel method (c) $S_1(n)$ and (d) $S_2(n)$ computed by TQWT-FB method (e) $S_1(n)$ and (f) $S_2(n)$ computed by proposed method

The two multi-component non-stationary signals and their obtained individual mono-components are by different methods at ∞ dB SNR are shown in Fig. 3. For $S_1(n)$, the mono-components are overlapped in the frequency domain, the Fourier Bessel method fails to separate the components so, the time order method is more suitable to separate them [14]. This can be verified by the Fig. 4 (a). The first and second mono-components of $S_1(n)$ are obtained by the time order method shown in Fig. 3 (b) and (c). The separated mono-components amplitude is lower in initial and end samples of $S_1(n)$ by time order method. Similarly, The first and second mono-components of $S_2(n)$ are obtained by the

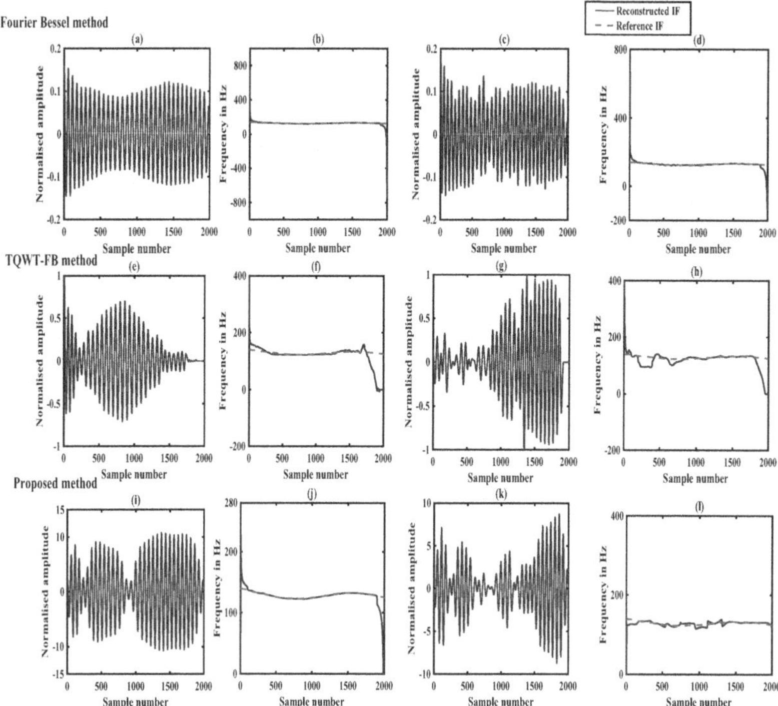

Fig. 5. Extracted FFC and IF of speech signals. At ∞ dB SNR (a) FFC (b) IF of FFC. At 10 dB SNR (c) FFC (d) IF of FFC by the Fourier Bessel method. At ∞ dB (e) FFC (f) IF of FFC. (c) At 10 dB SNR (g) FFC (h) IF of FFC by TQWT-FB method. At ∞ dB SNR (i) FFC (j) IF of FFC. At 10 dB SNR (k) FFC (l) IF of FFC by the proposed method.

Fourier Bessel, is represented in Fig. 3 (i) and (j) and the mono-components are well separated properly but the selection of the Fourier Bessel coefficient is done manually. Also, Fig. 3 (d)and (e) show the mono-components separated by the TQWT-FB method and the first component amplitude is lower and the separated component is less oscillatory in nature. TQWT-FB method cannot separate the mono-components properly at the end samples because both the mono-components lie in the same sub-band at the same time. Similarly, in Fig. 3 (k) and (l) the mono-components around the center lie in the same sub-band and are not separated properly. The Fig. 3 (f) (g) and (m) (n) show the mono-components of $S_1(n)$ and $S_2(n)$ obtained by the proposed method. The DQVWT appropriately separates the individual mono-components compared to the Fourier Bessel/time order and TQWT-FB method without setting any manual parameters. Also, the mono-components are reconstructed perfectly and exhibit a good oscillatory nature by the proposed method (Fig. 5).

The estimation of the IF of $S_1(n)$ and $S_2(n)$ by different methods are shown in Fig. 4. The Fourier Bessel/time order, TQWT-FB and the proposed methodologies are used for the computation of IF. The reference IF along with the computed IF is shown in Fig. 4. The reference IF is computed by feeding individual mono-components from to the IF computation block of the proposed method. From Fig. 4, it can be observed that the IF obtained by the proposed tracks the reference IF closely for signal $S_1(n)$. The variation in the IF obtained by the time order method and TQWT-FB method is due to the improper reconstruction of the mono-components. In the time order method, the reconstruction of the mono-components depends on the choice of the window length [14]. In TQWT-FB the mono-component reconstruction depends on the Q value of the wavelet used for signal decomposition [11]. In TQWT-FB method, the selection of the Q value to design the filter bank is independent of the nature of the signal, whereas in the proposed DQVWT, the Q value is selected dynamically based on the center frequency and bandwidth of the component.

For $S_2(n)$, the Fourier Bessel method and the proposed methods track the IF closely. The TQWT-FB method fails to track IF between sample numbers 200 and 300 because both mono-component lies in the same sub-band in these samples. Hence, it is impossible to separate them in TQWT-FB method. The Fourier-Bessel method tracks the IF of both mono-components accurately. However, in the Fourier Bessel method, the Fourier Bessel coefficient is set manually to separate the mono-components [15].

The application of the proposed method has been shown to estimate the IF of the fundamental frequency component (FFC) of speech signals. The speech signal with ID 10004 from the CMU-Arctic database [15,16], is used in the simulation. The speech signal is decimated by a factor of four and then the voiced region between sample numbers 12001 and 14000 is used in the simulation. The dataset also provides the electroglottograph (EGG) signal which is used to compute the reference IF of FFC.

The glottal closure instants (GCIs) is the measure of instant excitation of the vocal tract system [17]. The reference IF is computed by determining the GCI location's differenced region of the voiced signal. Figure 4 shows the extracted FFC by the Fourier Bessel, TQWT-FB and the proposed methods and estimated IF of FFC at ∞ dB SNR, 10 dB SNR, and 0 dB SNR when the speech is corrupted by the AWGN. The IF of FFC estimated by the proposed method tracks reference IF at ∞ dB SNR and 10 dB SNR case. The estimated IF by the Fourier-Bessel method tracks the reference IF in a better way because the sub-bands are selected manually. The estimated IF of FFC of speech signal can be used for emotion identification in the wireless body area network (WBAN) [9].

4.1 Performance Evaluation

The performance of different methods is evaluated in terms of MSE and their comparison is shown in the Table 1. The MSE is computed under three different cases at 0 dB SNR, 10 dB SNR and ∞ dB SNR.

Table 1. Computed MSE in dB at different SNRs using Fourier Bessel/time order, TQWT-FB and proposed method for two different signals.

Signal	SNR	Fourier Bessel/time order	TQWT-FB	Proposed method
$S_1(n)$	∞ dB	−243.2953	−239.846	−326.3743
	10 dB	−219.1015	−194.2821	−242.68125
	0 dB	−172.8264	−121.9412	−202.55014
$S_2(n)$	∞ dB	−335.0083	−189.9126	−262.8338
	10 dB	−190.2858	−178.0407	−221.90157
	0 dB	−114.2198	−138.7953	−159.28839

For the TQWT-FB method, the manual threshold values for the time domain are set. The possible values of the threshold for best MSEs for signal 1 are 0.4, 0.45, and 0.5 at ∞ dB, 10 dB, and 0 dB SNRs respectively. For the second signal, the threshold values are 0.1, 0.2, and 0.3 for ∞ dB, 10 dB, and 0 dB SNRs. The threshold value increases with an increase in noise level. The average MSE is computed by the execution of the program a hundred times for noise cases. From Table 1, it can be observed that the MSE obtained by the proposed method is always minimum in the noisy condition. For $S_1(n)$, the obtained MSE by the proposed method is lower than the MSE computed by other methods in the ∞ dB SNR. For $S_2(n)$ at the ∞ dB SNR, the MSE obtained by the Fourier Bessel method is minimal. This is because $S_2(n)$ mono-components are separable in the frequency domain and Fourier Bessel coefficients are set manually to separate them. However, in the proposed method, no manual setting is needed.

To compute MSE, the IF corresponding to the initial 25 samples and the last 25 samples are not considered as the computed reference IF dispersed in the frequency domain. This is because the mono-components fed to the IF computation block are terminated abruptly at the starting and ending samples. In this paper our objective is to estimate the IF of the multi-component non-stationary signals, however, the computational complexity of the proposed method is directly proportional to the length of the signal. If the length of the signal increases the computation time will also increase. If the length increases the number of TQWT arrays will increase which may lead to an increase in the computation time. The computational complexity of the proposed method can be given as $T_1 + L(T_2 + T_3 + T_4 + 2(M \times O(r \times L \times log_2 L))) + T_5 + P \times T_6$. Where $O \times (r \times L \times log_2 L)$ is the computational cost of radix-2 TQWT and ITQWT of L points length with redundancy of r [13]. There are on an average, a total M number of TQWT blocks at each iteration i $(1 \leq i \leq L)$ and the total time of TQWT computation will become $(M \times O(r \times L \times log_2 L))$ [11]. Also, the T_1 is the average time taken to window the signal, and T_2 is the average time for the Gaussian window centered at i to window the signal. Similarly, T_3 is the average time taken for the cutoff frequency computation block and T_4 is the average time for the TQWT parameters computation block. T_5 and T_6 are the time for mono-component generation and computation of the IF respectively. The average time taken for the computation of TQWT and ITQWT is the same so, the total time for the computation of TQWT array will become twice. There are total P number of mono-components so the total time for IF computation becomes $P \times T6$. The total computation time for signal $S_1(n)$ is 2.695391 s and 2.522347 s for $S_2(n)$. The system used for the computation is DESKTOP-CURT81D processor Intel(R) core(TM) i7-14700K with 64-bit operating system, x64- based processor.

The proposed method for accurately detecting the boundaries of the IF sample by sample movement of the Gaussian window is applied. However, in future, the computation time of the proposed method can be reduced by the sliding of the Gaussian window by V number of samples where $V > 1$. In some cases, V might depend on the average time period of the signal. The trade-off is that if the sliding of the Gaussian window by V number of samples the accurate IF may not be estimated at each sample.

5 Conclusion and Future Works

This paper, a novel method for the separation of the mono-components of a non-stationary signal based on DQVWT and the computation of their IF is proposed. The proposed method computes the Q value dynamically to separate the components of the signal at each sample instant. The separated components are added together to generate mono-components, whose IF is computed. Also, the performance of existing methods like Fourier Bessel/time-order, and TQWT-FB methods to compute IF are compared with the proposed method in terms of MSE at different SNRs. The proposed method has been tested on non-stationary signals consisting of LFM and NLFM mono-components and its application has been shown on a speech signal.

In future, the proposed method will be used to analyze different non-stationary signals such as biomedical signals, seismic signals, etc. Additionally, future work can be extended to reduce the computational complexity of the proposed method for the real-time application.

References

1. Boashash, B.: Time-Frequency Signal Analysis and Processing: A Comprehensive Reference. Academic Press (2015)
2. Tüske, Z., Drepper, F.R., Schlüter, R.: Non-stationary signal processing and its application in speech recognition. In: SAPA-SCALE Conference (2012)
3. Boashash, B.: Estimating and interpreting the instantaneous frequency of a signal. I. Fundamentals. Proc. IEEE **80**(4), 520–538 (1992)
4. Mathur, A., Choudhary, N., Upadhyay, A., Pachori, R.B.: Detection of glottal closure instants from voiced speech signals using the Fourier-Bessel series expansion. In: 2015 International Conference on Communications and Signal Processing (ICCSP), pp. 0474–0478. IEEE, April 2015

5. Movassaghi, S., Abolhasan, M., Lipman, J., Smith, D., Jamalipour, A.: Wireless body area networks: a survey. IEEE Commun. Surv. Tutorials **16**(3), 1658–1686 (2014)
6. Pachori, R.B., Sircar, P.: Time-frequency analysis using time-order representation and Wigner distribution. In: TENCON 2008-2008 IEEE Region 10 Conference, pp. 1–6. IEEE, November 2008
7. Huang, N.E., et al.: The empirical mode decomposition and the Hilbert spectrum for nonlinear and non-stationary time series analysis. Proc. Roy. Soc. London Ser. A Math. Phys. Eng. Sci. **454**(1971), 903–995 (1998)
8. Gilles, J.: Empirical wavelet transform. IEEE Trans. Signal Process. **61**(16), 3999–4010 (2013)
9. Dragomiretskiy, K., Zosso, D.: Variational mode decomposition. IEEE Trans. Signal Process. **62**(3), 531–544 (2013)
10. Pachori, R.B., Sircar, P.: A new technique to reduce cross terms in the Wigner distribution. Digit. Sig. Process. **17**(2), 466–474 (2007)
11. Pachori, R.B., Nishad, A.: Cross-terms reduction in the Wigner-Ville distribution using tunable-Q wavelet transform. Sig. Process. **120**, 288–304 (2016)
12. Nishad, A., Pachori, R.B.: Instantaneous fundamental frequency estimation of speech signals using tunable-Q wavelet transform. In: 2018 International Conference on Signal Processing and Communications (SPCOM), pp. 157–161. IEEE, July 2018
13. Selesnick, I.W.: Wavelet transform with tunable Q-factor. IEEE Trans. Sig. Process. **59**(8), 3560–3575 (2011)
14. Plazenet, T., Boileau, T., Caironi, C., Nahid-Mobarakeh, B.: Signal processing tools for non-stationary signals detection. In: 2018 IEEE International Conference on Industrial Technology (ICIT), pp. 1849–1853. IEEE, February 2018
15. Kominek, J.: CMU arctic databases for speech synthesis. CMU-LTI (2003)
16. Kominek, J., Black, A.W.: The CMU Arctic speech databases. In: Fifth ISCA Workshop on Speech Synthesis (2004)
17. Plumpe, M.D., Quatieri, T.F., Reynolds, D.A.: Modeling of the glottal flow derivative waveform with application to speaker identification. IEEE Trans. Speech Audio Process. **7**(5), 569–586 (1999)

High Frequency Response Pulse Detection and Pulse Width Measurement for the Radiation

Aryan Singh[1], Navaneeth Nampoothiri[1], Rishi Kundar[1], Rushikesh Suryawanshi[1], Anant Kulkarni[1(✉)], Mini Namboothiripad[1], Irfan Mirza[2], and Shashikant Dugad[2]

[1] Fr. C. Rodrigues Institute of Technology, Navi Mumbai, India
ar4013si-s@student.lu.se, anant.kulkarni@nirmauni.ac.in
[2] Tata Institute of Fundamental Research, Mumbai, India

Abstract. The need to efficiently detect and measure radiation is critical in various fields. This paper addresses the challenge of developing a fast, portable, and user-friendly radiation monitoring system. The proposed system utilizes plastic scintillating fibers (PSF) for radiation detection. A silicon photo-multiplier (SiPM) detects the radioactive particles absorbed by the fibers and converts them into electrical signals. Due to their low amplitude, these pulses require amplification; thus, an amplifier is employed. The quantization of these pulses is achieved through a comparator circuit, which converts the continuous signal into a discrete digital signal. The system leverages a field-programmable gate array (FPGA) to count the quantized outputs, determine pulse width, and implement coincidence logic for accurate radiation detection. Finally, wireless universal asynchronous receiver/transmitter (UART) communication allows data transmission from the monitoring device to a mobile device accessible by authorized users. This system offers real-time radiation level monitoring with potential applications in nuclear safety, security, and emergency response scenarios.

Keywords: SiPM · UART · FPGA · ESP · PSF · Amplifier · Comparator · Coincidence logic · Pulse width · PLD

1 Introduction

Illegal trafficking of nuclear materials poses a grave threat which involves the unauthorized possession, use, and transfer of such materials. The very nature of nuclear materials makes them incredibly dangerous. Even under controlled circumstances, their transportation and possession necessitate extreme caution. Irresponsible handling, accidental or intentional, can be catastrophic. Therefore, this technology would be a critical safeguard in ensuring global security and protecting the wellbeing of countless lives [3].

Supported by Tata Institute of Fundamental Research.

K. Atul et al. (Eds.): BodyNets 2024, LNICST 666, pp. 550–558, 2026.
https://doi.org/10.1007/978-3-032-16099-7_44

The device consists of a PSF designed to detect high-energy radiations particles emitted during the decay of radioactive elements. Following PSF is a SiPM that converts the absorbed scintillation light pulses into small electric pulses [4]. Due to their low signal strength, the incoming pulses require amplification and conversion into a digital format for compatibility with the FPGA module. This is achieved through a two-step process. First, an amplifier increases the magnitude of the pulses, making them easier to work with and less vulnerable to noise. Following this amplification, a comparator precisely qunatizes the signal to a critical threshold. The quantized output is then fed to the FPGA module, where pulse width and coincidence logic are determined. The pulse width is calculated by considering the internal clock frequency and the frequency of the quantized output, allowing for the measurement of pulse width in microseconds. The coincidence logic within the Radiation Monitoring system verifies if multiple detectors within the system have simultaneously detected a radiation event. The device transmits the desired result through a UART connection to a laptop or mobile device, notifying the user.

2 Literature Survey

It provides a comprehensive overview of all the research that was done for the proposed project and reviews the general conclusions that were made in order to help us carry out our tasks more successfully and effectively. The reader will be assisted in understanding the many factors highlighted by the study on various SiPM by the research overview. SiPMs have emerged as a new detector for low-density photon detection in applications like medical imaging and high-energy physics. They offer compact size, high gain, fast response, high photon detection efficiency, and magnetic field insensitivity. However, SiPMs have limitations like dark counts and after-pulsing, and their gain depends on biasing voltage and temperature. This paper explores power supply techniques for stable gain operation of SiPMs, including commercial and custom solutions. It concludes with recommendations for implementing the best approach for SiPM power supply [4]. SiPMs offer high gain and fast response for applications like TOF PET. Dedicated pre-amplifiers are essential to maintain optimal timing performance. Challenges include high sensor capacitance and oscillation issues. This article proposes a preamplifier concept using low-noise, high-speed transistors to address these challenges. It achieves a rise time of approximately 300 ps and enables precise timing measurements for 511 keV photon pairs coupled with specific crystals [1].

A plastic scintillator serves as the radiation detector, while the Silicon Photo Multiplier (SiPM) detects the scintillated photons generated during radiation interaction. This paper presents the system design of the proposed Radiation Detector and focuses on evaluating the performance of a high-frequency response front-end amplifier prototype. The fast response amplifier is designed using a bipolar junction transistor in a common base configuration. Various parameters including gain, bandwidth, and rise time are tested and the evaluation results are thoroughly discussed [3]. Current UART implementations typically rely on integrated circuits (ICs) within microcontrollers, often operating at a baud rate of 20 Mbps achieved with a 20 MHz clock [2]. This paper proposes a different process of using FPGAs and other programmable logic devices (PLDs) to implement UART functionality. By designing the transmitter, receiver, and core functions using VHDL, this approach offers several advantages. Firstly, it overcomes the limitations inherent in traditional methods. Secondly, it leads to a more compact, stable, and reliable design. Most importantly, implementing UART with programmable logic allows for customization based on specific needs, providing a level of flexibility unmatched by dedicated control chips.

Nuclear power plants, like many other industries, are undergoing a significant shift from traditional wired sensor networks to modern wireless technology. This transformation offers several advantages, including increased flexibility, reduced installation costs, and easier maintenance. The authors of paper [5] discuss a similar trend, highlighting the growing adoption of wireless sensor networks in nuclear facilities.

For building the GUI, Tkinter is a popular choice for building GUIs in Python. This book [8] delves into creating well-organized, functional, and responsive GUI applications using Tkinter.

3 System Components

3.1 FPGA

An FPGA is an integrated circuit that can be programmed by a user for a specific purpose after manufacturing. It consists of logical modules connected by routing channels. Due to its higher processing speed compared to a microcontroller, an FPGA can provide more accurate results. In this design, a Digilent Nexys 3 FPGA board is utilized [6]. The operating frequency of the FPGA is 100 MHz. The FPGA is employed to measure the pulse width of the incoming frequency, allowing for the determination of the time period in microseconds through specific calculations. Using the FPGA, unknown frequencies can be detected using coincidence logic.

3.2 ESP-Wroom-32

The ESP32 is a micro-controller with an integrated 2.4 GHz Wi-Fi Bluetooth module, utilizing TMSC ultra-low 40 nm technology. The Wi-Fi standard employed is 802.11n (2.4 GHz). In this design, the ESP32 is utilized to establish wireless communication between the device and the laptop/PC. Acting as an intermediate component, the ESP32 facilitates the transmission of processed data between the FPGA and the laptop/PC. The UART protocol is used for communication between the ESP and FPGA, while the Transmission Control Protocol (TCP) is employed for communication between the ESP and the laptop/PC.

4 Implementation

It comprises of all the research that was done for the work and reviews the general conclusion that were made in order to help us carry out our task more successfully and effectively. The reader will be assisted in understanding the many issues highlighted by the study on SiPM module by this research overview.

4.1 Pulse Width Modulation

The function of the Pulse Width Measuring module is to find the pulse width of unknown square pulses of fixed width and length coming from the front end of the radiation monitoring system. The longer the pulse width, the longer the scintillation light pulse, indicating a more radioactive material [4]. This is because a more radioactive material will produce more scintillation photons, which take longer to be collected by the SIPM and converted into electrical signals. Therefore, this information can be used to determine various properties of the radioactive material, such as its concentration. Figure 1 shows the block diagram for the pulse width measurement module. The FPGA performs a logical AND operation on the square pulse signals from the front end of the system and the internal clock. The resulting signal contains pulses with the same pulse width as the internal clock signal. The pulses are present when the square pulse signals have a high value and absent when they are low.

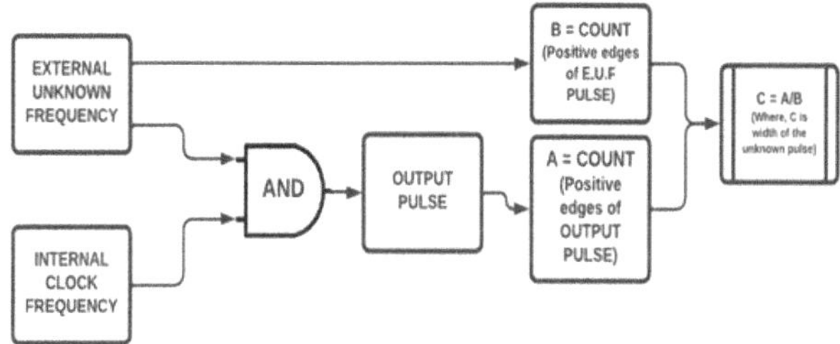

Fig. 1. Pulse Width Counter Block Diagram.

By calculating the number of pulses present when the square pulse signal is high and then multiplying that number by the positive half-time period of the internal clock, the width of the signal can be determined. The resultant pulses obtained after executing the AND operation and the square pulses are counted for a period of 1 s. Once this time period has passed, the number of pulses in the signal obtained after the AND operation and the square pulses is divided, giving the number of clock pulses present when the square pulse is high.

4.2 Coincidence Logic

The function of the coincidence logic in a radiation monitoring system is to determine whether multiple detectors within the system have detected a radiation event simultaneously. The coincidence logic helps filter out background noise or random events that may trigger individual detectors independently. By requiring multiple detectors to register a simultaneous event, it increases the system's sensitivity and reduces false alarms. This is especially important in radiation monitoring systems where accurate and reliable detection of radiation sources is crucial for safety and security purposes. Additionally, this module can also measure the frequency of the incoming signals. The proposed system employs the use of 8 scintillators that constantly monitor radiation. By creating an algorithm where the entire module is activated only after a set number of scintillators detect any radiation event of a certain frequency, the coincidence logic can be used to trigger the monitoring system. Figure 2 shows the block diagram for the coincidence logic.

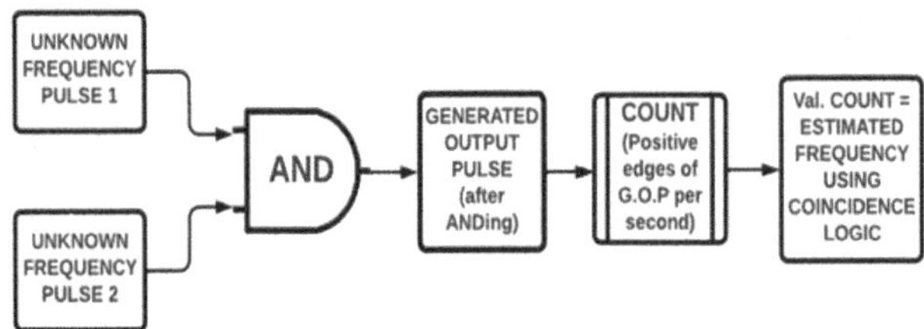

Fig. 2. Coincidence Logic Block Diagram.

The square pulses from the front end of the system (signals detected by the multiple scintillators used in the system) are given as input to the FPGA, where it performs a logical AND operation on the signals and generates an output signal. The frequency and pulse width of the generated pulse result from the AND operation of the incoming signals. Once the output signal is generated, the FPGA measures its frequency by counting the rising edges of the signal for a period of 1 s. The number of pulses counted within this time period corresponds to the frequency of the resultant signal.

4.3 FPGA - PC Communication

The value of the number of pulses or the frequency value of the signal is communicated from the FPGA to the PC using an ESP32 WROOM module [7], and the data from the FPGA to the ESP is sent through UART communication. The communication between the ESP and the PC works on the client-server communication module, where the PC functions as the client, and the ESP functions as the server. The client initiates a connection request with the server, and once the server accepts the request, a secure link is established between the client and the server through which the data is shared. Figure 2 shows the block diagram for establishing the communication between ESP and PC using the client server communication model (Fig. 3).

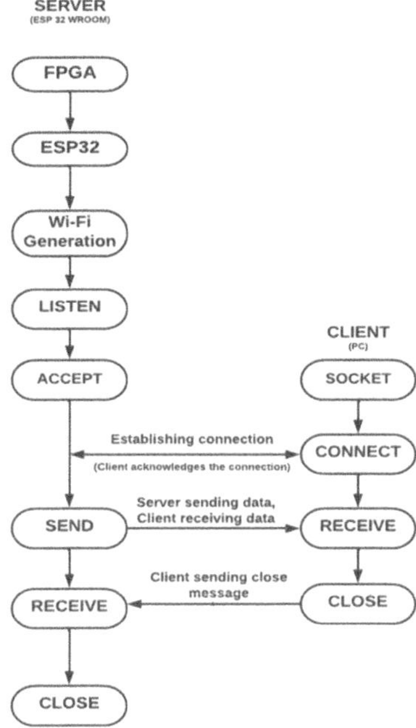

Fig. 3. Client - Server model between ESP and PC.

5 Results

It is during the implementation of this system where the input signal from a function generator is given to the FPGA board. Frequencies are varying from 5.00008 KHz–12.5 MHz for pulse width measurement and 52 KHz–60 KHz for coincidence logic. The outputs for both functions are displayed on the terminal and in a .csv file, which includes the time stamp and the desired results, such as the time period and the frequency.

As part of the process in determining whether or not the frequency of the photons collected is of a radioactive material, the pulse-width of the external frequency is measured Table 1 contains the practical and the calculated time-period (PO, CO) obtained as we increased the external frequency using the pulse width measurement logic. As we increased the external frequency the number of pulses obtained and the time-period/pulse-width was decreasing.

$$PracticalOutput(nsec) = PulseObtained * (\tau) \tag{1}$$

Table 1. .

External Input (KHz)	Pulses Obtained	PO (nSec)	CO (nsec)
5.00008	999	99990	99990
7	7141	71410	71420
10	5001	50010	50000
48	1042	10420	10416
50	1000	10000	10000
52	962	9620	9615
54	926	9260	9259
56	893	8930	8928
58	862	8620	8620
60	834	8340	8333
100	501	5010	5000
1000	51	510	500
5000	11	110	100
10000	6	60	50
12500	5	50	40

$$CalculatedOutput(nsec) = \frac{1}{ExternalFreuquency * 2} \tag{2}$$

In order to calculate the Practical output of the external frequency, Eq. (1) was used. Equation (1) consists of a product of the pulses acquired and the pulse width of the internal clock of the FPGA (τ). Calculated output has been obtained using Eq. (2), a frequency-time equation that has been divided by two, which will give us the ideal time period based on the calculations (Fig. 4).

A combination of hardware modules and algorithms effectively measured the pulse width of an unknown frequency signal. However, a one-pulse discrepancy emerged in the final value. Interestingly, this error became more prominent as the signal frequency increased. Conversely, as the frequency approached the utilized limit of 100 MHz, the one-pulse discrepancy became less significant. At lower frequencies, the measured value closely matched the actual value, indicating a minimal effect from the discrepancy. To determine the frequency of an unknown source, our team devised a system based on coincidence logic. The measurement process started by taking input from a specific number of SiPM modules. By performing an AND operation on two signals, we effectively measured the coincidence rate, which is proportional to the frequency of the input signal from the two sources. This approach yielded successful frequency measurements in the range of 50–60 kHz. In a separate aspect of the paper, we utilized socket programming to establish wireless transmission between an ESP32 microcontroller and a remote device. The ESP32 acted as the server, while a PC served as the client. The data transmission, with the server sending data and the client receiv-

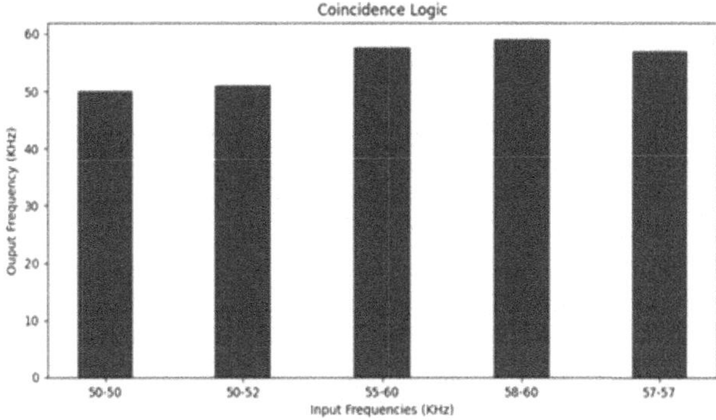

Fig. 4. Client - Server model between ESP and PC.

ing it, functioned flawlessly. Sockets enabled efficient and secure data transfer between the devices. Furthermore, to visualize the results, we created a basic GUI using the Tkinter module in Python to display the frequency and pulse width.

6 Conclusion

A combination of hardware modules and algorithms effectively measured the pulse width of an unknown frequency signal. However, a one-pulse discrepancy emerged in the final value. Interestingly, this error became more prominent as the signal frequency increased. Conversely, as the frequency approached the utilized limit of 100 MHz, the one-pulse discrepancy became less significant. At lower frequencies, the measured value closely matched the actual value, indicating a minimal effect from the discrepancy.

To determine the frequency of an unknown source, our team devised a system based on coincidence logic. The measurement process started by taking input from a specific number of SiPM modules. By performing an AND operation on two signals, we effectively measured the coincidence rate, which is proportional to the frequency of the input signal from the two sources. This approach yielded successful frequency measurements in the range of 50–60 kHz.

In a separate aspect of the project, we utilized socket programming to establish wireless transmission between an ESP32 microcontroller and a remote device. The ESP32 acted as the server, while a PC served as the client. The data transmission, with the server sending data and the client receiving it, functioned flawlessly. Sockets enabled efficient and secure data transfer between the devices. Furthermore, to visualize the results, we created a basic GUI using the Tkinter module in Python to display the frequency and pulse width.

Acknowledgment. The authors Would like to thank Tata Institute of fundamental Research, Mumbai for providing the opportunity to be a part of this work.

References

1. Benito, J., García-Díez, M., Sanchez-Tembleque, V., Fraile, L.M., Udías, J.M.: Performance study of plastic scintillators coupled to SiPM for fast-timing measurements. In: IEEE Nuclear Science Symposium and Medical Imaging Conference (NSS/MIC), Piscataway, NJ, USA, pp. 1–3 (2021). https://doi.org/10.1109/NSS/MIC44867.2021.9875794
2. Sowmya, K.B., Gomes, S., Tadiparthi, V.R.: Design of UART module using ASMD technique. In: 5th International Conference on Communication and Electronics Systems (ICCES), Coimbatore, India, pp. 176–181 (2020). https://doi.org/10.1109/ICCES48766.2020.9138098
3. Neha, V.B., Mohanty, B., Basu, A., Shaikh, M.S., Bonda, S., Mirza, I.: High frequency response pulse processing front-end for the radiation detector. In: Second International Conference on Advances in Electrical, Computing, Communication and Sustainable Technologies (ICAECT), Bhilai, India, pp. 1–4 (2022). https://doi.org/10.1109/ICAECT54875.2022.9807851
4. Shukla, R., et al.: A survey of power supply techniques for silicon photo-multiplier biasing. Int. J. Eng. Res. Gen. Sci. **2**(4), 1–5 (2014). https://api.semanticscholar.org/CorpusID:212590009. Accessed 20 Apr 2023
5. Ebenezer, J., Murty, S.S.: Deployment of wireless sensor network for radiation monitoring. In: International Conference on Computing and Network Communications (CoCoNet), Trivandrum, India, pp. 27–32 (2015). https://doi.org/10.1109/CoCoNet.2015.7411163
6. Nexys 3 FPGA Board Reference Manual, Revised 11 April 2016. This manual applies to the Nexys 3rev. B. https://digilent.com/reference/programmable-logic/nexys-3/reference-manual. Accessed 25 Apr 2023
7. ESP32 Microcontrollers with Wi-Fi and dual mode bluetooth, Espressif Systems (Shanghai). https://www.espressif.com/sites/default/files/documentation/esp32datasheeten.pdf. Accessed 13 Mar 2023
8. Moore, A.D.: Python GUI Programming with Tkinter: Design and Build Functional and User-Friendly GUI Applications. Packt Publishing (2021)

Metamaterial-Inspired Electromagnetic Sensor for Non-invasive Glucose Detection in Biological Samples

Debarati Dutta, Preeti Tiwari, and Anirban Sarkar(✉)

School of Computing and Electrical Engineering, IIT Mandi, Mandi, India
{s22005,d23257}@students.iitmandi.ac.in, anirban@iitmandi.ac.in

Abstract. This paper presents the development of advanced electromagnetic (EM) sensor utilizing novel metamaterial-inspired modified dual-SRR based resonators for non-invasive detection of glucose levels in biological samples. The sensor resonator employs a dual-SRR along with two SRRs to detect glucose concentration in physiological solution mimicking human blood. The best-suited optimized dimensions for the proposed sensor resonator structure is carried out using the Genetic-Algorithm within the framework of the CST Microwave-Studio. Leveraging frequency-shifting properties this sensor resonator prototyped on FR-4 substrate, detects a significant shift of 1 GHz in resonant frequency for 100 mg/dL and 200 mg/dL glucose-DI water physiological solution. This proposed sensor is compact, robust, inexpensive and sensitive makes it a good alternative in non-invasive blood glucose detection in biomedical industries.

Keywords: EM sensing · non-invasive sensing · blood glucose

1 Introduction

Diabetes is a devastating and growing problem in modern society and its harmful impact is escalating day by day. According to the International Diabetes Federation (IDF) Diabetes Atlas (2021), 10.5% of the adult population aged 20–79 years has diabetes, with nearly half of these individuals unaware of their condition. By 2045, IDF projections indicate that 1 in 8 adults, approximately 783 million people, will have diabetes, representing a 46% increase [1]. Diabetes is a chronic condition that arises when the pancreas fails to produce sufficient insulin or when the body is unable to effectively utilize the insulin it produces. Over time, diabetes can damage blood vessels in the heart, eyes, kidneys, and nerves, increasing the risk of serious health problems such as heart attack, stroke, and kidney failure, but continuous monitoring of blood glucose levels can help patients achieve the desired glycemic control and potentially prevent these complications. Regular monitoring of blood glucose levels can help prevent dangerous hyperglycemia (above 230 mg/dL) and hypoglycemia (below 65 mg/dL), thereby mitigating potentially fatal outcomes [2].

K. Atul et al. (Eds.): BodyNets 2024, LNICST 666, pp. 559–567, 2026.
https://doi.org/10.1007/978-3-032-16099-7_45

The most common method for measuring blood glucose levels involves using commercially available finger-pricking devices. This method is invasive, painful with limited measurements per day and provides a snapshot of blood glucose level at a specific moment. Consequently, their readings do not capture long-term patterns or trends in glucose fluctuations influenced by lifestyle, dietary habits, or medication used. Therefore, there is a growing demand for non-invasive, pain-free blood glucose monitors to encourage more frequent glucose monitoring, thereby making a significant contribution to diabetes care and prevention efforts [3]. Over the past decade, significant research has explored alternative methods for non-invasive glucose detection (NGD), such as optical techniques. These methods utilize optical parameters like optical coherence tomography (OCT), Raman spectroscopy, and fluorescence spectroscopy to identify glucose concentrations [4–6]. However, these glucose detection methods, such as absorbance spectroscopy using red/near-infrared and mid-infrared wavelengths, analyze light scattering on biological tissue but often require bulky, expensive instruments and are highly sensitive to physiological and environmental changes [7]. Enzyme-based electrochemical methods have been explored to measure glucose levels indirectly by analyzing sweat and interstitial fluid (ISF), then correlating these readings to blood glucose levels. While these methods offer good sensitivity, the time lag between glucose changes in sweat, ISF, and blood remains a challenge [8]. Among the various approaches, RF/microwave sensing techniques appear more promising, as they utilize electromagnetic waves (EM) that penetrate biological tissues without the harmful effects associated with ionizing radiation like X-rays. These techniques rely on dielectric characterization, where the dielectric permittivity and conductivity of blood are significantly influenced by glucose content, allowing for the development of a reliable correlation model [9–15]. The Debye and Cole-Cole models are frequency dependent analytical method in non-invasive blood glucose detection by accurately describing the dielectric properties of biological tissue and correlating them with the blood glucose level [16] Non-planar glucose monitoring sensors are bulky, less portable, and challenging to conform comfortably to the body's natural curvature. These limitations can make them less practical for everyday use. The development of wearable and attachable health monitoring systems is aimed at enhancing comfort and providing real-time health monitoring, both in clinical diagnoses and in daily life . During blood glucose measurement using microwave sensors, several challenges need to be addressed to ensure accurate and reliable readings: (a) The variability in biological tissue properties, such as skin thickness and composition, which can differ based on factors like gender, age, ethnicity, physical health, and fitness status, makes it challenging to isolate the sensed response to blood glucose concentration, (b) Additionally, uncertainty in the actual dielectric properties and thicknesses of biological tissues, which vary from person to person, further complicates accurate glucose measurement. Since blood permittivity changes minimally with glucose concentration, using EM sensors to monitor glucose variation heavily depends on selecting the precise frequency range, ensuring that the reflected and transmitted waves from the sensor to the blood capillary specifically capture information related to blood glucose levels.

In this work, a non-invasive robust electromagnetic resonator sensor is proposed on FR-4 substrate with dielectric constant of 4.4 and loss tangent 0.0025, which works on X band to monitor changes in blood glucose levels within the clinically relevant range of 100–200 mg/dL for Type-2 diabetes. A synthetic human blood model with accurate permittivity and loss tangent is prepared, which disrupt the electric field distribution around the sensor. This disruption allows the sensor to detect different glucose levels by tracking changes in the amplitude and frequency of the reflected signals at a specific frequency band. The first order Debye model is used analytically to correlate the measured glucose levels in aqueous solutions with the three key parameters of the Debye model. This proposed sensor resonator shows a significant resonant frequency shift of 1 GHz for the different glucose level proves its utility in biomedical sensing application.

2 Proposed Design Methodology and Analysis

2.1 Sensor Designing, Optimization and Validation of Metamaterial Property

The proposed metamaterial based sensor resonator is evolved through multiple stages where initially, a dual-SRR is placed at the center. To get a better resonance depth two SRRs are placed on the two sides of the dual-SRR. This arrangement gives a resonant frequency at 10.54 GHz with a resonance depth of -48.41 dB. The reflection and transmission response of the sensor resonator is depicted in Fig. 1. The proposed dual-SRR based final design is shown in Fig. 2(a) and (b) depicting all the optimized design parameters as follows W, L, g_1, g_2, w_1, w_2, w_3, w_4, w_5, l_1, l_2, l_3, l_4, h_1, h_2, h_3, h_4, r_1, r_2 which are listed in Table 1. To validate the metamaterial property of the proposed modified SRR sensor resonator, the real and imaginary part of the permeability and permittivity have been extracted as shown in Fig. 3. (a)-(b) and (c)-(d), respectively. The permittivity and permeability are dependent on impedance (Z) and refractive index (η), which are functions of reflection coefficient (S_{11}) and transmission

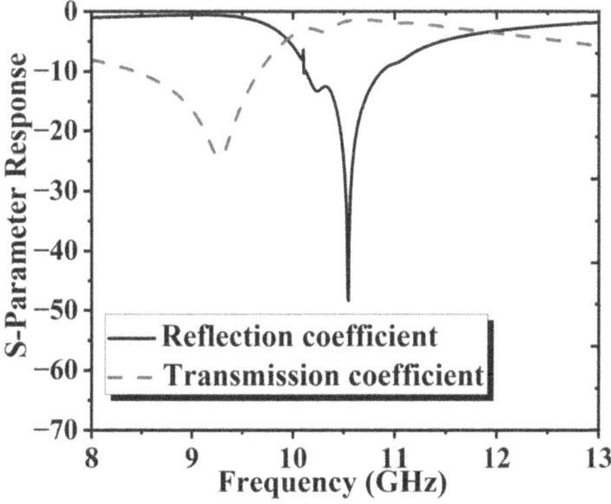

Fig. 1. S-parameter response of the proposed sensor resonator.

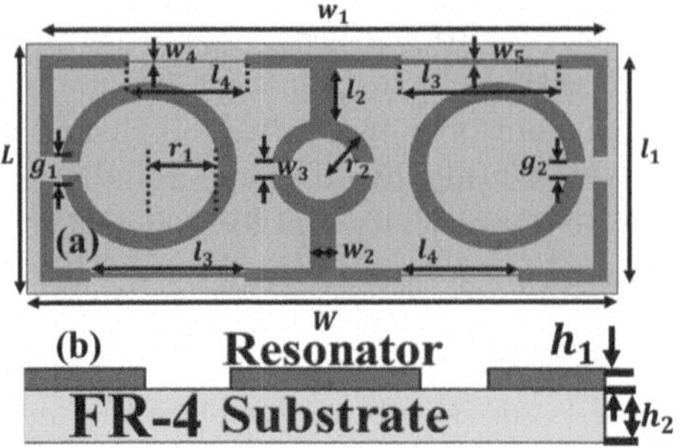

Fig. 2. Parameterized geometry of the proposed sensor resonator (a) top view, (b) layered side view.

Table 1. VALUES OF GEOMETRIC VARIABLES

Parameter	Dimension (mm)	Parameter	Dimension (mm)
W	22.84	L	10.18
w_1	21.84	l_1	9.18
w_2	1	l_2	2.143
l_3	6	l_4	4.5
w_3	0.5	g_1	1
w_4	0.2	w_5	0.1
r_1	2.7	g_2	0.5
r_2	2	h_1	0.035
h_2	1.5		

coefficient (S_{21}). The parameters are determined based on the following Eqs. (1), (2) [17]:

$$\mu = \eta Z \tag{1}$$

$$\epsilon = \frac{\eta}{Z} \tag{2}$$

where the impedance (Z) and refractive index (η) are obtained from the below Eqs. (3) and (4):

$$Z = \pm\sqrt{\frac{(1+S_{11})^2 - S_{21}^2}{(1-S_{11})^2 - S_{21}^2}} \tag{3}$$

$$\eta = \frac{1}{k_0 d}\left[\left[\ln\left(e^{ink_0 d}\right)\right]'' - i\left[\ln\left(e^{ink_0 d}\right)\right]'\right] \tag{4}$$

Here, The exponential term in Eq. (4), is represented by $e^{ink_0 d} = \frac{S_{21}}{1-S_{11}\frac{Z-1}{Z+1}}$, where $[\ln(e^{ink_0 d})']$ represents the real component, $[\ln(e^{ink_0 d})'']$ denotes the imaginary component of the complex number, k_0 denotes the wave-number and d represents the maximum length of the unit cell. As the figure suggested, Fig. 3, the proposed sensor resonator structure exhibits dual-negative metamaterial properties within the operating frequency range 10–11 GHz.

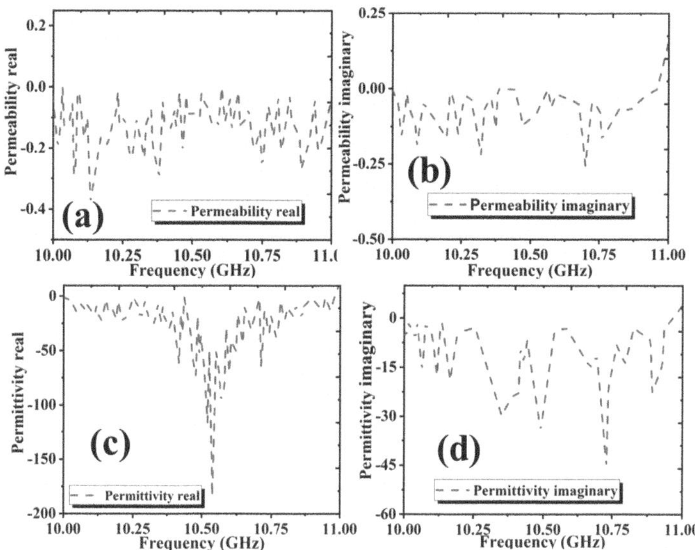

Fig. 3. Permeability and permittivity profile of the proposed metamaterial sensor resonator with highlighted operational dual-frequency band (a) real values of permeability, (b) imaginary values of permeability, (c) real values of permittivity, (d) imaginary values of permittivity.

2.2 Sensitivity Analysis

To analyze the sensitivity of the proposed sensor resonator geometry, the field properties of the structure at different modes are needed to be examined. Figure 4(a) shows the magnitude of electric field distribution of the proposed structure for the operational band. Figure 4 depicts the field distribution across the entire resonator surface operating at 10.54 GHz where the electric field is distributed across the resonator structure. According to the perturbation theory, the section with a high electric field density is more sensitive than a section with lesser density of electric field. Hence, it is evident that the entire resonator structure is sensitive and suitable for material under test (MUT) placement. The sensitivity of a sensor refers to the shift in resonant frequency per unit change in the permittivity of the loaded sample. The ability to detect the change in the output if there is a small change in the input, hence, high-sensitivity is always a crucial demand in designing advanced sensors.

3 Validation of Sensing Performance Using Cole-Cole Complex Permittivity Model

3.1 Performance Validation: Sample Preparation

The estimation of blood glucose in the human body is validated using a mimicked human blood model, which consists of a solution of deionized water (DI)

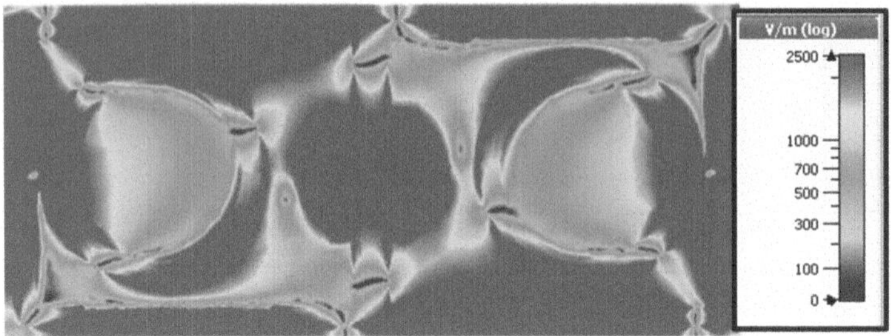

Fig. 4. Distribution of electric field within proposed sensor resonator at 10.54 GHz.

and dextrorotatory glucose (D-glucose). D-glucose, a naturally occurring form of glucose, is commonly found in the human body and is used in the solution to accurately replicate physiological conditions. To mimic various blood glucose concentrations, D-glucose solutions are prepared at different concentrations in DI water. Two different concentrations of D-glucose; 100 mg, 200 mg and 300mg are mixed with 100 mL of water to mimic 100 mg/dL, 200 mg/dL solution, respectively. To solely observe the effects of glucose in human blood; no other constituents are added to make the fluid more physiological relevant. These lab-made polar solutions are then tested using the 07039 Keysight Dielectric Probe Kit for determining the complex dielectric constant.

3.2 Complex Dielectric Constant Measurement Using Dielectric Probe Kit

The calibration of the dielectric probe kit for the complex permittivity measurement of DI water-D-glucose solution, is a crucial process that involves three key steps: open air calibration, shorted block calibration, and calibration with commercial drinking water. After the final calibration with commercial water the permittivity value is obtained to be 73 Typically the permittivity of water is usually between 70–80. The calibration with drinking water is essential because it serves as a standard reference with a known permittivity which ensuring the accuracy and reliability of subsequent measurements. Once the final step of water calibration is completed the complex permittivity measurements are conducted on samples with varying concentrations of D-glucose in fixed volume of deionized (DI) water. The real and imaginary permittivity values are obtained using the Agilent Vector Network Analyzer in the software 85070.

3.3 Validation of Cole-Cole Model

The general method of calculating complex permittivity by treating the real part and imaginary part assumes that the permittivity remains constant across frequencies. However, this method does not capture the frequency-dependent behavior of permittivity, which is crucial in complex materials like biological tissues. The Cole-Cole model addresses this by incorporating relaxation time and a distribution parameter to accurately represent how permittivity changes with frequency, making it a more precise approach for such materials. The complex permittivity values for a polar solution can be calculated using the Cole-Cole Eq. (5) [18].

$$\epsilon^*(\omega) = \epsilon_\infty + \frac{\epsilon_s - \epsilon_\infty}{1 + (j\omega\tau)^{(1-\alpha)}} \tag{5}$$

Here, ϵ_∞ is the permittivity at infinite frequency, ϵ_s is the permittivity at low frequency, τ is the relaxation time and α is the distribution parameter ($0 \leq \alpha < 1$) and when $\alpha = 0$ the equation simplifies to the Debye model. Polar solutions like glucose-water can be modeled using this way. The measured complex permittivity values are fitted to the Debye model to obtain the necessary parameters as a function of the glucose concentration (mg/dL). These parameters serve as indicators of glucose concentration, enabling non-invasive monitoring and accurate assessment of glucose levels based on dielectric properties. The experimental analysis to correlate the Debye model parameters with glucose concentration (mg/dL) find to be a first-order polynomial function. The empirical equations are mentioned in Eq. (6):

$$\epsilon_s = 1.78*10^{-16}*C+80, \quad \epsilon_{inft} = 1.12^{-17}*C+4.9, \quad \tau = 3.71^{-27}*C+10e-10 \tag{6}$$

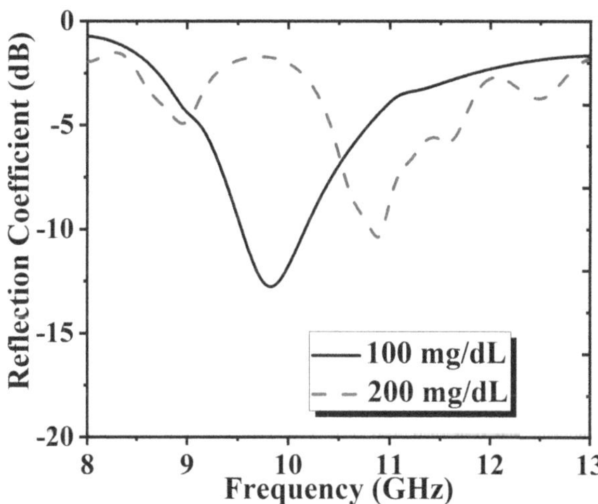

Fig. 5. Reflection co-efficient response for two different blood glucose concentrations.

Here, C is the concentration of glucose in mg/dL. The Debye model can be experimentally verified by placing a sample holder on the top of proposed sensor resonator and by adding a solution of DI water and D-glucose of specified amount.

In order to hold the prepared samples on the top of the sensor, a Polylactic acid (PLA) (ϵ_r = 2.4–2.6) sample holder of dimension 22.84 × 10.18 × 1.5 mm^3, has been positioned on the top of the sensor. The dielectric constant and electrical conductivity values for 100 mg/dL is 58.46, 1.40 S/m and 200 mg/dL blood glucose level these values are 50.02 and 1.4250 S/m, respectively [19]. The reflection response for the two different glucose solutions are depicted in Fig. 5. A frequency shift of 1 GHz can be seen due to the different concentration of glucose.

4 Conclusion

In conclusion, this proposed sensor resonator, inspired by metamaterial property, presents a promising approach for non-invasive diabetes detection directly from the human body. The sensor's ability to squeeze electromagnetic waves within a specific area enhances its sensitivity. Through thorough performance evaluation, we have demonstrated that this sensor holds great potential for biosensing applications. Moreover, its planar characteristic makes it an excellent fit for modern microwave-based lab-on-chip systems, offering simplicity and compactness in its design. This novel sensor design paves the way for advancements in non-invasive medical diagnostics and provides a valuable contribution to the field of microwave-based bio-sensing technology.

References

1. https://idf.org/about-diabetes/diabetes-facts-figures
2. Alberti, K.G.M.M.: The Classification and Diagnosis of Diabetes Mellitus. John Wiley Sons, Ltd., Hoboken, ch. 2, pp. 24–30 (2010)
3. Henning, T.: Commercially Available Continuous Glucose Monitoring Systems. John Wiley Sons, Ltd., Hoboken, ch. 5, pp. 113–156 (2009). https://onlinelibrary.wiley.com/doi/abs/10.1002/9780470567319.ch5
4. Villena Gonzales, W., Mobashsher, A.T., Abbosh, A.: The progress of glucose monitoring–a review of invasive to minimally and non-invasive techniques, devices and sensors. Sensors **19**(4) (2019). https://www.mdpi.com/1424-8220/19/4/800
5. Spegazzini, N., et al.: Spectroscopic approach for dynamic bioanalyte tracking with minimal concentration information. Sci. Rep. **4**, 7013, 1–7 (2014)
6. Sim, J., Ahn, C.-G., Jeong, E.-J., Kim, B.: In vivo microscopic photoacoustic spectroscopy for non-invasive glucose monitoring invulnerable to skin secretion products. Sci. Rep. **8**, 01 (2018)
7. Hina, A., Saadeh, W.: A noninvasive glucose monitoring soc based on single wavelength photoplethysmography. IEEE Trans. Biomed. Circuits Syst. **PP**, 1 (2020)
8. Daboss, E., Shcherbacheva, E., Galushin, A., Vokhmyanina, D., Karyakina, E., Karyakin, A.: Noninvasive diabetes monitoring through continuous analysis of sweat using flow-through glucose biosensor. Anal. Chem. **91**, 02 (2019)
9. Karacolak, T., Moreland, E., Topsakal, E.: Cole-cole model for glucose- dependent dielectric properties of blood plasma for continuous glucose monitoring. Microw. Opt. Technol. Lett. **55**, 05 (2013)

10. Dobson, R., Wu, R., Callaghan, P.: Blood glucose monitoring using microwave cavity perturbation. Electron. Lett. **48**, 905–906 (2012)
11. Hofmann, M., Fersch, T., Weigel, R., Fischer, G., Kissinger, D.: A novel approach to non-invasive blood glucose measurement based on rf transmission, 2011
12. Saha, S., et al.: A glucose sensing system based on transmission measurements at millimetre waves using micro strip patch antennas. Sci. Rep. **7** (2017)
13. Hussain, A., Kumar, A., Akhtar, M.J.: Design of csrr based planar sensor for non-invasive measurement of complex permittivity. Sens. J. IEEE **15**, 7181–7189 (2015)
14. Gabriel, S.M., Lau, R.W., Gabriel, C.: The dielectric properties of biological tissues: III. parametric models for the dielectric spectrum of tissues. Phys. Med. Biol. **41**(11), 2271–93 (1996). https://api.semanticscholar.org/CorpusID:25252313
15. Omer, A.E., et al.: Low-cost portable microwave sensor for non-invasive monitoring of blood glucose level: novel design utilizing a four-cell csrr hexagonal configuration. Nature **10**, 09 (2020)
16. Turgul, V., Kale, I.: Characterization of the complex permittivity of glucose/water solutions for noninvasive rf/microwave blood glucose sensing, pp. 1–5, 2016
17. Abdulkarim, Y., et al.: Design and study of a metamaterial-based sensor for the application of liquid chemicals detection. J. Mater. Res. Technol. **9** (2020)
18. Cole, K.S., Cole, R.H.: Dispersion and absorption in dielectrics I. Altern. Curr. Charact. **9**(4), 341–351 (1941)
19. Affendi, F., et al.: RF remote blood glucose sensor and a microfluidic vascular phantom for sensor validation. Biosensors **11**, 494 (2021)

Optimization of Clock Frequency Performance for Gnss Positioning

B. R. Sanjeeva Reddy, Muddavath Srikanth(✉), and M. Mani Chanda Goud

B V Raju Institute of Technology, Narsapur, Medak, India
{sanjeeva.reddy,22211D5503,21211D5502}@bvrit.ac.in

Abstract. Global Navigation Satellite system (GNSS) facilitate Earth based mapping via orbiting Satellite network. GNSS receivers calculate distance to these Satellites allowing users to Precisely determine their location. GNSS encompass multiple constellations providing global coverage. In order for GNSS systems to operate nowadays, high-precision atomic clock data must be transmitted from satellites to receivers, which requires massive bandwidth. The notion that each satellite transmits its own time information for this data redundancy. Current GNSSs rely on ground networks to monitor and correct satellite clocks. This project work discusses about how optical clocks are becoming more accurate timepieces than atomic clocks for wireless transmitter applications.

An introduction to optical clock technology, including its history and features, is given at the beginning of the text. The Allan Deviation (ADEV) method is then used to evaluate clock stability, and a stability analysis is performed by comparing optical clocks with the current Global Navigation Satellite System (GNSS) satellite clocks. The results indicate that on board GNSS satellites, optical clocks are more stable than atomic clocks. To achieve spacecraft payload requirements, additional technological developments might be required. Optical clocks, as opposed to the current atomic clocks on board GNSS satellites, may provide sub-millimeter range inaccuracy and far better timing performance in the GNSS location. The Study Specifically Pinpoints the atomic of the Galileo satellites.

Keywords: Positioning Navigation and Timing (PNT) satellites atomic clocks · optical clocks · clock stability research Allan deviation and GNSS

1 Introduction

Global Navigation Satellite System (GNSS) encompass System such as GPS, GLONASS, GALILEO, and Bei Dou, providing ubiquitous and accurate positing, Navigation and timing (PNT) services These systems operate through a constellation of satellites that broadcast signals to ground receivers, enabling precise location determination. GNSS technology relies on the accurate timing information provided by satellite

K. Atul et al. (Eds.): BodyNets 2024, LNICST 666, pp. 568–580, 2026.
https://doi.org/10.1007/978-3-032-16099-7_46

clocks and the known positions of the satellites in their orbits. The performance of GNSS is often evaluated based on the signal-in-space range error (SISRE), which impacts the achievable positioning accuracy. GNSS supports various applications, from personal navigation and geospatial mapping to critical scientific research and military operations. The integration of multiple GNSS constellations enhances positioning accuracy and reliability, as users can access signals from a larger number of satellites, reducing the impact of signal blockages and atmospheric disturbances.

Optimal clocks are designed to provide highly stable and accurate timekeeping by minimizing noise and systematic errors. These clocks are essential for applications requiring precise time synchronization, such as GNSS, telecommunications, and scientific research. The development of optimal clocks involves improving the stability of local oscillators and their synchronization to atomic transitions. Techniques like laser cooling and trapping of atoms, along with the use of optical frequency combs, enhance the performance of these clocks. The stability of an optimal clock is often quantified in terms of its frequency instability and systematic uncertainty. In advanced applications, optimal clocks can achieve stability levels that allow for measurements of physical phenomena with unprecedented precision, such as monitoring variations in the Earth's gravitational field or conducting fundamental tests of physical theories.

Atomic clocks are the cornerstone of precise timekeeping and frequency standards, using the consistent frequency of atomic transitions to maintain accuracy. Cesium atomic clocks, for instance, define the second based on the hyperfine transition frequency of cesium-133 atoms. These clocks are crucial for applications requiring high precision, such as GNSS, network synchronization, and scientific experiments. Advances in atomic clock technology have led to the development of optical clocks, which utilize transitions in optical ranges, providing higher frequencies and better precision compared to traditional microwave-based clocks. Optical clocks achieve remarkable stability by locking a laser to the atomic transition frequency and using an optical frequency comb to measure the frequency. This level of precision allows atomic clocks to serve as primary standards for time and frequency, enabling advancements in technology and science.

2 Literature Survey

2.1 Related Work

Extensive research has been conducted on enhancing the performance and reliability of Global Navigation Satellite Systems (GNSS). Multiple GNSS constellations such as GPS, GLONASS, Galileo, and Bidou have been developed to provide global coverage and improved accuracy [1]. Studies have focused on the integration of signals from these constellations to enhance positioning accuracy and robustness. Research by Misra and Enge (2006) delves into the fundamentals of GNSS, providing a comprehensive overview of system design and performance metrics [2]. Advances in GNSS receiver technology, as discussed by Kaplan and Hegarty (2005), have also contributed to improved signal processing capabilities and error mitigation techniques. Recent work by Montenbruck et al. (2017) highlights the benefits of multi-GNSS integration, demonstrating significant improvements in positioning accuracy and reliability [3]. Future research is focusing on mitigating signal interference and enhancing signal integrity to support emerging applications like autonomous vehicles and precision agriculture [4] Optimal clocks, which aim to minimize noise and systematic errors, are critical for applications requiring precise time synchronization. Research in this area has focused on enhancing the stability and accuracy of these clocks [5]. Techniques such as laser cooling and trapping of atoms, as explored by Katori et al. (2003), have significantly improved the performance of optical frequency standards. The development of optical frequency combs, as detailed by Udemy et al. (2002), has enabled precise measurement and control of optical frequencies, leading to unprecedented levels of clock stability. Recent advancements in optical lattice clocks, as discussed by Ludlow et al. (2015), have demonstrated remarkable frequency stability and accuracy, paving the way for redefining the second based on optical transitions. Ongoing research is addressing challenges like environmental sensitivity and technical complexity to further enhance the usability and performance of optimal clocks in practical settings [6] Atomic clocks are fundamental to precision time keeping and have seen substantial advancements over the years. Early work by Essen and Parry (1955) established the cesium atomic clock as the primary standard for time and frequency. Subsequent research has focused on improving the accuracy and stability of these clocks [7]. Developments in hydrogen masers, as discussed by Ramsey (1990), provided enhanced long-term stability for atomic clocks. The advent of optical clocks [8], as reviewed by Ludlow et al. (2015), marked a significant leap in clock performance, utilizing high-frequency optical transitions for superior accuracy. Recent research by Huntsman et al. (2016) and Brewer et al. (2019) has demonstrated optical clocks with fractional frequency uncertainties at the 10^-18 level, highlighting their potential for redefining the SI second and supporting advanced scientific and technological applications [9]. Current research aims to integrate these clocks into a broader range of practical applications, addressing challenges related to environmental robustness and miniaturization for field deployment. Incorporating these additional elements can provide a more detailed and forward-looking perspective in paper [10] (Fig. 1).

Paper Name	Author	Advantages	Challenges
Optical atomic clocks	Andrew D. Ludlow [2015].	Accurate data signal transmission over a lower Period	In This optical clocks Frequency Standards are very low
Compact Rb optical frequency standard with 10−15 stability	Shengnan Zhang [2017].	Rb optical frequency is Versatility and Potential for Future Applications	Power Broadening Effects
The CIPM list of recommended frequency standard values: guidelines and procedures	Fritz Riehle [2018].	Improved Time Scales and High Accuracy with Stability of Optical Clocks.	Initial High Uncertainty and Complexity.
Atomic Clocks for Geodesy	Tanja E. Mehlstäubler [2018].	Superior Short-Time Stability	Interferometer Phase Noise
20 years of developments in optical frequency comb technology and applications	Tara Fortier [2019].	Faster Acquisition Times	Low Power per Optical Mode
On a definition of the SI second with a set of optical clock transitions	Jérôme Lodewick [2019].	The proposed frequency unit based on multiple optical clock transitions	Dependence on Frequency Ratio Measurements.

Fig. 1. Table no Literature table

		can achieve a lower uncertainty compared to the current cesium-based definition	
Future GNSS constellations with optical inter-satellite links. Preliminary space segment analyses.	Gabriele Giorgi [2019].	Improved Precision in Orbit Determination	Limited Ground Infrastructure Adaptation
A User's View on GNSS Performance	Oliver Montenbruck [2020].	GNSS supports a variety of precise positioning techniques, such as Precise Point Positioning (PPP), which can achieve cm-level accuracy.	In This we are overcome for the clock frequency but Data Rate getting errors
GNSS-grade space atomic frequency standards: Current status and ongoing developments	Etienne Batori [2020].	improvement in the quality and availability of navigation signals that greatly benefit the positioning performance and robustness.	integrating different signals and managing the complexities of multi-GNSS receiver technology
Evaluation optical clock performance for GNSS position	Enkhtuvshin Boldbaatar [2023].	Optical clock performance for the GPS and using Galileo	The Data speed is slow and getting errors in the Atmosphere

Fig. 1. *(continued)*

3 Methodology

3.1 Atomic Frequency Standards

Atomic Frequence Standards rely on the consistent vibration of atom to measure time with extraordinary precision. These Standards are fundamental to various application from global positioning system (GPS) to telecommunication and scientific research Atom clock which utilize these standards are among the most accurate timekeeping devices available. Capable of maintaining time to within a few billionths of a second.

The importance of atom frequence standards cannot be overstated. They provide the foundation for synchronization in communication network. Ensure the accuracy of navigation system and support scientific experiments that require precise timing. The deification of the frequence of transition between two hyper fine level of the ground state of the cesium-133atom highlight the critical role of atom frequences standards in the Modern metrology.

The concept of atomic frequence standards emerged in the mid-20th century, revolutionizing time keeping by utilizing the consistent vibration of atom. The development of the first atom clock by Harold Lyons in 1949 marked the beginning of this revolution.

Atomic clock

An atom clock is an exceptionally accurate timekeeping device that uses the vibration of atom to measure time. The most widely used kind of atomic clock makes use of cesium-133 atom These clocks work on the basis of monitoring the microwave signals that atoms' electrons release when their energy levels change The International System of Units (SI) defines a second as having a precise frequency of 9,192,631,770 cycles per second, which is the resonance of caesium atoms in clocks.

Atomic clocks on GNSS satellites are critical for time and frequency information used in navigation signal generation. Accuracy of these clocks impacts the overall performance of GNSS systems, with clock stability being a major factor.

Clock stability is measured using Allan Deviation (ADEV), indicating the standard deviation of the fractional frequency error over predefined intervals.

Optical clock

An optical clock is a type of atomic clock that uses the frequency of light emitted or absorbed by atom as its timing element. These clocks operate on the principles of quantum mechanics and are extremely precise, often surpassing the accuracy of traditional microwave-based atomic clocks.

Integrating optical clocks with GNSS systems could offer significant improvements in timing accuracy and precision for various applications, including navigation, telecommunications, and scientific research.

Allan Variance

Allan Variance is a statistical method used to analyse the stability of frequence signal over time. It quantifies the frequency Stability of oscillator clock and other time keeping devices by comparing the difference in the frequence between successive time intervals.

$$\sigma_y^2(T) : \frac{1}{2M^2T^2}(N - 2M + 1) \tag{1}$$

- M is the number of averaging intervals
- T is the averaging time

Frequence Bands

The Band Frequence are select on the required on the required compounds like "cs" and "sr" which are using in the GPS and Galileo System. In the we are having Difference of Frequences and Bands there are L1, L2, L5 (Fig. 2).

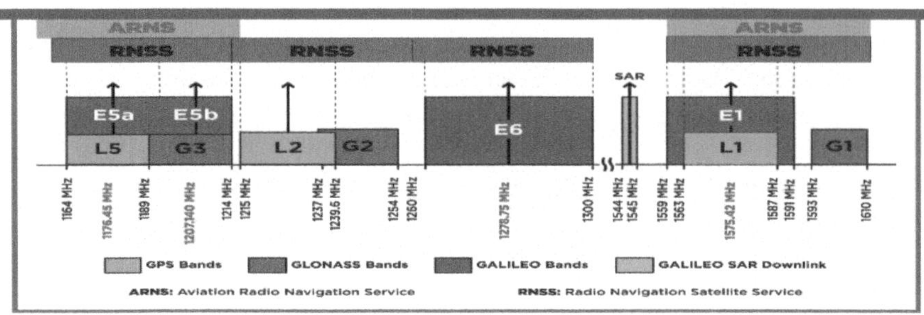

Fig. 2. no1 Frequence Bands

Nearly every civilian (consumer and enterprise) receiver support GPS L1 signal at 1575.74 MHz, which includes the Course/Acquisition (C/A) code, as well the encrypted Precision (P(Y)) code, which is only authorized users can access. In the future, the L1 signal will be augmented with increased availability for civilian users and L1M for military users.

GPS's L2P(Y) signal at 1227.6 MHz has long been used for precision military applications. Civilian users also can use it in a "codeless" fashion, where the receiver finds the L1 signal first and then uses some of the L2 signal's information to improve accuracy.

As with L1, the GPS modernization program is adding two L2 signals which is not high precision but rather a stronger and slower signal designed to be available in more challenging environments. A receiver can access L2C without first receiving L1. The other new signal, L2M, is available only to authorized users.

L5 signal at 1176.45 MHz was developed for aviation safety. It's the most advanced civilian signal available from GPS because it's faster like the precision codes at L1 and L2, and for its higher power and lower frequency. L5 currently is widely available (from 12 satellites) and is expected to be fully available (24 satellites) in 2024.

In this we are using the 1 × 10–14 frequence in the L1 band to Transmitter a single for the basics station.

$$y(t) = \frac{1}{2\pi v_0}\frac{\mathrm{d}^{\emptyset}(t)}{\mathrm{d}t} = \frac{\phi(t)}{2\pi y_0} \tag{2}$$

- Y(t) = Normalized frequency
- V0 = Nominal frequency
- ϕ = radians

- $2\pi v0$ = phase Frequency

Modulation Techniques

GNSS (Global Navigation Satellite System) transmission system are designed to provide accurate position navigation and timing information. These System include GPS, Galileo, Each GNSS consist of a constellation of satellites transmitting signals to receiver on the ground GNSS signals are transmitted on multiple frequencies, such as L1, L2, and L5 for GPS or E1, E5, and E6 for Galileo. These signals use various modulation techniques like Binary Phase Shift Keying (BPSK), Quadrature Phase Shift Keying (QPSK), and Binary Offset Carrier (BOC) to encode navigation data and spread spectrum codes. The data rates typically range from 50 bps to 250 bps, ensuring robust signal transmission even in challenging environments.

Binary Phase Shift Keying (BPSK) is one of the simplest and most widely used modulation schemes in digital communication systems. It is a form of phase modulation that uses two distinct phases to represent binary data. These two phases are typically separated by 180 degrees, which correspond to the binary digits 0 and 1 (Fig. 3).

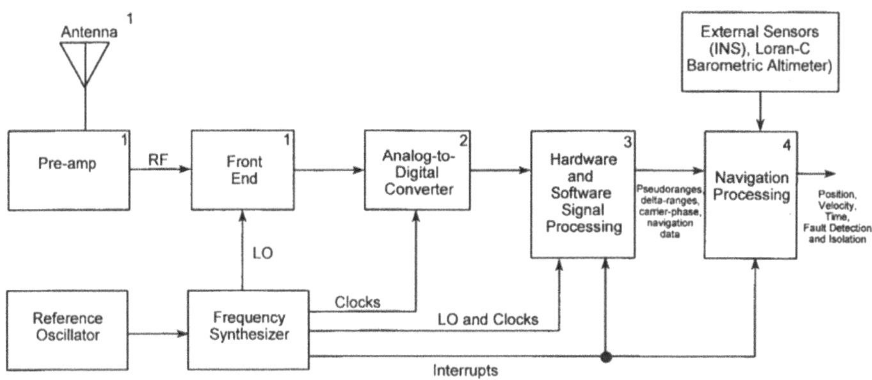

Fig. 3. Block diagram of modulation of Bpsk

The performance of BPSK can be evaluated in terms of its bit error rate (BER), which is a measure of the likelihood that a bit will be incorrectly received. The BER of BPSK is primarily influenced by the signal-to-noise ratio (SNR) of the communication channel. In an ideal noiseless environment, BPSK can achieve error-free transmission.

The design of the BPSK transmitter and receiver also involves several practical considerations. The transmitter must generate a stable and precise carrier signal, and the phase modulation must be accurately controlled to ensure the correct representation of the binary data.

One of the challenges in BPSK systems is phase ambiguity. Since BPSK uses only two phases, a 180-degree phase shift in the received signal can lead to incorrect data interpretation. To address this issue, differential encoding can be used, where each transmitted bit is encoded relative to the previous bit. This approach eliminates the phase ambiguity problem, ensuring that the receiver can correctly interpret the transmitted data even in the presence of phase shifts.

Precise Point Positioning (PPP) is a satellite-based navigation technique that allows for the determination of accurate and precise positions anywhere on Earth using Global Navigation Satellite Systems (GNSS). PPP provides centimetre-level accuracy by utilizing precise satellite orbit and clock data, along with advanced error correction models. This makes it an attractive solution for applications requiring high precision without the need for a local reference station, unlike traditional differential GNSS (DGNSS) methods. PPP relies on signals from multiple GNSS constellations, such as GPS, Galileo It uses precise satellite orbit and clock information, typically provided by organizations like the International GNSS Service (IGS).

PPP relies on signals from multiple GNSS constellations, such as GPS, Galileo It uses precise satellite orbit and clock information, typically provided by organizations like the International GNSS Service (IGS) (Fig. 4).

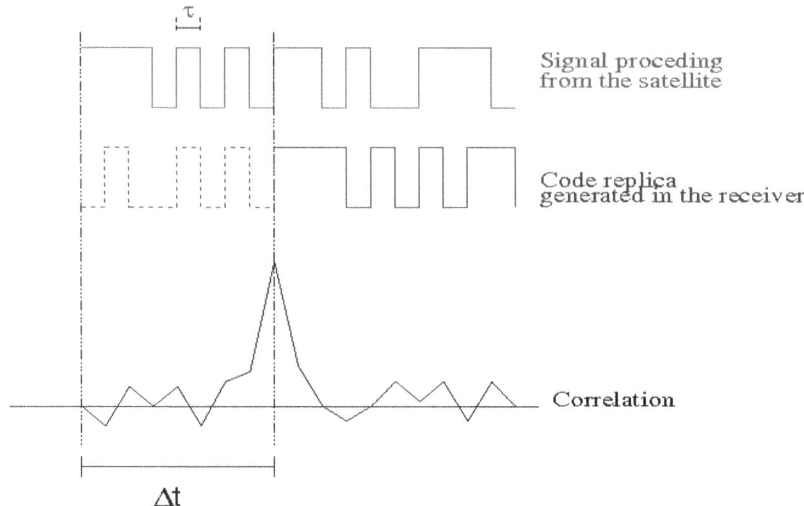

Fig. 4. Waves of signal proceding from the Ground to satellite

Speciation Densities are related by the equations for phase and frequency

$$s_x(f) = \frac{1}{(2\pi v_0)} s\phi(f) \tag{3}$$

$$sy(f) = \frac{f^2}{v_0} s_\emptyset(f) \tag{4}$$

s(x)and s(y) are the axis to Calculate the frequencies and correlation.

In the correlation we are using difference types of frequences and taking the calculation of Data pack which are transamination for the Ground stations to Satellites.

Mapping in the context of GNSS typically refers to the process of using satellite positioning data to create maps or spatial representations of geographic features. GNSS systems, such as GPS, GLONASS, Galileo, provide accurate location information that can be used for various mapping applications.

Mapping with GNSS involves collecting position data from satellites using receivers on the ground or on mobile devices. This data can then be used to create maps that show the locations of various points of interest, landmarks, terrain features, or other geographic information.

Modern GPS systems depend on atomic clocks to synchronize satellite signals, enabling accurate position determination. This technology has become integral to various industries, including transportation, telecommunications, and military operations.

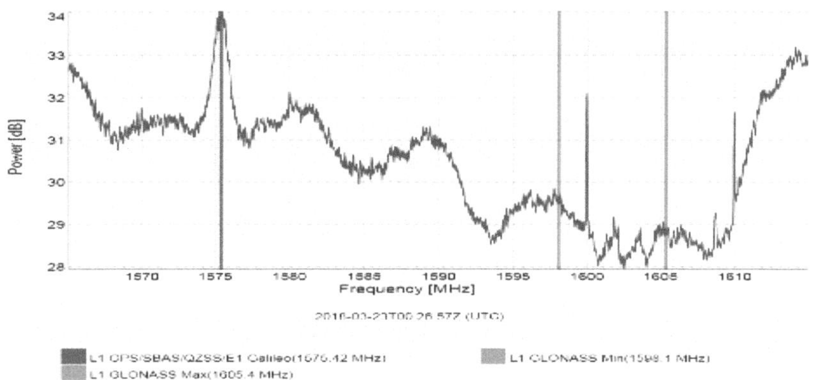

Transmitted data single for the source to satellite for location (Fig. 5).

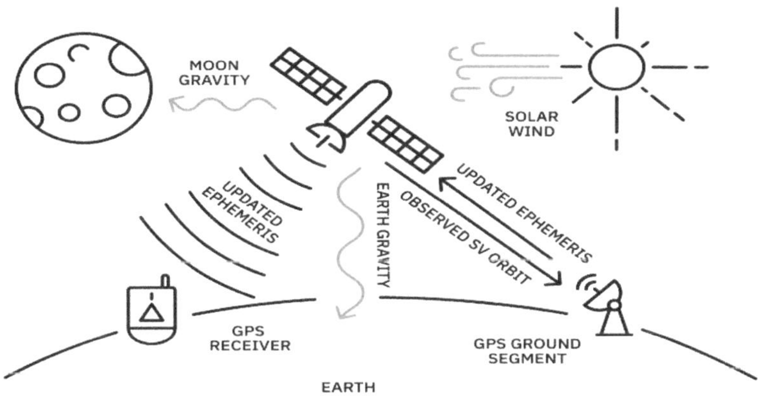

Fig. 5. Mapping for the locations

Frequences Data: Frequency is affected by the atmosphere and getting the error at the frequency 1*10^-13 finding the frequency's there below fig. (Fig. 6).

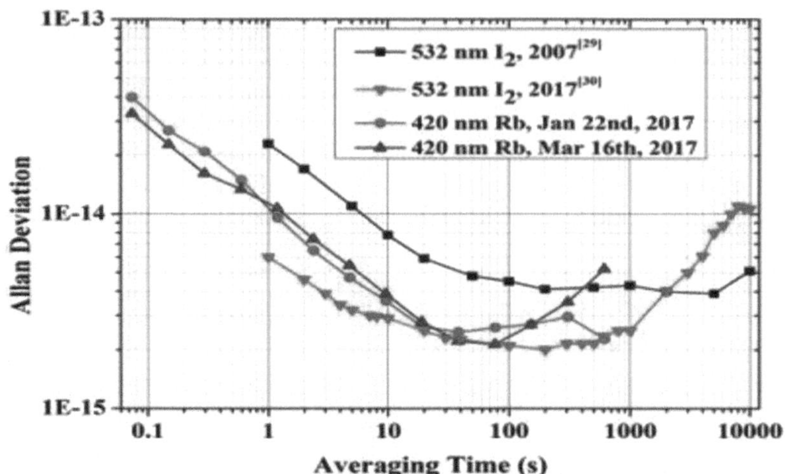

Fig. 6. Difference types of frequences

Accurate timekeeping has always been vital for navigation. Early navigators relied on celestial observations and mechanical clocks to determine their position. The advent of atomic clocks revolutionized navigation by providing precise timing for GPS systems.

Modern GPS systems depend on atomic clocks to synchronize satellite signals, enabling accurate position determination. This technology has become integral to various industries, including transportation, telecommunications, and military operations.

Ground Stations.

To find the Basic Station we are using Longitude,latitude and Angle to find a Base station to Transmit a Data from Ground Station to Satellite.

In the practical output in showing the data rate which is transmission for the ground stations The Data speed(x)is bits per second and Time period (y).

In this below figure we can see the output of modulation technique and output of the BPSK modulation techniques (Fig. 7).

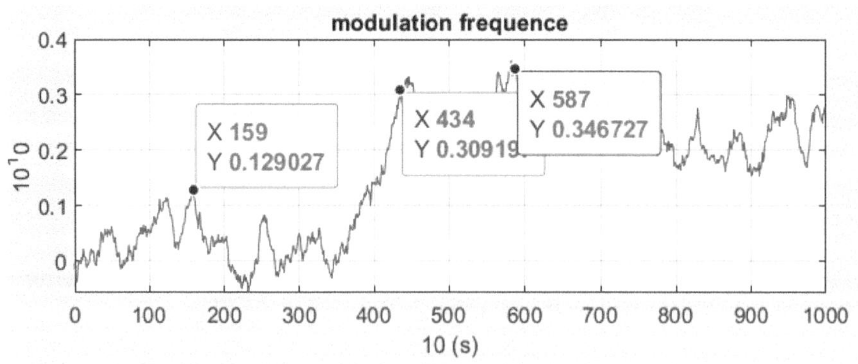

Fig. 7. Wave of output modulation Technique

In this figure we are varying the Data speed (x) in bits per second and Time period(y) accordingly so output is observed that data transmission is in less than 15 s.

To find the Basic station we are using Longitude, Latitude and Angle to find a Base station to Transmit a Data from Ground Station to Satellite.

In the process we can see the speed of the data transmission in the packed for the ground Satiation to differenced types of satellite to communication between them to find Data rate.

4 Conclusion

In Conclusion the advancements in frequence Standards and atom frequence measurement have transformed moder time keeping from early developments to cutting-edge optical clocks, these technologies play a crucial role in various applications, including navigation, Telecommunications, and scientific research. Continued research and innovation in this field promise even greater precision and new opportunities for discovery. Optical clocks have demonstrated a remarkable potential to surpass atomic clocks in terms of stability and accuracy, particularly for applications in satellite-based positioning, navigation, and timing systems. This project has highlighted the superior performance of optical clocks, particularly in the context of GNSS satellites, where they offer enhanced timing precision and reduced range inaccuracy.

The transition from atomic to optical clocks on GNSS satellites could lead to significant improvements in global navigation and positioning accuracy, with implications for a wide range of applications, from everyday navigation to advanced scientific research. However, achieving this transition will require continued technological advancements, integration efforts, and cost-reduction strategies.

In conclusion, while there are challenges to overcome, the future of optical clocks is promising. With further research and development, optical clocks could become the new standard in high-precision timekeeping, driving innovation and enhancing the performance of critical systems worldwide.

5 Future Scope

The development of optical clock technology represents a significant advancement in timekeeping and has the potential to revolutionize various applications, especially in the realm of wireless transmitter applications and satellite-based navigation systems. Future research and development efforts in this field could focus.

Technological Integration: To fully leverage the benefits of optical clocks, further integration with existing satellite systems, such as GNSS, will be crucial. This includes addressing the challenges related to power consumption, size, and environmental robustness.

Miniaturization and Robustness: Developing compact and robust optical clock systems that can withstand the harsh conditions of space is essential. Advances in materials science and engineering could play a pivotal role in achieving this goal.

Cost Reduction: Currently, the high cost of optical clocks is a barrier to widespread adoption. Future research should aim at reducing manufacturing costs through innovative production techniques and economies of scale.

Improved Accuracy and Stability: While optical clocks already offer superior accuracy and stability compared to atomic clocks, ongoing research could further enhance these attributes. This might involve refining the laser stabilization methods and improving the control over environmental factors.

Expanded Applications: Beyond GNSS and PNT applications, optical clocks could be explored for use in other fields such as telecommunications, financial systems, and fundamental physics research. Understanding and expanding the potential use cases will drive further innovation.

Regulatory and Standardization Efforts: As optical clocks become more prevalent, establishing international standards and regulations will be important to ensure compatibility and interoperability across different systems and countries.

References

1. Evaluating of Optical atomic clocks. https://doi.org/10.1103/RevModPhys.87.637
2. Compact Rb optical frequency standard with 10−15 stability. https://doi.org/10.1063/1.5006962
3. The CIPM list of recommended frequency standard values: guidelines and procedures. https://doi.org/10.1088/1681-7575/aaa302
4. Atomic Clocks for Geodesy. https://doi.org/10.1088/1361-6633/aab409
5. Fortier, T., Baumann, E.: 20 years of developments in optical frequency comb technology and applications. Commun. Phys. **2**, 153 (2019). https://doi.org/10.1038/s42005-019-0249
6. On a definition of the SI second with a set of optical clock transitions. https://doi.org/10.1088/1681-7575/ab3a82
7. Giorgi, G., Kroese, B., Michalak, G.: Future GNSS constellations with optical inter-satellite links. Preliminary space segment analyses. In: 2019 IEEE Aerospace Conference, Big Sky, MT, USA, pp. 1–13, 2019. Future GNSS constellations with optical inter-satellite links. Preliminary space segment analyses. https://doi.org/10.1109/AERO.2019.8742105
8. Montenbruck, O., Steigenberger, P., Hauschild, A.: Comparing the 'Big 4' - A User's View on GNSS Performance. In: 2020 IEEE/ION Position, Location and Navigation Symposium (PLANS), Port-land, OR, USA, pp. 407–418, 2020. A User's View on GNSS Performance. https://doi.org/10.1109/PLANS46316.2020.9110208
9. Batori, E., Almat, N., Affolderbach, C., Mileti, G.: GNSS-grade space atomic frequency standards: current status and ongoing developments. Adv. Space Res. https://doi.org/10.1016/j.asr.2020.09.012
10. Boldbaatar, E., Grant, D., Choy, S., Zaminpardaz, S., Holden, L.: Evaluating optical clock performance for GNSS positioning. Sensors **23**(13), 5998 (2023). Evaluation optical clock performance for GNSS position. https://doi.org/10.3390/s23135998

Performance Analysis of GFDM System Using DGT-Based Filter over FTR mmWave Channels

Manpreet Kaur(✉) and Hem Dutt Joshi

Thapar Institute of Engineering and Technology, Bhadson Road, Patiala 147001, Punjab, India
{mkaur_phd17,hemdutt.joshi}@thapar.edu

Abstract. Next-generation wireless communication systems will face various demands, including exponentially increasing data rates, ensuring ultra low power consumption for battery-operated communication sensors, and providing extremely short response times critical for control applications. To meet these flexible requirements, a unified physical layer waveform has been proposed, known as Generalized Frequency Division Multiplexing (GFDM), designed for beyond $5G$ (B5G) communication systems. One of the key features of GFDM is the use of flexible prototype pulse-shaping filters, which leads to improved performance. In this paper, the performance of the GFDM system is analysed for the Discrete Gabor Transform (DGT) based filter over fluctuating two-ray (FTR) fading channel with zero forcing (ZF) receiver. The GFDM performance is analysed in terms of average symbol error rate (ASER) and Noise Enhancement Factor (NEF) for 16 QAM modulation scheme.

Keywords: Average symbol error rate · Fluctuating two-ray mmWave channels · GFDM · Noise Enhancement Factor

1 Introduction

The introduction of 5G technology has revolutionized wireless communication systems, providing unparalleled speeds, ultra-low latency, extensive device connectivity, and exceptional network capacity. As the global community seeks to redefine future wireless communication systems, the focus on developing beyond 5G (B5G) is intensifying. The diverse requirements for B5G standards include data rates of 1 Gb/s, device densities of up to 10^7 devices/km^2, support for high mobility up to 1000 km/h, and latency ranging from 10 to 100 ms [23]. B5G networks are anticipated to play a crucial role in numerous future applications, including e-health services, fully autonomous vehicles, the Internet of Things (IoT), and virtual and augmented reality [22].

To meet the evolving demands of future communication systems, GFDM has emerged as a non-orthogonal waveform with several advantageous features, positioning it as a promising candidate for next-generation networks like B5G and

K. Atul et al. (Eds.): BodyNets 2024, LNICST 666, pp. 581–591, 2026.
https://doi.org/10.1007/978-3-032-16099-7_47

6G. GFDM provides better spectral efficiency since only a single CP is added to the entire GFDM block [15]. Additionally, GFDM reduces out-of-band emissions by utilizing circularly shifted prototype filters [10]. GFDM is particularly well-suited for scenarios like machine-type communication (MTC) due to its enhanced robustness against synchronization errors [16]. Despite these advantageous features, GFDM has certain limitations like higher implementation complexity and increased intersymbol and inter-carrier interference due to sub-carrier filtering. However, utilizing effective receiver techniques and appropriate pulse-shaping filters can reduce this interference, leading to enhanced SER performance in the GFDM system [15]. The GFDM system provides flexibility in filter selection based on specific applications, allowing it to support a variety of filter types without limitations. Consequently, filter selection plays a critical role in determining key factors such as out-of-band (OOB) radiation, SER performance, and interference mitigation in the GFDM system.

From a physical layer perspective, the primary challenge is to choose an appropriate waveform and channel model that can meet the diverse demands of B5G networks. Many studies in the literature have concentrated on optimizing filter design to enhance GFDM systems, specifically in terms of reducing out-of-band emissions, improving SER performance, and mitigating interference. In 2016, Atul Kumar et al. developed an enhanced Nyquist pulse-shaping filter for the GFDM system by incorporating the Meyer auxiliary function [9]. Subsequently in 2017, the performance of "Better than Nyquist" pulse-shaping filters was assessed for a 16-QAM scheme over an AWGN channel with a zero-forcing (ZF) receiver [11]. Further, in [2], Po-Chih Chen et al. proposed an algorithm for filter optimization using characteristic matrices, this approach effectively reduced out-of-band radiation while preserving SER performance. In 2019, a novel pulse shape was developed by linearly combining two distinct pulses, and its performance analysis revealed a trade-off between SER performance and OOB radiation [6]. Recently, in 2023, a prototype filter was developed to reduce OOB emissions by incorporating constraints such as boundary conditions, energy constraints, and spectral density energy concentration degree (SDECD) [13]. In the same year, a novel pulse-shaping filter was designed using the discrete Gabor transform to enhance both SER performance and power spectral density [8].

Modeling the channel is essential for evaluating the statistical performance of any wireless communication system. As a result, research has increasingly focused on exploring higher frequency bands, such as the millimeter-wave (mmWave) range (30–300 GHz) [5,18,21]. This research suggests that the FTR fading model more accurately captures the characteristics of small-scale fading in outdoor mm-wave channels operating at 28 GHz. In 2017, Romero-Jerez et al. introduced the FTR fading model [19], which was subsequently enhanced by M. Lopez-Benitez et al. in 2021 [14]. In [3,20], the performance over the FTR fading channel is assessed in terms of the ASER for multihop detect-and-forward and amplify-and-forward relaying systems. Further in [1,12,17] also, the ASER performance analyses over the FTR fading channel for both the maximum ratio combining (MRC) and the selection combining (SC) techniques are presented.

Recently, in 2023, the ASER performance of the GFDM and STC-GFDM systems under imperfect channel estimation over the FTR fading channel was presented [7].

The paper provides a performance analysis of GFDM systems operating over the FTR fading channel, using a DGT-based pulse-shaping filter for the μ-QAM modulation technique, the asymptotic analysis is also provided for the GFDM system.

1.1 Notations

Previously, vectors were represented using an arrow over the letter. In this work, vectors are represented using bold lowercase letters.

2 System and Channel Models

2.1 GFDM System Model

The GFDM system contains K sub-carriers and M sub-symbols. At the transmitter side, the input binary data is first mapped into a complex data vector $\boldsymbol{d}$ using μ-QAM technique. This data vector $\boldsymbol{d}$ is decompose into K sub-carriers with M sub-symbols on each sub-carrier (i.e.$N = KM$). Now, the output of the GFDM modulator can be presented as $\boldsymbol{x} = \mathbf{A}\boldsymbol{d}$. Here $\mathbf{A}$ is a $KM \times KM$ transmitter matrix, defined as $\mathbf{A} = (\boldsymbol{g}_{0,0}, \cdots \boldsymbol{g}_{K-1,0} \qquad \boldsymbol{g}_{0,M-1}, \cdots \boldsymbol{g}_{K-1,M-1})$, where, $\boldsymbol{g}_{k,m}$ is the frequency and time-shifted version of the prototype pulse shaping filter $\boldsymbol{g}$. A cyclic prefix (CP) of N_{cp} samples is then added to $\boldsymbol{x}$ to produce $\boldsymbol{x}_c$.

The modulated signal $\boldsymbol{x}_c$ is transmitted through a wireless fading channel. Assuming perfect synchronization and after removing the cyclic prefix, the received signal can be expressed as

$$\boldsymbol{y} = \mathbf{H}\boldsymbol{x} + \boldsymbol{w} \tag{1}$$

where, $\mathbf{H}$ is a $N \times N$ circulant channel matrix having impulse response $\boldsymbol{h}$ $(= [h_0, h_1, , h_2..., h_{L-1}]^T)$ and vector $\boldsymbol{w}$ denotes additive white Gaussian noise with zero mean and ${\varrho_w}^2$ variance. Considering perfect channel estimation and linear modulation, the received signal after channel equalization and linear demodulation can be written as

$$\boldsymbol{z} = \mathbf{B}\mathbf{A}\boldsymbol{d} + \mathbf{B}\mathbf{H}^{-1}\boldsymbol{w} \tag{2}$$

where $\mathbf{B}$ is the receiver matrix. Here, a zero-forcing receiver ($\mathbf{B} = \mathbf{A}^{-1}$) is used, which removes self-interference at the receiver but enhances the noise.

2.2 FTR Channel Model

The PDF of the instantaneous SNR γ per symbol of FTR distribution is given as [14]

$$f_{\gamma_t}(\gamma_t) = \frac{m^m}{\Gamma(m)} \sum_{r=0}^{\infty} \frac{K_f^r d_r}{r!} f_G(\gamma_t; r+1, 2\sigma^2) \tag{3}$$

where

$$f_G(\gamma_t; r+1, 2\sigma^2) = \frac{\gamma_t^r}{\Gamma(r+1)(2\sigma^2)^{(r+1)}} \exp\Big(-\frac{\gamma_t}{2\sigma^2}\Big) \tag{4}$$

and the coefficient d_r is given by

$$\begin{aligned} d_r = & \sum_{s=0}^{r} \binom{r}{s} \sum_{l=0}^{s} \binom{s}{l} \Gamma(r+m+2l-s)\ (m+K_f)^{-(r+m+2l-s)} \\ & \times\ K_f^{2l-s} \Big(\frac{\Delta}{2}\Big)^{2l} (-1)^{2l-s}\ R_{r+m}^{s-2l}\Big(\big[K_f \Delta/(m+K_f)\big]^2\Big). \end{aligned} \tag{5}$$

Here, $2\sigma^2 = \bar{\gamma}/(1+K_f)$ where $\bar{\gamma}$ is the average SNR at the GFDM receiver and $K_f = \frac{{C_1}^2+{C_2}^2}{2\sigma^2}$ is defined as the relative power between the dominant and reflected signals. Parameter $\Delta = \frac{2C_1C_2}{{C_1}^2+{C_2}^2} \in [0,1]$ is used to indicate the degree of similarity between the two primary waves and m determines the degree of fading in the channel, and the value of m should be an arbitrary positive real number. The function $R_v^\eta(x)$ in (5) is defined in [14] as

$$R_v^\eta(x) = \begin{cases} \left(\frac{v-\eta}{2}\right)_\eta \left(\frac{v-\eta+1}{2}\right)_\eta \frac{x^\eta}{\eta!}\ {}_2F_1\Big(\frac{v+\eta}{2}, \frac{v+\eta+1}{2}; 1+\eta; x\Big), \eta \in N^+ \\ {}_2F_1\big(\frac{v-\eta}{2}, \frac{v-\eta+1}{2}; 1-\eta; x\big)/(\Gamma(1-\eta)), \qquad \text{otherwise} \end{cases} \tag{6}$$

where, $(q)_n = \Gamma(q+n)/\Gamma(q)$ is the Pochhammer symbol, and ${}_2F_1$(u, v; w; x) is the Gauss hypergeometric function. The two-wave with diffused power (TWDP) model is in fact a specific case of the FTR model [19]. Moreover, the PDF of the one-sided Gaussian, Rayleigh, Rician, Hoyt, and Nakagami fading models are special cases of FTR PDF.

Table 1. Simulation parameters.

Parameters	Values
Sub-carriers (K)	64
Sub-symbols (M)	5
Filter	DGT based filter
Mapping	16 QAM
Cyclic Prefix	16
Receiver	Zero forcing (ZF)
Channel	FTR

3 ASER Analysis of GFDM System

3.1 Exact Analysis

This section presents an exact ASER analysis of the GFDM system operating over the FTR fading channel for 16-QAM modulation technique. A DGT based pulse shaping filter is used for analysing the ASER performance. The ASER for the GFDM system can be written as [7]

$$P(e) = \frac{R_0^{'}\Gamma(r+1)}{(2r+1)\sqrt{\pi}} \times {}_2F_1\left(r+\frac{1}{2}, r+1; r+\frac{3}{2}; \frac{-(1+K_f)}{\bar{\gamma}}\right) - \frac{R_0}{2}\left(1 - \frac{4}{\pi}\sum_{i=0}^{r}\frac{(1+K_f)^i}{\bar{\gamma}^i(2i+1)} \times {}_2F_1\left(i+\frac{1}{2}, i+1; i+\frac{3}{2}; \frac{-(1+K_f)}{\bar{\gamma}} - 1\right)\right). \quad (7)$$

where

$$R_0^{'} = \frac{R_0(1+K_f)^{(r+1)}}{\Gamma(r+1)\bar{\gamma}_t^{(r+1)}}, \quad (8)$$

$$R_0 = \sum_{r=0}^{\infty}\frac{2\,m^m}{\Gamma(m)}\frac{(p-1)K_f^r d_r}{pr!}. \quad (9)$$

and

$$\gamma = \frac{3R_T}{2(2^{\mu}-1)}\frac{E_s}{\xi N_o}, \quad (10)$$

$$R_T = \frac{KM}{KM + N_{cp} + N_{cs}}. \quad (11)$$

where, ξ is the noise enhancement factor (NEF), μ is the modulation order of QAM, E_s is the average energy per symbol, and $N_o/2$ is the power spectral density of noise. The function ${}_2F_1(a,b;c;z)$ is the Gauss hypergeometric function [4].

3.2 Asymptotic Analysis

This section presents the asymptotic performance of the GFDM system. The expression of asymptotic ASER of the GFDM system can be written as [7]

$$P^{\infty}(e) = \left(\frac{p-1}{p}\right)m^m(m+K_f)^{-m}{}_2F_1\left(\frac{m}{2}, \frac{(m+1)}{2}; 1; \frac{K_f\Delta}{m+K_f}\right) \times \left[\frac{2(1+K_f)}{\sqrt{\pi}\bar{\gamma}} - 1 + \frac{4}{\pi} \times {}_2F_1\left(\frac{1}{2}, 1; \frac{3}{2}; \frac{-(1+K_f)}{\bar{\gamma}}\right)\right]. \quad (12)$$

For asymptotic analysis, the higher values of average SNR are considered, due to which $2\sigma^2$ approaches infinity.

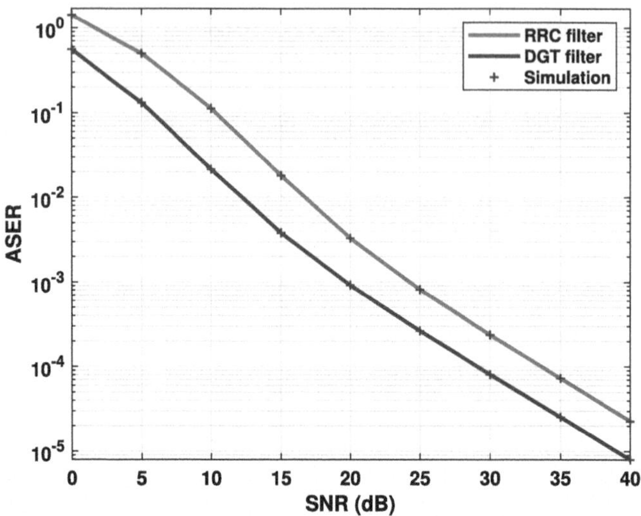

Fig. 1. ASER for 16 QAM GFDM system with $\alpha = 0.9$ for RRC and DGT based filters over FTR fading channel

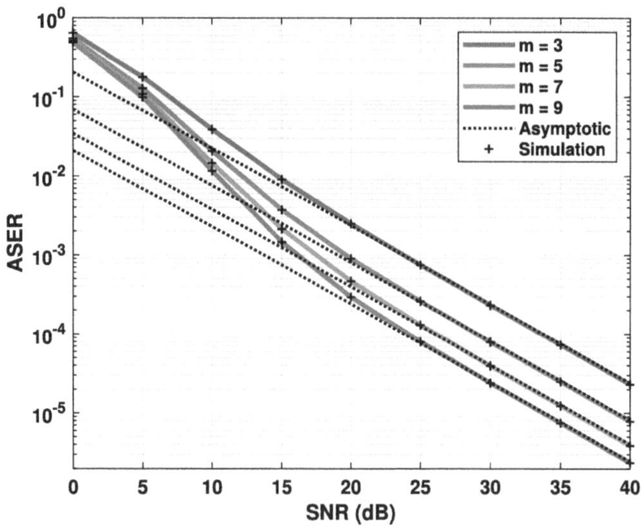

Fig. 2. Exact and asymptotic ASER for GFDM system in FTR channel for $K_f = 10$, $\Delta = 0.1$, $\alpha = 0.5$ and $m = 3, 5, 7$ & 9.

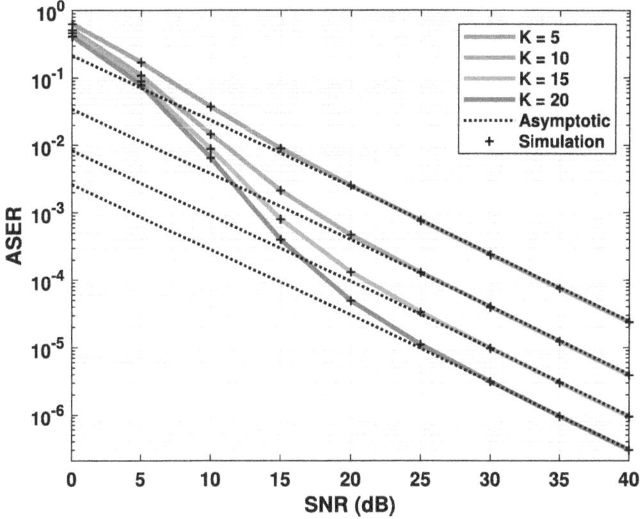

Fig. 3. Exact and asymptotic ASER for GFDM system in FTR channel for $m = 7$, $\Delta = 0.1$, and $K_f = 5, 10, 15$ & 20.

4 Results and Discussion

In this section, the performance of the GFDM system is analysed. The results obtained with the DGT-based filter are compared to those achieved with the conventional RRC pulse-shaping filter. The ZF receiver is employed, as it effectively eliminates self-interference while also amplifying noise, a behaviour influenced by the chosen pulse shape. The DGT-based filter significantly reduces the noise enhancement factor.

4.1 Symbol Error Rate

This section presents numerical results for the SER performance across FTR fading channels. The simulation results are given for $M = 5$ subsymbols, $K = 64$ subcarriers and a CP of 16. Table 1 lists the system parameters and values used to evaluate the results in this section.

Figure 1 shows the SER performance of the GFDM system with conventional RRC and DGT based filters over the FTR fading channel for the 16-QAM modulation scheme. The values of the FTR channel parameters considered for the analysis are $\Delta = 0.1$, $K_f = 10$, and $m = 5$ and roll off factor $\alpha = 0.9$. As shown in Fig. 1, the SER performance improves with the DGT-based filter compared to the conventional RRC filter. At SNR = 20 dB the SER value for the RRC filter is 3.297×10^-3, while for DGT based filter, it is 9.172×10^-4. The SER values indicate a significant performance improvement of the DGT filter-based GFDM system over the FTR fading channel.

The plot in Fig. 2 illustrates the relationship between the ASER and SNR for a GFDM system. The plot showcases ASER's exact and asymptotic behaviours for a GFDM system with specific parameters: $\Delta = 0.1$, $K_f = 10$, and $m = 3, 5, 7, 9$. The plots demonstrate how the ASER performance of a DGT filter based GFDM is affected by the channel parameter m variation. The figure shows that increasing the value of m from 3 (indicating heavy fluctuations) to 9 (indicating light fluctuations) reduces the impact of channel fluctuations, leading to improved ASER performance.

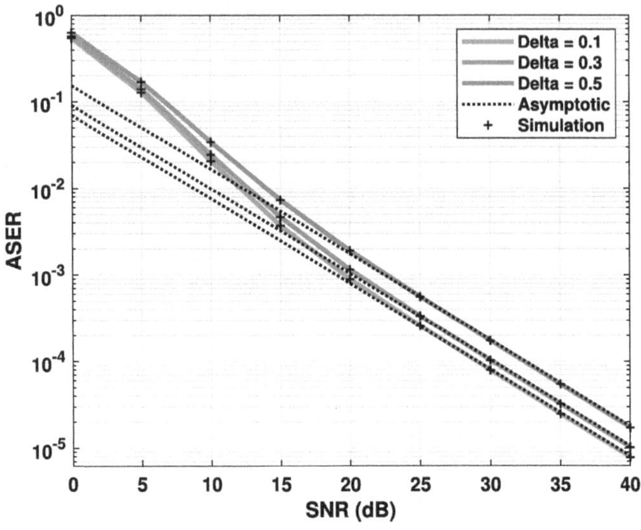

Fig. 4. Exact and asymptotic ASER for GFDM system in FTR channel for $m = 5$, $K_f = 10$, and $\Delta = 0.1, 0.3$ & 0.5.

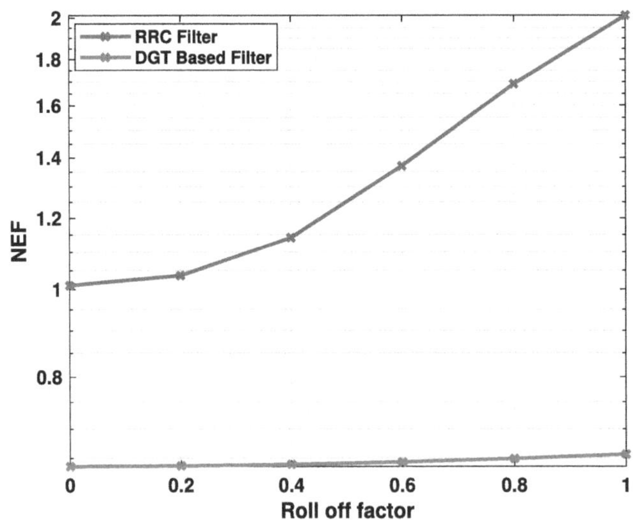

Fig. 5. NEF of GFDM with RRC and DGT based filter for different values of roll-off-factor α.

Figures 3 illustrate the impact of channel parameter K_f, on the ASER performance. These plots consider a $m = 7$, $\Delta = 0.1$ and $K_f = 3, 5, 7$ & 15. The curves clearly demonstrate an improvement in ASER for larger values of K_f. A higher value of K_f indicates that the total power of the dominant components is greater than the power of the scattered waves. This will ultimately reduce the fading effect of the channel. The plot demonstrates that the performance of GFDM improves with increasing value of parameter K_f.

Conversely, in Fig. 4, the ASER experiences a slight deterioration as Δ increases from 0.1 to 0.5. This occurs because an increase in Δ leads to a more significant phase difference between the two primary waves, ultimately intensifying the severity of channel fading. Figure 4 presents the ASER of the GFDM system for the channel parameters $m = 7$, $K_f = 10$, $\Delta = 0.1, 0.3$ & 0.5. As the figure depicts for a 16-QAM GFDM system at 30 dB SNR, the ASER increases from 2.61489×10^{-4} to 5.1567×10^{-4} as the value of Δ increases from 0.1 to 0.5. This happens because an increase in Δ results in a greater phase difference between the two main waves, which ultimately exacerbates the severity of channel fading.

4.2 Noise Enhancement Factor

The plot in Fig. 5 shows the graph between NEF and roll off factor α. The zero-forcing (ZF) receiver is employed for the analysis; while it eliminates interference (ISI and ICI), it can also lead to noise enhancement, which negatively impacts SINR performance. Since noise enhancement is influenced by pulse shaping, properly designing the prototype filter can improve SEP performance. For a roll-off factor of $\alpha = 0.4$, the NEF value is 1.1412 for the RRC filter and 0.6394 for the DGT-based filter. These NEF values clearly demonstrate that the DGT-based filter has a significantly lower NEF. When the DGT-based filter is used with a ZF receiver, the ZF receiver mitigates interference in the GFDM system, while the DGT-based filter helps to reduce the NEF.

5 Conclusion

This paper analyses the performance of the DGT filter based GFDM system in terms of ASER and NEF over the FTR fading channel. For this analysis, 16-QAM modulation scheme, ZF receiver, and varying channel parameters (m, K, δ) have been considered. The NEF is calculated and plotted for different values of roll off factor α for the performance comparison of the DGT based filter and the conventional RRC filter. The analysis results above demonstrate that the DGT-based filter enhances the performance of the GFDM system in the FTR fading channel. It significantly reduces the NEF for the ZF receiver, which ultimately improves the system's ASER and mitigates interference.

References

1. Al-Hmood, H., Al-Raweshidy, H.S.: Performance analysis of mmWave communications with selection combining over fluctuating-two ray fading model. IEEE Commun. Lett. **25**(8), 2531–2535 (2021)
2. Chen, P.C., Su, B.: Filter optimization of out-of-band radiation with performance constraints for GFDM systems. In: 2017 IEEE 18th International Workshop on Signal Processing Advances in Wireless Communications (SPAWC), pp. 1–5. IEEE (2017)
3. Dixit, D., Sahu, P.: Performance of multihop detect-and-forward relaying system over fluctuating two-ray fading channels. Trans. Emerg. Telecommun. Technol. **29**(8), e3423 (2018)
4. Gradshteyn, I., Ryzhik, I., Jeffrey, A., Zwillinger, D.: Table of integrals, series, and products. Table of Integrals (2007)
5. Hur, S., et al.: Proposal on millimeter-wave channel modeling for 5G cellular system. IEEE J. Sel. Top. Signal Process. **10**(3), 454–469 (2016)
6. Kalsotra, S., Kumar, A., Joshi, H.D., Singh, A.K., Dev, K., Magarini, M.: Impact of pulse shaping design on OOB emission and error probability of GFDM. In: 2019 IEEE 2nd 5G World Forum (5GWF), pp. 226–231. IEEE (2019)
7. Kaur, M., Joshi, H.D.: Performance of gfdm system with channel estimation error over ftr mmwave channels for 5G and beyond communication. AEU-Int. J. Electron. Commun. **172**, 154967 (2023)
8. Kaur, M., Joshi, H.D., Magarini, M., et al.: Dgt-based pulse shaping filter for generalized frequency division multiplexing system. Phys. Commun. **61**, 102227 (2023)
9. Kumar, A., Magarini, M.: Improved Nyquist pulse shaping filters for generalized frequency division multiplexing. In: 2016 8th IEEE Latin-American Conference on Communications (LATINCOM), pp. 1–7. IEEE (2016)
10. Kumar, A., Magarini, M.: On the modeling of inter-sub-symbol interference in GFDM transmission. IEEE Commun. Lett. **23**(10), 1730–1734 (2019)
11. Kumar, A., Magarini, M., Bregni, S.: Improving GFDM symbol error rate performance using "Better than Nyquist" pulse shaping filters. IEEE Lat. Am. Trans. **15**(7), 1244–1249 (2017)
12. Laishram, M.D., Aheibam, D.S.: Performance of dual-branch selection combining receiver over Fluctuating Two-Ray (FTR) fading channels for 5G mmWave communications. AEU-Int. J. Electron. Commun. **117**, 153093 (2020)
13. Liu, M., Xue, W., Gao, J., Jia, P., Xu, Y., Volvenko, S.V.: Prototype filter design for effectively suppressing out-of-band radiation in GFDM systems. IEEE Commun. Lett. **27**(2), 696–700 (2022)
14. López-Benítez, M., Zhang, J.: Comments and corrections to new results on the fluctuating two-ray model with arbitrary fading parameters and its applications. IEEE Trans. Veh. Technol. **70**(2), 1938–1940 (2021)
15. Michailow, N., et al.: Generalized frequency division multiplexing for 5th generation cellular networks. IEEE Trans. Commun. **62**(9), 3045–3061 (2014)
16. Nekovee, M.: Quantifying performance requirements of vehicle-to-vehicle communication protocols for rear-end collision avoidance. In: VTC Spring 2009-IEEE 69th Vehicular Technology Conference, pp. 1–5. IEEE (2009)
17. Olyaee, M., Eslami, M., Haghighat, J.: Performance of maximum ratio combining of fluctuating two-ray (ftr) mmwave channels for 5g and beyond communications. Trans. Emerg. Telecommun. Technol. **30**(10), e3601 (2019)

18. Rappaport, T.S., MacCartney, G.R., Samimi, M.K., Sun, S.: Wideband millimeter-wave propagation measurements and channel models for future wireless communication system design. IEEE Trans. Commun. **63**(9), 3029–3056 (2015)
19. Romero-Jerez, J.M., Lopez-Martinez, F.J., Paris, J.F., Goldsmith, A.J.: The fluctuating two-ray fading model: statistical characterization and performance analysis. IEEE Trans. Wirel. Commun. **16**(7), 4420–4432 (2017)
20. Singh, S., Mitra, D., Baghel, R.K.: Performance evaluation of relay assisted wireless powered network over fluctuating two ray fading channel with diversity reception. Wirel. Pers. Commun. **121**(3), 1739–1755 (2021). https://doi.org/10.1007/s11277-021-08718-3
21. Tan, Y., Wang, C.X., Nielsen, J.Ø., Pedersen, G.F., Zhu, Q.: A novel b5g frequency nonstationary wireless channel model. IEEE Trans. Antennas Propag. **69**(8), 4846–4860 (2021)
22. Zhang, C., Ueng, Y.L., Studer, C., Burg, A.: Artificial intelligence for 5G and beyond 5G: implementations, algorithms, and optimizations. IEEE J. Emerg. Sel. Top. Circuits and Syst. **10**(2), 149–163 (2020)
23. Zhang, Z., et al.: 6G wireless networks: vision, requirements, architecture, and key technologies. IEEE Veh. Technol. Mag. **14**(3), 28–41 (2019)

Author Index

K. Atul et al. (Eds.): BodyNets 2024, LNICST 666, pp. 593–595, 2026.
https://doi.org/10.1007/978-3-032-16099-7

The manufacturer's authorised representative in the EU is Springer Nature Customer Service Centre GmbH, Europaplatz 3, 69115 Heidelberg, Germany. If you have any concerns regarding our products, please contact ProductSafety@springernature.com

Printed and bound by CPI Group (UK) Ltd, Croydon, CR0 4YY
07/07/2026
02160906-0015